Praise for

Different Bodies, Different Diets

As a health and fitness educator and fat burning researcher, I am very impressed with Dr. Mein's work. *Different Bodies, Different Diets* is one of the most comprehensive books I have ever read. Anyone interested in learning the exact specifics about their body type and constitution should add this book to their library. I especially enjoyed the way she encourages everyone to eat ample quantities of *essential* fats and oils, and that high cholesterol levels are primarily due to *stress*, not egg yolks – thus destroying the low fat diet myth.

Thank you, Dr. Mein, for your landmark book. I truly feel that this world will greatly benefit from your health and nutritional wisdom.

-Jay Robb, Author of *The Fat Burning Diet*

This book is a genuine tribute to women. I highly recommend this material to every woman who pursues her health and well-being with consciousness and integrity.

-Caroline M. Myss, Ph.D., Author of *Anatomy of the Spirit*

An entire health care system that is unique, comprehensive and practical. Dr. Mein gives importance to the very basics which traditional medicine usually ignores. Its detailed inclusion of "how to" specifics makes it useful for creating a daily program that can be followed by any reader who is seeking to improve their health and longevity.

-David R. Hawkins, M.D., Ph.D., Author of *Power Versus Force*
and *Orthomolecular Psychiatry* (with Linus Pauling)

Congratulations on an excellent body of work "embodied" in your observations of different body types and dietary relationships.

-George J. Goodheart, D.C., Discoverer and Developer of Applied Kinesiology

Dr. Mein, after 20 years of observation and helping thousands of women regain their health, has produced a unique system of understanding metabolism.

-John F. Thie, B.S., D.C., Author and Founder of *Touch for Health*
Founding Chairman of the International College of Applied Kinesiology

I have been using body typing in my office for many years, but never to the extent and detail that Dr. Mein has brought forth in this book. Dr. Mein is to be congratulated for the tremendous work that went into putting this book together. I previously was often confronted with the problem that a patient didn't fit into an exact body type or was a mixture of the types I was using. Now, with the 25 types detailed as they are, the confusion is no longer present.

-Sheldon C. Deal, N.D., D.C., President, International College of Applied Kinesiology
Author of *Life Through Nutrition*

Personal Experiences

I have been following my Body Type diet from *The 25 Body Type System* for over five years and it works. Dr. Mein identified me as a Thyroid type and told me that the vegetarian diets I had been on for years were not supporting my body. Old habits don't change easily, but the difference in how I feel when I get protein, convinced me.

–Juawayne Hope, Founder of "Blisswork"

After spending years searching for "perfect health" and following many different diets, I still felt like there where gaping holes in my dietary program. I'm a Nervous System type. Dr. Mein's system provided me with a practical day-to-day meal schedule that I could follow.

-Barbara Summer, Health Clinic Personnel

The diet system that Dr. Mein recommended for me and my family has enlightened me. I used to be very concerned about my daughter's eating habits. She's a Kidney type. I'm a Gonadal type, who feels best eating a light lunch and a heavy dinner. My daughter does best with a heavy lunch and a light dinner. She does well with peanut butter, while I do well with strawberry yogurt. Even though we don't eat all the same foods, there are enough similarities between the "Frequently" and "Moderately" foods that I can prepare a meal plan that works for all of us.

-Linda Neff, Homemaker

Weight has been a problem all my life; I even gained weight just eating salad. In just 6 months on Dr. Mein's diet, I lost 40 pounds. Not once during this time did I feel that I was starving. As a Pancreas type, I learned to eat at the right times, rotate my foods, and include more variety in my diet.

-Darlene Smith, Medical Transcriptionist

I have a sensitive digestive system. My solution was to not eat, but that left me susceptible to everything that came along. I'm a Pineal type, so I need to eat the bulk of my protein before 2 p.m., since this is when my body can assimilate it. Eating this way makes all the difference in the world in how I feel.

-Judy Liu, M.F.C.C.

I travel extensively throughout the world, eating many meals in airplanes, restaurants, and hotels. Following my Stomach diet from The *25 Body Type System* has eliminated my allergy attacks and minimized my "jet lag". I am now able to maintain my weight without feeling deprived.

-Pepe Romero, Classical Guitarist

The 25 Body Type System

VisionWare Press
4118 Raya Way, San Diego, CA 92122

Printed in the United States of America
First Printing: April 1998

Carolyn L. Mein, D.C.
P.O. Box 8112
Rancho Santa Fe, CA 92067

Publisher's Cataloging-in-Publication
(Provided by Quality Books, Inc.)

Mein, Carolyn L.
Different bodies, different diets / Carolyn L. Mein --
Women's ed., 1st ed.
p. cm. -- (25 body type system series)
ISBN: 0-9661381-0-4

1. Chiropractic. 2. Women -- Nutrition.
3. Somatotypes. 4. Reducing diets.
I. Title

RZ242.M45 1998 613.2'082
LC 96-177957 QBI97-41437

Different Bodies Different Diets

Women's Edition

The 25 Body Type System

Dr. Carolyn L. Mein

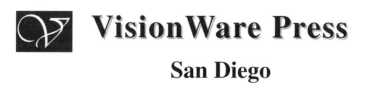

VisionWare Press

San Diego

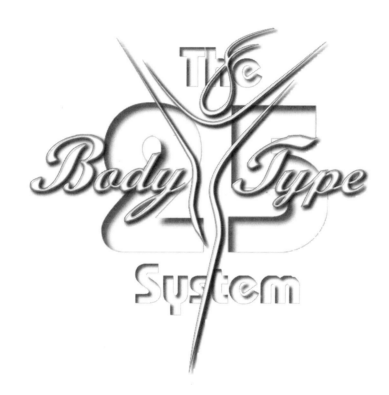

This book is

dedicated to:

All my wonderful patients, friends, participants and everyone who has ever searched for their ideal diet, or looked to better understand themselves and others.

Acknowledgements

I would like to express my gratitude and acknowledge everyone who has helped me in this endeavor. Special thanks to everyone who was photographed as part of this project, especially to those whose photos are in this book.

Most importantly, my deep heartfelt gratitude and appreciation to all my special patients and friends who so freely shared with me their experiences and insights during the developing and refining of the diets, menus, and psychological profiles. I am particularly grateful to those who so willingly revealed themselves and shared their personal awareness by answering my seemingly endless questions. For without them this work would never have been possible. I would like to specifically acknowledge:

George Goodheart, D.C., for developing muscle testing as an accurate means of communicating with the intelligence of the body.

Elliot Abravanel, M.D., for his *Body Type Diet and Lifetime Nutritional Plan* which opened the door for my research.

Leon F. Seltzer, Ph.D., whose expertise in English and Psychology was of great help as a consultant. For synthesizing the psychological profiles and scrutinizing them for accuracy and content.

Anthony W. Liu of VisionWare InterActive and his staff, especially Ian Hilton, Drew Goldstein, Jared Pollard, and Hobie Trivitte for doing the computer scanning and layout work for all the photographs, text, and developing the CD-ROM, Video, and Web site.

Nadine Mein, my mother, for her untiring patience and perseverance in typing, proofing and editing this book for accuracy and completeness and making sure it was easy to read and understand.

Carol Kemp for her observant eye in helping me identify distinguishing characteristics among types; her assistance with photo selection, layout, captions, and questionnaires; and for her support throughout this extensive undertaking.

My office staff, Renee Bergeron, Elaine Hoover, D.C., Terri Lew, Nancy Alaura, and Kathy Gunningham, for their dedication in taking photos, interviewing participants, and organizing data. Special thanks to Renee for her consistency and assistance with revisions.

Wayne Mein, my brother, for his many hours of dedicated assistance with typing and working with photos.

Maxine Seltzer for her library research in checking sources and citations as well as for her suggestions on tables and charts in the text.

Tatiana Popova for her research and verification of other diet plans for the "Advanced Dietary Guide".

Vladimer Verhovskoy for his formatting ideas and legal expertise.

Juawayne Hope, developer of "Blisswork", for the use of her studio during photography sessions, and for her support and enthusiastic recommendation of the body type diet to her many students.

My appreciation to everyone who, after applying the diet designed for their type, provided me with valuable feedback and menu ideas.

My thanks and love to all of you!

Contents

Preface

You've probably seen lots of diets, and if you're like most people, you've tried more than you'd care to mention. I'll bet you've even blamed yourself for not having the will power to stay with a diet long enough to see results. The diets seemed logical enough and they worked for others, so the problem must be you, right? I don't think so. *Why should one diet be right for everyone?* We don't all look the same, and we don't even like the same foods, so why should everyone lose weight on the same diet? Besides, if the diet really supported you, why was it so difficult to stay on it? In working with patients for over 20 years, I have never found the "ideal diet". I have found certain diets that worked for certain people, but these same diets either didn't work or caused problems for others; and in some cases they were actually harmful. While there certainly are universal guidelines, I have never found a single dietary plan that was appropriate for everyone.

It's when these universal principles are brought down into the specific day-to-day application, that problems arise. "Exactly how much fat, protein, and fruit should I eat?", "When is it best for me to eat fruit or protein?" and "Why do I feel tired after eating?" are just a few of the questions patients asked. Unfortunately, there's no single answer, since the answer varies with the individual. However, there is some commonality among people and it is based on similar body chemistry. This is what lead me to discover 25 distinct body types – each with their own nutritional requirements – and develop an outline of the ideal diet for each individual; regardless of whether their goal was to *lose*, *gain*, or *maintain* an optimal weight.

About 12 years ago, a patient brought me Abravanel's book on body typing. I was thrilled; this was the first diet book that made sense! It took into account that there were dietary differences based on a person's dominant glandular system. Because the principles were right for me, I thought I had found the answer. But as I worked with Abravanel's typing system, I found its use limited. Like other typing systems I had tested in the past, I began to see too many people who seemed to be a blend of more than one type. Needless to say, working with someone who is a blend of several types is almost as time consuming as having no typing system, because everything still needed to be individually tested. The question that every diet conscious person wants to know is, "What should I eat?" While I could use muscle testing to discover the ideal foods for my patients, this was extremely time consuming and impractical.

With degrees in Chiropractic, Acupuncture,Clinical Nutrition, Bio-Nutrition, and Applied Kinesiology, I had the tools to directly access the body's innate wisdom about its function and nutritional requirements. I was intrigued by the idea of an accurate body-typing system, and began discovering the missing types. One-by-one they appeared until, about 6 years ago, I reached a total of 25 separate types. In addition to dietary similarities, I also became aware of certain physical and psychological similarities that were type consistent. Each type has its own specific dietary needs, food cravings, key supporting foods, foods to avoid, and even timing and scheduling of meals. I have tested these nutrition plans with thousands of patients with consistent responses and results. Developing a specific dietary plan for an individual is now very simple. The answer lies in identifying their specific body type.

The basis of my body type system is that every person has a dominant gland, organ or system. This is the one that is stronger (or more dominant) than the rest. It is present at birth, determines certain physical characteristics and psychological traits, is the first to be called upon when the body is under stress, and remains constant throughout one's life. (For simplicity's sake, when I refer to a person's dominant gland, this will also include the dominant organs and systems.)

Since every gland has its own unique function, it stands to reason that it would have its own specific nutritional requirements. So, I identified the foods that best supported each gland, as well as the ones that produced the greatest amount of stress. These foods are listed as the "Frequently" and "Rarely" foods for each type. The key to "The Body Type System" is correctly identifying your body type. You have several options, and may use one or ultimately all of these methods.

1. Physical characteristics
2. Psychological profiles
3. Points of awareness
4. The body's response to foods
5. Diet recognition

Some of the initial feedback I received from people when they first saw this book was that it was overwhelming. Although the book itself is large, the information you need is contained in about 200 pages. The remaining 300 pages pertain to the other types. In essence, this is a guide to all diets. It simplifies the vast field of diet and nutrition, by putting all the 25 categories of diets into one book.

Diets in general are confusing because of all the contradictions. The reality is that each diet is valuable to someone. The question is how much of the information applies to you. Since it's your dominant gland that determines what nutrients and eating plan is right for you, the answer lies in knowing your body type.

1. My intention is to make it easy for you to confidently identify your own specific body type using the photographs and data provided in Chapter 2.
2. As soon as you identify your body type, you can start incorporating the foods and food combinations most nurturing to your system.
3. Reading the text information that explains the basic dietary principles behind this system will give you a greater understanding of how to get the most from your ideal food plan.
4. Once you've determined your own body type, you will probably want to discover the body types of your family and friends. We also invite you to participate in our further research.

For additional assistance in determining the body types of your loved ones, included in this series is the Men's edition. The Children's edition is in process. In the meantime, it is important to know that women, men and children all have the same 25 body types. The dietary information, food lists, menus and much of the psychological profile is basically the same. Children are especially sensitive to what they eat, so body typing your children can reap tremendous rewards. Such childhood problems as irritability, mood swings, hyperactivity, depression, and fatigue can result from consuming food that places too much of a strain on a child's delicate system.

Once a child's body type has been identified, parents can choose a diet that can reduce, and at times even eradicate, a variety of behavioral difficulties. Rarely is everyone in a family the same body type. The difference in body types often explains the differences in personalities. Knowing a child's psychological profile can be of tremendous assistance in helping them develop and understand themselves. While each diet is different, there are similarities, so rearranging diets to support all the members of the family is easy.

As a comprehensive guide, this book offers you (and your family and friends) tailor-made recommendations for permanent eating plans based on your body's very particular nutritional needs. These individualized recommendations include:

- a detailed list of foods that offer maximum nutritional support for your system,
- advice as to the *frequency* with which different foods are best eaten,
- the *time(s) of day* that your body can best digest these foods, specifically when the largest meal is best consumed,
- menus and food *combinations* that best support your body,
- special programs for weight control, whether your goal is to *lose* or *gain* weight and then to maintain your ideal weight in the safest, most effective way. Following the correct diet allows you to lose weight in the appropriate areas.

The Psychological Profile contains valuable insights into greater understanding of one's self and others. Not only does the dominant gland have specific effects on the physical body, it has a specific psychological effect. This is reflected in the personality through characteristic traits. Each type has its particular challenges that result in an underlying motivation. How well each person is doing with their challenges is reflected in the "At Worst" and "At Best". The "At Best" provides direction and a realistic, achievable goal. The Psychological Profile answers the questions of, "Who am I? Why do I act the way I do? What's my lesson?" and "How well am I doing?" The first step toward harmonious relationships is understanding – both of self and others.

A future book will discuss in depth the mental, emotional and spiritual dimensions of each body type, as well as the most successful ways members of each type have found to overcome their challenges. This additional information can help you create even greater health in your life and relationships.

Thank you for selecting this book. My purpose in writing it is to provide you with the tools to take control of your dietary habits and lifestyle. The Psychological Profiles are written to help you become more aware of who you are and to help you improve your life and relationships. This book is designed to be stimulating and informative. I hope you enjoy it and that the quality of your life is better because of it.

Carolyn L. Mein, D.C.
San Diego, California
October, 1997

CHAPTER 1

BODY TYPES –WHAT ARE THEY?

THE NEED FOR BODY TYPING

Everyone knows that following the right diet is essential to good health, but which diet? Most people go through a process of trial and error, meaning they try one diet after another – with moderate success – or give up and go back to the diet they were raised on as children. This, as you will later discover, may or may not be right for them.

Many people try to get the vitamins and minerals they need by enhancing their diets with nutritional supplements. Unfortunately, they often lack a way of knowing what is really right for their particular body, and eventually discover that what has worked so well for someone else has done little for them.

Sound familiar? Are you still looking for solutions? Body typing has the answer to these questions and many more.

After years of researching this subject, I identified 25 specific body types based on a person's dominant gland, organ, or system.

Identifying your body type can open doors to nutritional awareness, self-awareness – and personal empowerment. In a nutshell, it shows the way to obtain perfect body weight and optimum health.

I am constantly shown the value of this program when people I have body typed several years earlier come back to tell me what a difference it's made in their lives. This is why I feel compelled to share it with you.

Like so many others, Barbara came to me after spending years searching for the secrets to "perfect health." She tried programs that included diet, exercise, meditation, fasting, juicing, and colonics. With the Ayurvedic system, she learned that she needed dense protein in her diet. Following the program was difficult for her, as it left too many questions unanswered. Not being able to find the missing factors, she felt dissatisfied because she had once again failed in her quest to achieve good health.

Seeking a personal approach to solving her health problems, Barbara came to me for body typing. After filling out the questionnaire and testing her body's response to certain foods, we determined that she was a Nervous System body type, meaning her dominant gland or system was her nervous system.

When Barbara and I went over the diet she would be following, she realized that she had not been eating enough of the kinds of protein that her body needed. Through her tendency toward vegetarianism, she had been making food choices that seemed healthy, but were not properly supporting her system.

After following her new body type diet for several weeks, Barbara reported back to me that she was feeling better than ever. She felt she was finally on the road to the "perfect health" she had been seeking for so long. What had happened was that her system had begun to come back into balance and, as a result, her health and well-being were improving.

WHY DOES BODY TYPING WORK?

The basic principle of body typing is that each individual body type needs a different set of "rules to play by". In other words, what works for one type does not necessarily work for another. The reason people experience such contradictory results with diets is that not everyone reacts the same way to the same foods or food combinations.

Just because a diet regimen consists of whole, healthy foods, doesn't make it right or beneficial for your particular body type. Therefore, it's important to learn how to recognize which foods affect your individual body positively.

All foods contain certain nutrients that support or stimulate specific glands, organs, and systems of the body. For example, dates support the adrenals but supply a lot of sugar which stimulates the thyroid gland. So if the thyroid is your dominant gland, dates should be avoided, but included if your type is Adrenal. Since each body type has strengths and weaknesses in different areas, each one has different nutritional needs.

Advantages of Body Typing

The value of knowing your type is more than being able to lose weight. *Once you determine your body type you will learn which foods to eat to sustain your body for maximum health and vitality.* By eating the foods that *support* your body, you will find that you will be able to reach and/or maintain your proper weight.

As you know, your general health determines how you feel. Therefore, the more you know about your body, the more you can ensure your own happiness and sense of well-being. Knowing what problems or illnesses your particular type is prone to can be vital in preventing them.

Diet can be as simple as eating the foods that support your body and avoiding those that create unnecessary stress. By giving your body what it needs, food cravings disappear and your energy increases.

Since each type has its own characteristic shape, knowing your body type will lead to a more realistic expectation of your appearance. All too often, women think they need to make their bodies look like the current model, who in reality just happens to have the body type that is most flattered by the current fashion styles. It's time we establish our *own identity.*

Included in the photos of each type are examples of someone who is underweight, overweight, and at their ideal weight. You will see that certain characteristics, such as the prominent buttocks of the Gonadal and Kidney, will always be present regardless of weight. Some types like the Heart and Pancreas tend to be round while others have a long, slender appearance.

Your type-related psychological profile will provide you with insights allowing for greater self-understanding, as well as compassion and expanded awareness of the strengths and challenges of others. The knowledge and perception of deep-seated tendencies, concerns, and motivations can offer you a greater sense of direction and acceptance of yourself and those around you.

BENEFITS OF THE RIGHT DIET

One of the first indications that your body is under excessive stress is an imbalance in your weight, either over or under. While weight gain is generally the most common symptom of the body being out of balance, so is weight loss.

Maintaining your ideal weight and energy level is the goal of this program. Even if you have no desire to lose or gain weight, body typing can help you achieve and maintain optimal health. This is done through meeting the specific needs for your body.

From here on, *diet means: the consumption of foods chosen to support your body.* By choosing the foods your particular body most needs, you can:

- promote clearer thinking, better concentration, and improved memory;
- reduce susceptibility to depression, mood swings, irritability, hyperactivity, and fatigue;
- help eliminate digestive distress, intestinal gas and bloating; and
- improve appetite, or help curb the tendency to eat certain foods at times when they are not supportive.

To identify your ideal diet, you need to determine your dominant gland, organ, or system (which will be referred to for simplicity's sake as your dominant gland). **Your dominant gland is the strongest gland, and it has the greatest influence on your body.** This gland is what determines your shape, appearance, and areas of weight gain. Like your fingerprints, your body type is present at birth and remains constant throughout your life.

WEIGHT AS A SIGNAL

When you begin to notice either weight gain or loss, your body is signaling you that it's time to restore its balance. The easiest way to assist your body is by changing your diet to include the foods it needs most and eliminate those that are stressful.

Even minor dietary changes can have amazing results, meaning you don't have to do everything before you see a difference. Simply by creating more variety in their weekly menus, or eating certain foods at specific times of the day, people have been able to increase their health and sense of well-being as well as attain and maintain their proper weight.

Often women with long histories of yo-yo dieting or who have battled weight all their lives, including those who were "born heavy" or started the battle in their teens, have finally been able to rid themselves of unwanted pounds and inches by sticking to the diet plan that is tailor-made for their body type. And what they really appreciate with this body typing program is that they can keep the weight off!

Chronic Weight Problems

Darlene battled a weight problem since her teens. Her thick waist and heavy thighs prompted her to try every diet that came along. She was thoroughly familiar with the grapefruit diet, Slim Fast™, Dexatrim™, etc., etc., etc. She had even resorted to trying a tablespoon of vinegar every day to see if that could possibly help her lose weight. **Exercise didn't work either!** She tried every routine to exhaustion that might help get her waist thin again so she wouldn't be embarrassed in a bathing suit.

When she came to me, Darlene weighed 173 pounds. Her body type was Pancreas, and her weight gain was due to her overstressed dominant gland. I also discovered that everything she had been doing to lose weight was counterproductive for her body type. I outlined a dietary plan that would be nutritionally supportive and would help her lose the excess pounds.

After only six months, faithfully following her eating plan, Darlene had lost 38 pounds. When she began to follow the diet that was right for her body type, she lost weight easily and consistently. As she got into it, she became creative in rotating her foods and including a wide variety. Darlene was finally able to enjoy life because of better health, vitality, self-esteem, and increased energy.

Since your body type is something that you are born with, it has a "blueprint" for how you gain weight and what you must do to take it off. When you understand your body's specific needs, it helps eliminate any guilt you might feel in not trying the diet that is working for your friends or relatives. You will know what you need!

In using this plan to improve your health and increase your well-being, you will find that your body begins to function at a highly efficient level. When you know what feeling good is like, you will begin to know which foods have the best, or the worst, effect on you.

As you become more aware of your body's response to what you eat, you will also be more conscious of other things in life. You may have greater sensitivity to external things like smells, temperature, or the moods of others, and perhaps to energies around you. Your body's new balance can also balance other aspects of your being, allowing you to live a much fuller and richer life.

HOW IT ALL BEGAN

My personal experience with diet began, like most of you, by eating what my mother served. She fixed what my father wanted and since he was raised on a farm, dinner usually consisted of beef or chicken and potatoes, bread, and a vegetable or salad. As a child, I was usually somewhat bloated, suffered from periodic intestinal gas, and carried a few extra pounds around my waist and lower abdomen.

While in chiropractic college, I began to experiment with my diet. I stopped eating red meat and started eating brown rice and vegetables. That was great! I lost the extra weight I was carrying and the gas and bloating disappeared. Over the years, I began to notice that when chicken was served, I ate more than my share. My main protein sources were cheese, yogurt, and cottage cheese. After a while, I noticed that I was gaining weight in my thighs.

Throughout my studies of diet and nutrition, I acquired more practical knowledge through muscle testing than by any other method. Muscle testing is a simple, accurate way of communicating directly with the body through a strong or weak muscle response. It is a way of by-passing the conscious mind and communicating directly with the unconscious, the part that runs the body and carries out all automatic functions, such as digestion and assimilation.

Even though I was using muscle testing to determine the most supportive brands and varieties of what I was eating, I didn't think to ask if I was getting enough of the kind of protein I needed. When I met my husband, continuing with a vegetarian diet was no longer practical, so I conceded to including fish, eggs, and chicken. By making this change to my diet, and doing a few limited floor exercises, I lost the extra eight pounds I had accumulated over the previous ten years of being a vegetarian.

It was just after this experience that a patient brought in *Dr. Abravanel's Body Type Diet and Lifetime Nutritional Plan*, by Elliot D. Abravanel, M.D. and Elizabeth A. King (1983). According to this book, I was a Thyroid and needed to eat dense protein, which was exactly what I had done; and I had the results to prove that it worked!

This was the first diet book I'd seen that made sense. It was based on a person's dominant gland, that determined the foods that best supported that gland, the best time of day to eat the largest meal, and weight gain patterns for each body type.

EVOLVING THE BODY TYPE SYSTEM

Dr. Abravanel's book opened a door for me. At last there was a way to make diet and nutrition make sense. It's the glands that determine your basic shape – like flat or prominent buttocks, muscle tone, body build (including wide or narrow hips), where you gain weight, and the foods you crave to give you the greatest energy boost.

I liked the basic premise, and I had proven it to be accurate; however, the diet for the Thyroid type had to be modified to best support me. As I read through the diets for the other types, I realized they also needed modification if the patients I saw were going to be able to use them.

There was something about the book that bothered me. Abravanel had identified four body types for women: the Adrenal, Thyroid, Pituitary, and Gonadal. But only three of these types applied to men, and the one that was missing was the Gonadal. Now I just couldn't believe that, in at least some men, the gonads were not their dominant gland.

Still, the book had a lot of merit, so I continued to incorporate it into my practice and taught classes at the community education adult school on body typing. As I worked with it, I started to find people who didn't fit the four types identified, but seemed instead to be a combination.

DISCOVERY! ADDITIONAL TYPES

In the spring of 1987, I attended a workshop by Richard and Laura Power, nutritionists from Bethesda, Maryland. They had developed a system of eight body types, also based on a person's dominant gland. These types were anthropologically and genetically determined and consisted of: Adrenal, Thyroid, Pituitary, Gonadal, Thymus, Pineal, Pancreas, and Balanced (meaning no single gland was dominant).

To determine type, they used a checklist that included both structural and psychological items, physical measurements, and blood type. They too had discovered people who didn't fit in even their expanded types, so to accommodate the misfits they proposed "combination types" (such as Gonadal-Thyroid), with the first gland being the one that exerted the primary influence.

I was thrilled to learn that there were four more types. I was especially fascinated by one type, the Pineal, that Power described as having a small head and a rather delicate or slight body build. The descriptive information was very sketchy, and the dietary material was practically non-existent.

I compiled what other data I could find on the pineal gland, including both its physical and metaphysical attributes. It is commonly associated with intuition and intuitive guidance. Physically, it is known to secrete hormones, is associated with the menstrual cycle, and is activated by sunlight. This is the gland that is responsible for the depression common in individuals who live in cloudy or overcast areas like Seattle, or regions where there are long periods of darkness like Alaska. The Pineal body type is extremely sensitive to the presence or lack of sunlight, and will often feel depressed when the sun doesn't shine.

To determine the appropriate diet, meaning the one that would be indigenous, and therefore most supportive for the Pineal type, I considered the lifestyle and diet that would be typical for a South Sea Island native, as this is where Power had placed their genetic origin. Available foods would be fresh fruits and vegetables, coconuts, and freshly caught fish. Since they would have had no refrigeration or electricity, fish would be caught in the morning, brought in and immediately cooked for the midday meal. With the climate being temperate, personal energy would generally be higher in the early part of the day, and lifestyle would revolve around available sunlight.

With these factors in mind, I wondered if some of my patients might be Pineals. I started by using the muscle response test (described in the *"Muscle Testing"* booklet) to determine how they responded to island foods. I noticed that many of those who were having digestive problems tested very well for fish, coconut, and fresh (rather than dried) fruit.

I wondered if the time of day they ate fruit or protein made a difference. It did. They all had difficulty digesting protein for the evening meal, but had no problem when they ate protein around noon.

Their body structure, weight gain pattern, and food cravings were similar to, but not exactly like, the Gonadal and Thyroid. The Pineal type seemed like a blend of these two types.

Pineal Type

Over time, a clear psychological profile emerged for the Pineal. As a group, these individuals are high-strung, yet perceptive, and unusually intuitive. Since the pineal gland is the reception point for intuition, these types take in vast amounts of data, so much so that most Pineals have difficulty distilling it into concise usable information.

Over and over again I observed the difficulty Pineals had in translating this intuitive, unfocused information into "earth terms", or something applicable to daily living. Most of them are very talkative and talk as a way of distilling the vast amount of raw data that they are constantly barraged with into something they can apply or pass on to someone else. Quick and bright, they are stimulated by learning, particularly when it involves personal growth and awareness. Bringing in light seems to be a central theme that is reflected both in their personality and surroundings.

Typically, the homes they select, or renovate, are full of large windows and skylights. While most of us enjoy the sun, but can tolerate cloudy, overcast days, Pineals can't. When the sun doesn't shine, they tend to be seriously vulnerable to moodiness and depression. "Sun worshippers" by nature, as well as one of the most physically sensitive types, their skin often reveals the damage done by overexposure to the otherwise nurturing rays of the sun they so much crave.

One of my Pineal patients, Sue, decided she would move from San Diego to a less populated region in Washington state. She wanted to "commune" with nature and selected a picturesque area that appealed to her spiritually. In a very short time, she discovered that the rainy climate and frequent cloudy, overcast days made her feel moody and irritable. So, she returned to San Diego. Even though she wasn't thrilled to go back into a region that was so congested, she realized she had to have the sunlight to function.

A New Type

My discovery of additional types started with a twelve year-old patient, Mary. I began with her weight gain pattern which, like the Gonadal type, was buttocks and thighs. When I tested her body's response to the "Frequently" and "Rarely" foods of the Gonadal, the answers didn't match. I then tested her response to the "Key Indicator Foods By Type" for each of the other seven known types, but nothing fit.

Her general body structure and muscle mass were stronger and more dense than the Thyroid – more like the Adrenal, but not quite. I had before me someone who had the general weight gain pattern of the Gonadal, with physical characteristics similar to the Adrenal,

If I followed the rules of other systems, I had a person who fell between two types, or was a blend of the two. For me, this was not an acceptable answer. Dietarily, a blended type is only slightly more useful than having no type.

Then I asked Mary what foods she liked and tested her body's response to them. I thought her answers were typical for a teenager – pizza, peanut butter sandwiches, and mint chocolate ice cream. I was amazed when she tested strong for pizza, but even more so when peanut butter on whole wheat bread was weak but strong on enriched white bread – hardly the result her mother or I would have preferred. The next surprise came when I tested her for cherries – weak for fresh, strong for cherry pie.

By this time, her mother and I were looking at each other in amazement; this didn't fit what either of us (her mother being a nutritionist) had been taught was a healthy diet. We even started to speculate as to whether the bodies of the younger generation had finally adapted to "junky" diets and if so, what organ would have to be especially strong to handle the additional stress. The kidney seemed a logical choice and fit with Mary's medical history as being her strongest organ.

Kidney Type

Mary's physical characteristics included a distinct waist, with no weight gain across her lower back in the kidney region. She had a medium bone structure, dense solid musculature and a strong constitution. Given the foods that best supported her body, her physical characteristics, medical history, weight gain pattern, and location of her dominant energy focus, I concluded and verified that her kidneys were her dominant organ and, consequently, her body type.

I tested the food profile I had compiled for Mary on other children and found that the ones with similar physical characteristics responded well to the same foods. I continued to expand this list with others, including the time of day foods were best eaten and the best combinations, then I checked Mary's response to the new information. This way I was able to determine what was true to type and what was unique to the individual.

This is the procedure I used to discover and develop the rest of the types. Essentially, when I was presented with someone who didn't fit into any of my known types, I started checking their body's response to foods. This eventually lead me to the identification of a new type. During the discovery stage, the longest time I went between new types was six months, and the last type to appear was the Eye, which also happened to be my brother and father's type.

BASIC CONCEPT OF BODY TYPING

We are all different. What works for me does not necessarily work for you. While there are basic similarities, it's the differences that make us unique. This is particularly true when it comes to food and diets. The problem with most diets is the "one size fits all" theory. Unfortunately, with diets as in clothing, this one size can never be form fitting.

But if I had to check all the foods, combinations, and eating schedules for every person, it would be very time consuming and, consequently, impractical. Knowing a person's body type is like knowing their clothing size; from here all that was necessary to do was to make minor alterations.

While there are 25 distinct types, there are similarities between types. The glands that are known for having the greatest influence on the body are the adrenals, pituitary, and thyroid. You can find some of this early research in *Food Is Your Best Medicine*, by Dr. Henry Bieler (1966).

THE FUNDAMENTALS OF BODY TYPING

Glands determine physical characteristics as well as the location of weight gain. We can divide the 25 body types into three categories based on area of weight gain. **Women gain weight predominantly in their upper body, lower body, or all over.** Most types fall in the lower body weight gain group. Within this group, some gain in their lower abdomen, but not in their buttocks while others are just the opposite, gaining in their buttocks but not in their lower abdomen. These are the first physical characteristics to observe when determining body type.

These characteristics are illustrated in three contrasting types.The Adrenal type is a classic example of weight gain in the upper body. The Pituitary type gains weight throughout the entire body, or all over, while the Thyroid type gains mainly in the lower body.

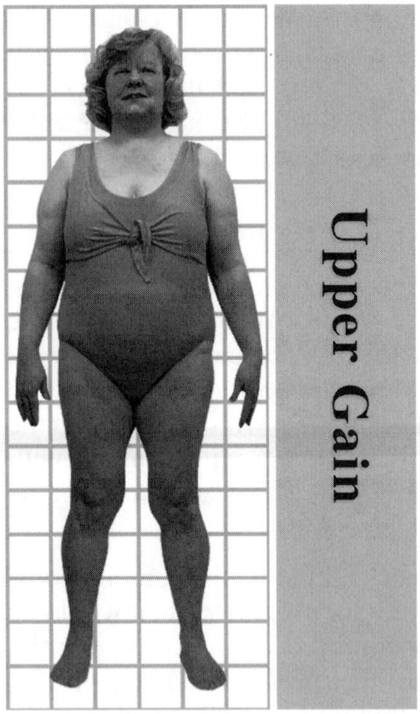

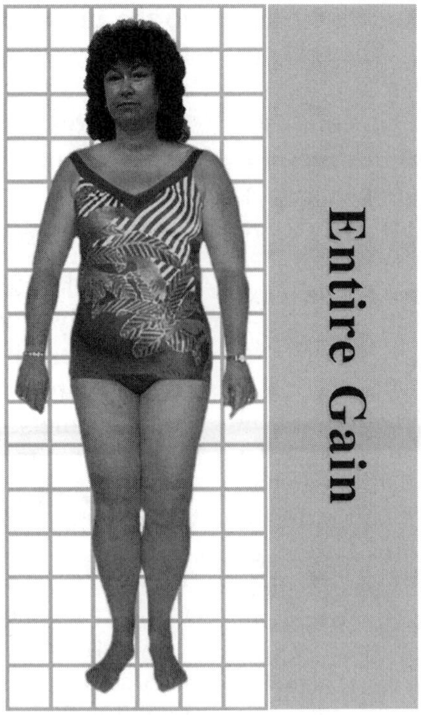

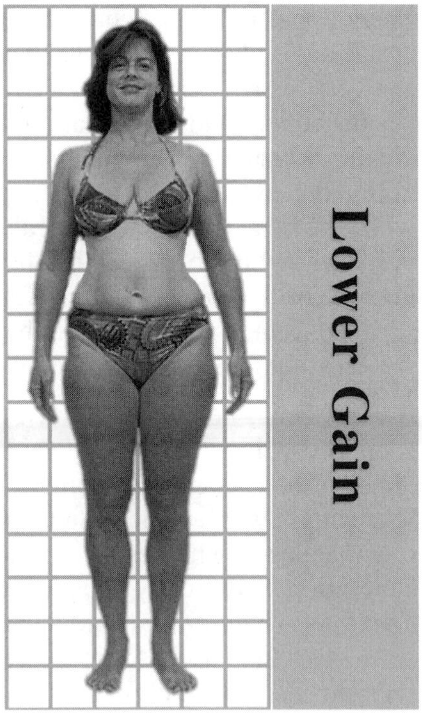

Not only do these types have different weight gain patterns, they have different personalities, health challenges, and dietary requirements. Understanding these three types will give you a good concept of the differences between body types and why one diet can't possibly be right for everyone.

Even though the Adrenal and Pituitary often have similar physical characteristics, their dietary needs are opposite. Adrenals require a light breakfast and heavy meal at dinner, while Pituitaries need a heavy breakfast and light early dinner. When Adrenals eat a large breakfast, they want to eat

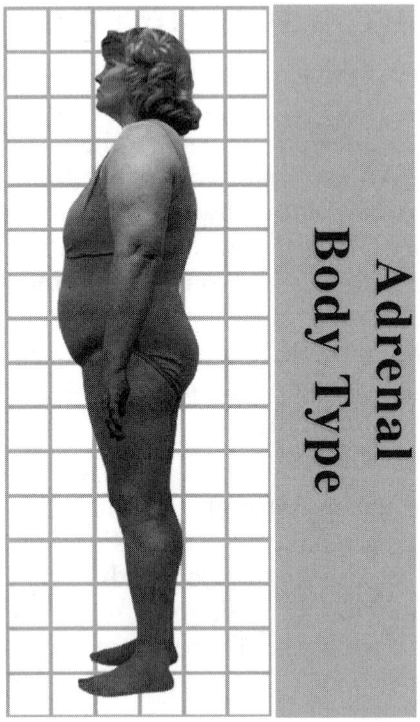

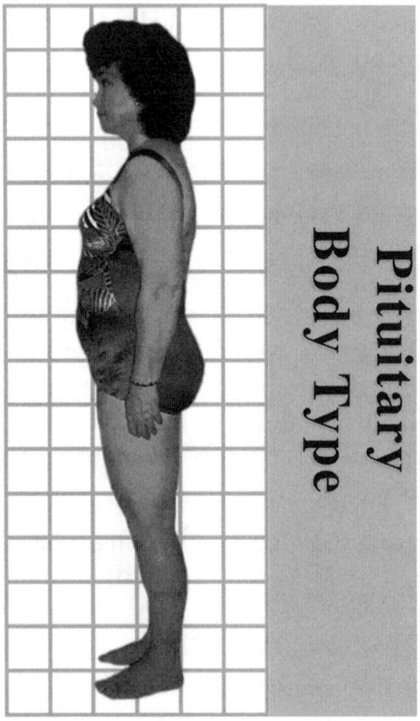

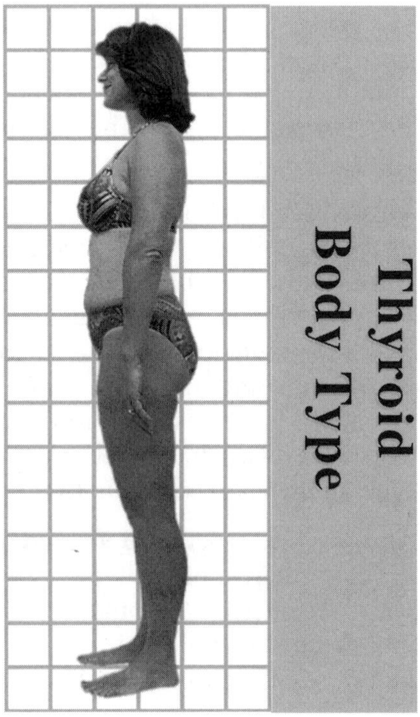

all day long. Pituitaries would prefer to skip breakfast, but need it to get their energy moving down in their body, which eating does. Adrenals need to emphasize dairy, as dairy stimulates the pituitary and gets the energy moving into the head. Pituitaries need to avoid dairy as it provides too much stimulation to an already overactive gland. Red meat stimulates the adrenal glands, so Adrenals need to avoid it, while Pituitaries need the adrenal stimulation; so steak and eggs for breakfast is ideal for them.

Not only are they dietary opposites, but physically Adrenals have a dense, solid musculature, while Pituitaries have a layer of softness that covers their muscles, giving them a soft appearance. Adrenals are physically strong, with high energy and a need for exercise. Pituitaries are sensitive and prefer mental to physical activity.

Equally opposite are the Adrenal and Thyroid types. Since the thyroid and pituitary glands are located relatively close, with the thyroid in the throat and the pituitary in the head, these types resemble each other more than either one does to the Adrenal. Like the Pituitary, the Thyroid type needs a moderate to heavy breakfast. Food earlier in the day provides a sustaining energy, of which Thyroids need a continuous supply.

CONTRASTING TYPES: ADRENAL AND THYROID

Sally and Lisa had been friends for years, and they recently began to get together frequently, doing things they both enjoyed. But Lisa found she was having difficulty keeping the pace that her aggressive, robust friend would set for them. She came to me complaining of being tired all the time and having digestive problems that seemed to bother her only after she and Sally had been out to eat. She was afraid her friend was having an adverse effect on her after all these years, and it was a concern for her.

I determined Lisa's dominant gland and found that she was a Thyroid, one of the more delicate body types. I asked her about her friend, Sally, and what kind of activities and events they attended. I also inquired as to the kinds of foods they ate when they were out. I felt that Sally might be an Adrenal, a stronger, more physically robust type. If this were true, it could be that Lisa was trying to match her lifestyle to Sally's, and because she wasn't supporting her own needs, it was beginning to wear her down.

I asked if Sally would come in for body typing. When she did, I found my suspicions were true; she was indeed an Adrenal type. In their friendship, Sally was the pacesetter: energetic, enthusiastic, and physically oriented. She loved to eat steaks, spicy Mexican or Italian food, and those Double Whoppers™ at the local hamburger place. She also liked participant sports and activities that challenged her physically. Sally was never happier than when she found a new challenge and could "go for it" with all she had. It never dawned on her that Lisa wasn't enjoying these things just as much as she was.

Adrenals are characterized by their strong, heavy musculature in the torso, arms, and legs and medium-to-large bone structure. They are physically oriented, with naturally high energy and stamina. A classic example of an Adrenal man is a football linebacker. Adrenal women have a "boyish" figure, with a straight, poorly defined waistline. They are easily excited and generally throw themselves into new experiences with great enthusiasm. They show an exuberance when in pursuit of a goal, and can exhibit a great deal of physical presence. Sally fit the picture perfectly.

Thyroids, in contrast, have a more delicate appearance with long, slender hands and feet and a medium bone structure. They are slighter in appearance and less muscular than their Adrenal counterparts.

Thyroid women have a well-defined waist that gives them an hourglass figure. They are physically less active than the Adrenals and are much more reserved. In pursuing their goals, Thyroid types generally show a great deal of persistence and dedication to whatever project they have undertaken, doing things in a quiet, orderly manner.

Lisa, normally quite reserved, was becoming exhausted trying to keep up with the activities of her friend, Sally. When she came to me, she knew something about her life needed changing as her lifestyle was affecting her health.

Most types have low energy periods. The body's automatic response during this time is to crave those foods that supply the greatest stimulation for the dominant gland or organ. For Adrenals, the low point usually occurs in the early evening, and the foods craved are beef, including hamburger, and/or salty foods like peanuts, chips, and pretzels. Sally preferred a salty snack followed by strenuous physical activity. Later she wanted a moderate to large dinner that included meat or spicy food.

Lisa's idea of a nice time was to have a Chinese dinner, see a good movie, and then stop afterwards for a gooey dessert. But Sally liked to play tennis or run so she could work off her stress for the day, and then have a big steak dinner, Mexican or Italian food. Being the less forceful of the two, Lisa usually gave in to her friend, and suffered the consequences. Neither of them could know that the disparity in their desired activity and eating habits was due to the differences in their body types.

DIETARY DIFFERENCES BETWEEN ADRENAL AND THYROID

Adrenals and Thyroids can eat together at the same table and at the same time. But there is quite a difference in the foods you're apt to find on their plates. The Thyroid type is more likely to be eating fish or chicken, with vegetables and rice, while the Adrenal will want a big juicy steak with baked potato, sour cream, and a lettuce salad.

Strong types like the Adrenal can manage to stay healthy on a diet of red meat and salty foods in younger years, but as they age this kind of indulgence could be disastrous. The Adrenal types, particularly men, are prone to suffering from a fatal heart attack with no obvious warning.

Adrenals are also prone to high cholesterol levels, and tend to eat foods like eggs and red meat that often aggravate the problem. The American Heart Association designed its dietary recommendations for this group of people. Each of the 25 body types has a certain predisposition to some kind of disease, and for the Adrenal it is heart disease.

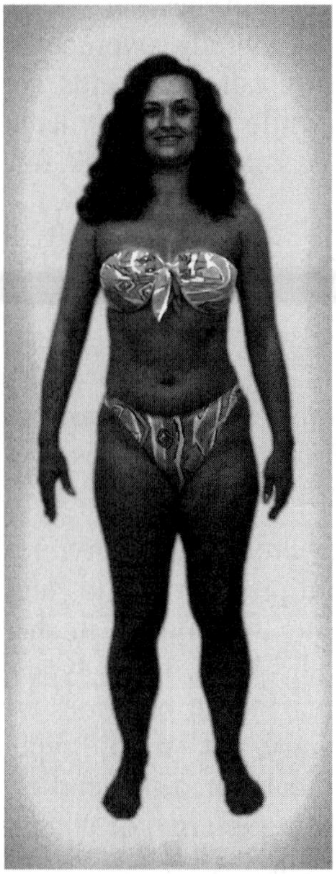

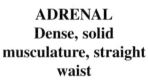

ADRENAL
Dense, solid musculature, straight waist

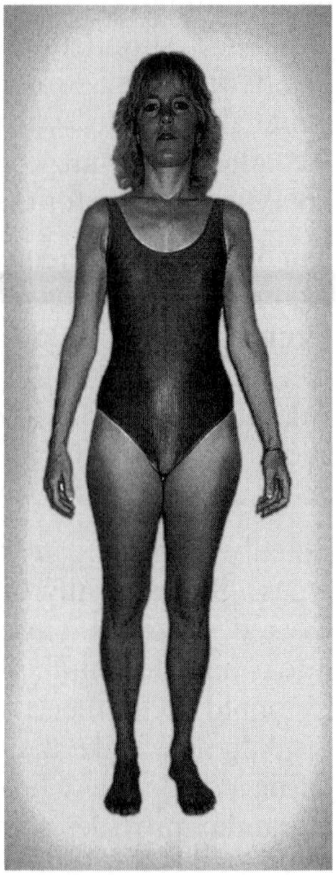

THYROID
Average, elongated musculature, well-defined waist

Since diet has been proven to compound cholesterol problems, it makes sense for the Adrenal types to watch their food intake and eat a healthy, well-balanced diet. The body manufactures 70-90% of the total cholesterol and uses it to make antibodies, enzymes, and hormones. High cholesterol levels are stress related, particularly in the Adrenal types. These types can relieve the stress on their dominant gland by stimulating the opposite glands, the thyroid and pituitary. This is done by eating sweet fruits and dairy products. Eating raw vegetables and avoiding salt, red meat, and eggs (stimulants for the adrenal gland) can lower cholesterol and help promote necessary weight loss.

While Adrenals lose weight easily, it is equally easy for them to regain those pounds. Because weight is such an issue for them, they are always gaining weight and then losing it. Adrenal types are the "dieting experts." Many weight loss diets offered to the public appear to have the Adrenal type in mind, as these programs seem specifically designed for them. In fact, the cornerstone of diets, Weight Watchers™, was designed around and for the Adrenal type

The "classic diet" consisting of raw fruits and vegetables, yogurt, and cottage cheese was designed and is perfect for the Adrenals. Unfortunately, the results for many other body types on this diet is anything but ideal.

Diets that don't work are those that cause you to gain weight where you desire to lose it and lose weight in the places you need to keep it. Inability to stay on a diet because you're constantly hungry or tired means you are not getting sufficient energy from the foods you are eating, so the diet you are following is not supporting you. The wrong foods are often difficult to digest and "sit" in your stomach, causing you to feel sluggish or ill.

Food's Effect on Areas of Weight Loss

Losing weight is not simply about losing pounds, but losing them in the right places. Adrenals gain their weight in the upper body, while most other types, like the Thyroid, put on weight in the lower body. The "classic" weight loss diet does not support Thyroid types. Thyroid women tend to carry all of their excess weight in their lower abdomen and thighs, with minimal weight gain in the upper body. Weight loss above the waist is rarely their desired goal.

"Classic" diets cause the dieter to lose weight from the upper body and to gain it in the lower body. Body chemistry is regulated by a person's dominant gland and determines what nutrients their body requires. Lack of essential nutrients is what accounts for weight loss in the wrong places and is why the "classic" diet is unacceptable for most types.

Chemically speaking, Adrenals and Thyroids are at opposite ends of the scale. Adrenals are naturally high in sodium and low in potassium, while Thyroids are just the reverse.

Sodium/potassium ratios are affected by eating vegetables that are either raw or cooked. Cooking increases the sodium content of vegetables. Since raw vegetables contain a higher potassium-to-sodium ratio than cooked, Adrenals can benefit by eating the larger percentage of their vegetables raw. Raw vegetables contain more potassium and since the Adrenal body is naturally high in sodium, increasing potassium helps balance this ratio, allowing the system to eliminate excess fluid, resulting in weight loss.

Nutrient-rich foods generally achieve a better balance than simply taking nutritional supplements. Thyroid types, who are naturally high in potassium, can throw their systems out of balance with too much potassium from raw vegetables. The result is weight loss in the upper body, which Thyroids don't need.

An important point to remember is: different food groups affect different areas of the body causing weight gain or loss in specific regions. Raw vegetables affect the upper body or torso, and dairy products affect the lower body, particularly the thighs.

Fruits recommended in classic diets pose a problem for Thyroid types. Sweet fruits, like bananas and oranges, stimulate the thyroid gland just like the sweets and pastries the Thyroids crave. An excess of these fruits overstimulates their dominant gland and stresses their bodies as if they had eaten refined sugar.

Stimulation of a gland or organ should not always be avoided. There are times when it is appropriate, as mentioned earlier in the case of the Adrenal needing to stimulate the thyroid gland to help restore balance. However, in an overstressed system, excessive stimulation of the dominant gland can destroy the body's balance.

In stimulating a gland, energy is directed into an area of the body, causing increased activity. Too much stimulation causes fatigue, resulting in diminished function of the gland and imbalance in the body. The first clue to imbalance is weight gain in the area characteristic of the body type, but not necessarily in the same location as the dominant gland. For example, in the Thyroid and Pineal types, weight gain is in the lower body, not the head or throat. This is because the energy is predominately in the head, but doesn't move as freely in the lower body.

When the body is in crisis or overstressed, it will crave the foods that provide the greatest relief in the quickest way possible by stimulating the dominant gland. When the dominant gland is functioning poorly due to the fatigue of overstimulation, the body continues to crave foods to further stimulate its activity. But, by satisfying this craving, the gland is depleted even further, and eventually becomes totally exhausted. The resulting imbalance causes more weight gain. Losing the excess weight requires taking the stress off the body, giving the dominant gland a rest, and rebuilding the complementary glands. In the case of Thyroids, the adrenal glands are complementary.

Adrenals crave red meats and salty foods to stimulate their adrenal glands, and Thyroids want carbohydrates and sweets to stimulate their thyroid glands. Avoiding these foods can eliminate the overstimulation of the dominant gland and give it time to recover.

For the dominant gland to recover from being overstressed, it needs to be given a rest. This is where the stimulation of an opposite strong and healthy gland can relieve strain on the fatigued gland. For example, Adrenal types need to stimulate the thyroid gland to take over for the adrenal glands, which can be done by eating sweet fruits.

The Thyroid type, on the other hand, should avoid red meat and salty foods because these foods stimulate rather than rebuild. To rebuild the adrenal glands, they need to include dense protein like chicken, fish, and eggs, and avoid sugar as well as sweet fruits. This takes the stress off the thyroid gland and allows it to recover. These protein foods will rebuild the adrenal glands which eliminates the craving for sweets.

The remaining diet for the Thyroid should consist of vegetables, of which 70% should be steamed or baked, and whole grains like rice and oats. Breads should be eliminated because the combination of grain, yeast, and sweetener is hard to digest and promotes weight gain in the lower abdomen, a major problem area for Thyroids.

Breakfast is vital to the Thyroid type, and so is eating regular meals during the day. This is because the Thyroid's energy level usually increases after eating, unless they have overeaten or consumed foods that were not right for their body type, thereby creating more stress.

BEYOND 3 TYPES

Now that you have had a chance to become familiar with three types, unless you happened to be one of them, you probably noticed some things that fit and others that did not. While there is a certain amount of overlapping in parts of the diet, each type has its own unique diet. If by any chance you should feel that you might have difficulty differentiating between two types, the types usually in question are generally so close that even if you followed the diet that wasn't specifically for your type, following either diet will still be beneficial.

A couple of types that are very similar to the Thyroid are the Lymph and Thalamus. In the past they would have been considered variations of the Thyroid type; as you will see, each one is different.

Since each type is so unique, the psychological profile is often the easiest way to differentiate your body type. Not only does your dominant gland control your physical body, it plays an important role in your psychological make-up as well. It determines basic characteristics and motivates you to act the way you do. Knowing what motivates you can even be helpful in finding the job that is most appropriate.

Understanding your basic nature allows you to look at your personal challenges from a new perspective. Seeing what these traits are like when expressed at their best provides insights into how to overcome the challenges. Observing whether your current behavior patterns fall closer to the "At Worst" or "At Best" provides a developmental guidepost.

Realizing that everyone else with your same body type has had to face these same challenges provides a sense of comfort. You know that you are not alone, and your challenges are the opportunities that connect you to your strengths. Identifying what is most important to you aids in self-identity.

MODIFIED THYROIDS: LYMPH AND THALAMUS

From all appearances Sharon did not have a weight problem, but she did tend to be heavier below the waist than above it. When she came to me she was concerned about the excess weight on her thighs. In her quest for a more balanced body, she had tried several diets and always lost in her face, neck, and upper abdomen. But, try as she might, nothing seemed to work for her in slimming down her thighs. Her answers to my first few questions gave me the impression, before body typing her, that she might be a Thyroid. However, I discovered that she was not a Thyroid at all, but one that resembles this type very closely.

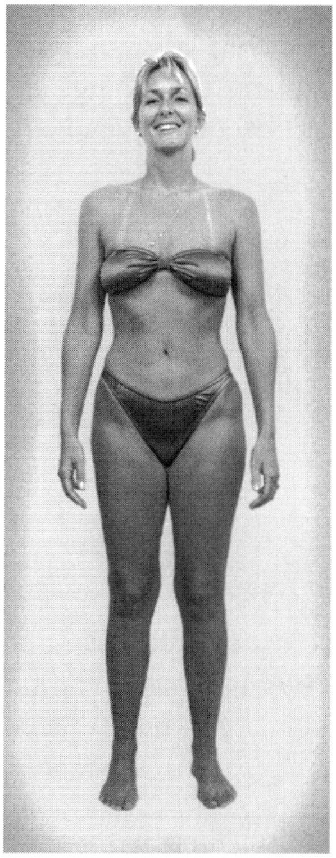

LYMPH
Broad shoulders

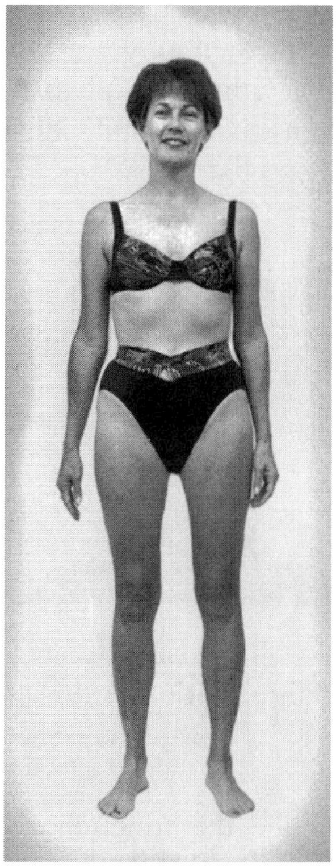

THYROID
Shoulders and hips relatively even

A number of body types are similar to the Thyroid, in that they have several things in common. Body structure, build, weight-gain areas, dietary sensitivities, and psychological make-up are some specific similarities. Two of these types are Lymph and Thalamus.

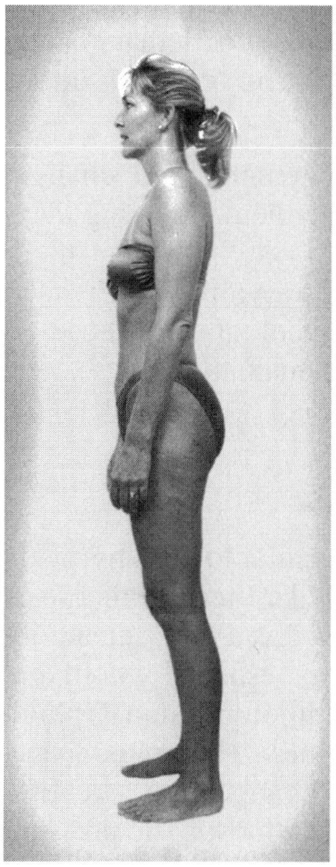

LYMPH
Prominent buttocks
Flat abdomen

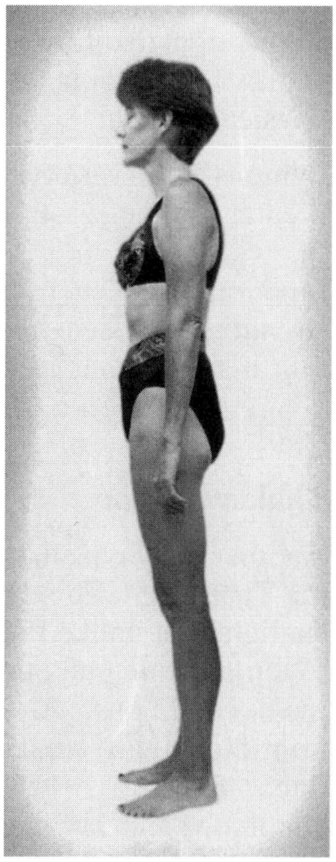

THYROID
Relatively flat buttocks
Lower abdominal bulge

Sharon is a Lymph type and is very much like the Thyroid in that she is delicate in appearance and gains excess weight in her thighs. However, she doesn't have the Thyroid's lower abdominal bulge problem and has nicely defined buttocks as contrasted to the Thyroid's minimal derriere. Both male and female Lymphs have the same body characteristics of broad shoulders, narrow hips, and strong abdominal muscles.

Lymphs need to eat protein, but they are especially sensitive to any meat that has been fed hormones or antibiotics. Their best protein source is wild game or non-domesticated fowl such as wild duck, goose, or Cornish game hens. Spicy foods stimulate their lymphatic system, as does physical movement and drinking adequate amounts of water. While this stimulation can activate a sluggish system, like anything else it can be overdone, so one should avoid going to extremes. The lymphatic system does not move on its own, but is activated by muscle movement. Likewise the Lymph body type requires outside stimulation to prevent stagnation, lethargy, and depression. This stimulation can be either physical or mental.

Lymphs like variety, excitement, and change. Mental challenges stimulate them, allowing them to feel alive and alert which keeps them functioning at their best. Lymph types need strenuous physical movement and, because of this, many become professional athletes.

Thalamus Type

Another body type that is similar to the Thyroid is the Thalamus. This type, like the Pineal, craves sunlight, but unlike Pineals, has a high sensitivity to temperature and humidity, especially cold and moist conditions. Air conditioning, rain, or high humidity can make the Thalamus very uncomfortable. Also, changes in weather conditions and variations in atmospheric pressure can cause them to suffer from headaches, body aches, sinusitis, depression, mood swings, or a general irritability.

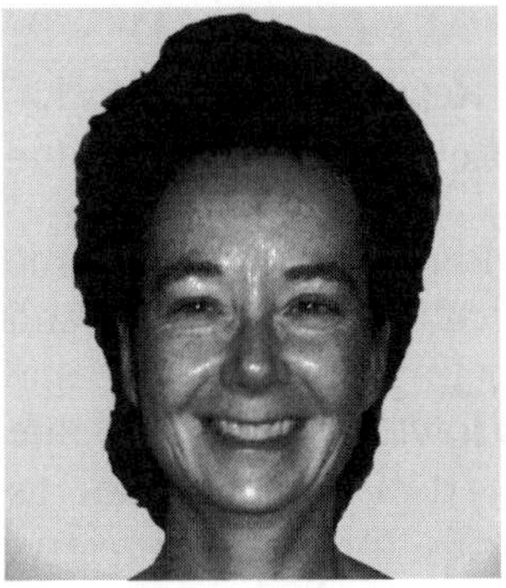

THALAMUS
High, wide dominant forehead

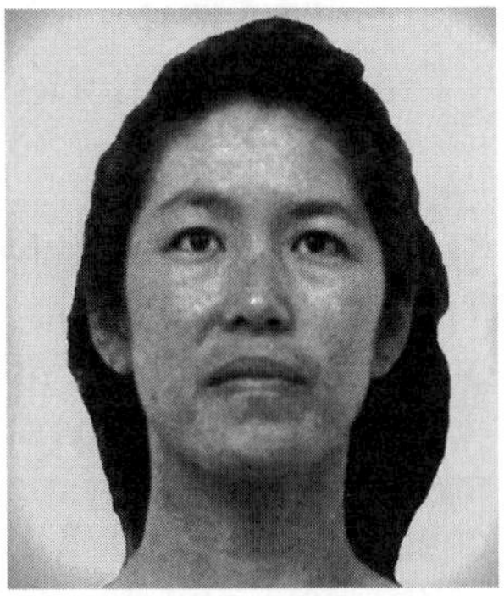

THYROID
Average, proportional forehead

Since their dominant gland is located in the head, so too is the greatest focus of their energy. Consequently, this is where your attention is often drawn. Identifying physical characteristics of the Thalamus are a high, wide dominant forehead, narrow chin, and long, slender face. They are usually average-to-tall in height, slender, and delicate in appearance with a well-proportioned body.

As children, Thalamuses frequently have protruding ears, which often is an area of great concern for their parents. But as they mature, they are generally not noticeable. While some parents consider corrective surgery for these children, it is rarely necessary as they normally "grow into" their ears.

Their ears are the physical expression of their innate ability to listen and their sensitivity to sound, particularly music. More so than any other type, they will keenly observe and be aware of both their physical and emotional surroundings. Thalamuses tend to be relatively easygoing, are sensitive to and considerate of others, and are good listeners.

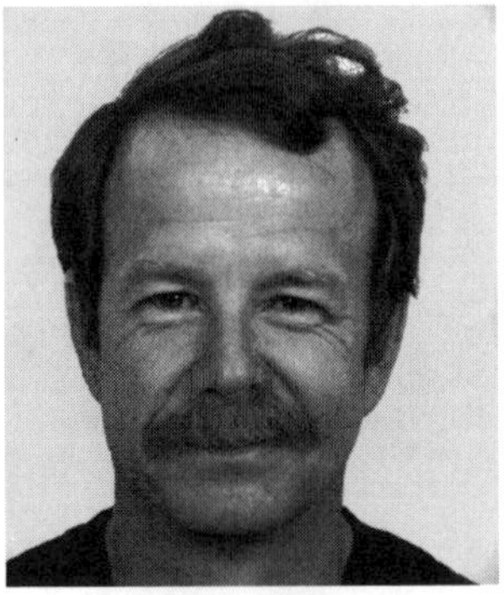

THALAMUS
High, wide dominant forehead

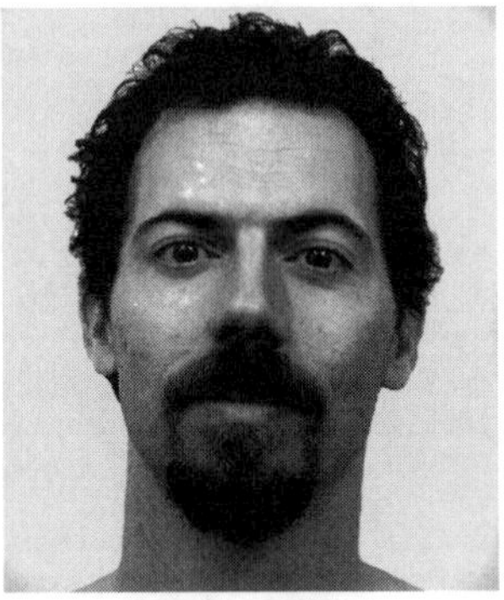

THYROID
Average, proportional forehead

Since the function of the thalamus gland is to collect, sort, and send incoming information to the appropriate areas of the brain, it seems appropriate that the most obvious distinguishing feature of the Thalamus body type is their high, wide dominant forehead. They are more mental than emotional and will typically deliberate a long time over different aspects of a problem before arriving at their final decision. However, when they are under stress, they may become tense or anxious and have difficulty organizing their thoughts and quieting their minds.

Always striving for excellence, Thalamus types tend to work best by themselves and at their own pace. They are exceptionally well-suited for such professions as scientists and researchers.

The Thalamus body type, like the Pineal type, should eat their largest meal of the day at lunch; but unlike Pineals, they can have protein at dinner as well. They digest most protein quite well, including beef, cashews, and sunflower seeds, but surprisingly, not almonds or oysters.

While the Thalamus can eat protein and grains any time of the day, fruits should be consumed only in the morning. It is best to save other kinds of sweets until later in the day and eat them as bedtime snacks.

One of my Thalamus patients told me that she ate almonds on a regular basis because she had heard that the almond was the best nut to eat. I told her that eating almonds was stressful for her particular body and could be the source of the headaches and digestive upsets she was having. Once she eliminated almonds from her diet these symptoms quickly vanished.

WHY SO MANY TYPES?

A system that is complete enough to identify all the types makes knowing what to eat and when to eat it simple. With so many types, it's no wonder people have thrown up their hands and concluded that we're all different. But if this were the case, why do we constantly see diets that are supposed to work for everyone? And it's true, many diets work for a number of people. But then why don't they work for everyone?

There had to be an answer that would bring some order into the dietary jungle. The concept of body typing made sense. I could certainly see the reasoning behind creating general categories, but that didn't solve the practical problem of sorting out the details necessary to answer the question, "What exactly should I eat, doctor?"

By having an individual type, rather than a combination, I can be extremely specific concerning dietary information, characteristics, recommendations, and even a psychological profile. Having all this information allows me to provide you with a basis to work from that gives you a lifetime guide for your body.

Being as specific as possible allows you to get rid of the last few pounds and to keep the weight off once you have lost it. The diet that is right for you is compatible with your body, so it's easy to maintain and incorporate into your lifestyle.

The obvious question is, "How many types are there and have all the types in all the races been discovered?" Do different races have different body types?

I am satisfied that there are only 25 types. The last one (the Eye) was discovered in 1991. Prior to that the longest time between discovering a new type was six months. To make sure I hadn't missed a type, I did complementary body typing sessions for the general public for three years. I also typed everyone in my practice and worked extensively with their diets.

I went to Japan specifically to see if certain cultures were predominantly one body type. I found the same 25 types in the Asian population as I did in the Western world. Everyone I have evaluated has been one of the 25 types.

The following two pages illustrate all 25 body types at their ideal weight. As you become more familiar with each type by studying the three-view photos of the eight people per type, you will begin to notice similarities that will enable you to identify the body type of people you know.

DIFFERENT BODIES
DIFFERENT DIETS

The Body Type System

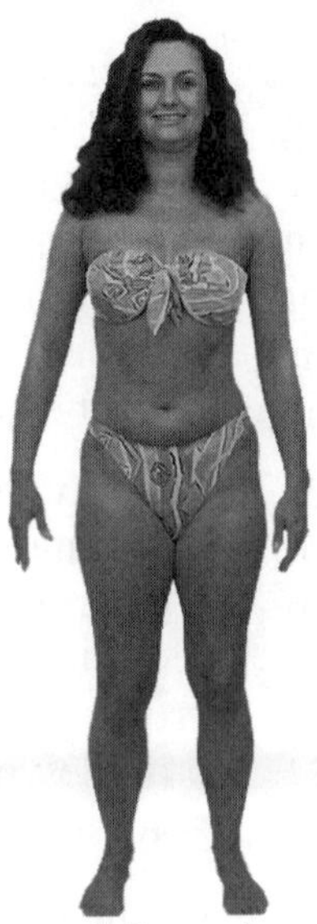
Adrenal

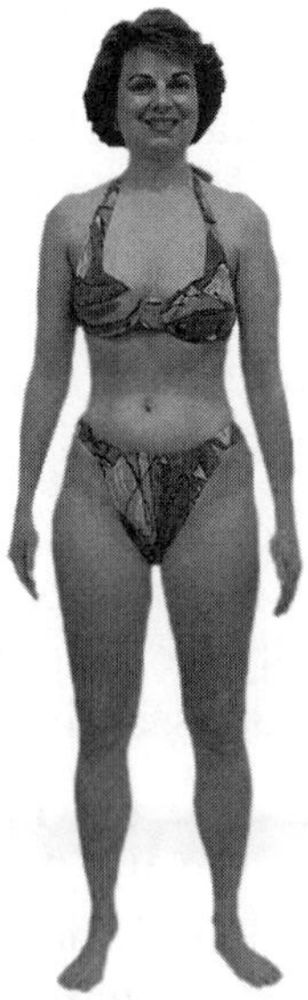
Balanced

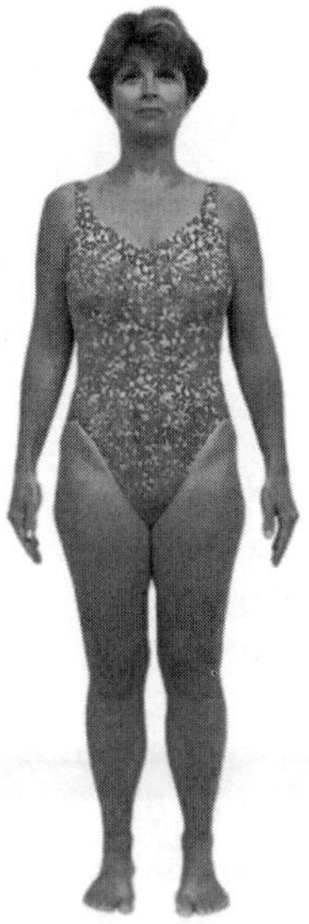
Blood

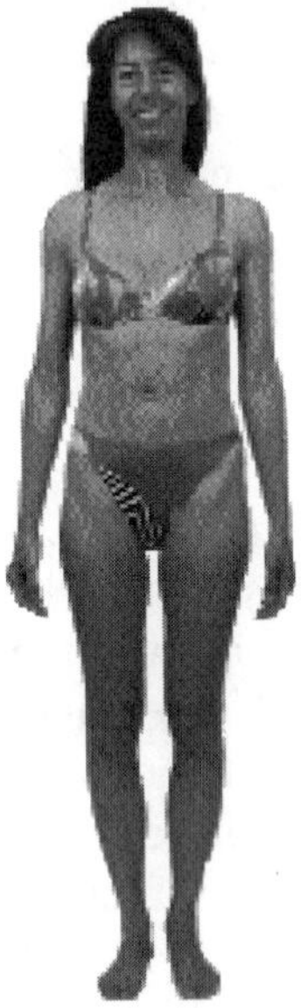
Hypothalamus

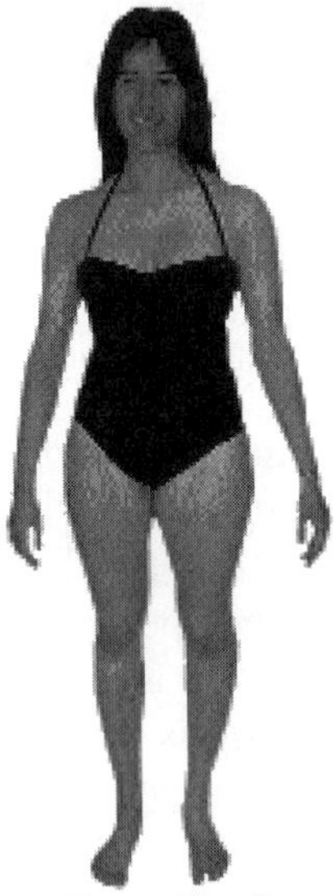
Intestinal

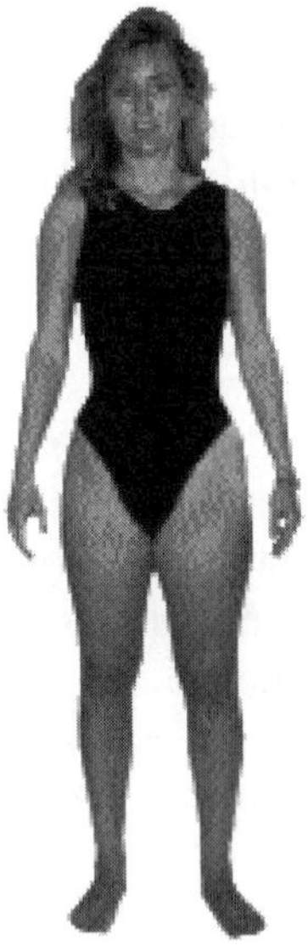
Kidney

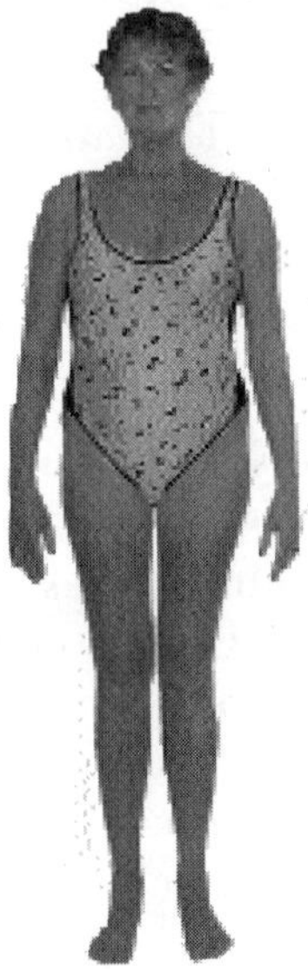
Liver

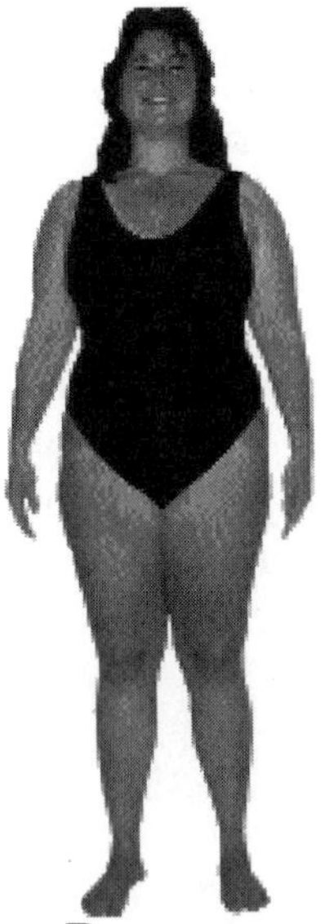
Pancreas

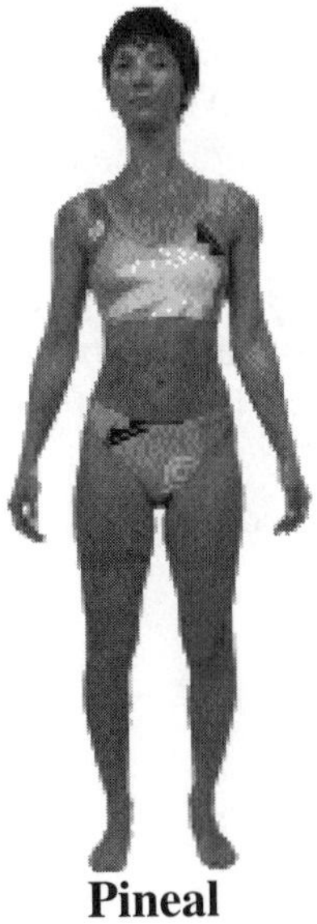
Pineal

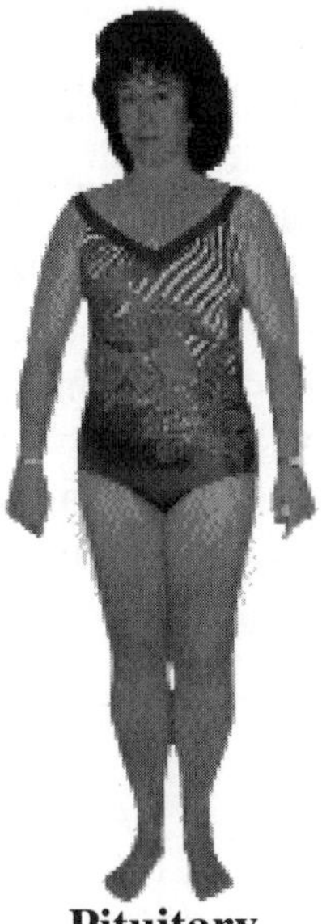
Pituitary

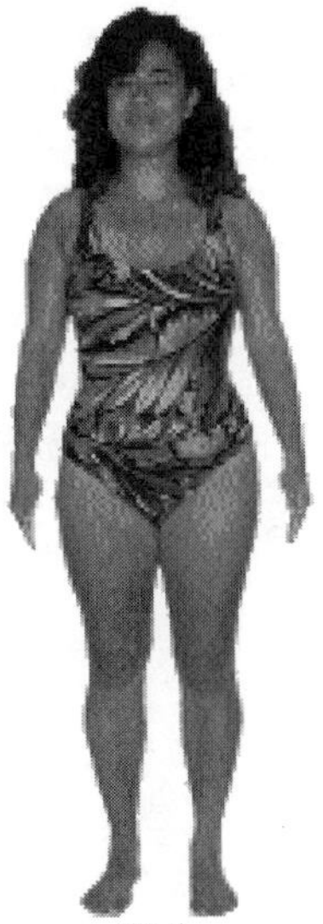
Skin

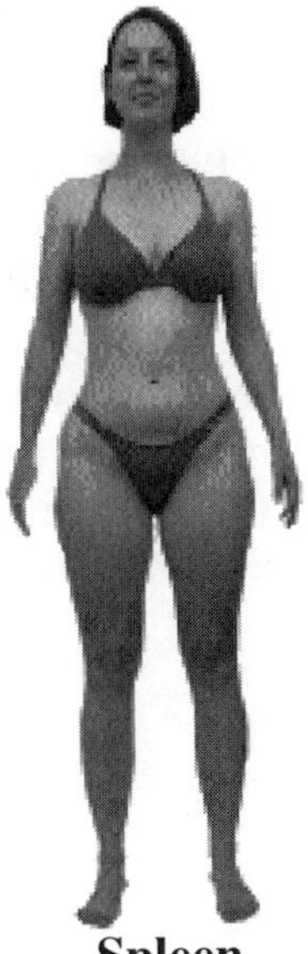
Spleen

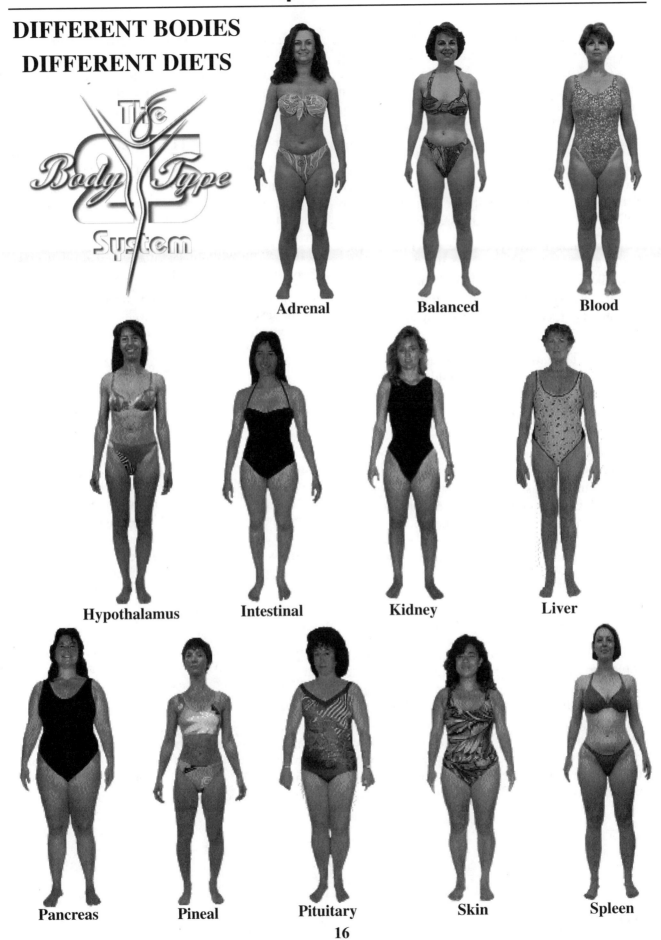

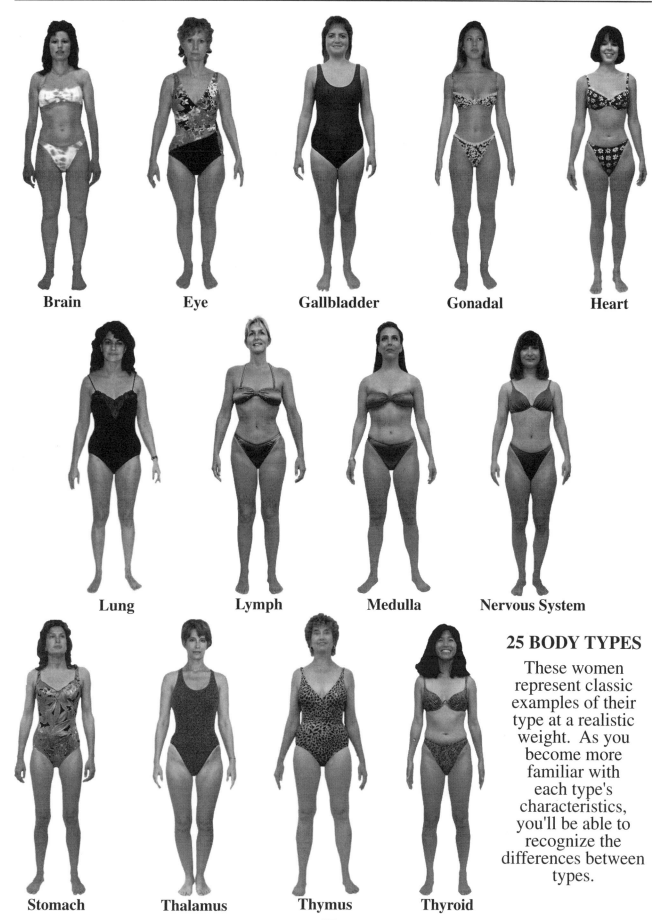

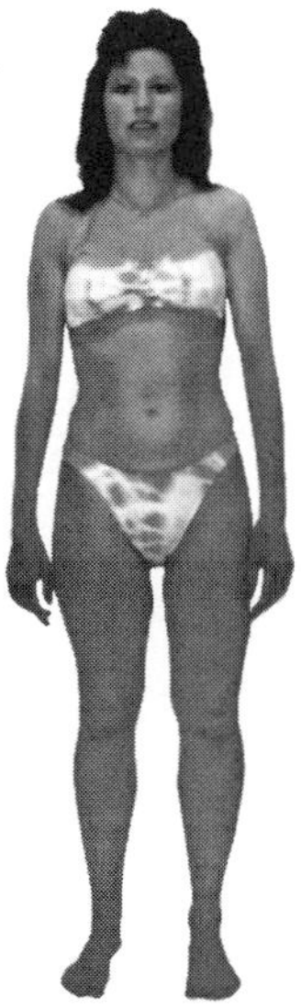

Brain

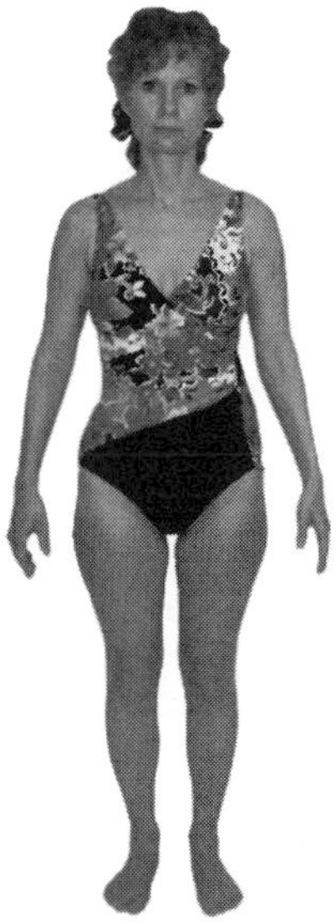

Eye

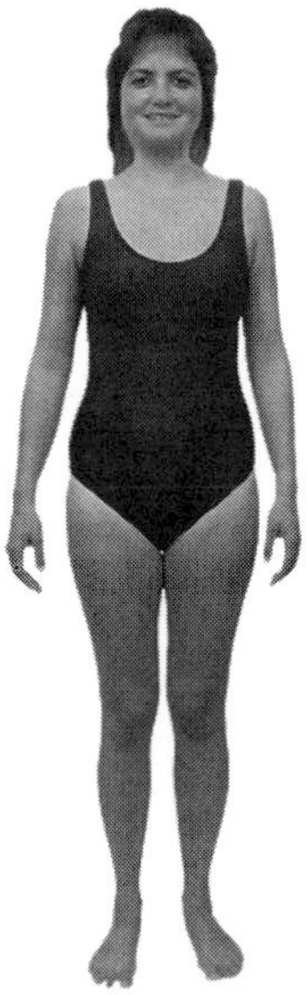

Gallbladder

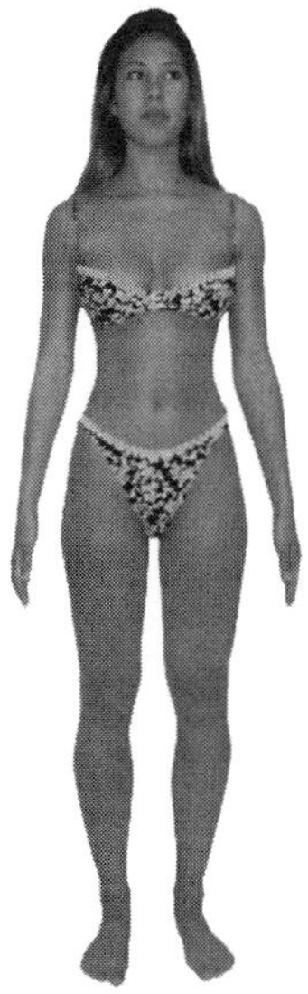

Gonadal

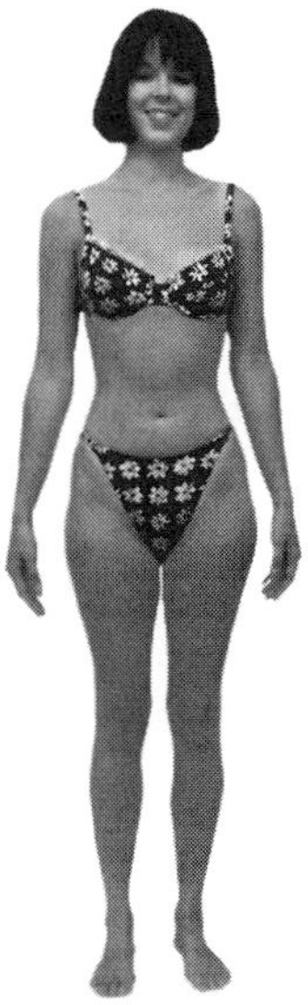

Heart

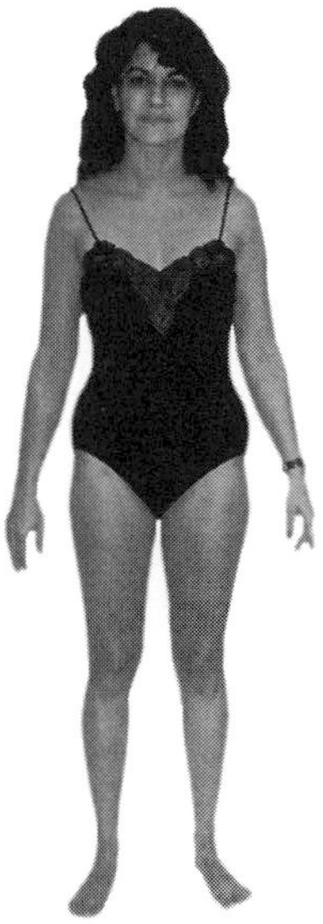

Lung

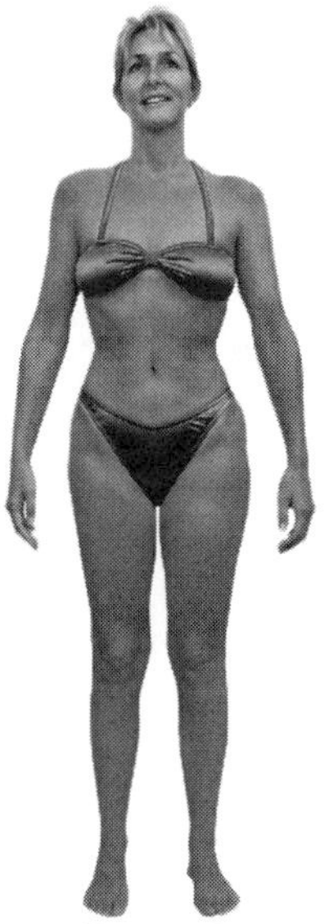

Lymph

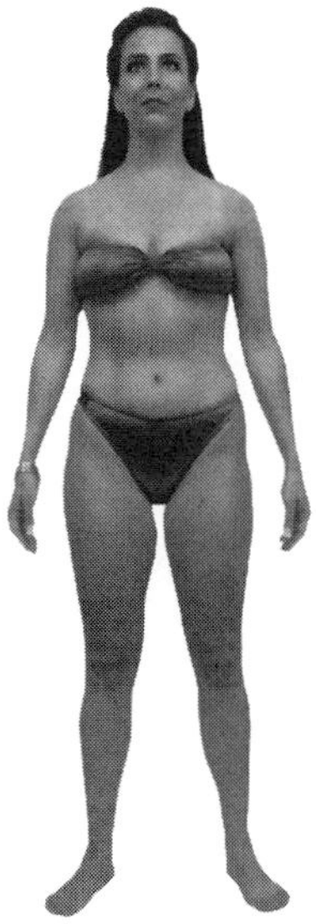

Medulla

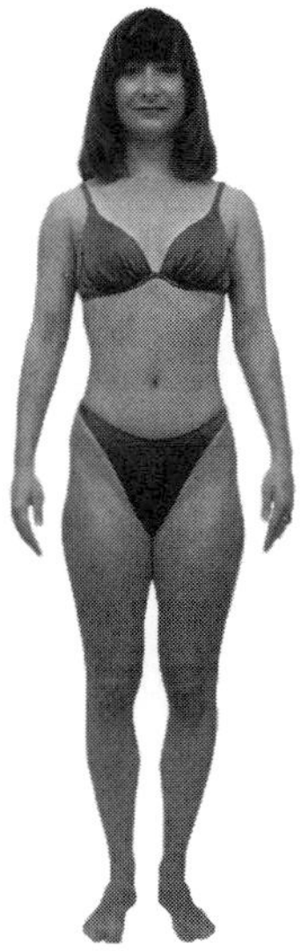

Nervous System

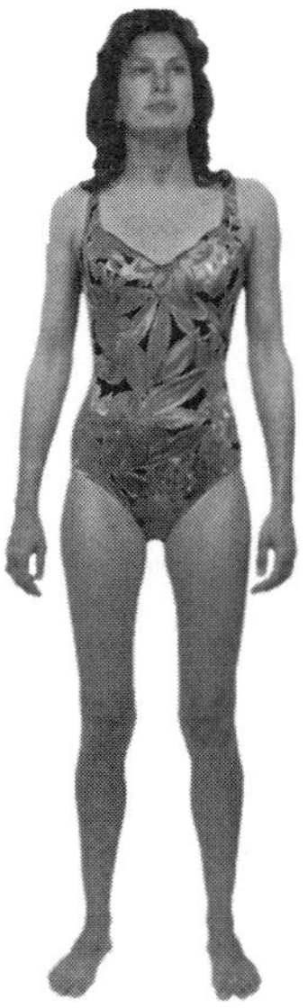

Stomach

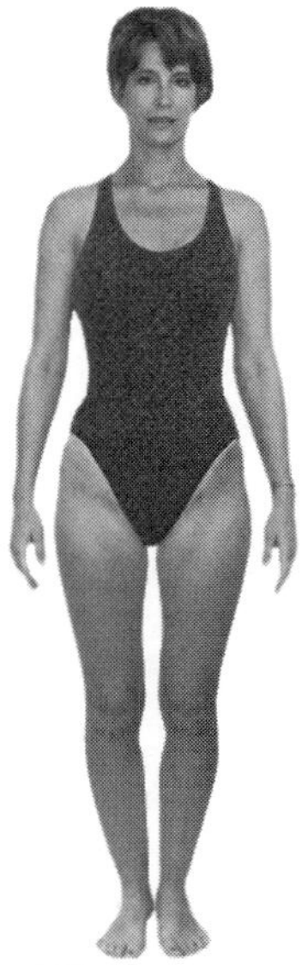

Thalamus

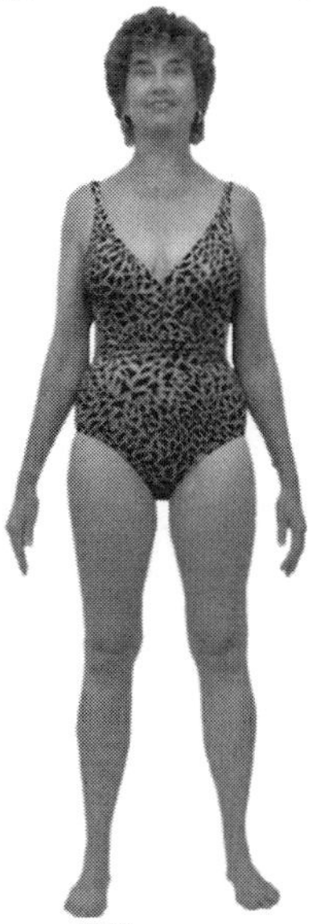

Thymus

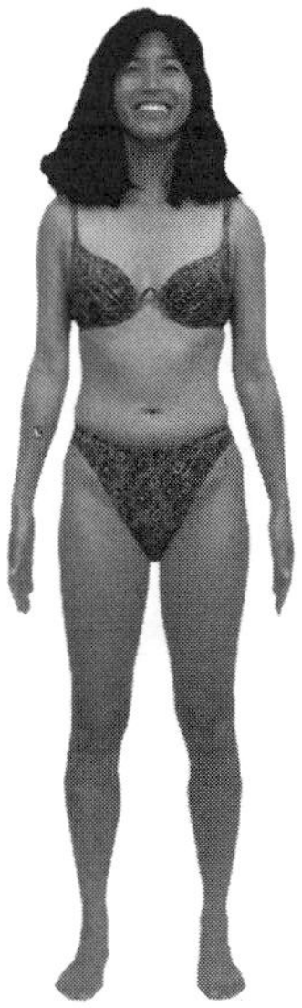

Thyroid

25 BODY TYPES

These women represent classic examples of their type at a realistic weight. As you become more familiar with each type's characteristics, you'll be able to recognize the differences between types.

CHAPTER 2

WHAT IS YOUR BODY TYPE?

Have you recognized yourself in any of the body types mentioned so far? You may have seen yourself in several, but there will be only one type that is truly "you". Your body type is determined by your dominant gland, which greatly influences your general appearance, including your body shape and structure, weight gain pattern and metabolism.

Each of the 25 distinct body types has different nutritional requirements. This is why certain diets work well for some people but not for others. In fact, the wrong diet can actually push dieters farther away from their desired health and weight goals.

It's your dominant gland that determines the diet that is best for you. Just as certain foods stimulate a particular gland, other foods support or rebuild it. Since our dominant glands are different, we require different nutrients. This is because we deplete those used by our dominant gland first. Consequently, we need to eat the specific foods that replace these nutrients.

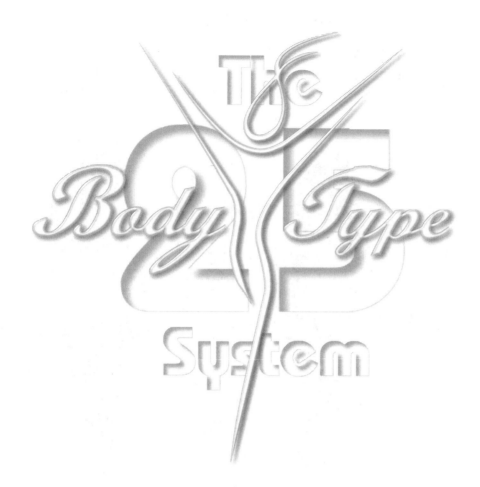

DETERMINING YOUR BODY TYPE

Look at the following 3 primary weight gain patterns and select the one that best describes you. Where is your main area of weight gain? This is the stubborn area, the hardest place to lose weight or the most difficult to keep toned.

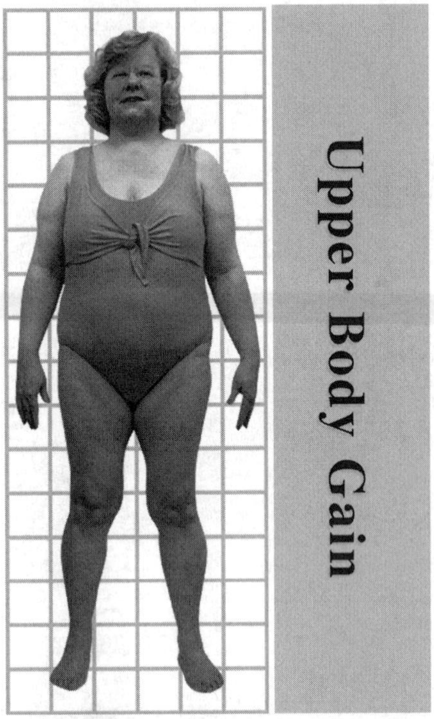

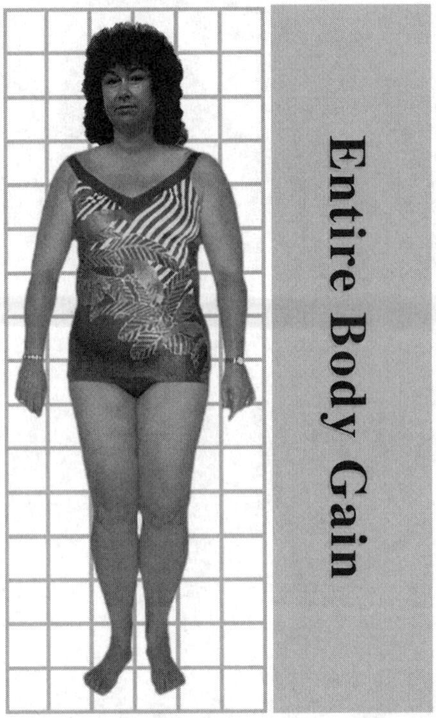

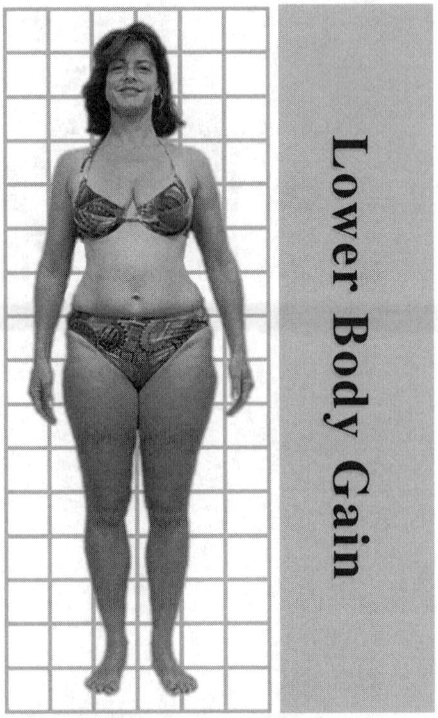

Upper body gain refers to the torso, particularly across your back. The first sign is your bras get too tight or blouses start to gap and won't stay buttoned.

Entire body gain is when it's hard to say where you gain, it's all over with no particular spot. Since your weight gain is so even, you can carry large amounts of weight without it being too apparent.

Lower body gain includes waist, lower abdomen, upper hips, lower hips, buttocks, and thighs. Not all of these areas will necessarily be a problem. You will usually notice weight gain first in either the lower abdomen or buttocks, thighs may or may not be involved.

- If the upper or entire body gain describes you, you've just narrowed your choices down to 6 or 7.
- Refer to the list on the following page for these types.
- Then look at their corresponding photos in the "25 Body Type Photos" section beginning on page 30.
- Pay particular attention to the captions with an asterisk (*).
- By eliminating the ones that don't fit you, you'll reduce your possibilities to 2 or 3.
- Read the corresponding one paragraph "Essence" beginning on page 82 and select the one that matches your personality.
- You've just identified your body type!

Once you have identified your body type, you may proceed directly to your specific "Profile and Diet".
Chapters 3 through 5 contain basic dietary information and explain how to best implement your diet.

Lower body is where most women gain weight so this group contains the greatest number of body types. To narrow this group down further, continue on to page 21. Do you gain weight predominantly in your buttocks and thighs, lower abdomen, or lower abdomen and thighs? **If buttocks and thighs, you're down to 3 choices, so you are ready to proceed directly to the photos and verify with the Essences.** If you gain in your lower abdomen, do you also gain in your thighs? If not, you are down to 6 choices, ready to proceed to the photos and then the "Essences".

Main Area of Weight Gain

Upper Body

Adrenal
Brain
Intestinal
Liver
Pancreas
Skin
Stomach

Go to Photos

Entire Body

Adrenal
Intestinal
Nervous System
Pituitary
Skin
Stomach

Go to Photos

Lower Body

Adrenal
Balanced
Blood
Brain
Eye
Gallbladder
Gonadal
Heart
Hypothalamus
Intestinal
Kidney
Lung
Lymph
Medulla
Nervous System
Pancreas
Pineal
Skin
Spleen
Stomach
Thalamus
Thymus
Thyroid

PRELIMINARY CATEGORIES

The first step in identifying your body type is to look at your area of weight gain as illustrated in one of these three lists. You will notice that some types appear in more than one area. This is because certain types can have more than one weight-gain pattern which can change during their lifetime.

The Adrenal type, for instance, gains weight in her thighs when she is primarily expressing her feminine personality and in her torso when expressing her masculinity. When Geraldine gave up her business and got married, she noticed her weight gain areas began to change. Within a few years, her weight gain completely shifted from her upper body to her thighs. While your weight pattern can change during your lifetime, your body type remains the same.

If you gain weight in either your upper body or all over, you have narrowed your type down to 6 or 7 body types. You will probably be able to identify your type simply by looking at the photos and then confirming your choice by reading the Essence from that type's psychological profile.

You will notice that almost all the types are listed under lower body gain. This doesn't mean that you are all Thyroids. To divide this group, look at where in your lower body you gain. Is your excess weight in your hips, thighs, and buttocks, but not your lower abdomen? If your lower abdomen is a problem, do you gain weight in your thighs?

Lower Body Weight Gain

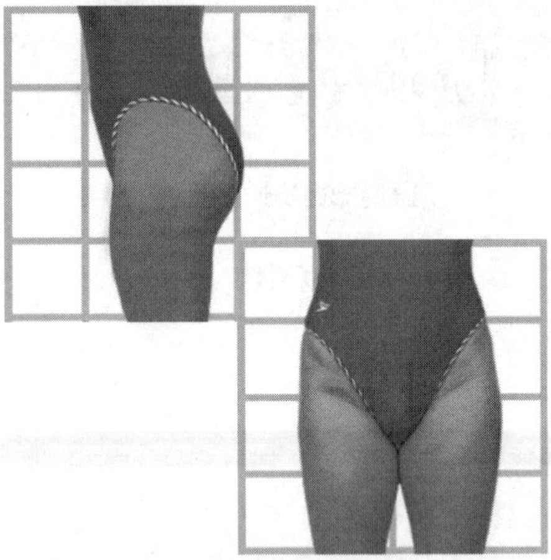

Buttocks & Thighs

Gonadal

Kidney

Lymph

Go to Photos

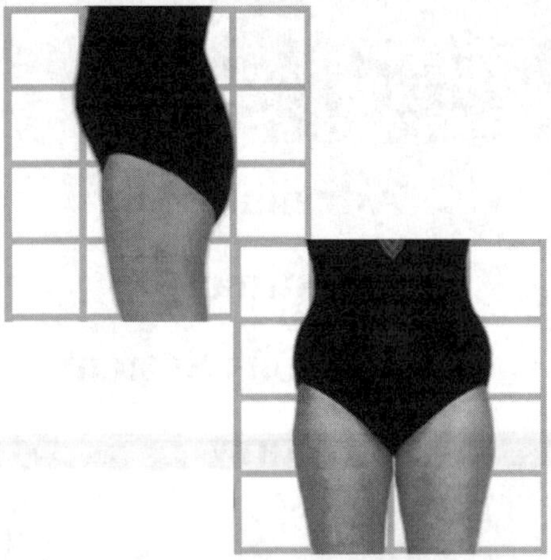

Lower Abdomen

Blood

Brain

Gallbladder

Intestinal

Lung

Pancreas

Go to Photos

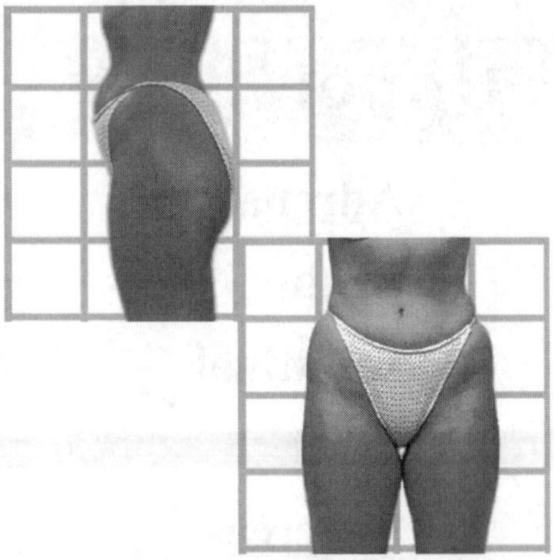

Lower Abdomen & Thighs

Adrenal

Balanced

Blood

Eye

Heart

Hypothalamus

Kidney

Lymph

Medulla

Nervous System

Pancreas

Pineal

Skin

Spleen

Stomach

Thalamus

Thymus

Thyroid

Go to Waist

If you are fortunate enough to gain in your buttocks rather than your lower abdomen, you've narrowed your type down to 3 choices. If you get depressed when you don't exercise, you're probably a Lymph. You can go directly to the Lymph photos and then read the "Essence" paragraph in the Lymph body type "Psychological Profile". If it fits, you've identified your type. If not, read the Gonadal and Kidney.

Since physical characteristics are often similar, you can ultimately identify your type by the psychological profile. When Gonadals get stressed or over-loaded, they look for "no-brainer" jobs. Kidneys will procrastinate until the last minute, then when under pressure force themselves to excel, often surprising themselves at what they can accomplish.

If you gain weight in your lower abdomen, but not in your thighs, you only have 6 types to evaluate. If you are in the largest group, you can further reduce your choices by looking at the shape of your waist.

Waist

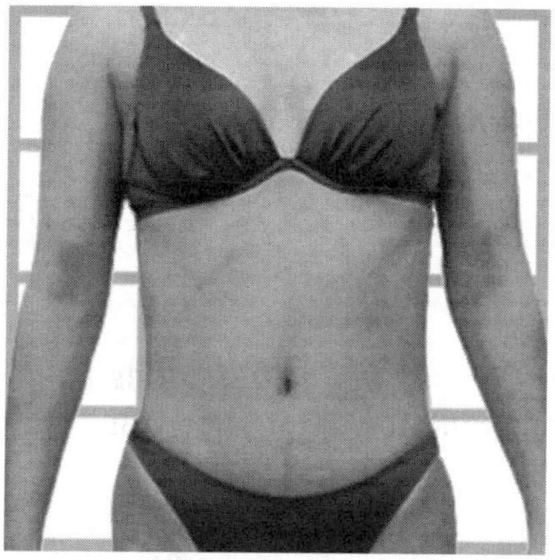

Straight

Adrenal
Blood
Eye
Hypothalamus
Medulla
Nervous System
Skin
Stomach
Thymus

Go to Photos

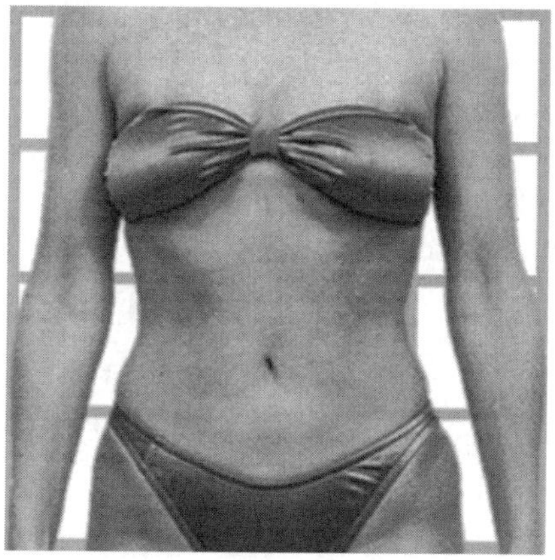

Defined

Balanced
Blood
Eye
Heart
Hypothalamus
Kidney
Lymph
Medulla
Nervous System
Pancreas
Pineal
Skin
Spleen
Stomach
Thalamus
Thymus
Thyroid

Go to Photos or continue on for additional physical charactertics.

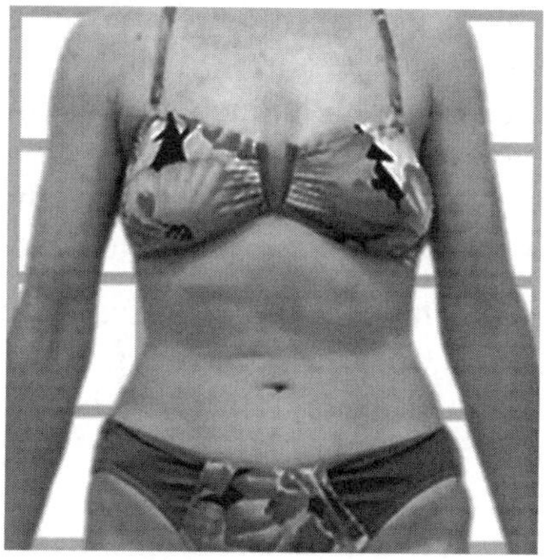

Well-Defined

Eye
Heart
Kidney
Pancreas
Spleen
Thyroid

Go to Photos

SHAPE OF WAIST
Look at the shape of your waist in relation to your hips. Regardless of your weight, is your waist straight, to where boy's jeans fit best; defined; or well-defined, creating an hourglass shape?

KEY PHYSICAL CHARACTERISTICS

Physical characteristics, including weight gain patterns, are important because they provide obvious clues to the dominant gland. There are some physical traits that are so distinctive that their presence alone can be enough to identify a type. While some types have characteristics that are quite obvious, others are more subtle or are identifiable by a composite of common features.

Reflected in the physical characteristics are family features, race or genetic traits, and even climate adaptations that have become characteristics of a race. There is also a secondary gland influence that is reflected in the physical characteristics which, while subtle or minimal in some people, can be pronounced in others. However, it's still your dominant gland, regardless of the strength of your secondary gland, that determines your ideal diet, so this is where you want to place your focus.

Because there are so many contributing factors, physical characteristics are only one part of accurate type determination. Their main purpose is to narrow the field of type selection. The more familiar you are with characteristics of particular types, the easier it will be for you to identify those types. While certain characteristics are typical of specific types, not everyone in that type will always have all the characteristics. Ultimately, it's the body's chemical response to certain foods that determines body type. Fortunately, the dominant gland influences many areas, resulting in the development of different ways to determine body type so anyone can accurately discover their own type.

Remember, the physical characteristics are guides, not absolutes, so don't rule out a type just because you don't have 100 per cent of all the possible characteristics.

"Buttocks, Back, and Abdomen"

In addition to being the most obvious, these characteristics are consistently the most indicative of type. While weight gain or loss will exaggerate, and exercise can help enhance or control these areas, the basic patterns are consistent. The photographs on the following page illustrate these characteristics:

1. Shape of the buttocks: relatively flat, rounded, or prominent.

2. Low back curvature: slight (identified as straight), moderate (average), or increased (swayed).

3. Abdomen: upper, lower, entire, minimal or no gain (giving a flat appearance).

"Hips and Thighs"

The next set of photographs shows the variations of weight gain in the upper and lower hips, as well as thighs.

Upper hips are defined as the area on the hips, from the waist to about five inches below the top of the hip bones. Lower hips extend around the widest part of the buttocks, about seven inches below the top of the hip bones. This is the indentation where the thigh bone connects to the hip bone.

Weight gain in the thighs can be described in the following ways:

1. No or insignificant weight gain in thighs, as seen in the Gallbladder body type.

2. No weight gain on outer thighs, with gain on entire inner, typical of Intestinal types.

3. Even weight distribution over entire thighs, often seen in the Pituitary body type.

4. Distinct upper/outer bulge on upper one-third only (saddlebags), a key identifying factor for the Eye type, especially when weight gain is found only in this thigh region.

5. Variation on the "saddlebags" bulge, continuous upper/outer weight gain on upper two-thirds of thighs, with main protrusion on upper one-third. Commonly found in Thyroids, as well as the majority of body types.

6. Bulge extending along entire thighs to the knees, as seen primarily in the Gonadal type.

"Shoulders, Back, and Waist"

These photos show the back view of weight gain in the upper hips; upper back, defined as the area under the arms; mid back, as the area just under

BUTTOCKS, BACK & ABDOMEN
Side View Shape Variations

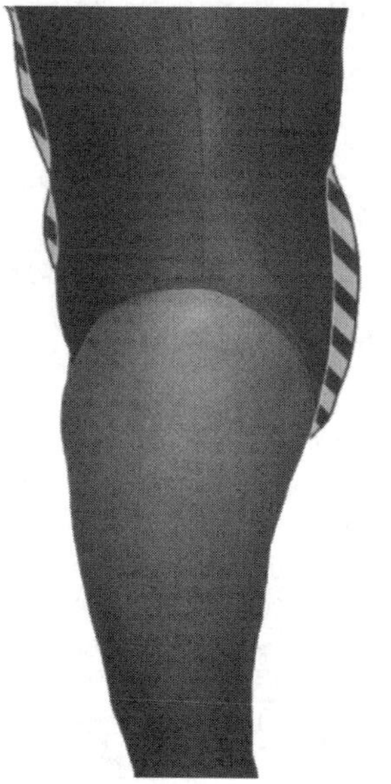

LIVER
BUTTOCKS: Relatively flat
LOW BACK CURVATURE: Straight
ABDOMEN: Upper, minimal in lower

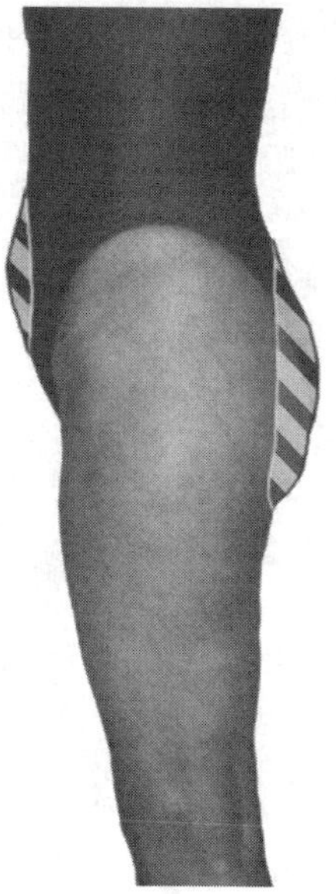

THYMUS
BUTTOCKS: Rounded
LOW BACK CURVATURE: Average
ABDOMEN: Lower

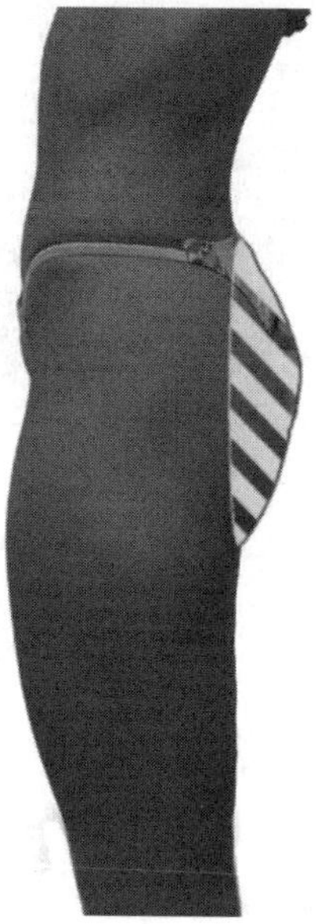

LYMPH
BUTTOCKS: Prominent
LOW BACK CURVATURE: Swayed
ABDOMEN: No gain

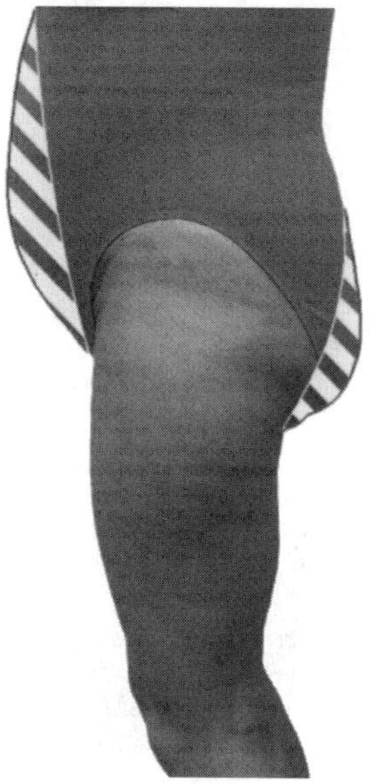

SKIN
BUTTOCKS: Relatively flat
LOW BACK CURVATURE: Straight
ABDOMEN: Entire

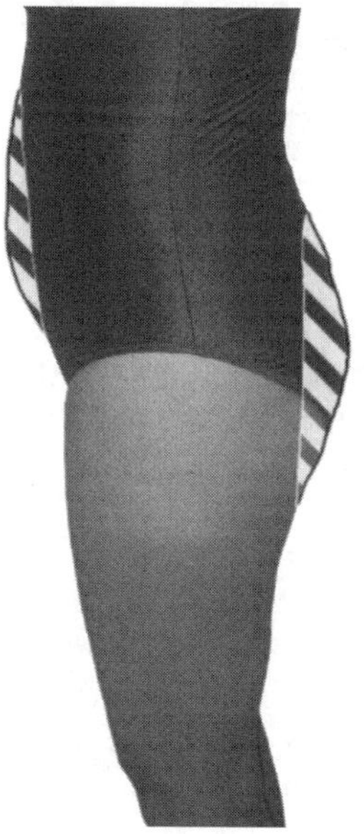

NERVOUS SYSTEM
BUTTOCKS: Rounded
LOW BACK CURVATURE: Average
ABDOMEN: Entire

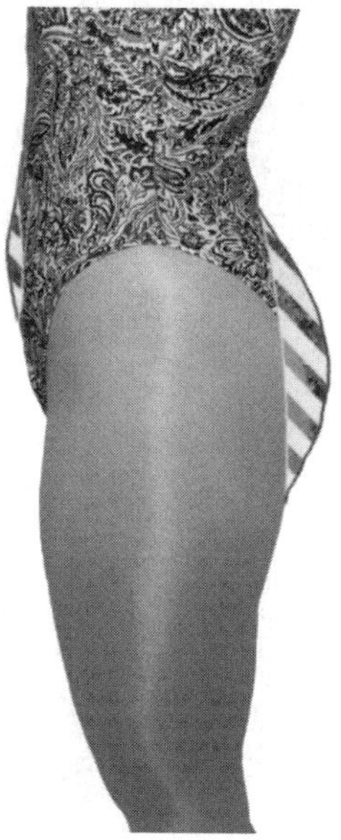

GONADAL
BUTTOCKS: Prominent
LOW BACK CURVATURE: Swayed
ABDOMEN: Minimal gain

HIPS & THIGHS
Weight Gain Variations

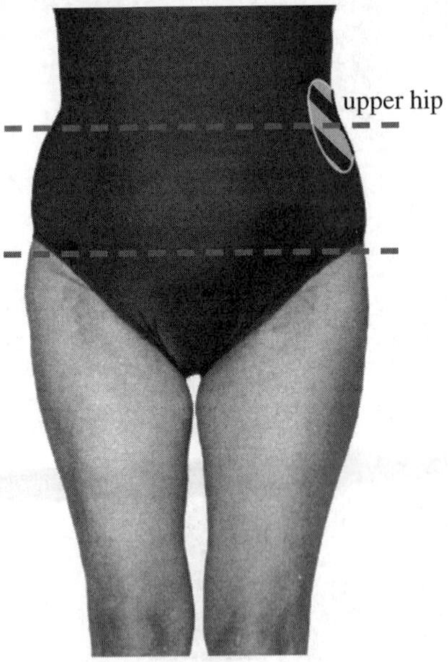

GALLBLADDER

HIPS: Upper hips

THIGHS: No or insignificant weight gain

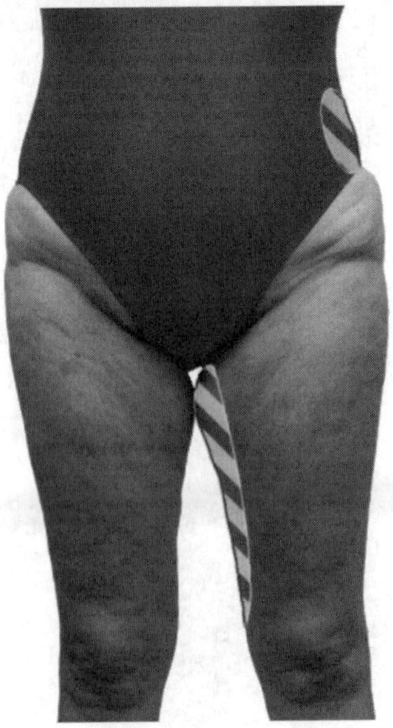

INTESTINAL

HIPS: Upper hips

THIGHS: Entire inner, with little gain on outer

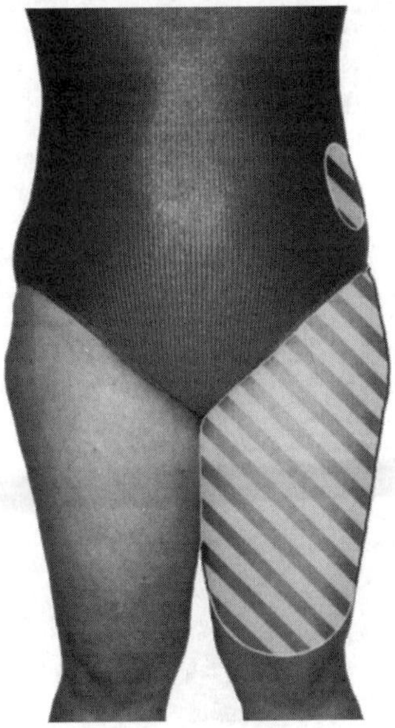

PITUITARY

HIPS: Upper hips

THIGHS: Entire thighs, even weight distribution to knees

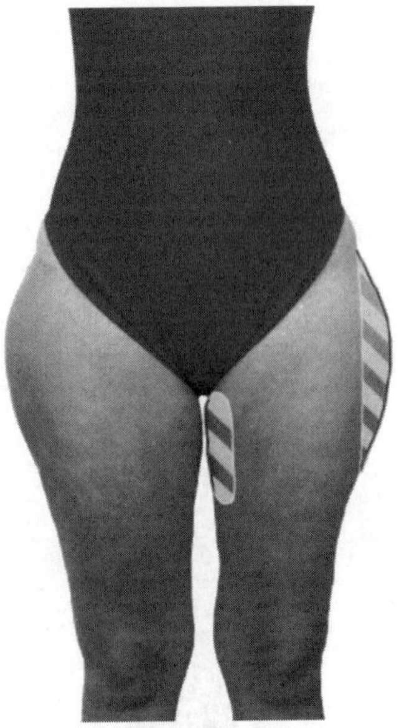

EYE

HIPS: Minimal gain

THIGHS: Characteristic gain in entire upper 1/3rd of thighs, particularly apparent on outer 1/3rd

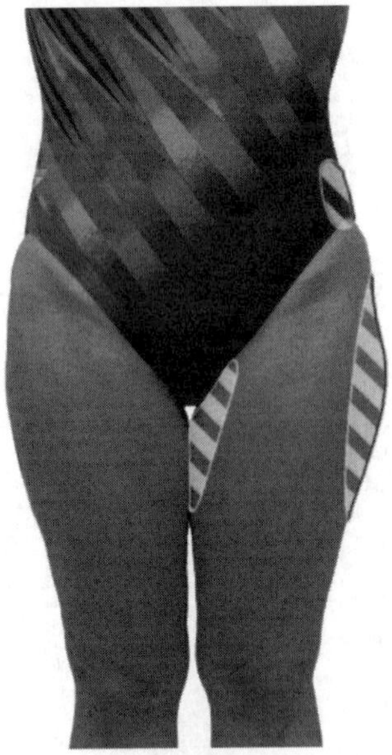

THYROID

HIP: Upper hips

THIGHS: Gain in entire upper 2/3rds, including upper inner thighs, particularly appparent on outer 2/3rds

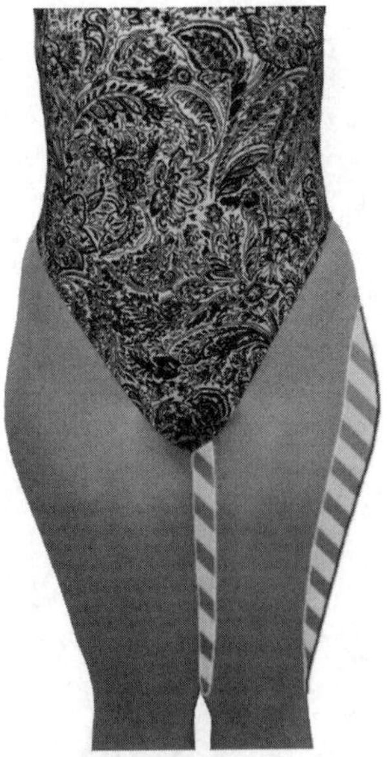

GONADAL

HIPS: Lower hips

THIGHS: Gain in entire thighs, with main protrusion on upper outer 1/3rd and entire inner, continuing to knees

SHOULDERS, BACK & WAIST

Weight Gain Variations in Back

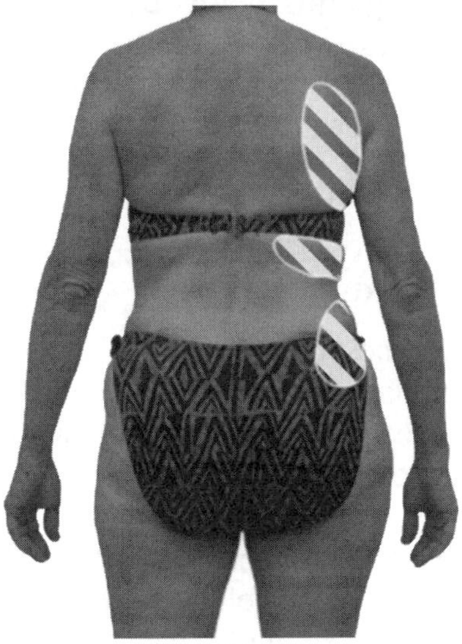

STOMACH

UPPER BACK: Weight gain

MID BACK: Minimal gain

UPPER HIPS: Weight gain

WAIST: Defined

SHOULDER WIDTH: Relatively even with hips

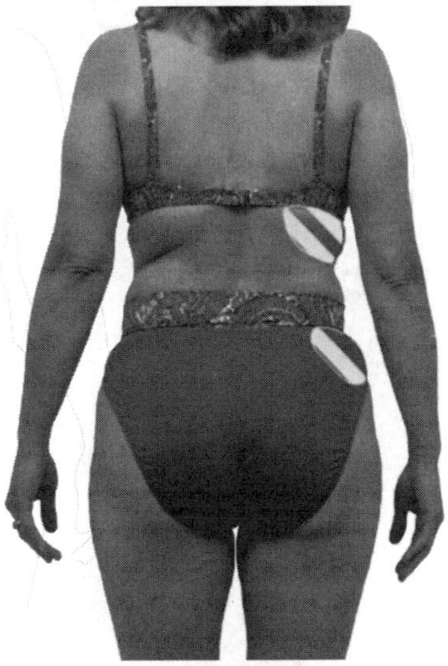

HEART

UPPER BACK: No weight gain

MID BACK: Weight gain

UPPER HIPS: Weight gain

WAIST: Defined

SHOULDER WIDTH: Relatively even with hips

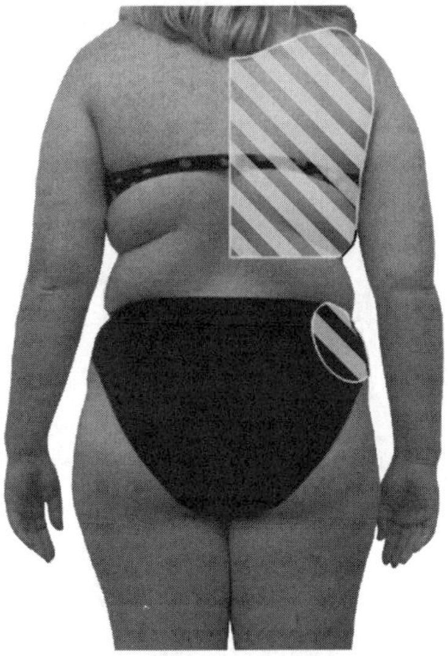

PITUITARY

ENTIRE BACK: Weight gain

UPPER HIPS: Weight gain

WAIST: Straight

SHOULDER WIDTH: Relatively even with hips

SHOULDER & HIP RELATIVITY

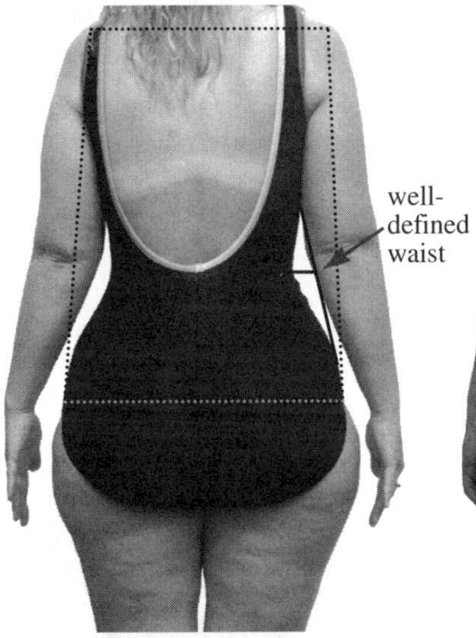

PANCREAS

SHOULDER WIDTH: Narrower than hips

ARMS: Gain in back of arms

ENTIRE BACK: No weight gain

UPPER HIPS: Some weight gain

LOWER HIPS: Weight gain

WAIST: Well-defined

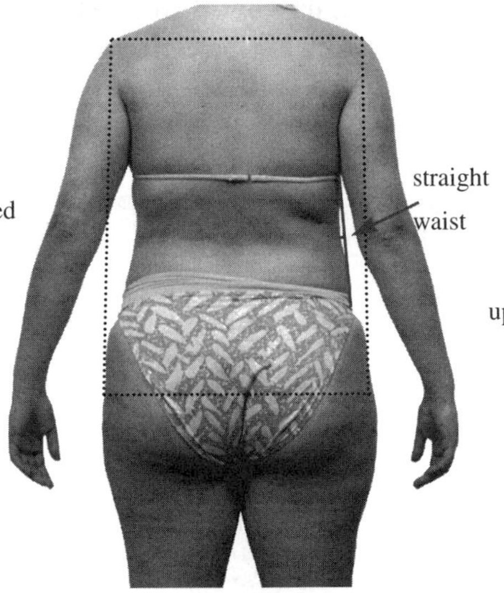

SKIN

SHOULDER WIDTH: Even with hips

ENTIRE BACK: Weight gain, square, flat upper back

UPPER HIPS: Weight gain

WAIST: Straight

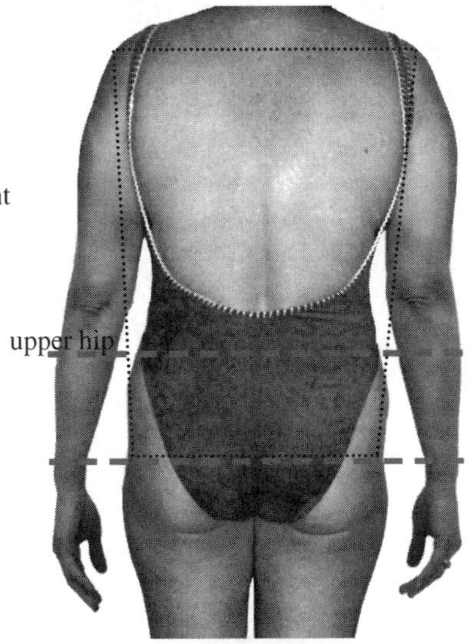

LIVER

SHOULDER WIDTH: Broader than hips

ENTIRE BACK: Weight gain

UPPER HIPS: Some weight gain

WAIST: Straight

ARMS

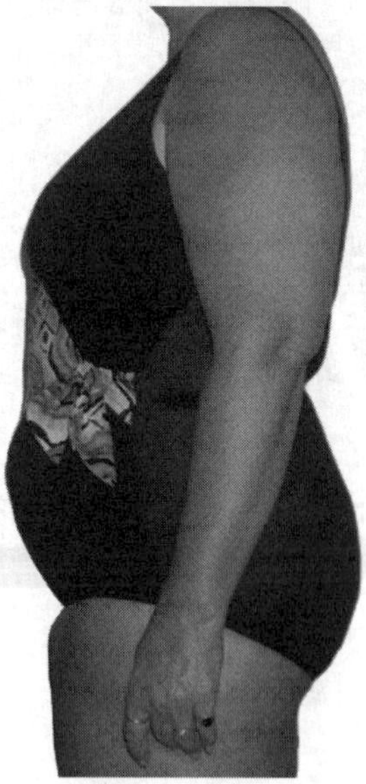

PANCREAS
Gain only in upper arm.

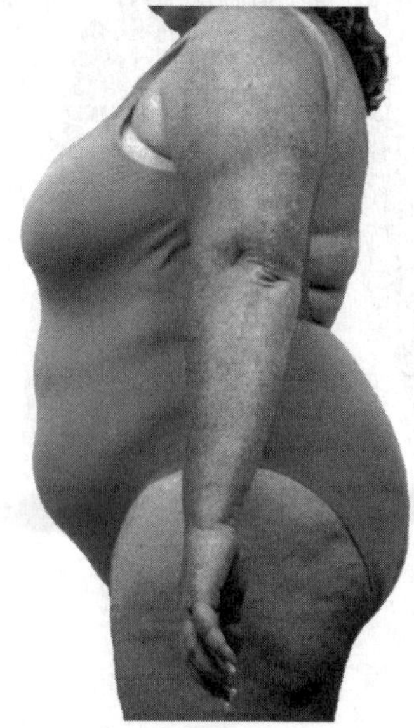

SKIN
Weight gain in entire arm.

the bra; and entire back. Shoulders are described as broader than, relatively even with, or narrower than, hips. The photos also show the contrasts between the well-defined waist, as in the Pancreas, and the thick, straight waist of the Skin, Liver, and Pituitary.

"Arms "

The photos above show variations of weight gain in the arms. The Pancreas has a unique weight gain in that they gain in the upper arm, but not in the lower arm. This is contrasted with the Skin's weight gain in the entire arm, which is typical of most types.

"Size and Shape of Head"

The photos below contrast the long, oval head of the Kidney, the small head of the Pineal, and the large head of the Pituitary.

"Hands "

For most body types, the hands are proportionate to the body and can be considered average. However, there are some types whose hands are a significant factor in determining their body type. The photos on the following page show the thick, wide hands of the Adrenal; the classic small hands of the Pancreas type; the broad, square palms with short fingers of the Eye; the puffy hands of the Skin; the knobby knuckles of the Medulla type; and the long, slender hands of the Thyroid. Even if you don't have the characteristic hands, you may still be one of these types. But, if your hands do match one of these descriptions, carefully look at this particular body type.

SIZE & SHAPE OF HEAD

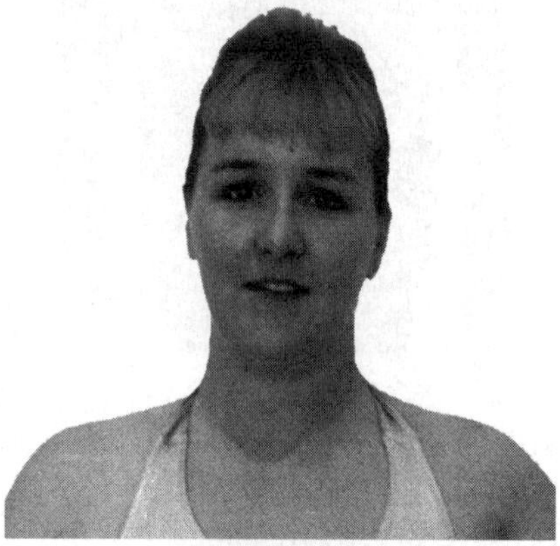

KIDNEY
Head proportionate to body.
Classic long, oval face.

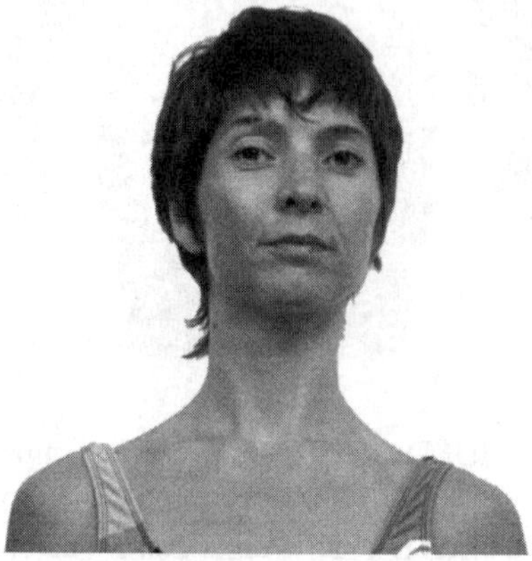

PINEAL
Small head compared to body.

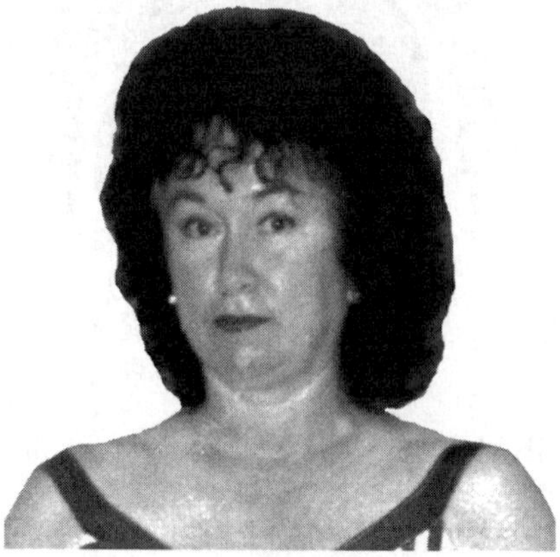

PITUITARY
Large head compared to body.

HANDS

If your hands match one of these, look specifically at that body type.

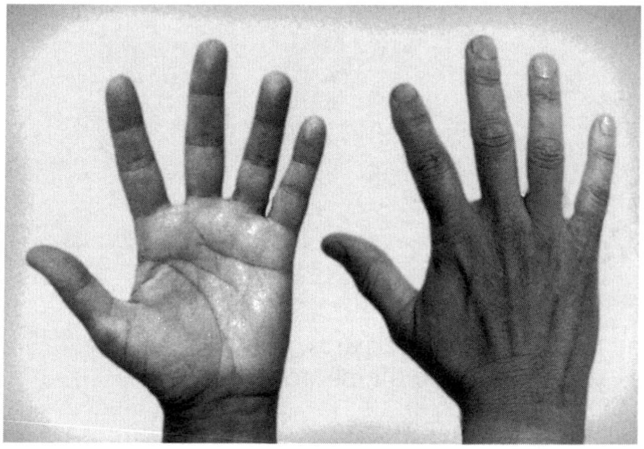

The thick, wide hands of the **Adrenal**

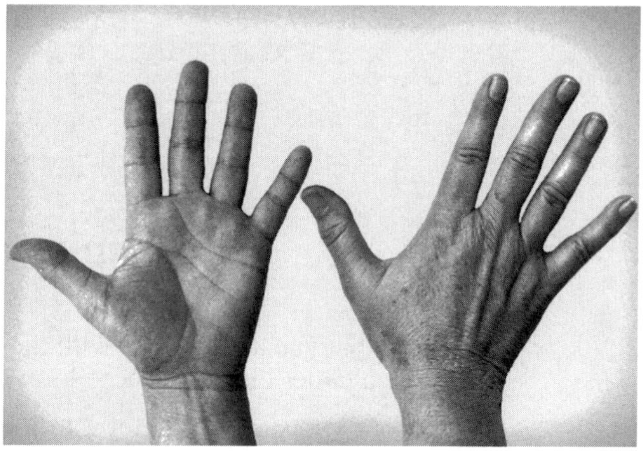

Classic small hands of the **Pancreas**

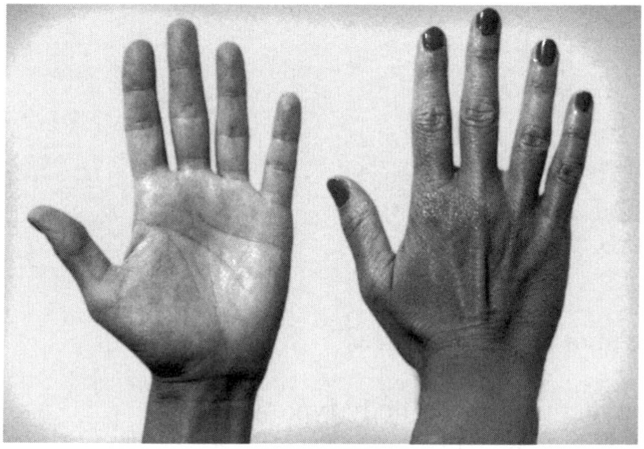

The wide hands with short fingers of the **Eye**

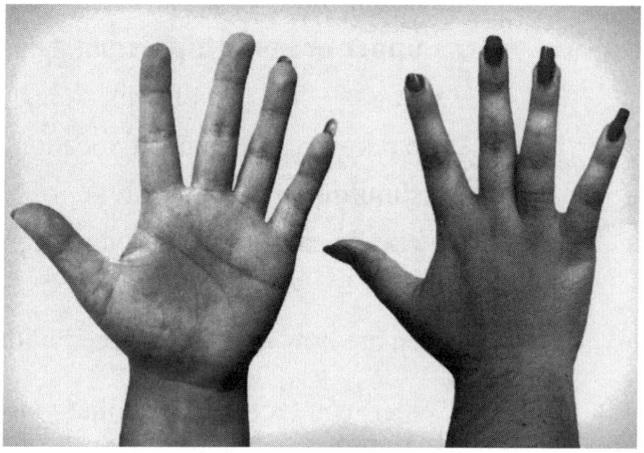

The puffy hands of the **Skin**

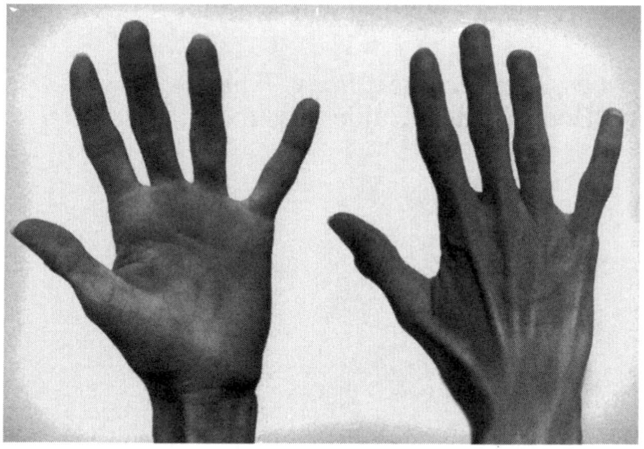

The knobby knuckles of the **Medulla**

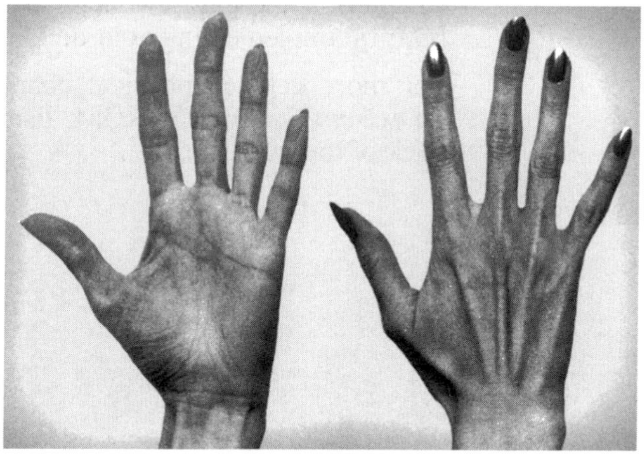

The long, slender hands of the **Thyroid**

Determining Your Type

Now that you are familiar with the basic physical characteristics, you'll have a better idea of what to look for as you go through the photos.

Before you start, it's helpful to look at yourself in a mirror or a photo, paying particular attention to your:

- **low back** curvature,
- **abdominal** weight gain,
- **upper or lower hip** weight gain,
- **thighs** – location of gain,
- **back** – weight gain and location,
- **shoulder** width, and any
- **classic characteristics** you might have.

You are now ready to proceed with the photos and "Essences".

When you feel confident that you have identified your body type, you may proceed directly to the "Profile and Diet" for your type.

If you have difficulty distinguishing between 2 or 3 types, read their complete "Psychological Profile".

Chapters 3 through 5 contain basic dietary information and helpful hints on implementing your diet.

For more detailed physical characteristics, refer to the "*Body Type Questionnaire*" or CD-ROM, listed in "Body Typing Guides" at the back of the book.

The following photos beginning on page 32 include eight women of each body type, with three full-body views showing front, back, and side. Each type includes examples of someone who is:

- **ideal** – at their optimal weight and fitness,
- **underweight** – types that have difficulty gaining or maintaining weight,
- **overweight** – showing initial and secondary weight gain,
- **classic** – characteristics typical of a type,
- **variations** – sometimes there is a range of characteristics within a type including an alternative weight gain pattern.

The photos illustrate the identifying physical characteristics, while the captions describe these along with other distinguishing features. Asterisks (*) highlight the most pronounced characteristics and initial weight gain areas as well as those features most helpful in differentiating one type from another.

Adrenal

Balanced

Blood

Brain

Eye

Gallbladder

Gonadal

Heart

Hypothalamus

Intestinal

Kidney

Liver

Lung

Lymph

Medulla

Nervous System

Pancreas

Pineal

Pituitary

Skin

Spleen

Stomach

Thalamus

Thymus

Thyroid

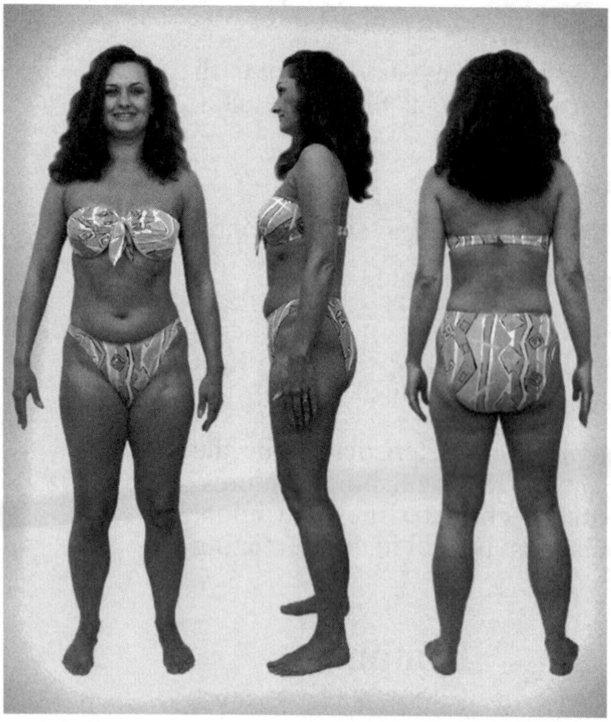

Personality tends to be expressed in one of two ways. The more feminine is gregarious and vivacious, outgoing and charming. Initial weight gain is in thighs.

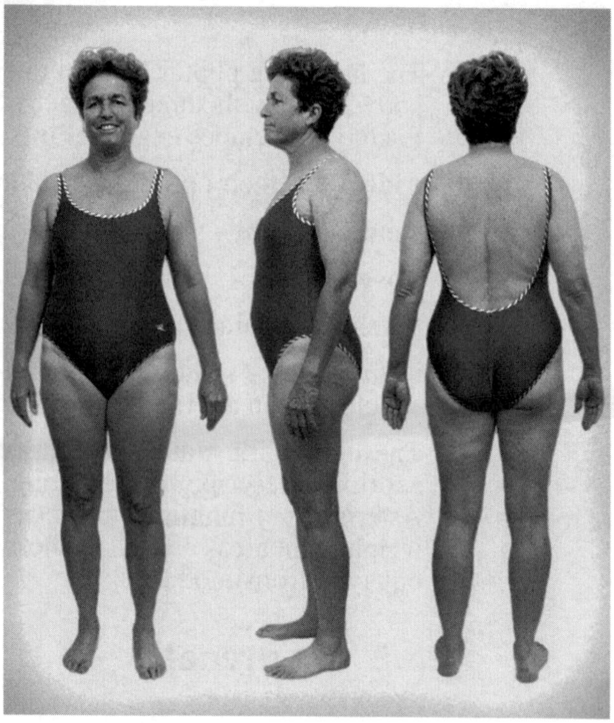

The more masculine is direct and strong-willed with a forceful presence. Weight gain is predominantly in torso. Inherently high energy, strength, and endurance.

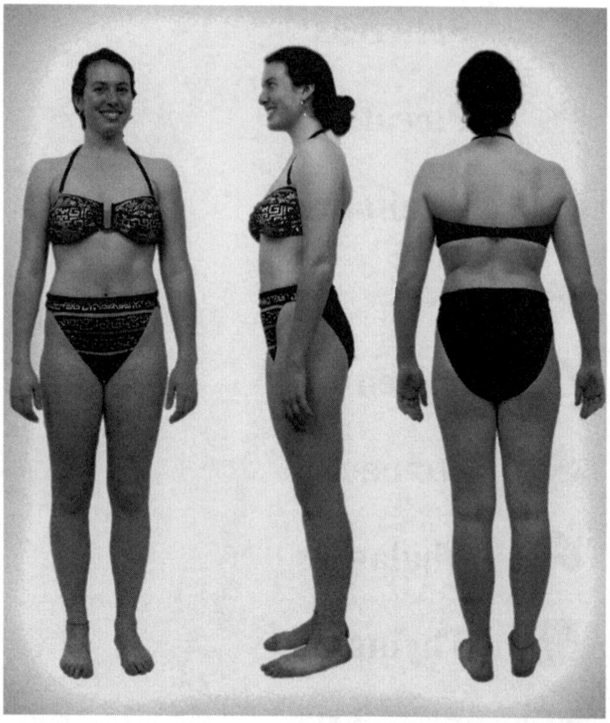

*"Boyish" figure with straight, poorly defined waist. Average to short-waisted. Dense, solid musculature throughout torso, arms, thighs, and calves.

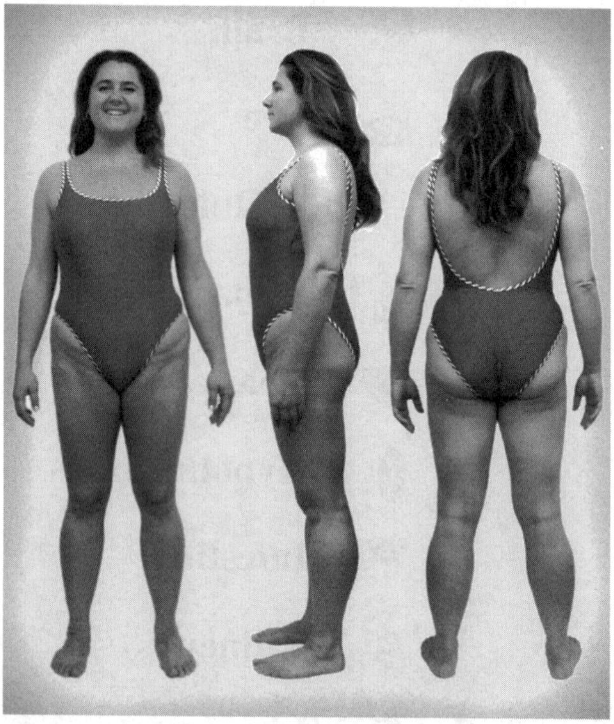

Wide, sturdy, grounded stance. Excess weight easy to gain and often fluctuates according to emotional state. Breasts average-to-large, depending on weight distribution.

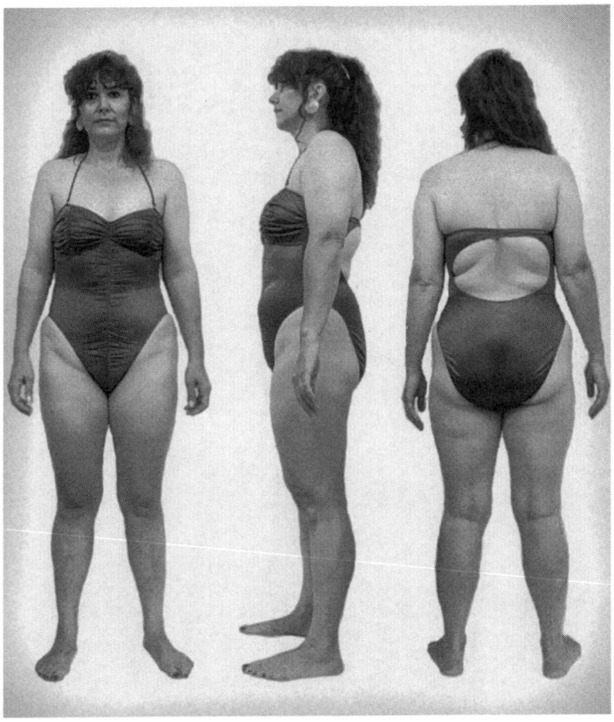

*Initial weight gain in abdomen; waist; upper, middle, and entire back; upper hips; upper arms; breasts; upper 2/3rds to entire thighs; and face. Bone structure medium-to-large.

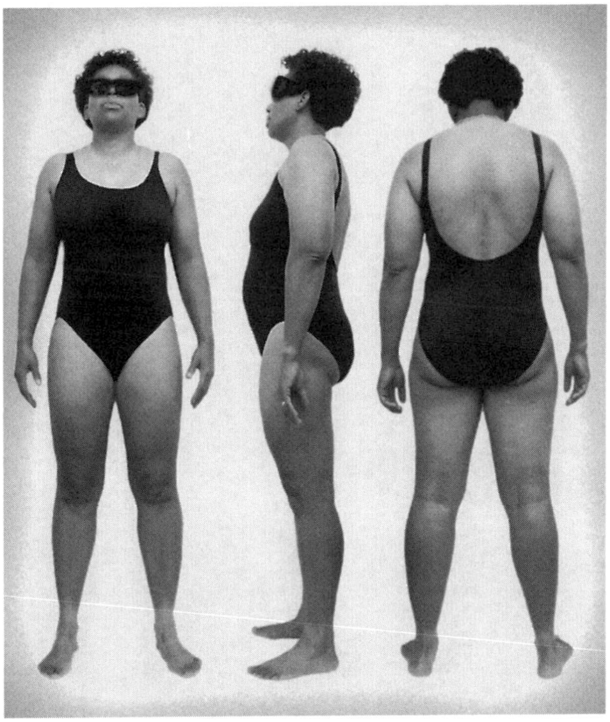

Low back curvature straight-to-average. Buttocks relatively flat-to-rounded. Shoulders and hips relatively even. Height generally average, but can range from very petite to tall.

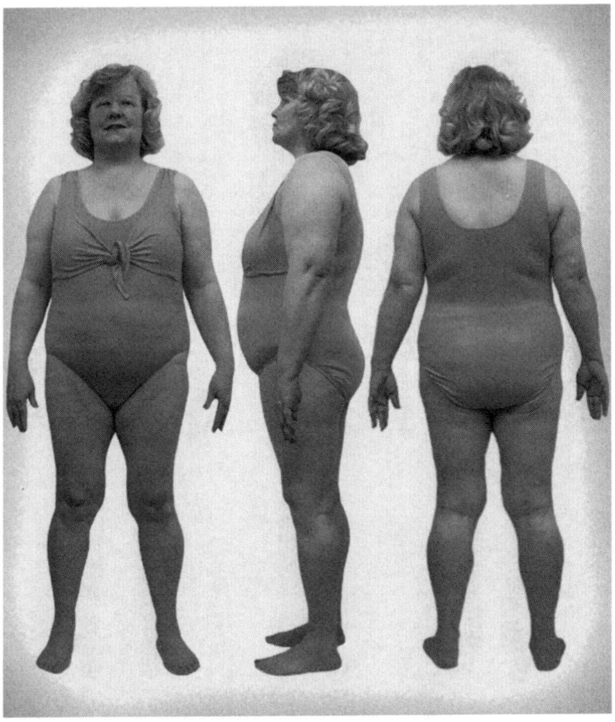

Alternative weight-gain pattern limits gain in thighs to upper inner, with predominant gain in upper body. Hands often large and/or wide, with strong, thick thumb muscle.

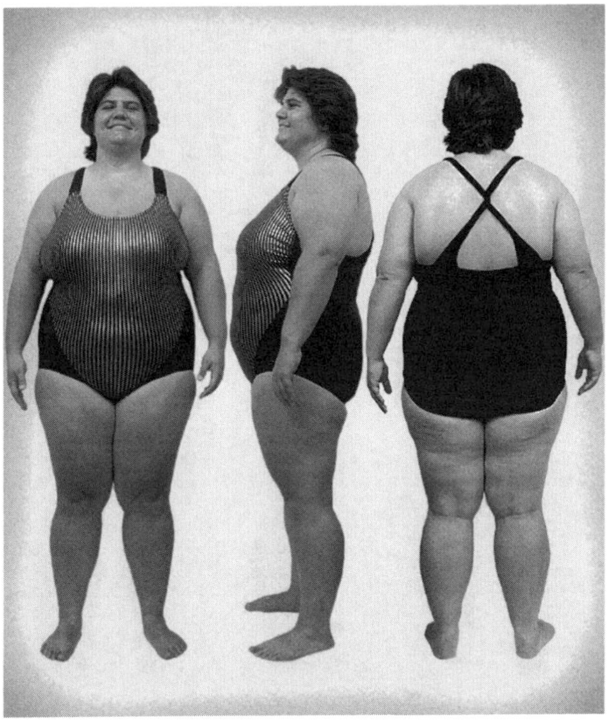

Secondary weight gain all over, including under chin, with large amounts of weight accumulating predominantly in entire abdomen, waist, and upper hips.

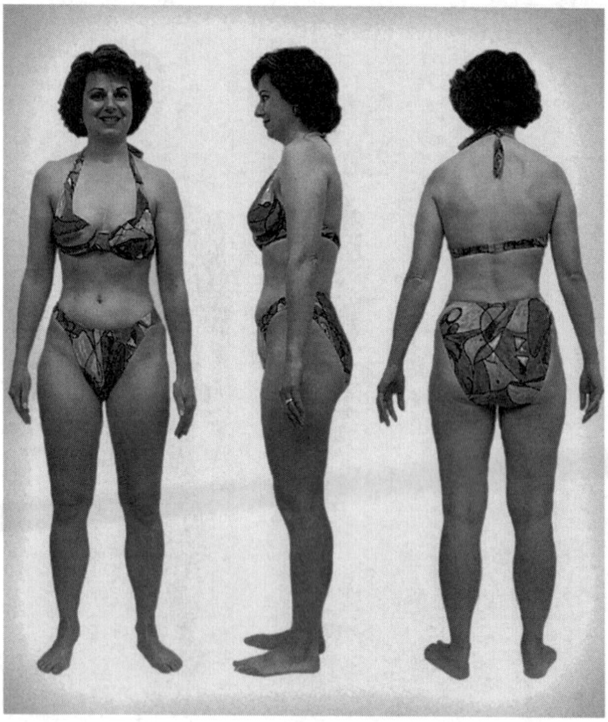

*Bright, sparkling eyes – especially when smiling. Essentially playful and adventurous, they embody the synergy that brings about balance.

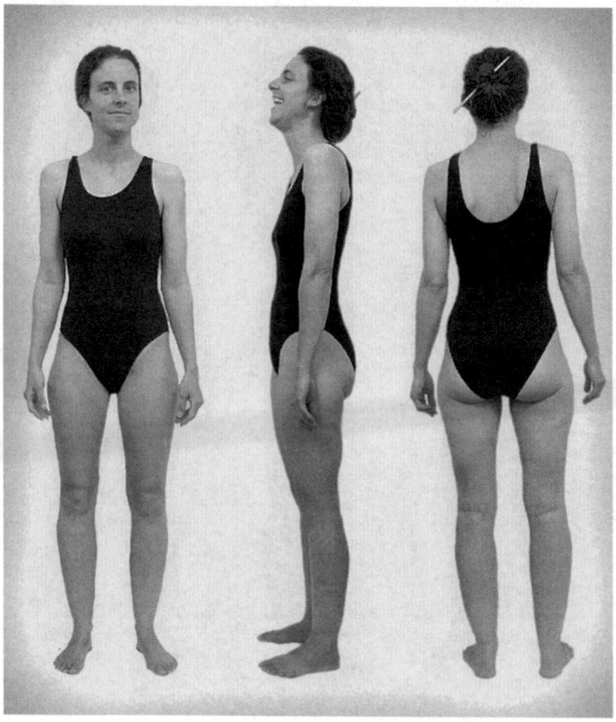

*Buttocks somewhat flat, due to blending into upper and outer thighs, creating a rather droopy appearance.

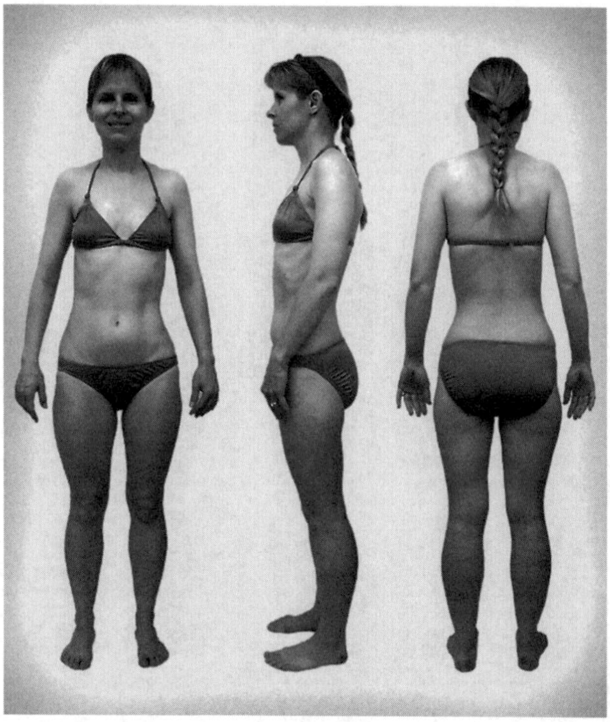

Long-waisted with short-to-average legs, or short-waisted with long legs. Defined waist. Average, elongated musculature.

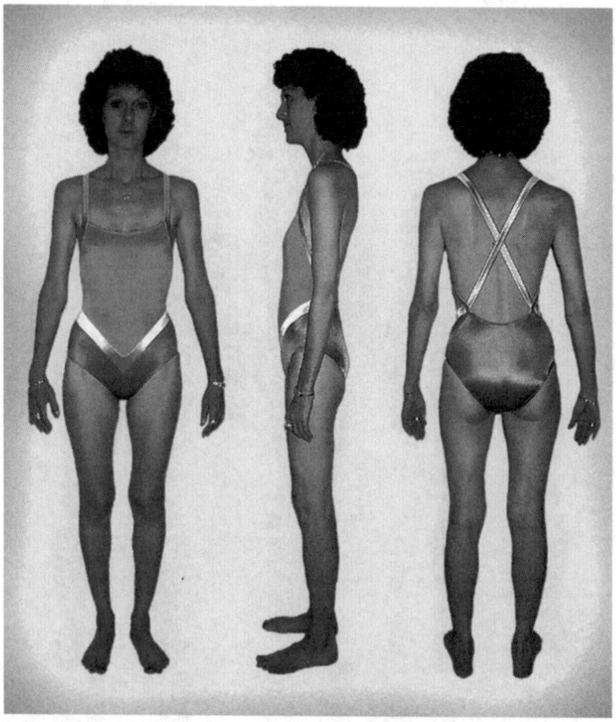

Shoulders relatively even with, to broader than, hips. Height generally average, but can range from petite-to-tall. Bone structure small-to-medium.

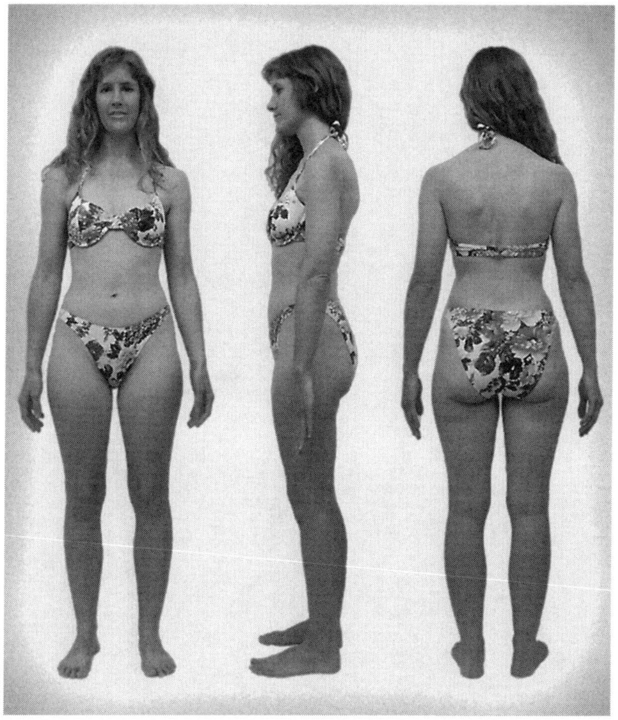

*Initial weight gain in entire upper 2/3rds of thighs including upper inner thighs extending into lower buttocks, lower abdomen, waist, upper and/or lower hips.

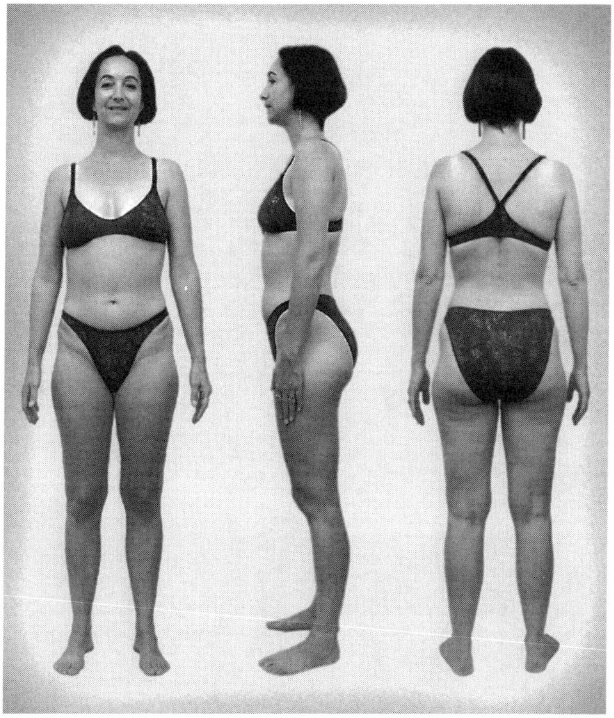

Average oval or rectangular face with high forehead; or heart-shaped, pixie-like face with V-shaped chin.

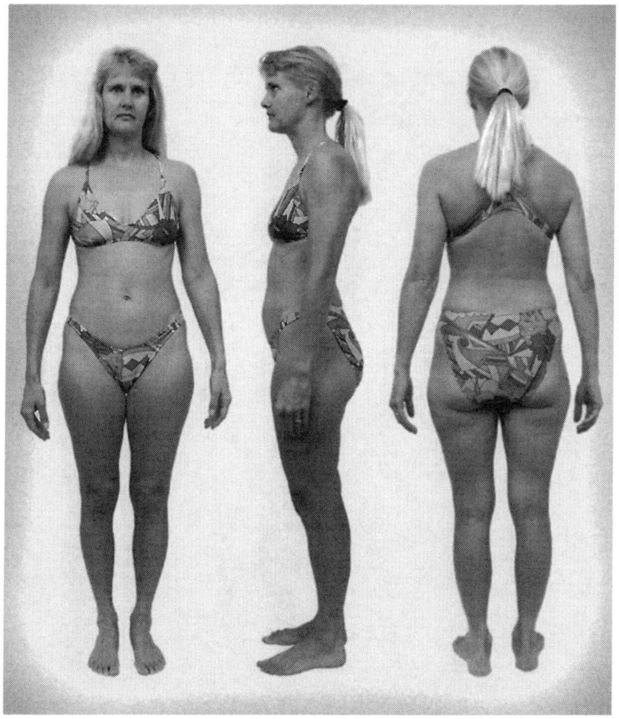

Breasts small-to-average. Low back curvature average-to-swayed. Rounded-to-prominent buttocks that appear flat.

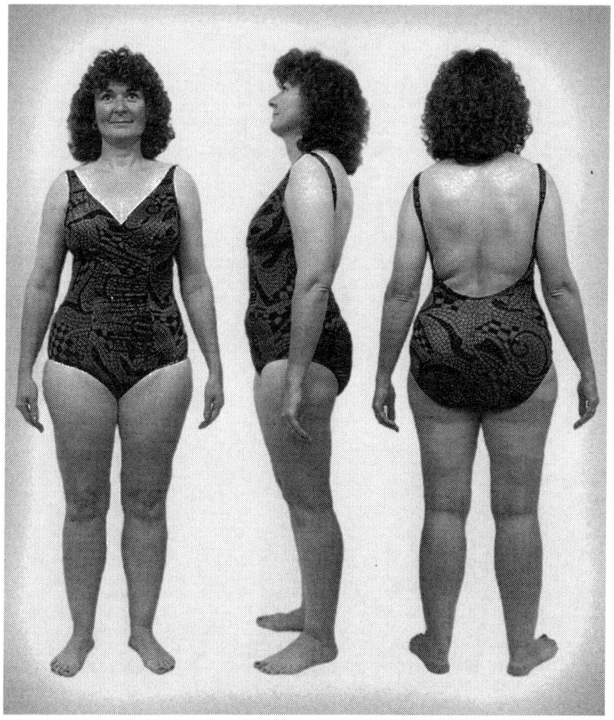

Secondary weight gain in entire thighs, eventually extending into entire abdomen, middle back, upper arms, and upper hips.

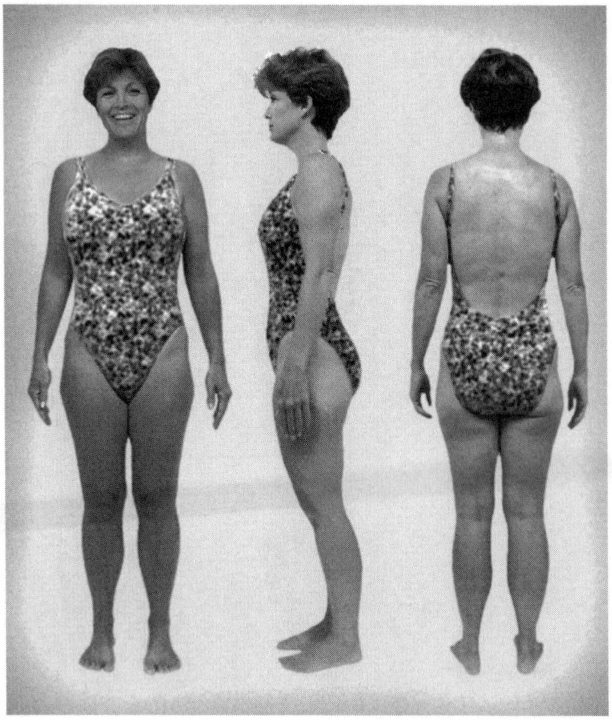

*Known for going to great lengths to maintain harmony. More than any other type, social and environmental harmony are essential to their health and well-being.

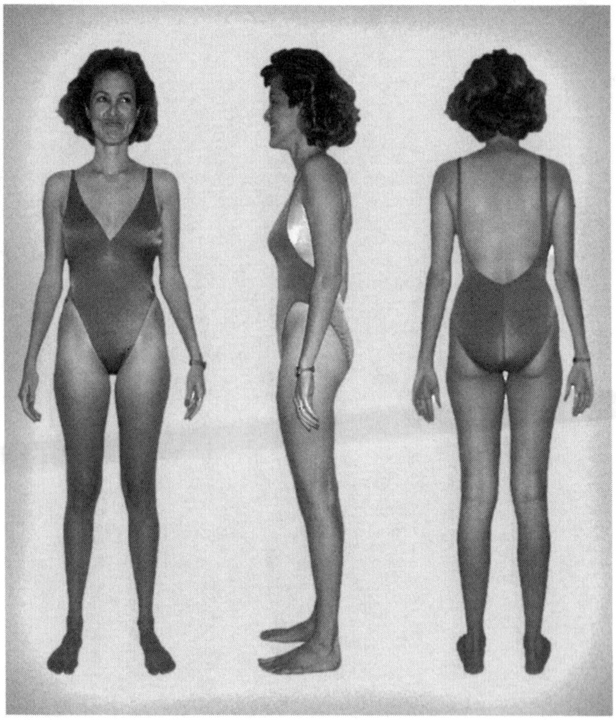

Expressive, receptive eyes that immediately draw attention to face. Average rectangular or oval face, often with low forehead.

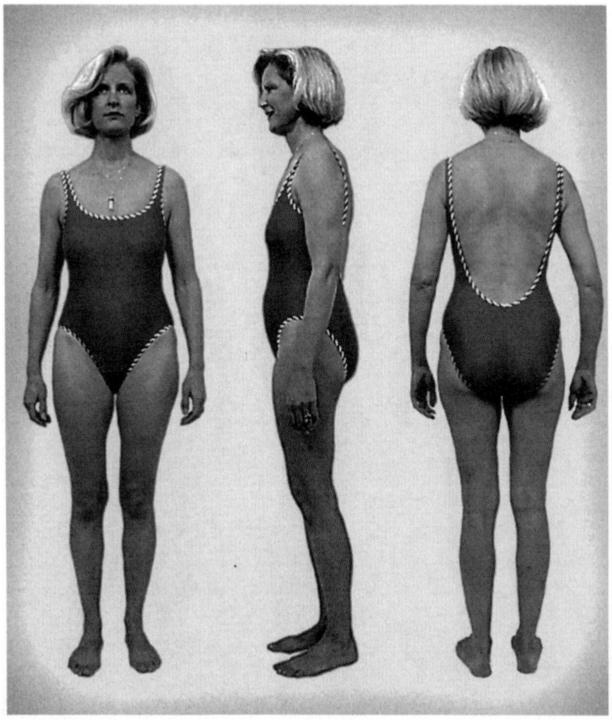

Height generally average, but can range from petite-to-tall. Bone structure typically medium, but can vary. Average or broad, square hands.

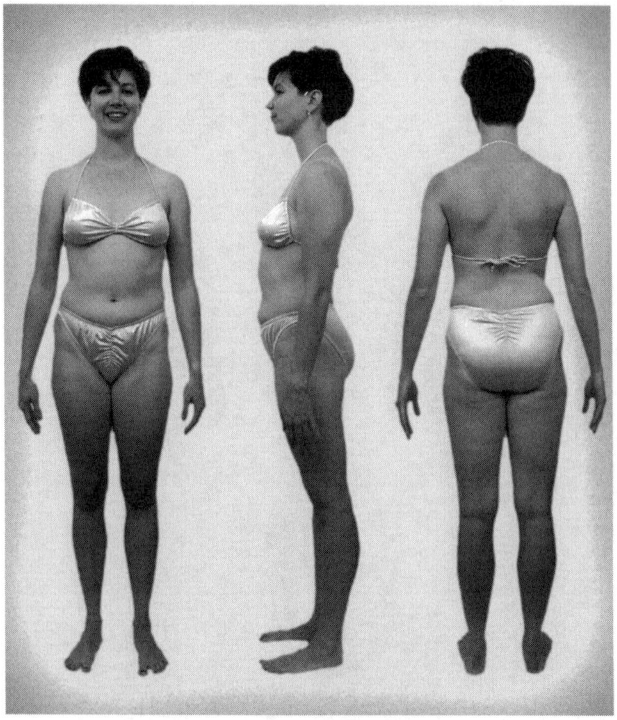

Torso solid with straight-to-defined waist, often short-waisted. Average, elongated musculature with little definition.

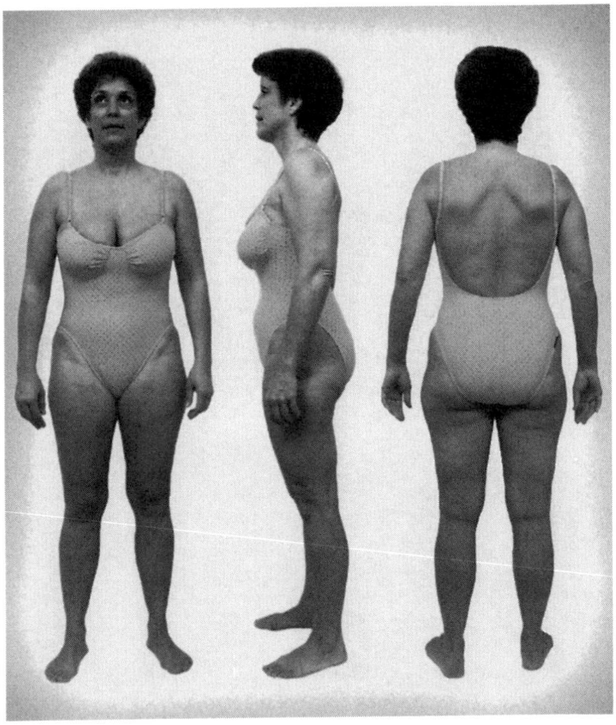

*Initial weight gain in lower abdomen, upper hips, waist, and upper inner to outer 2/3rds of thighs. Breasts average-to-large.

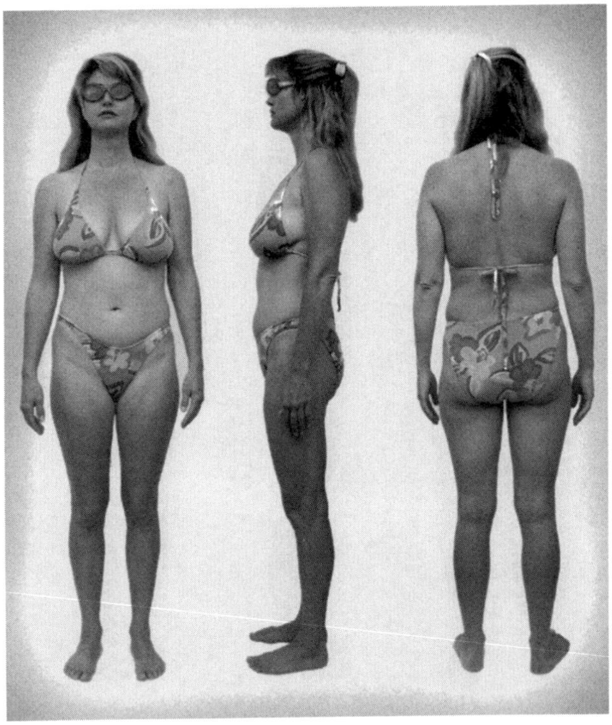

Low back curvature average-to-swayed. Buttocks relatively flat-to-rounded. Shoulders relatively even with hips.

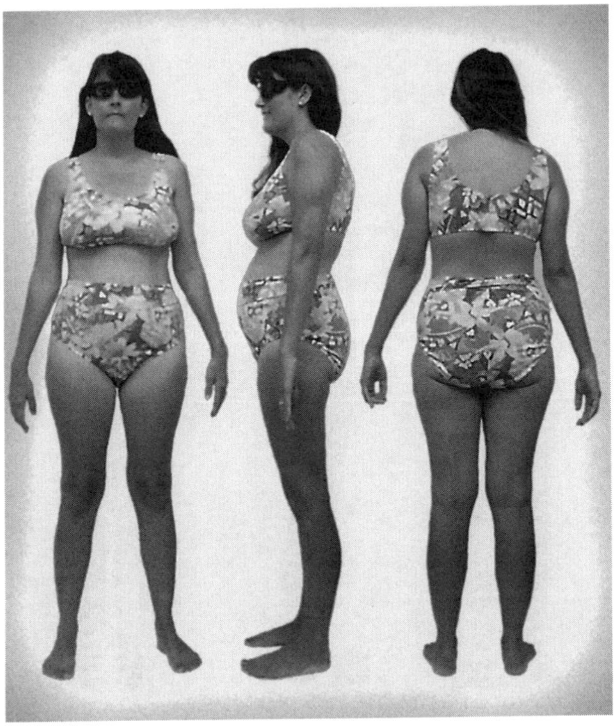

Weight gain of over 20 pounds is carried mainly in torso including entire back, but not lower hips.

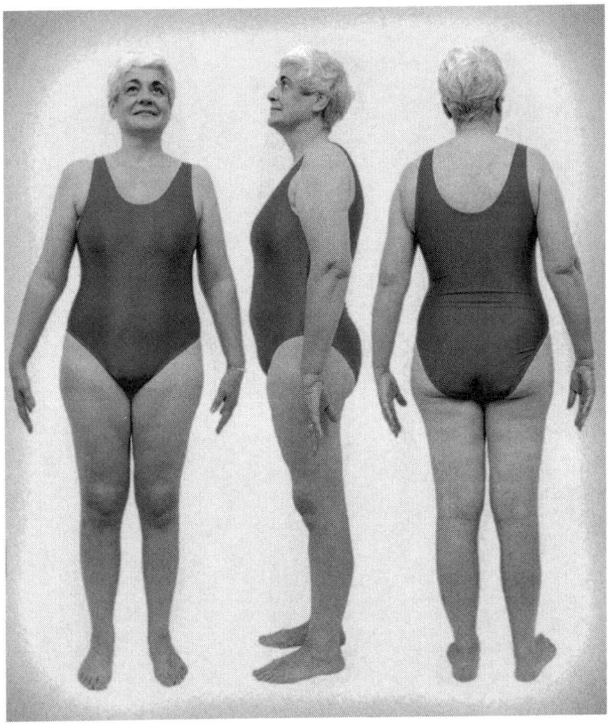

Secondary weight gain in entire upper 2/3rds of thighs, entire abdomen, buttocks, middle back, upper back under arms, upper arms, breasts, face, and under chin.

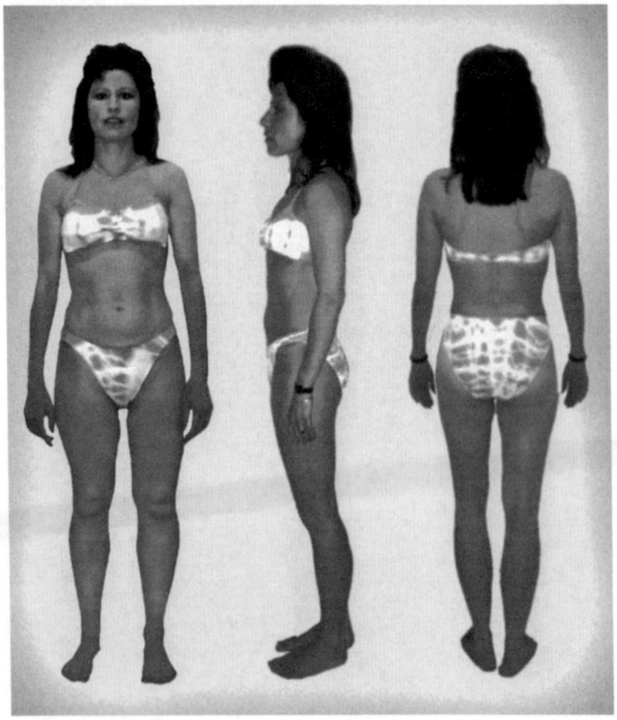

*Frequently have dominant striking face, with piercing or commanding eyes. Average oval or rectangular face.

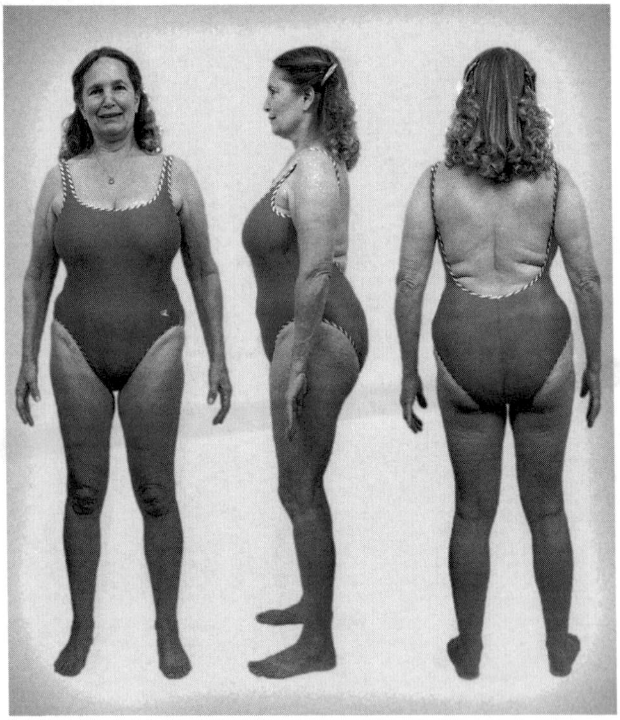

*Dominant forehead, often high. Usually endowed with large breasts, which are also area of initial weight gain.

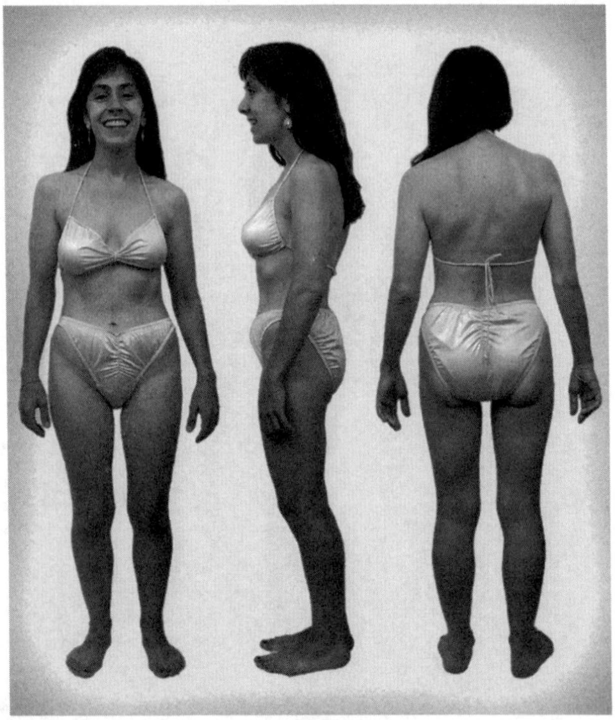

Known for intensely gathering information in detail. Precise in speech and actions with strong desire to do things right.

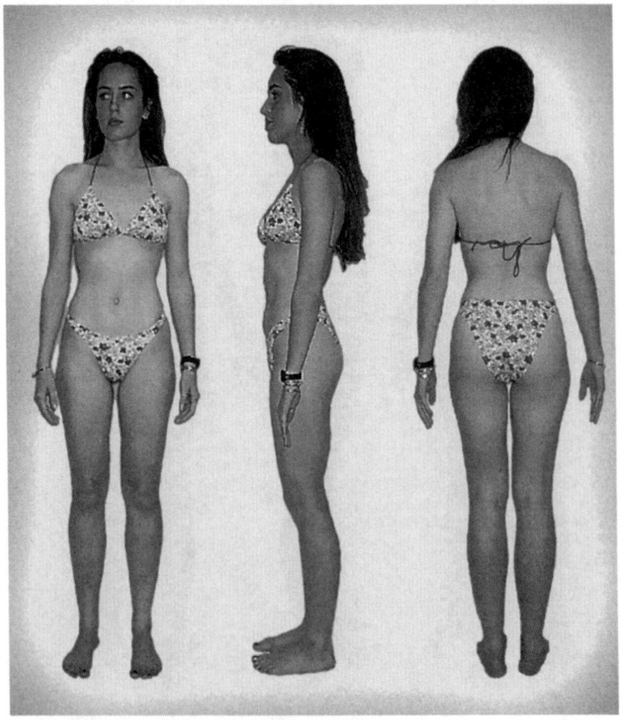

Relatively slender torso with average-to-large breasts. May have difficulty gaining or maintaining weight. Average to short-waisted.

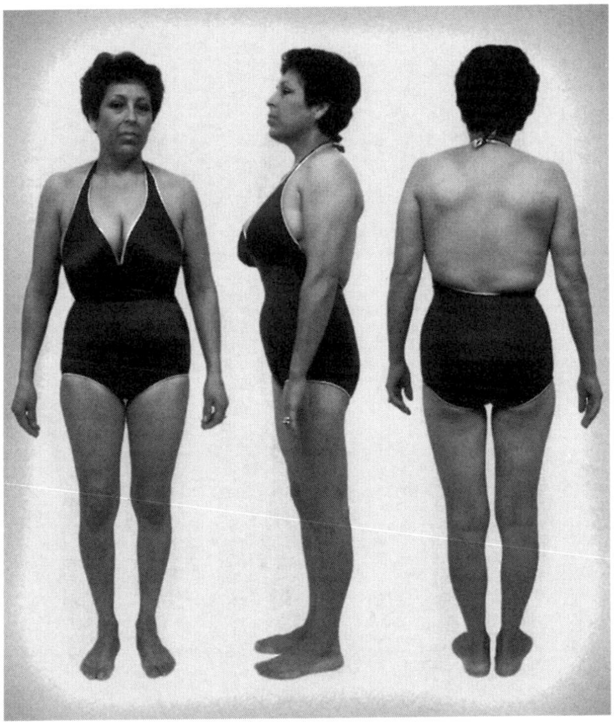

*Initial weight gain in breasts, upper hips, waist, lower abdomen and possibly upper inner thighs. Bone structure small-to-medium.

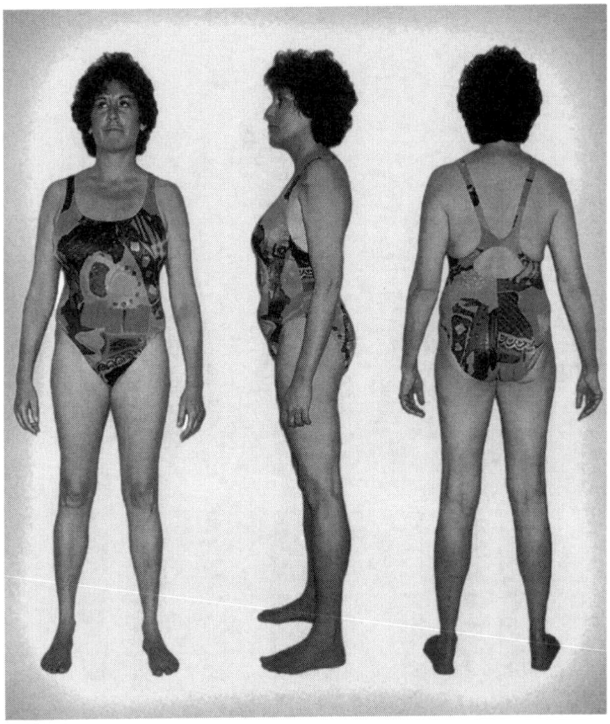

Shoulders relatively even with, to broader than, hips. Height petite-to-average. Average, elongated musculature. Slender legs.

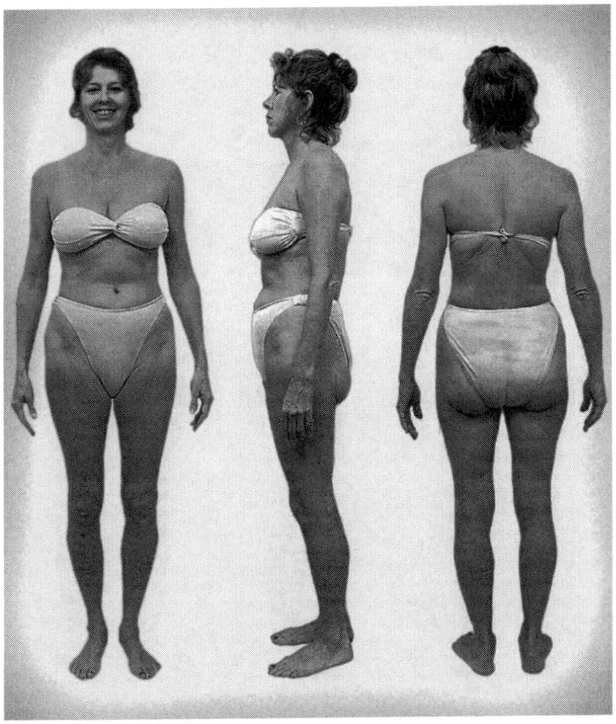

Buttocks relatively flat-to-rounded. Low back curvature can range from straight-to-swayed. Either straight or well-defined waist.

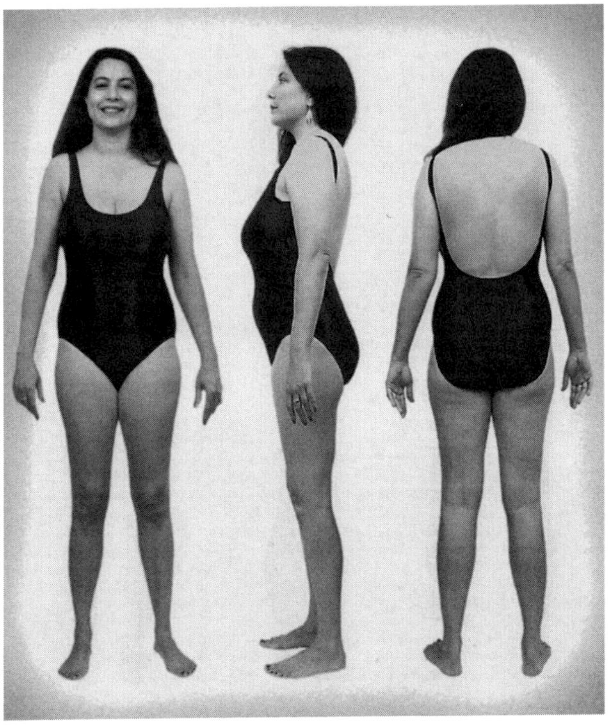

Secondary weight gain in entire back, buttocks, inner-to-entire upper 2/3rds of thighs, upper arms, face, under chin, then all over.

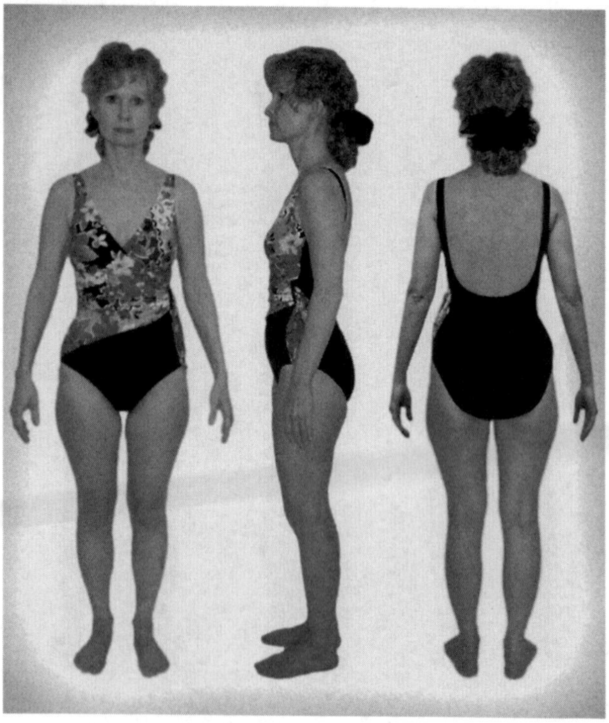

*Eyes dominant or hooded. Vision is dominant sense and can be reflected in excellent eyesight and/or the ability to see what others don't notice.

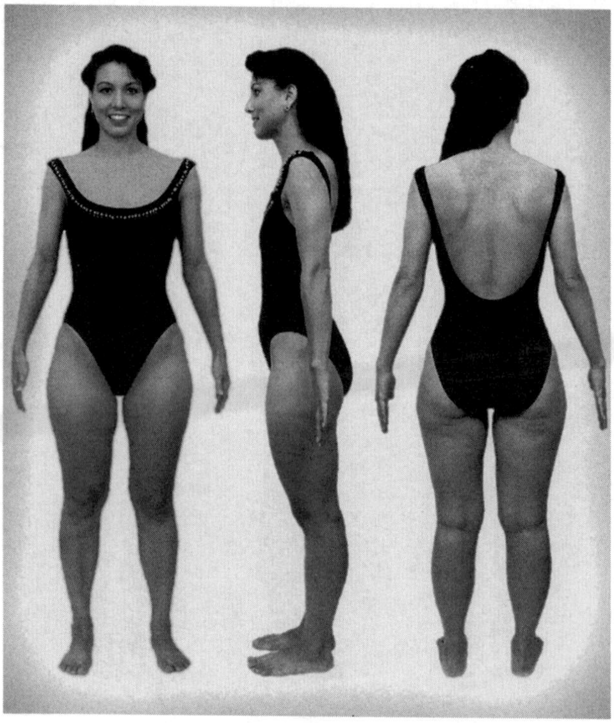

*Characteristic protrusion on upper 1/3rd of outer thighs. Body may be at least full size smaller above waist than below.

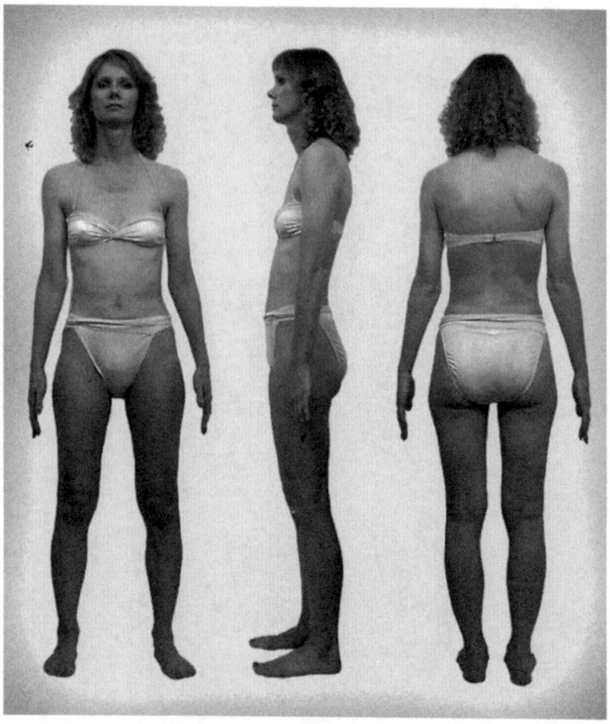

May have difficulty gaining or maintaining weight. Average, elongated musculature. Often have broad, square palms with short fingers.

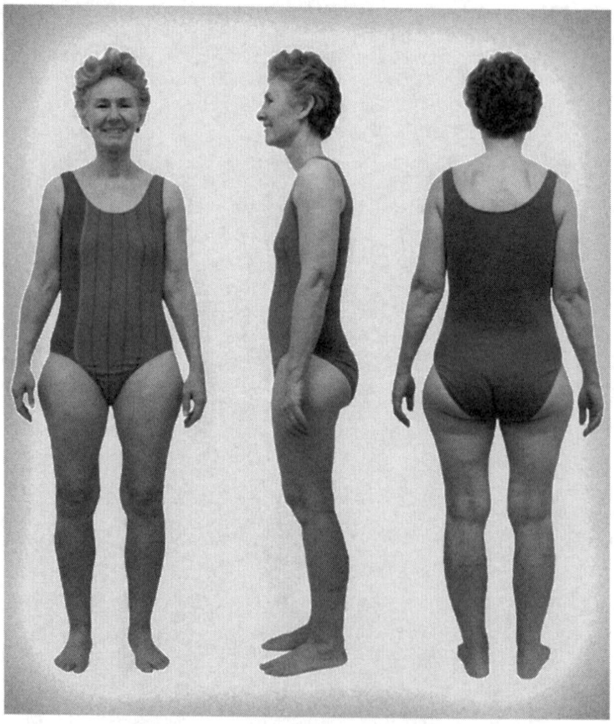

Shoulders narrower than, to relatively even with, hips. Height ranges from very petite to tall. Bone structure small-to-medium. Breasts small-to-average.

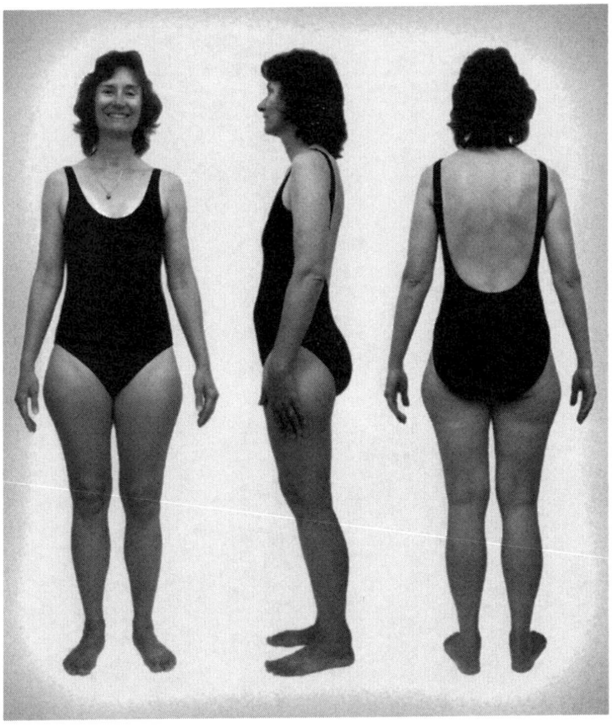

*Initial weight gain on upper 1/3rd of outer thighs, upper inner thighs, lower abdomen, and lower buttocks.

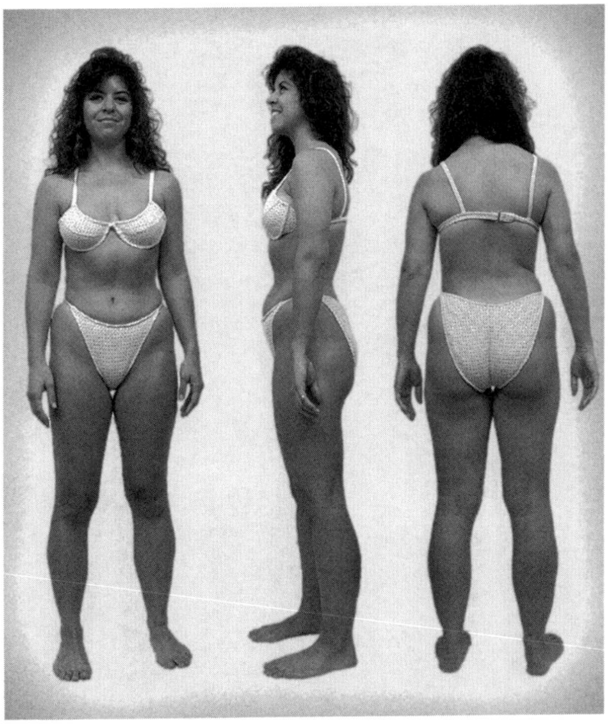

Alternative weight-gain pattern: minimal gain on upper 1/3rd of outer thighs with soft layer of fat covering entire body.

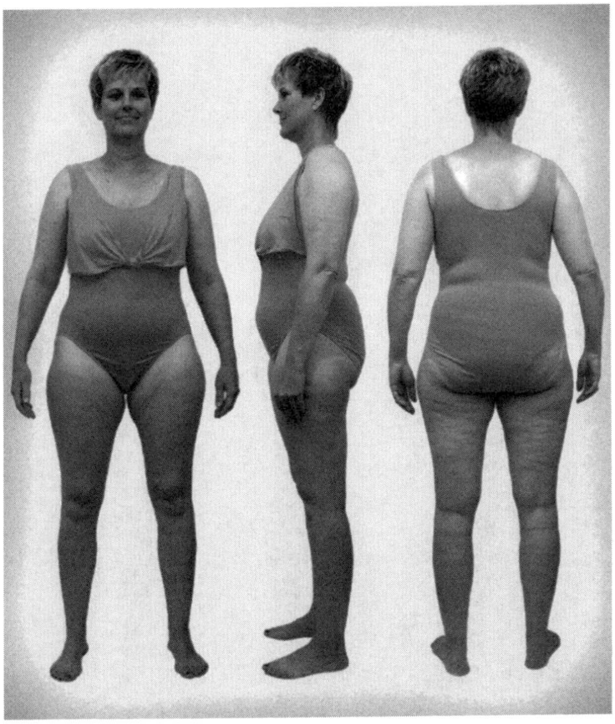

Low back curvature straight-to-average. Buttocks relatively flat-to-rounded. Average to long-waisted. Straight to well-defined waist.

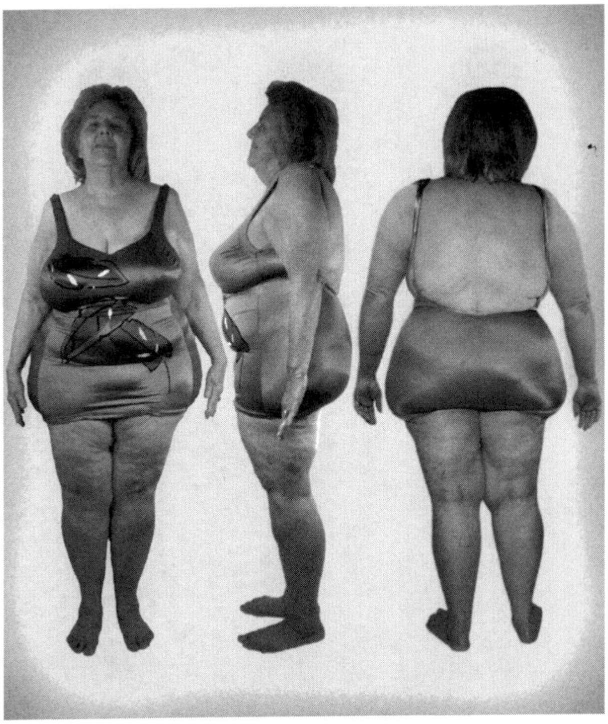

Secondary weight gain in face, under chin, upper arms, breasts, waist, upper and/or lower hips, and eventually entire back.

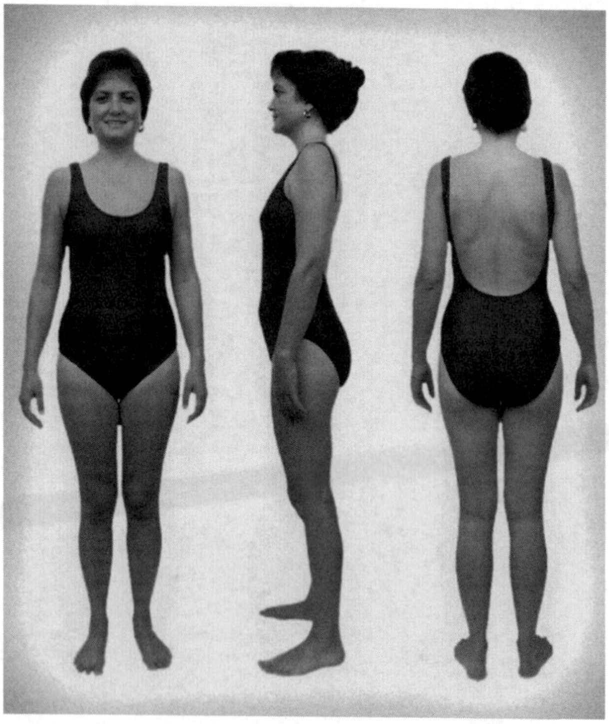

*Practical, helpful, down-to-earth personality. Consistent, reliable, and dependable. Often timid, preferring to work behind the scenes.

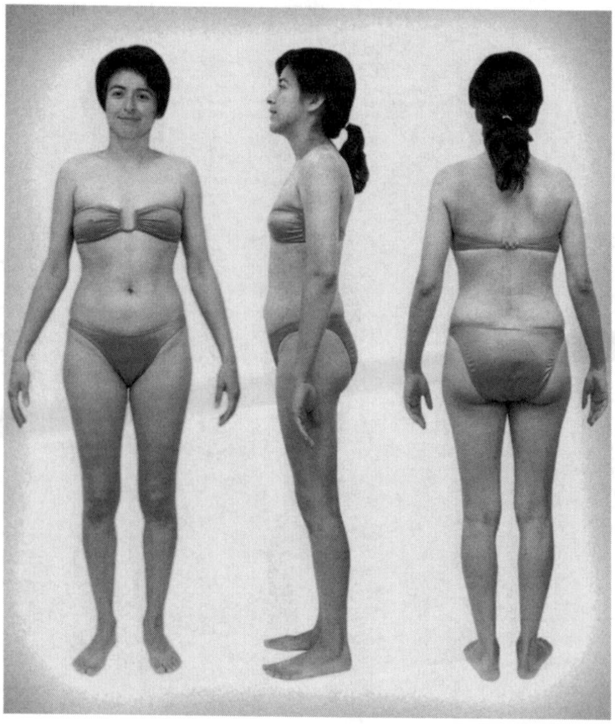

Solid torso with most of weight gain in lower abdomen. Shoulders relatively even with hips. Height petite-to-average.

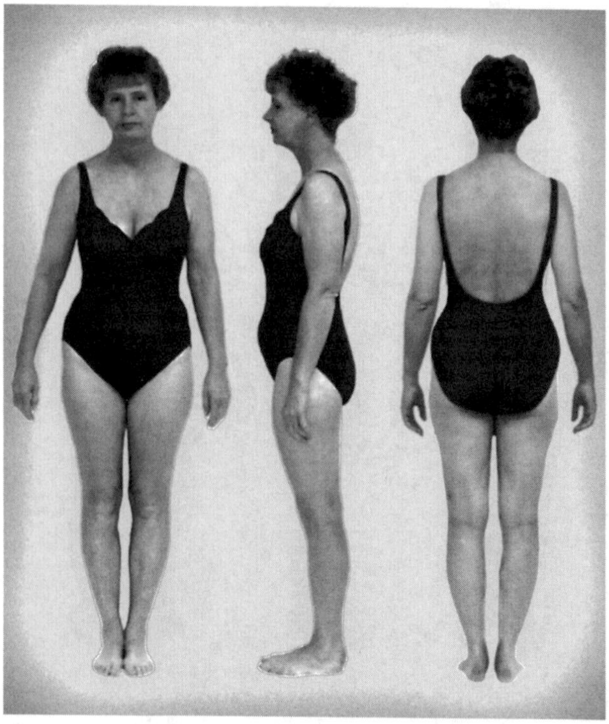

Oval or rectangular head. May have small, deep-set eyes. Straight-to-defined waist. Average to short-waisted.

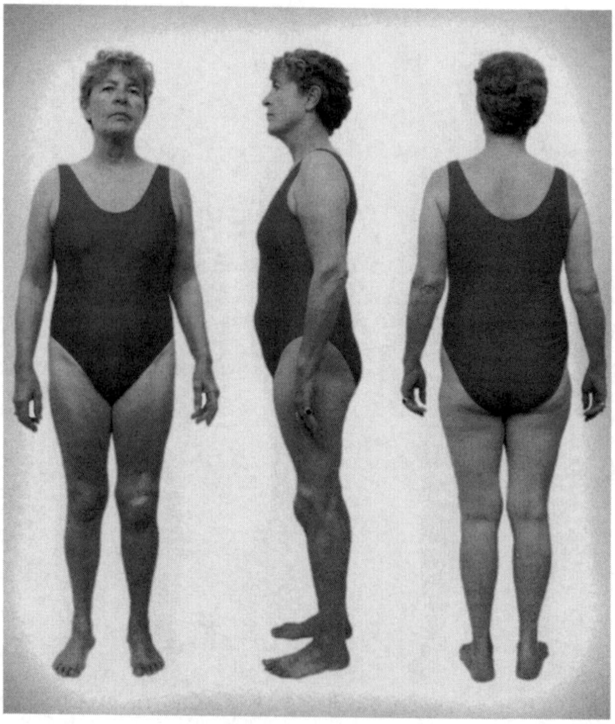

Calves thin-to-muscular. Low back curvature straight-to-average. Buttocks relatively flat-to-rounded. Hands average.

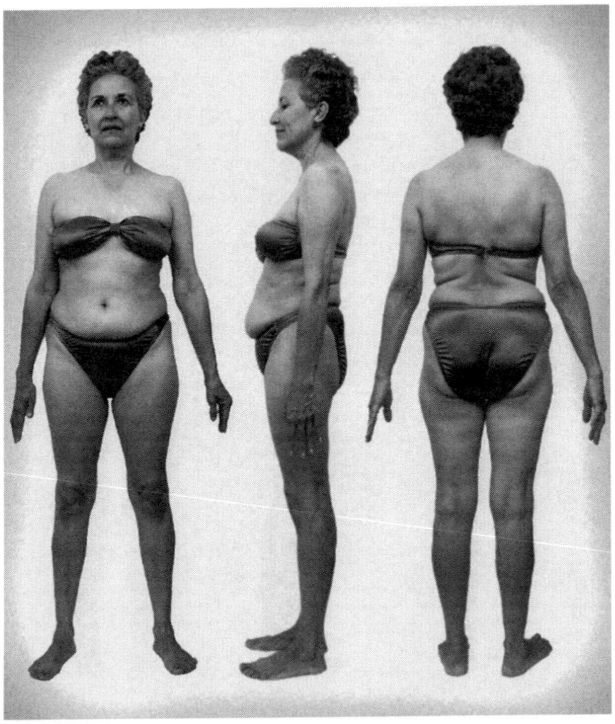

*Initial weight gain in lower abdomen, waist, and upper hips with little or no gain in thighs, legs, lower hips, and buttocks.

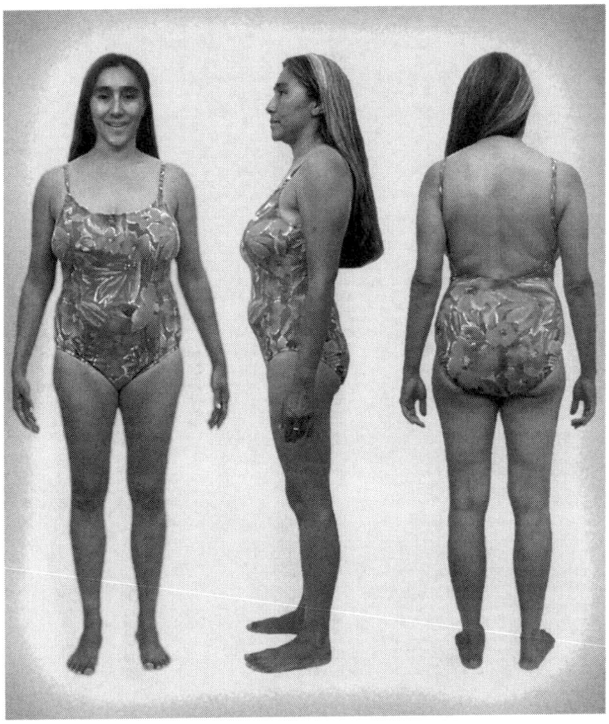

Breasts small-to-large. When weight gain is over 5 pounds, breasts may also increase, only to decrease when weight is lost.

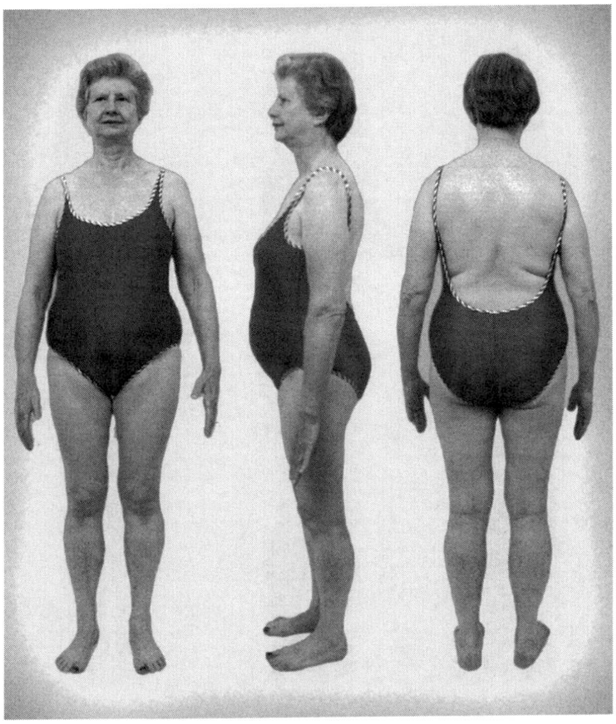

Bone structure small-to-medium. Average, elongated musculature. Slender legs with little or no weight gain in thighs except upper inner.

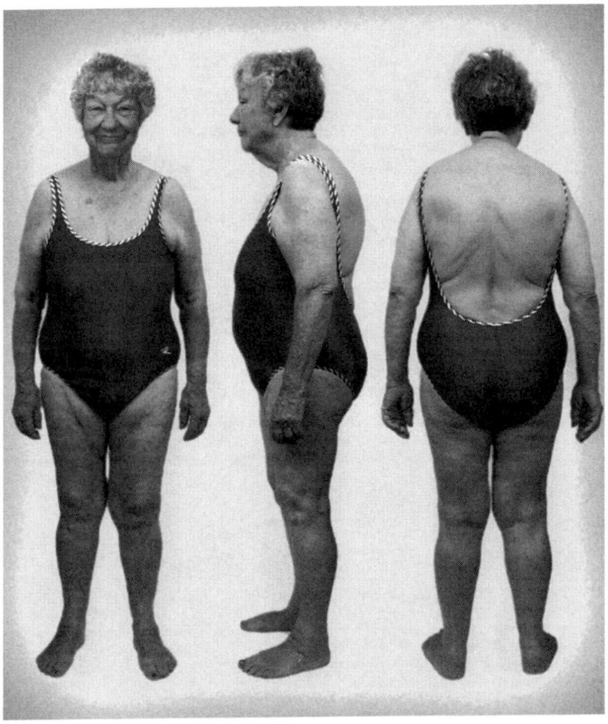

Secondary weight gain in torso as general thickening, face, under chin, breasts, upper arms, entire abdomen, and middle back.

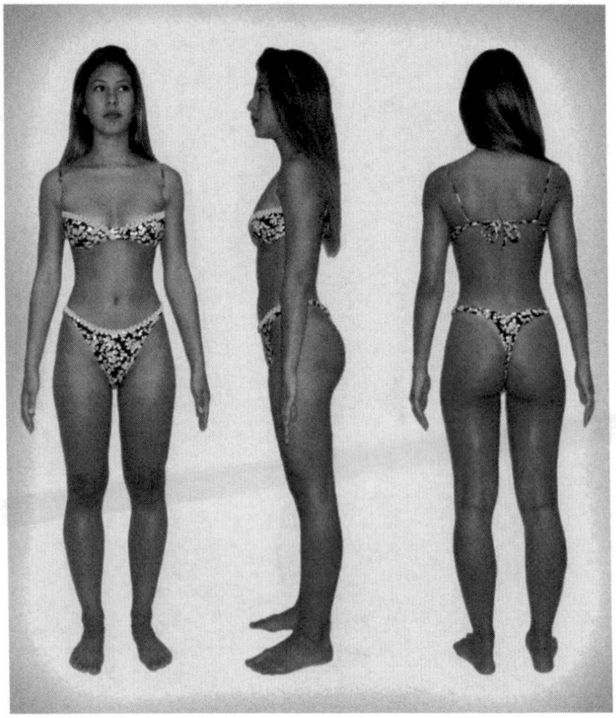

*Prominent muscular buttocks, often with sway back, and relatively flat stomach. Characteristic muscular thighs that appear developed to the knees.

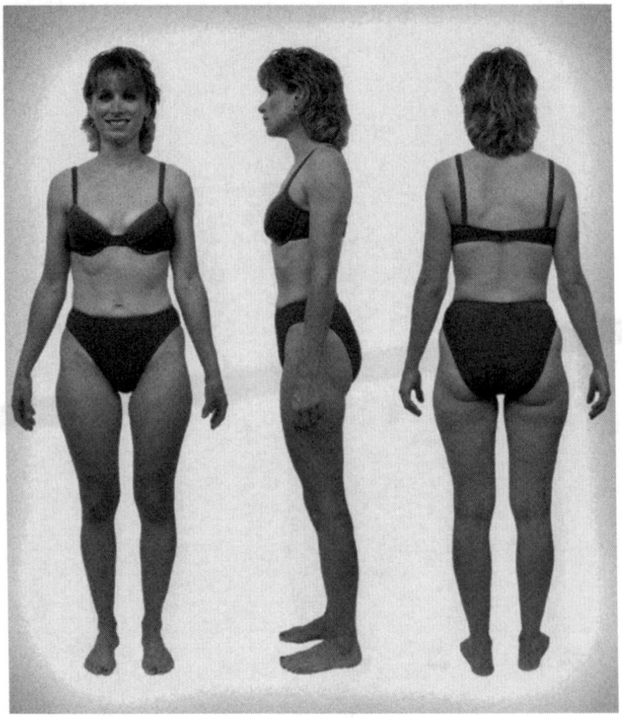

When loses mental clarity will do “no-brainer” jobs. Generally light and playful. Bright, attractive, oval or rectangular face, often with delicate features.

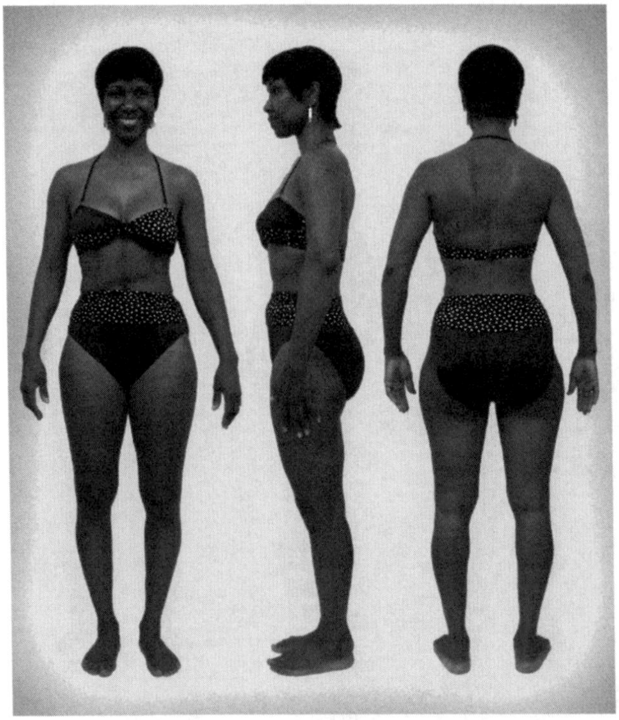

Hourglass figure with defined to well-defined waist. Average to long-waisted. Body often at least a full size smaller above waist than below.

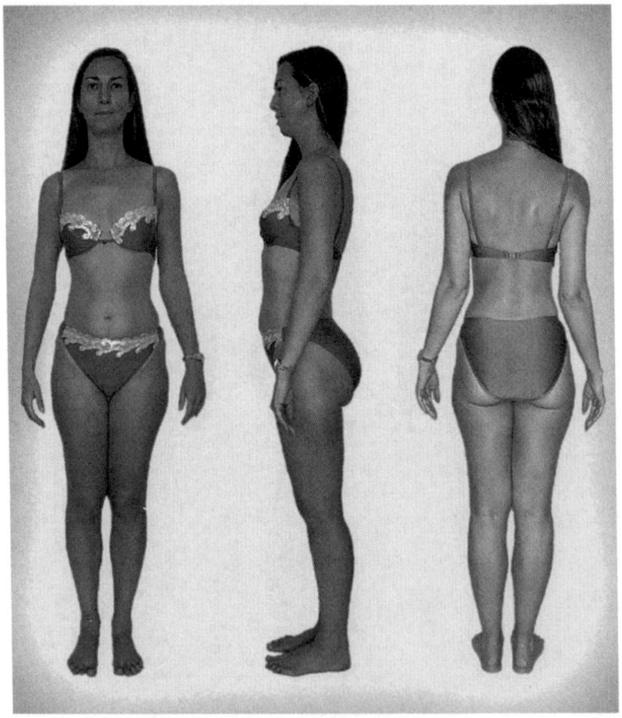

Buttocks prominent-to-rounded. Low back curvature average-to-swayed. Shoulders narrower than, to relatively even with, hips.

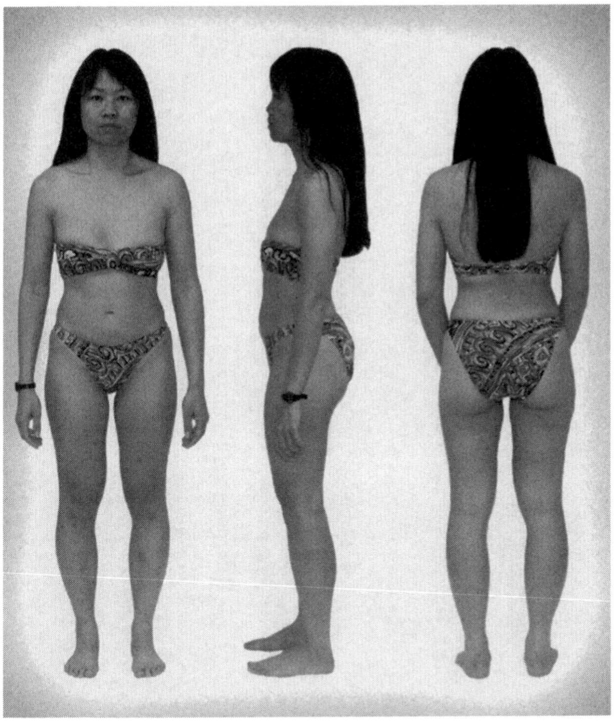

*Initial weight gain in buttocks, lower hips, and entire thighs with main protrusion on upper outer 1/3rd and entire inner thighs continuing to knees, inner knees, and possibly waist.

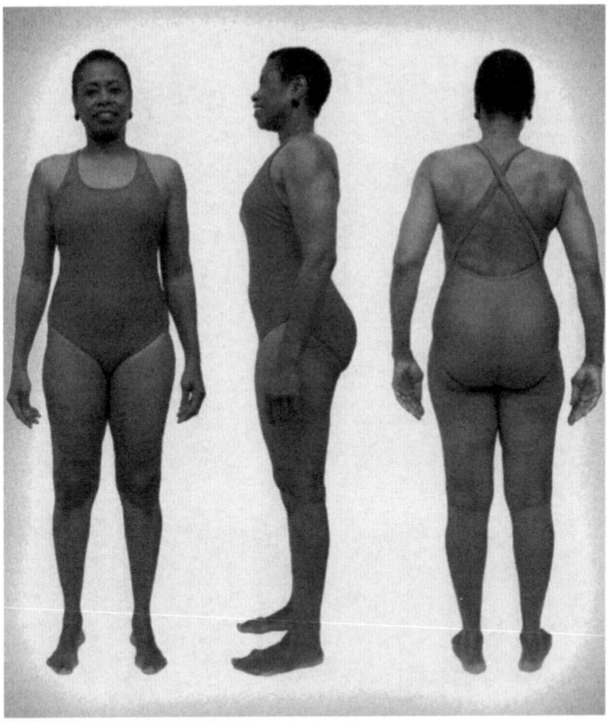

Weight often varies from 25 pounds overweight to 15 pounds underweight. Cellulite formation is common. Breasts small-to-average.

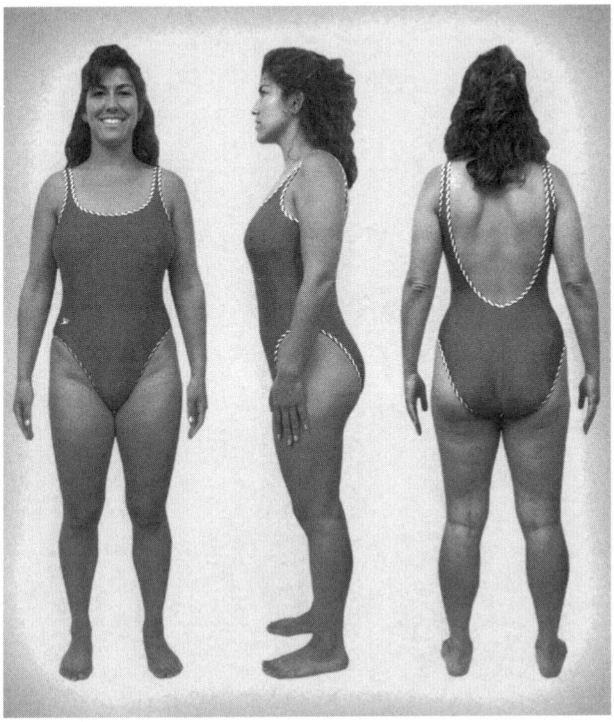

Bone structure small-to-medium. Average, elongated musculature. Height petite-to-average.

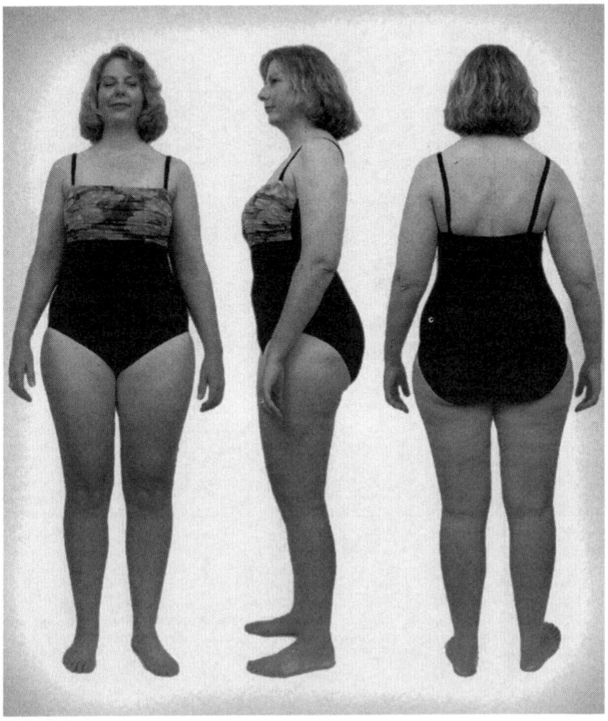

Secondary weight gain in upper arms, middle back, lower-to-entire abdomen, waist, breasts, face, under chin, and upper hips.

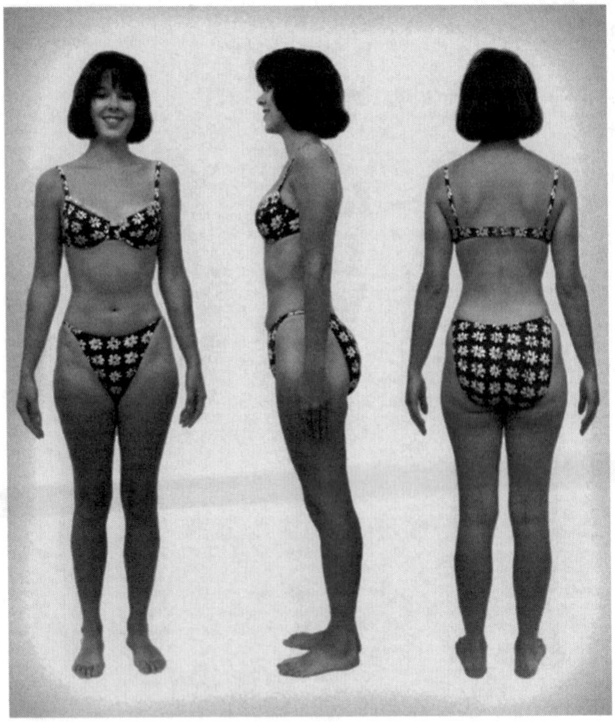

*Soft, round, heart-shaped appearance. Firm, shapely, rounded-to-prominent buttocks. Layer of softness covering muscle, resulting in little definition.

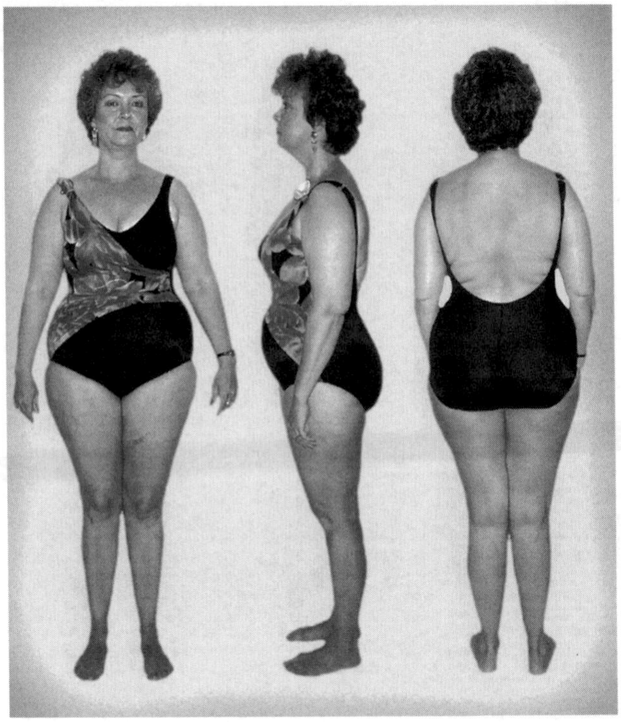

Like the heart, they bring their own rhythm or music to their environment, readily influencing others' moods.

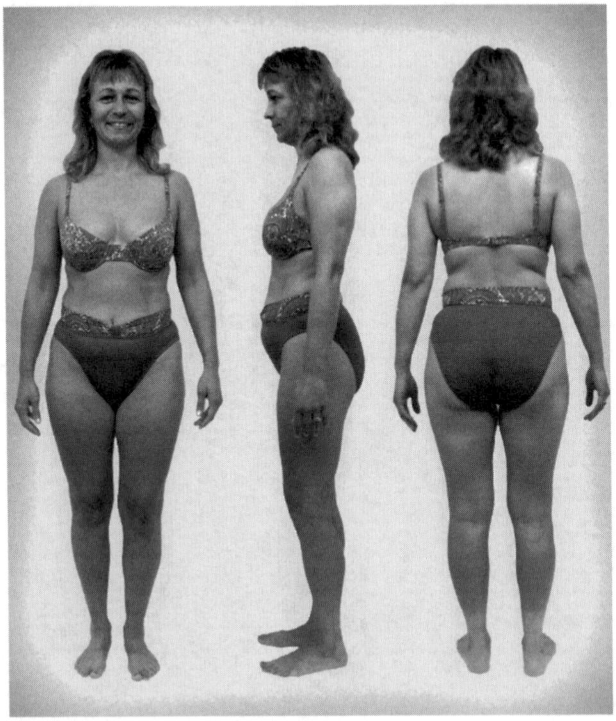

Breasts average-to-large. Low back curvature straight-to-swayed. Shoulders narrower than, to relatively even with, hips.

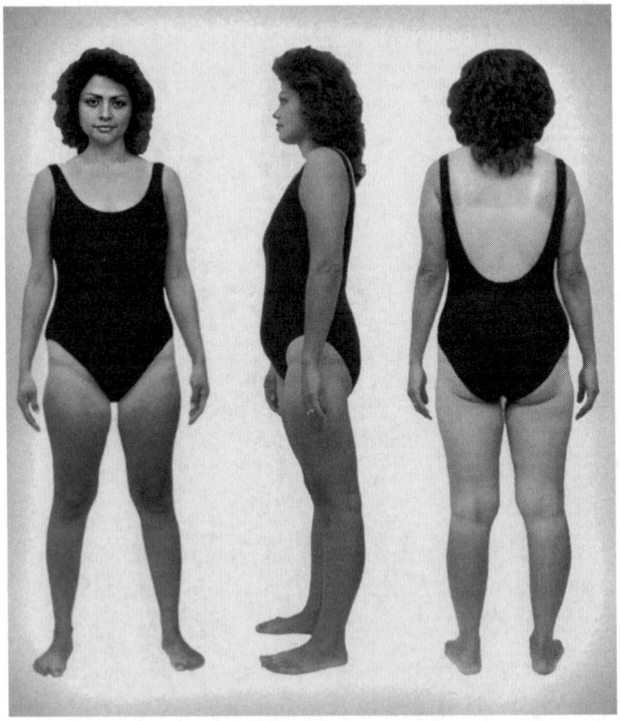

Height petite-to-average. Bone structure small-to-medium. Small-to-average hands and feet. Heart-shaped or oval, full face.

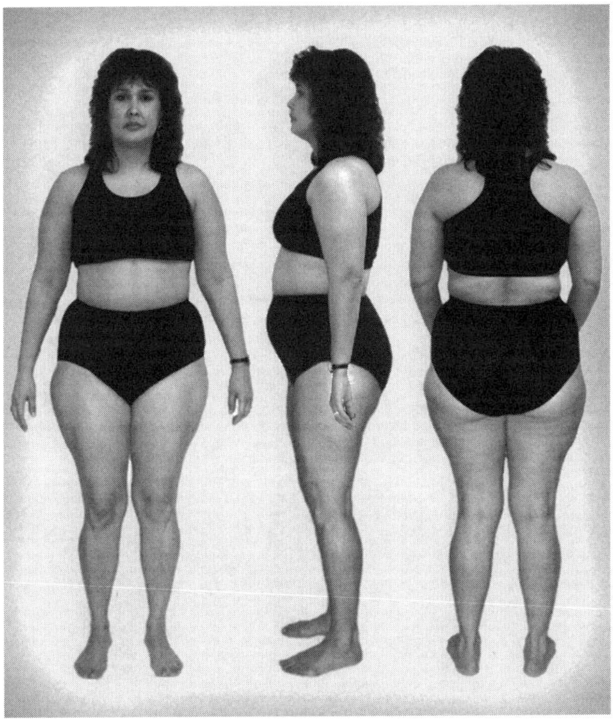

*Initial weight gain in lower abdomen, entire upper 2/3rds of thighs including upper inner thighs, inner knees, waist, middle back, and upper hips.

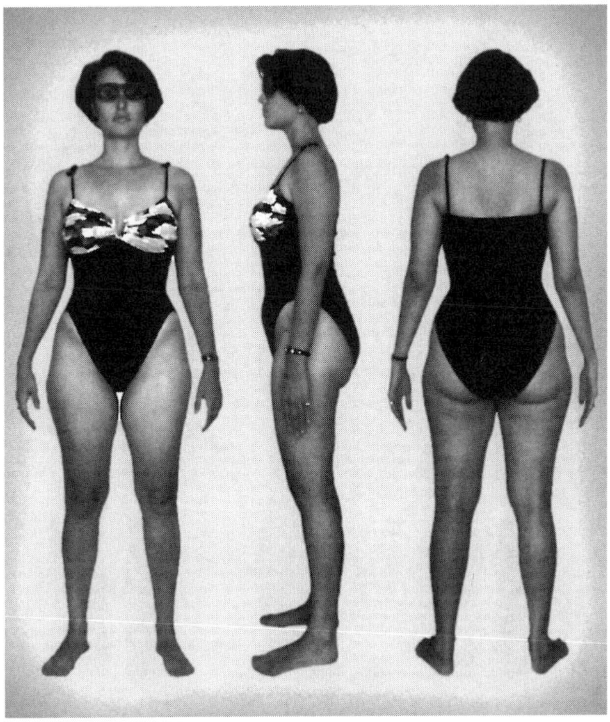

Alternative weight-gain pattern: lower abdomen, lower hips, and thighs. Generally sweet, gentle, warm, and approachable.

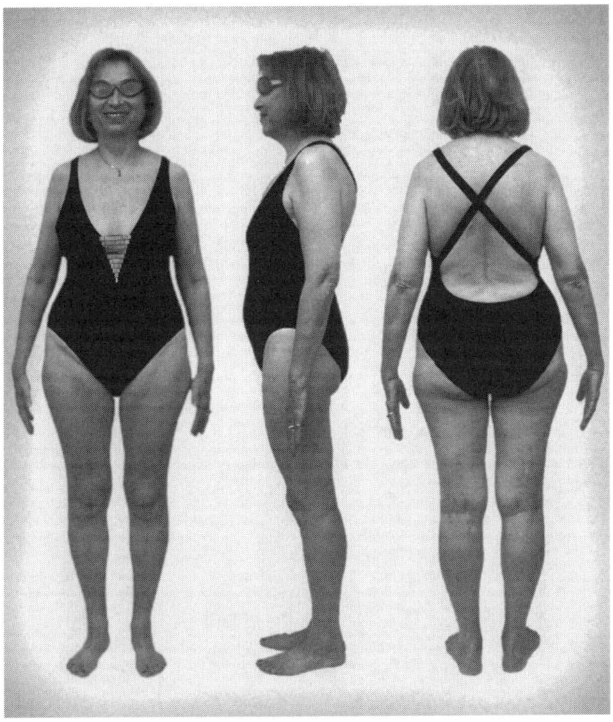

Body is often at least full size smaller above waist than below. Defined to well-defined waist. Average to short-waisted.

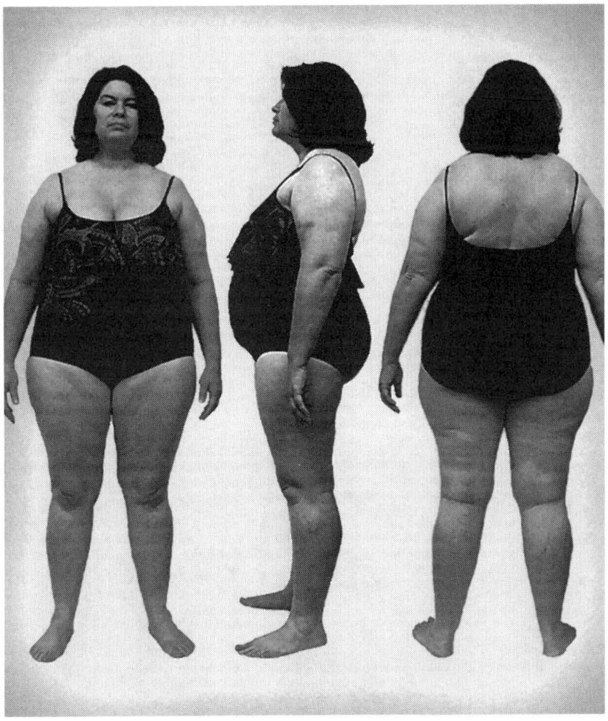

Secondary weight gain in face, under chin, upper arms, breasts, buttocks, and entire back, still maintaining a round, shapely appearance.

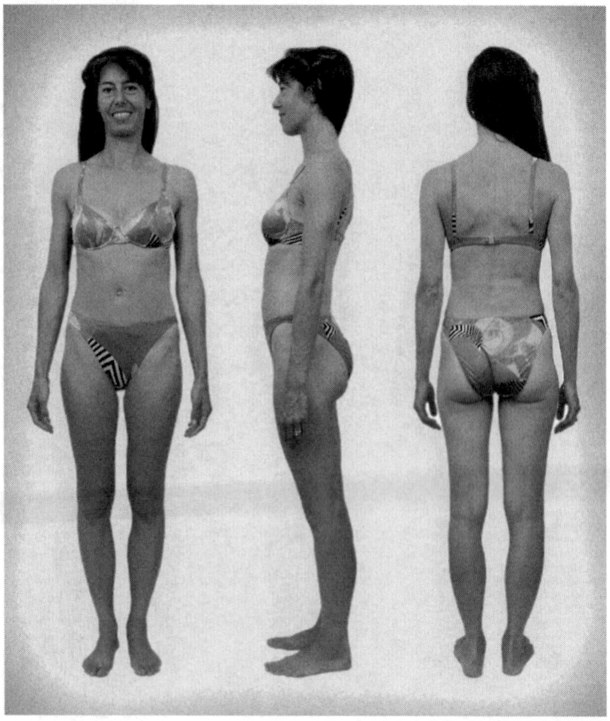

*Characterized by extremes: will completely immerse themselves in a project or endeavor, then transfer all their energy onto something else, as if going through phases.

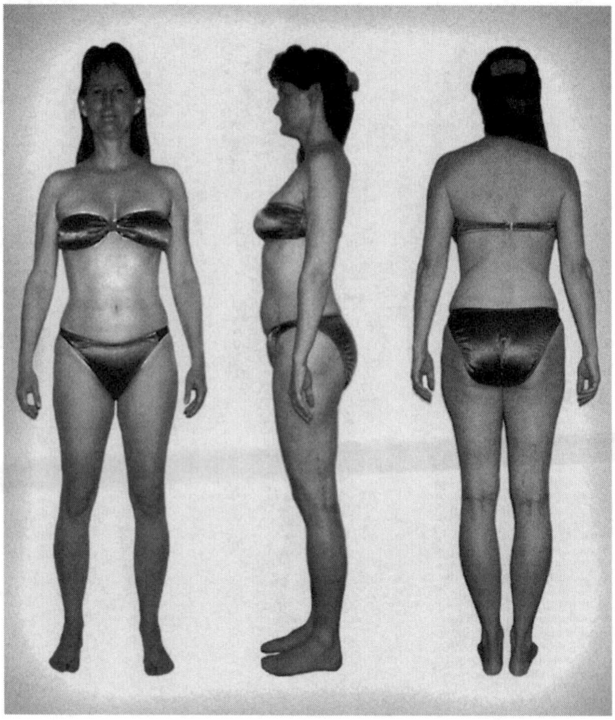

Height average to very tall. Bone structure medium. Generally prefer hot and dry to moderately humid, temperate climate or very cold weather.

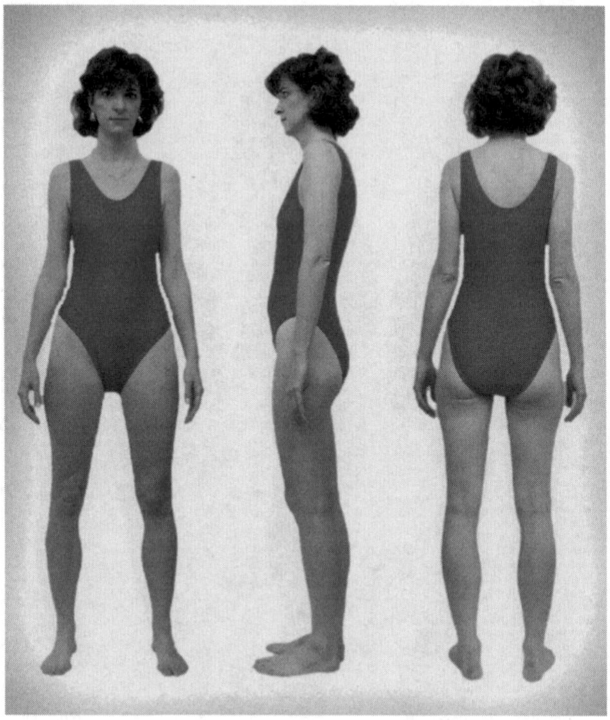

May have difficulty gaining or maintaining weight. Low back curvature straight-to-average. Buttocks relatively flat-to-rounded.

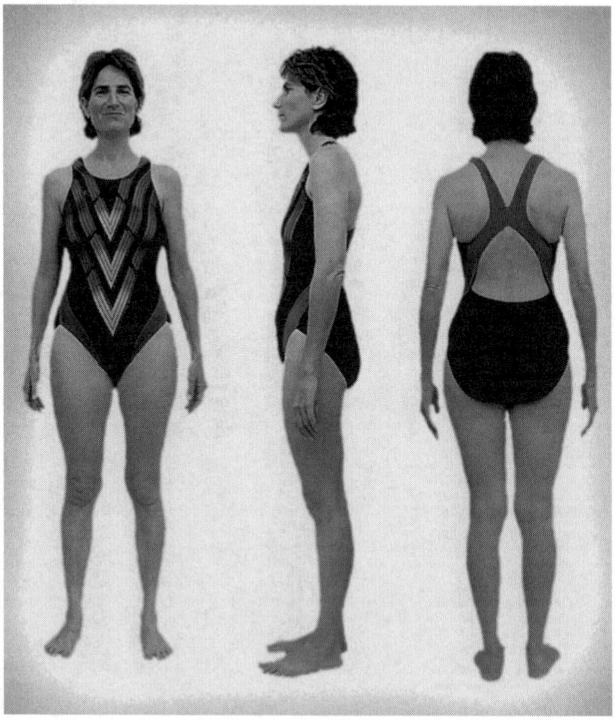

Shoulders narrower than, to relatively even with, hips. Often have long arms and legs. Average, elongated musculature. Waist straight-to-defined. Average to long-waisted.

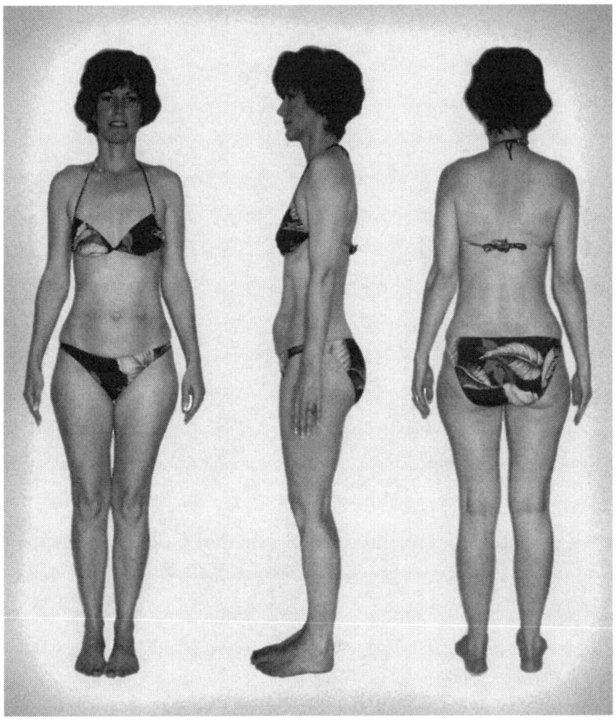

*Initial weight gain in lower abdomen, entire upper 2/3rds of thighs including upper inner thighs, buttocks, upper hips and waist. Long, slender torso.

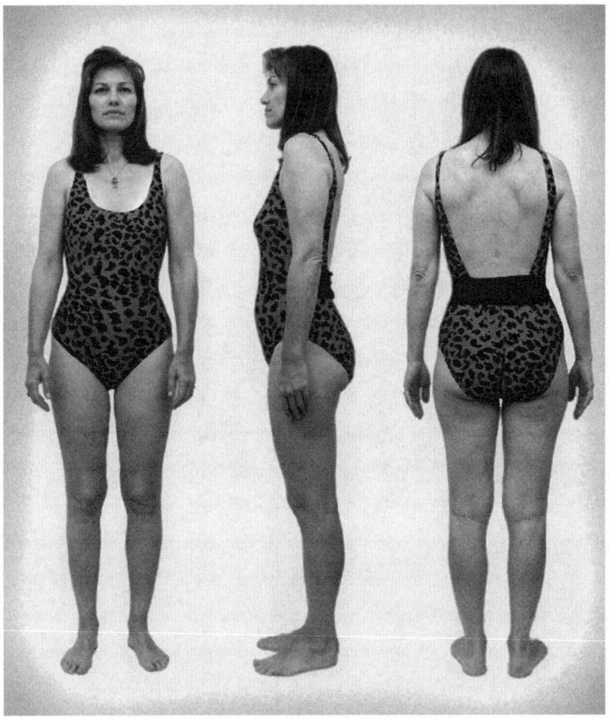

Often have wistful, distant look in eyes. Head small-to-average, with long, narrow, rectangular or oval face. Breasts small-to-average.

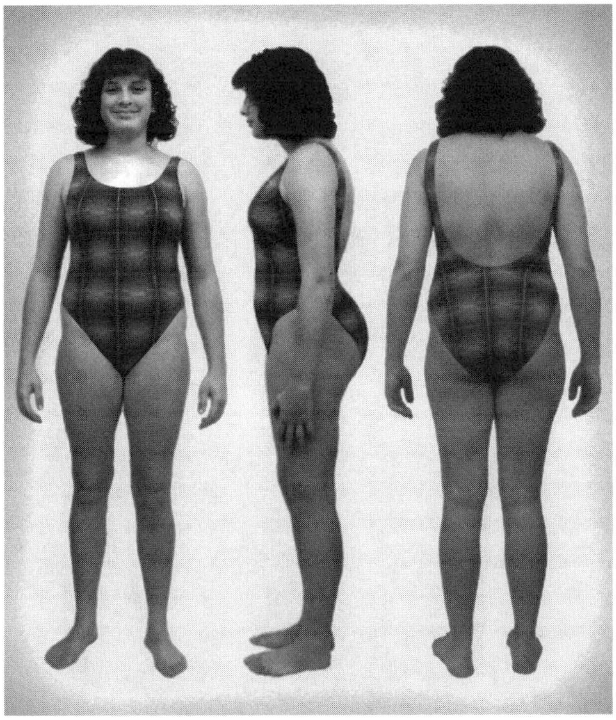

Alternative weight-gain pattern: entire abdomen, waist, upper hips, and buttocks. Broad chest and torso.

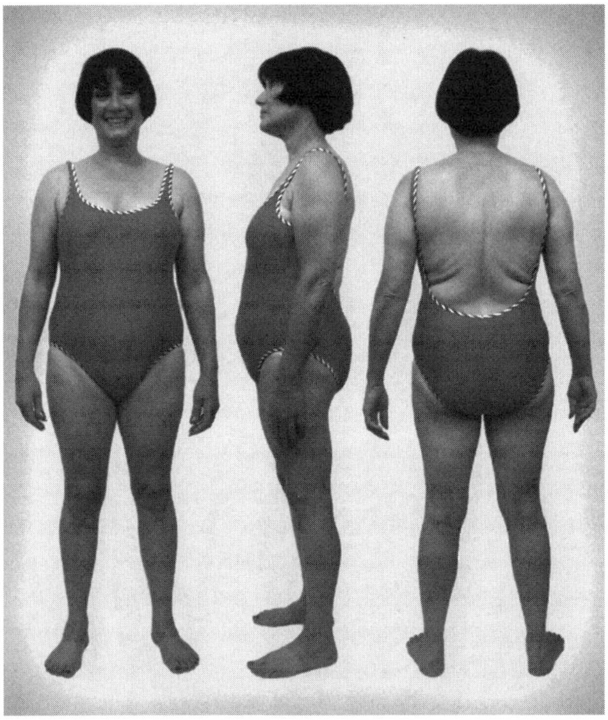

Secondary weight gain in entire abdomen, middle-to-entire back, breasts, upper arms, face, and under chin, with little gain in lower hips.

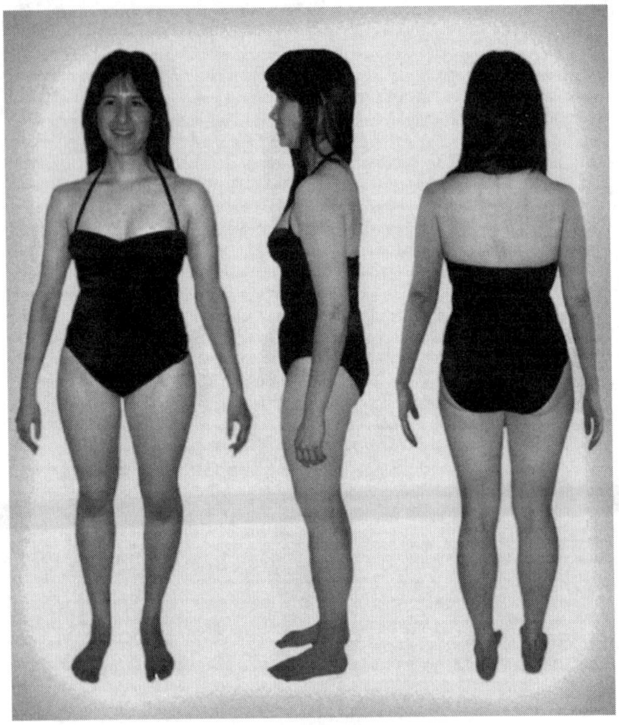

*Solid body with layer of softness covering muscle, reducing muscle definition. Often have muscle weakness under chin which gives rise to double chin.

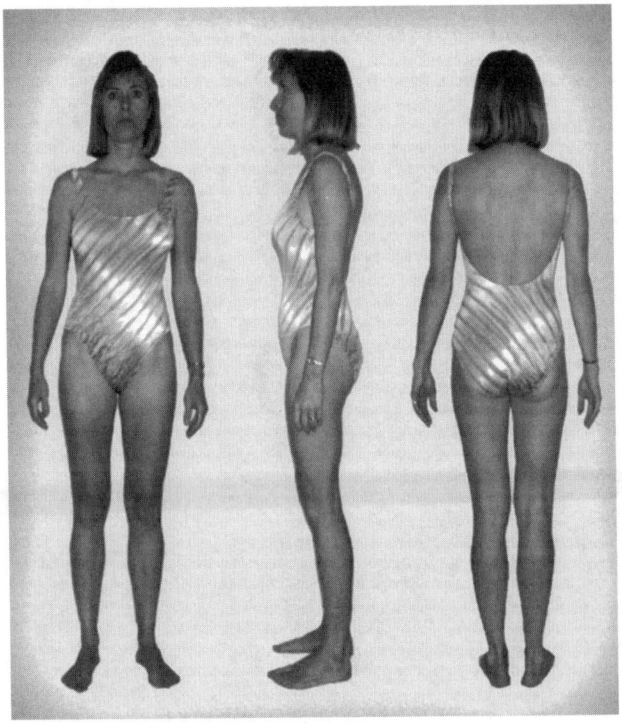

Emotionally sensitive with an open approach to life. Need new experiences to grow mentally, emotionally, or spiritually or will expand physically.

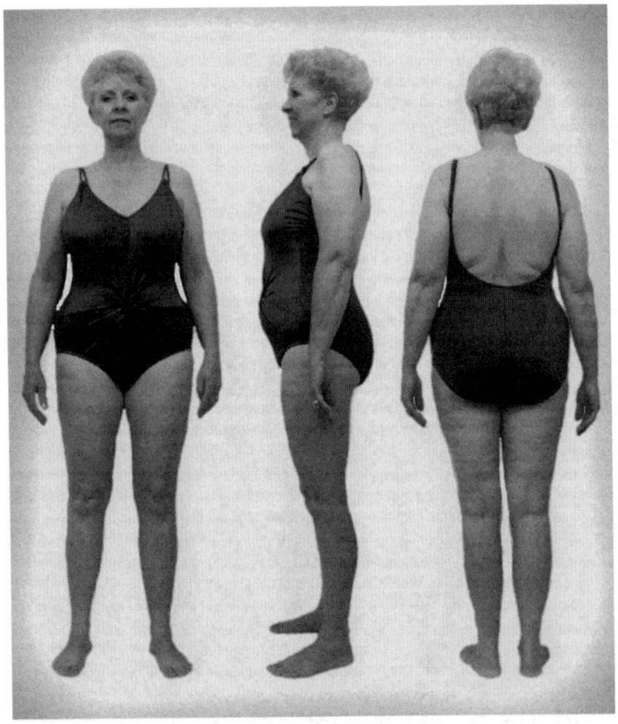

Weight accumulates primarily over intestinal region, in upper and lower abdomen, upper hips, and waist – more in front of body than back. Bone structure small-to-medium.

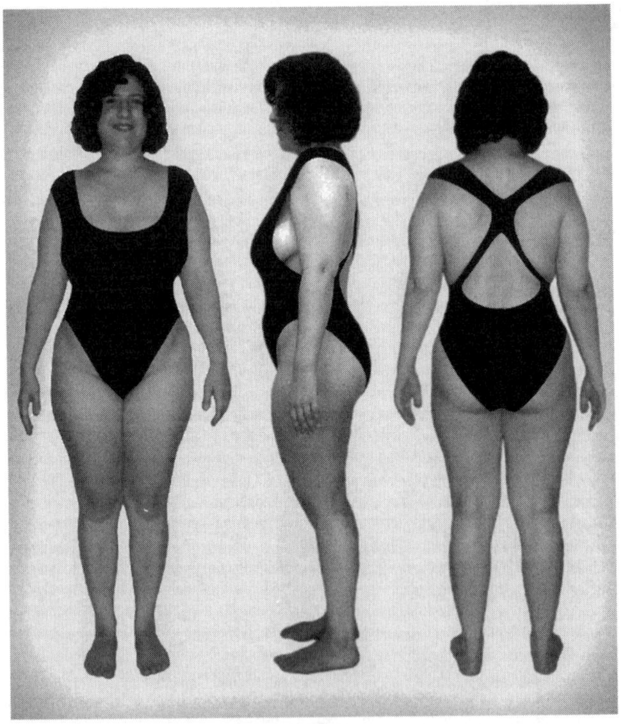

Height average, although can range from petite-to-very tall. Shoulders narrower than, to relatively even with, hips. Breasts average-to-large.

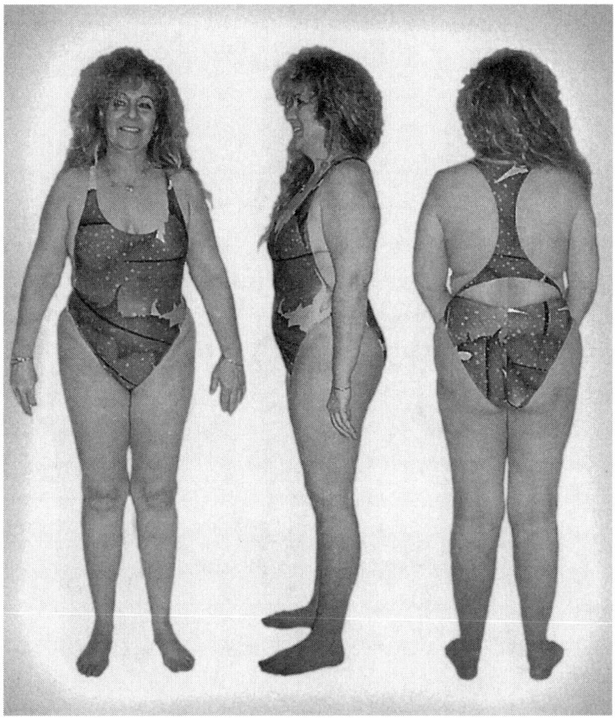

*Initial weight gain in lower-to-entire abdomen, waist, upper hips, inner knees, entire inner and possibly entire upper 2/3rds of thighs. May gain initially in breasts.

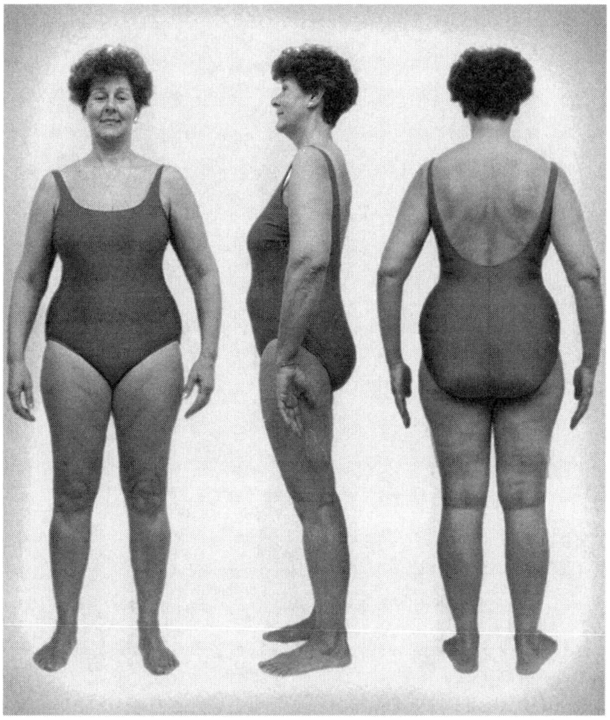

Buttocks relatively flat-to-rounded. Low back curvature straight-to-average. Waist straight-to-defined. Often have relatively straight calves. Average to short-waisted.

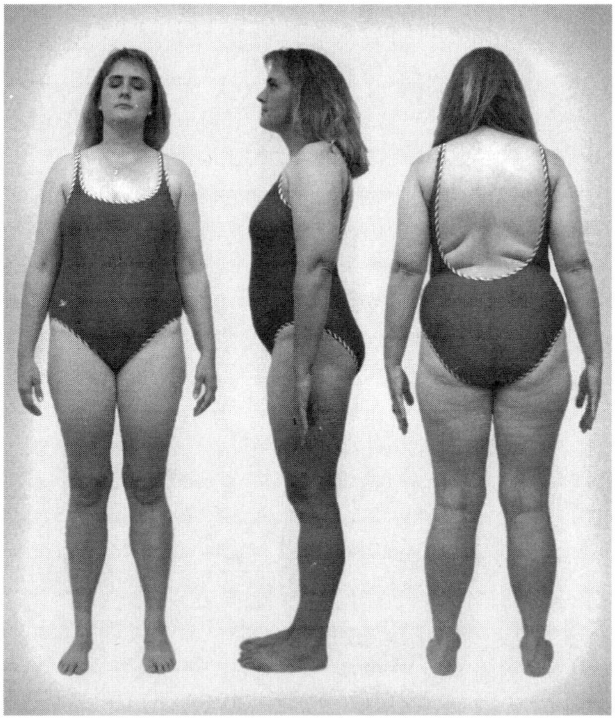

Capable of carrying large amounts of weight. While weight may be gained in thighs, it is disproportionately less than on abdomen.

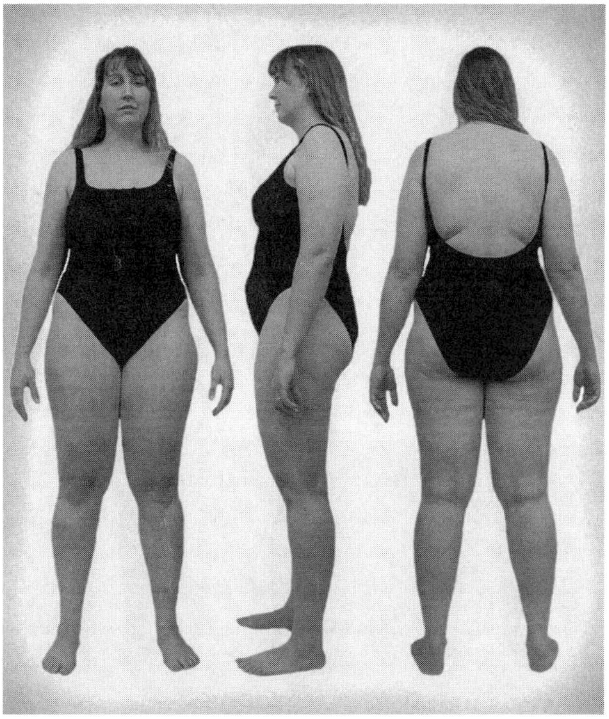

Secondary weight gain in face, under chin, upper arms, entire back, buttocks, and extending throughout entire thighs; then generally all over.

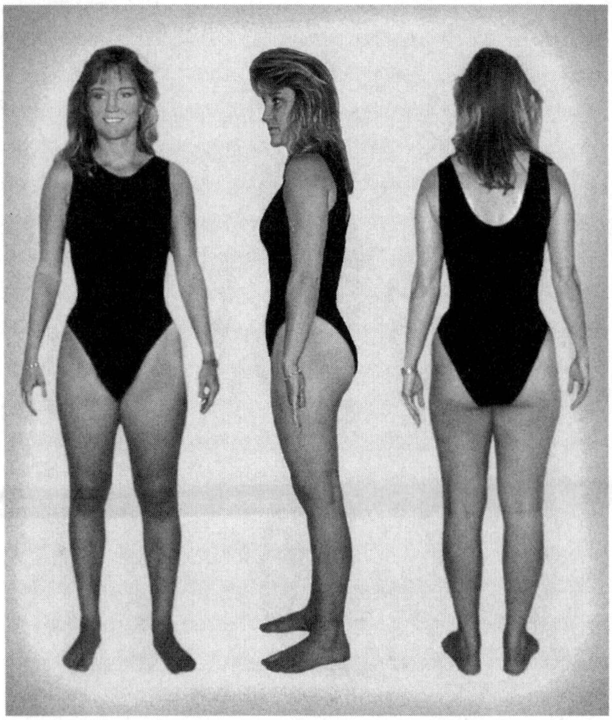

*Long, oval face with V-shaped chin and high forehead. Large, muscular thighs. Buttocks rounded-to-prominent. Low back curvature average-to-swayed.

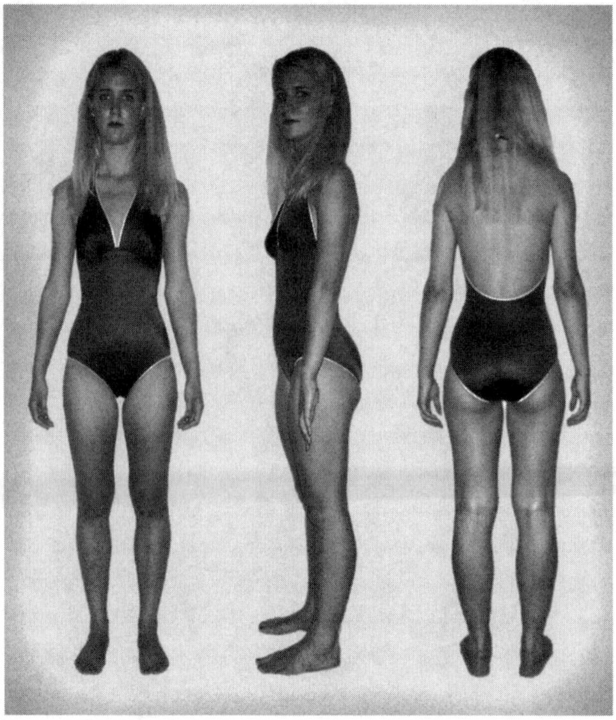

Tend to procrastinate, forcing themselves to excel when under pressure of deadlines, time, or performance.

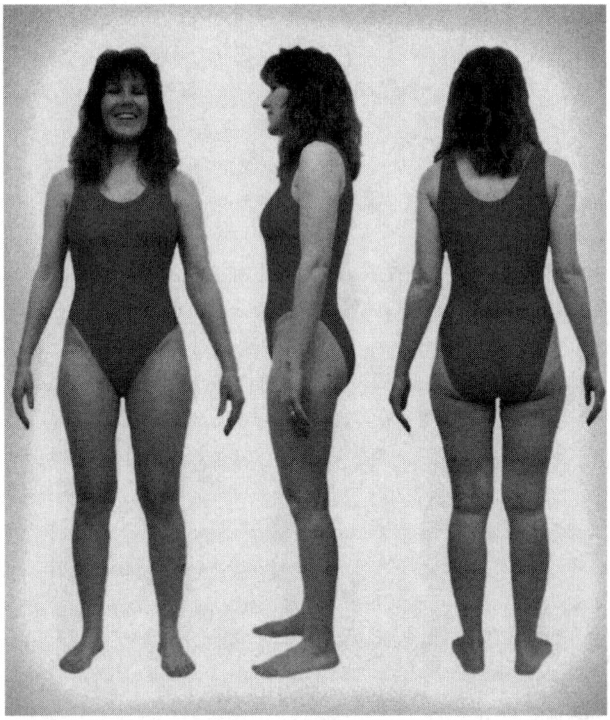

Height generally petite-to-average. Shoulders relatively even with hips. Average, elongated to dense, solid musculature.

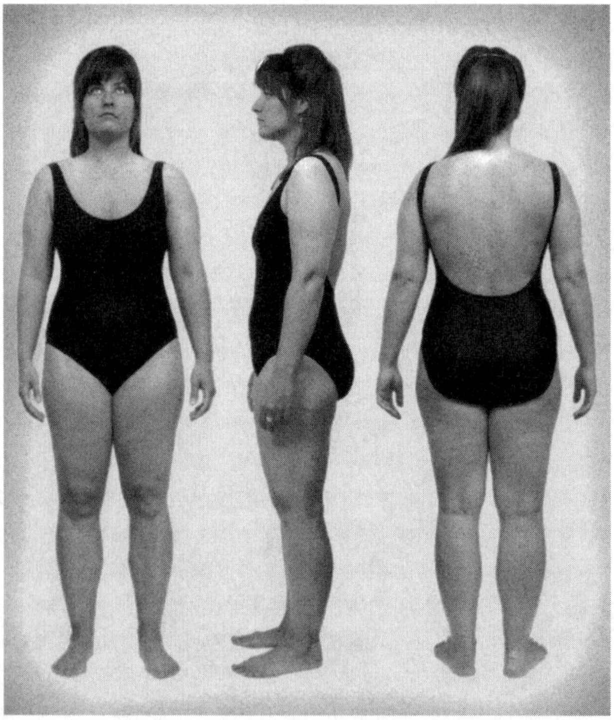

Bone structure medium. Hands often broad and square with short-to-average fingers. May have wide feet with short-to-average toes.

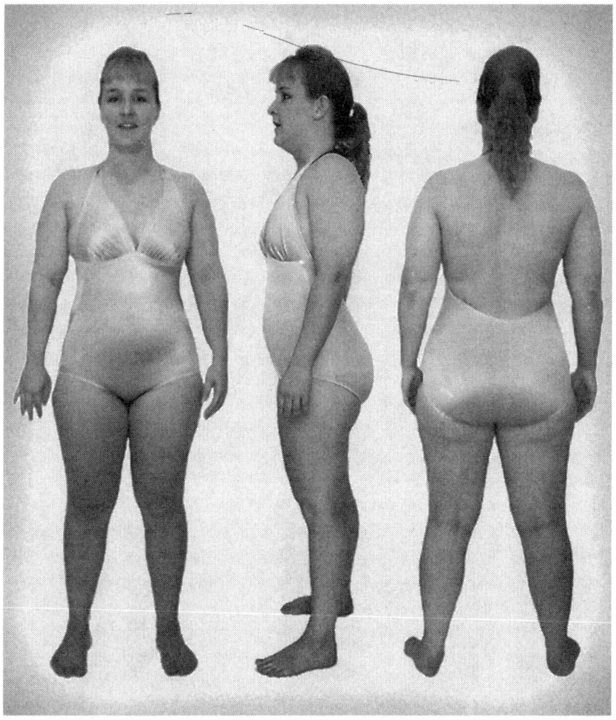

*Initial weight gain in entire upper 2/3rds of thighs including upper inner thighs which can extend to knees, inner knees, lower hips, buttocks, and minimally, if at all, in abdomen.

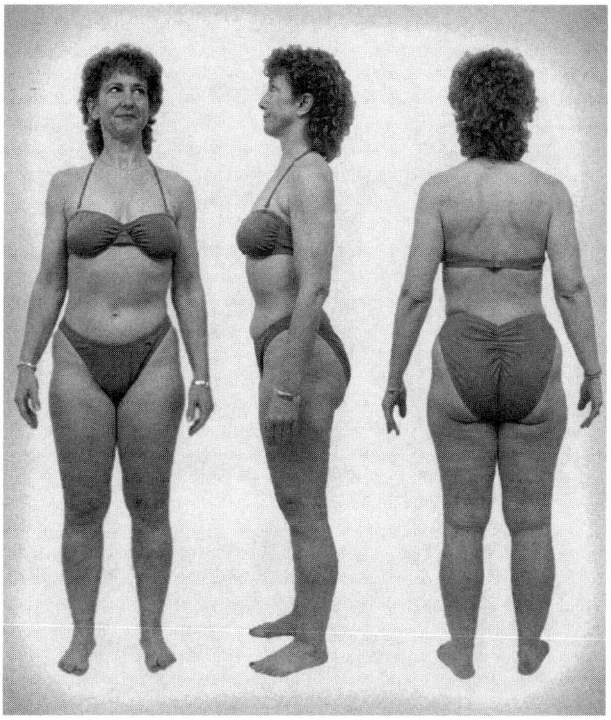

Average to long-waisted. Breasts small-to-average. Strong, sturdy body. Defined to well-defined waist.

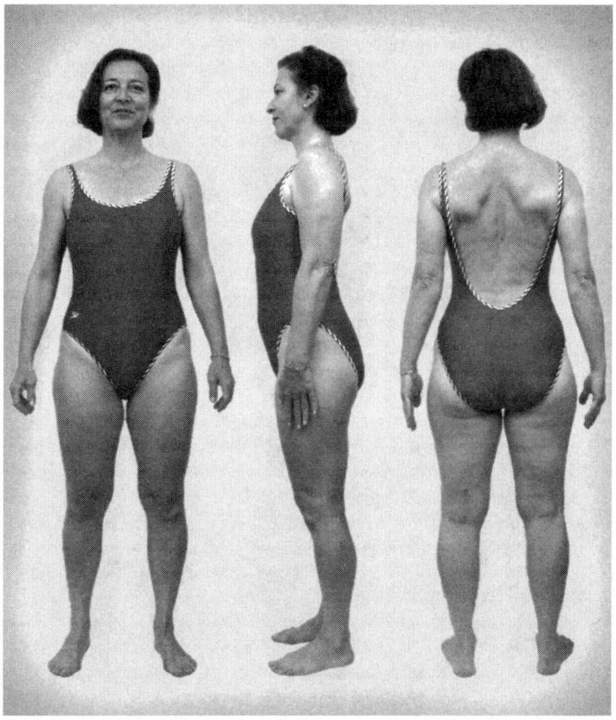

Main weight gain in buttocks and entire upper 2/3rds of thighs, which can continue to knees. Prone to developing cellulite.

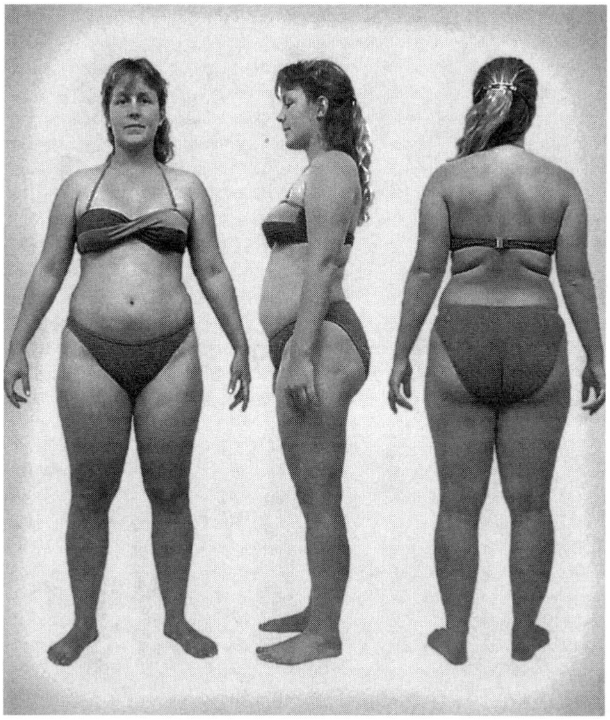

Secondary weight gain in legs (including calves and ankles), lower-to-entire abdomen, waist, upper hips, upper arms, face, and middle back.

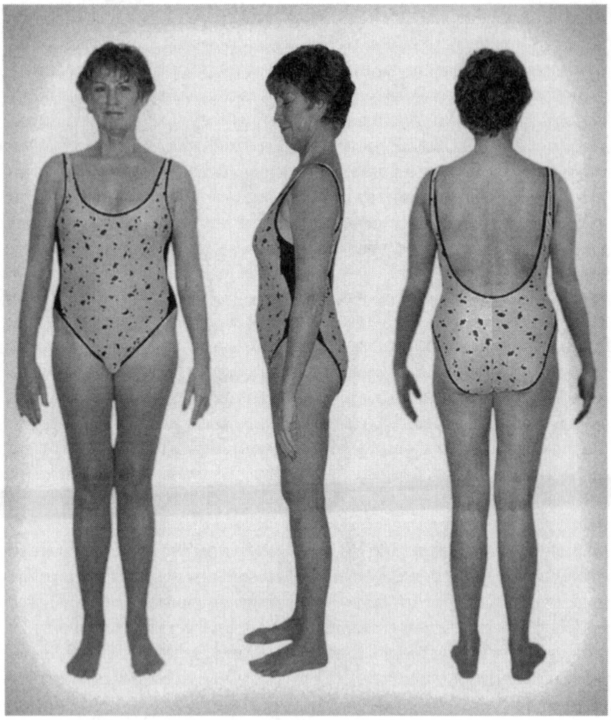

*Broad, thick torso with little weight gain in thighs. Shoulders relatively even with, to broader than, hips. Buttocks relatively flat-to-rounded.

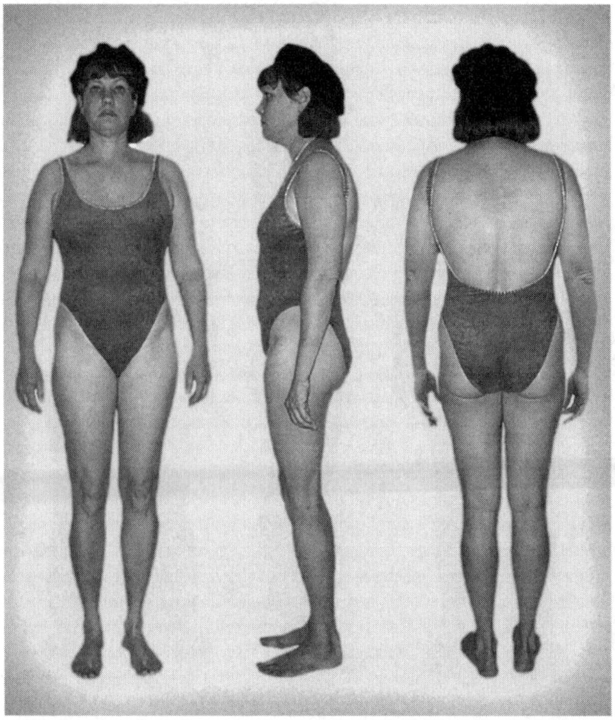

Typically smaller lower body with narrow hips. May wear two sizes of clothes, with top larger than bottom. Height generally average, although can range from petite to very tall.

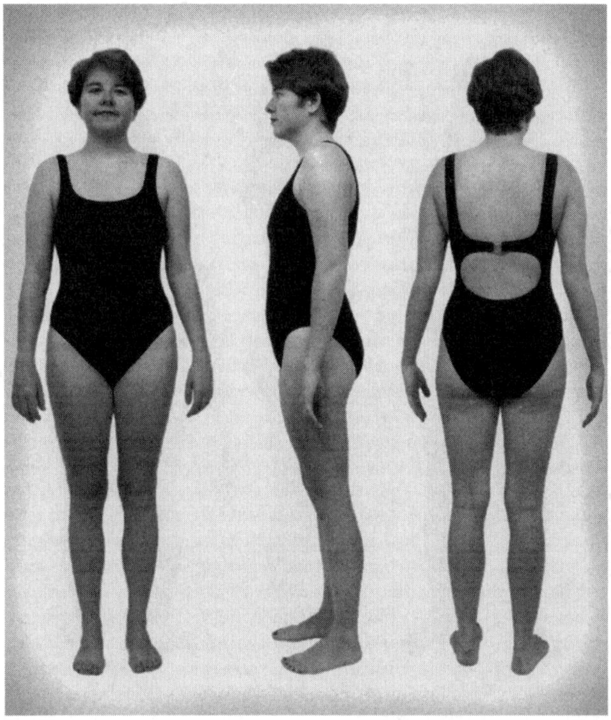

Exceptionally loyal and family oriented. Good teachers. Tend to put things together so they flow. Low back curvature straight-to-average.

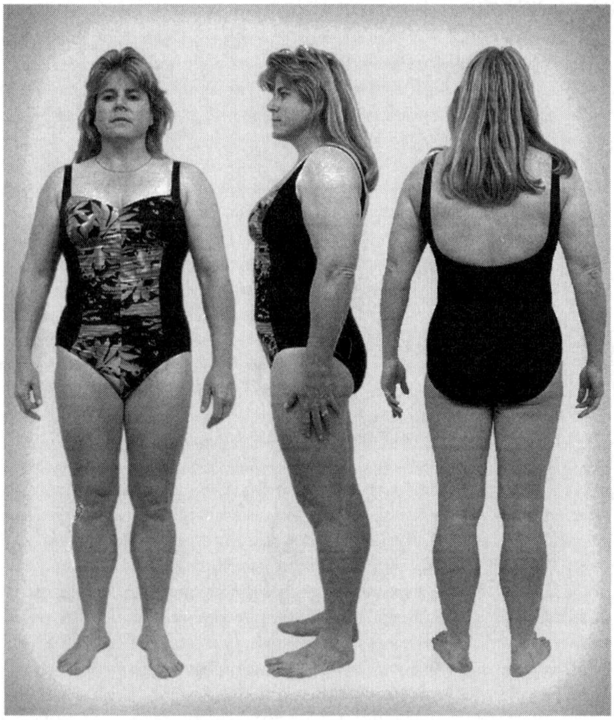

Strong, solid body with sturdy appearance. Dense, solid musculature, often with well-defined muscular calves. Average-to-thick or wide hands and feet.

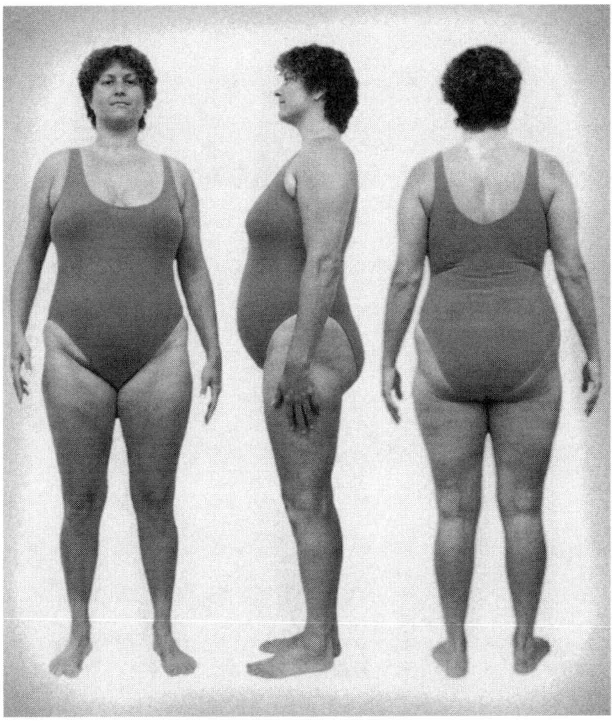

*Initial weight gain in lower-to-entire abdomen; waist; upper, middle and entire back; upper hips; and upper inner thighs, with slight gain in entire upper 2/3rds of thighs.

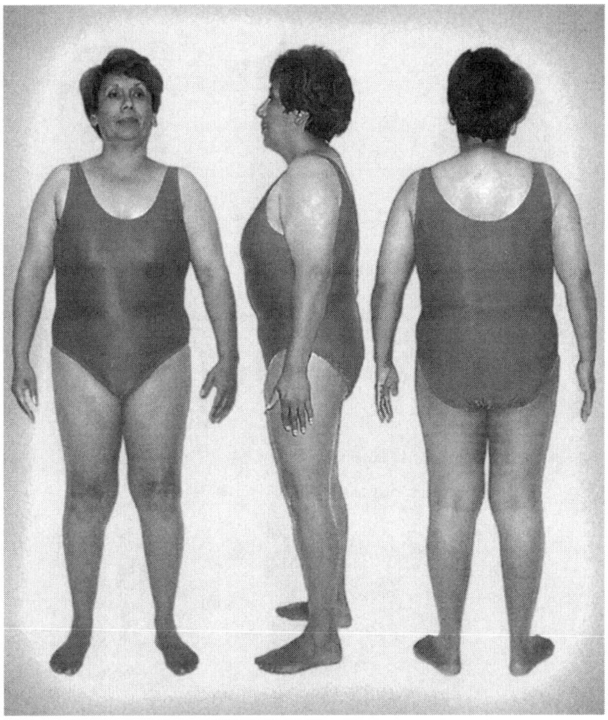

Alternative weight-gain pattern: upper abdomen, waist, entire back, upper hips, upper inner thighs, upper arms, and face.

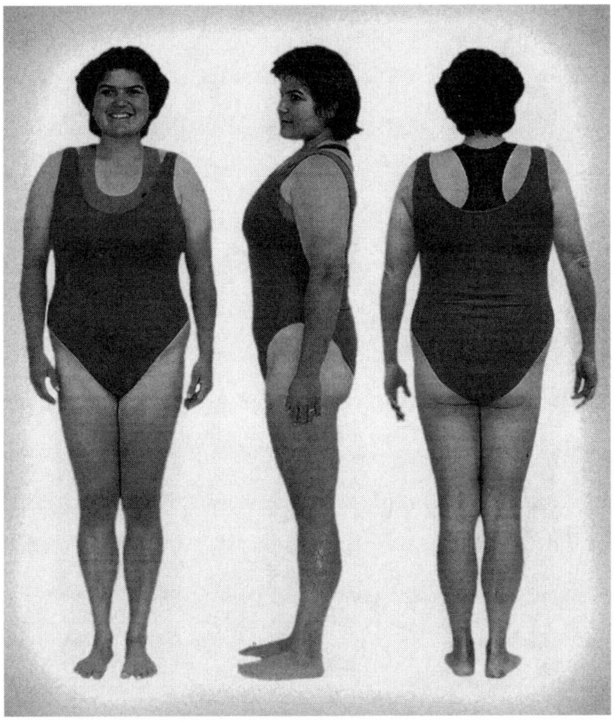

Bone structure small-to-large. Breasts average-to-large. Straight-to-defined waist. Average- to short-waisted.

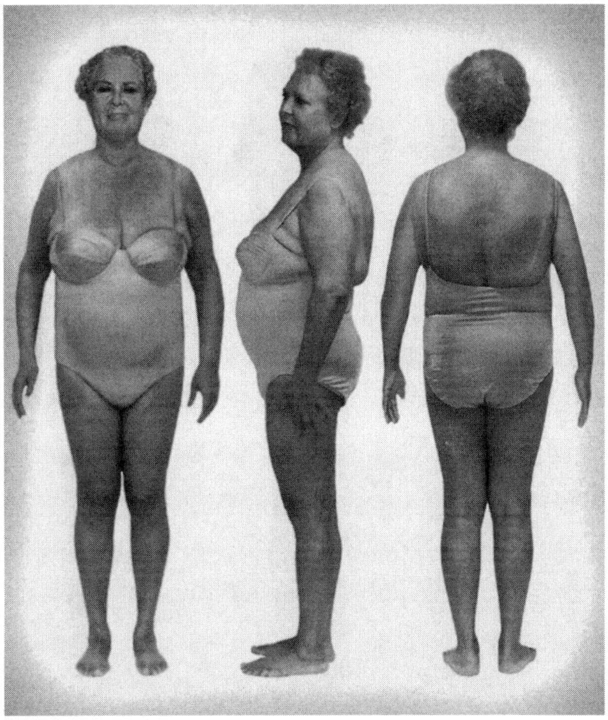

Secondary weight gain as solid thickening in upper abdomen, upper and entire back, upper arms, entire inner and outer thighs, under chin, and breasts.

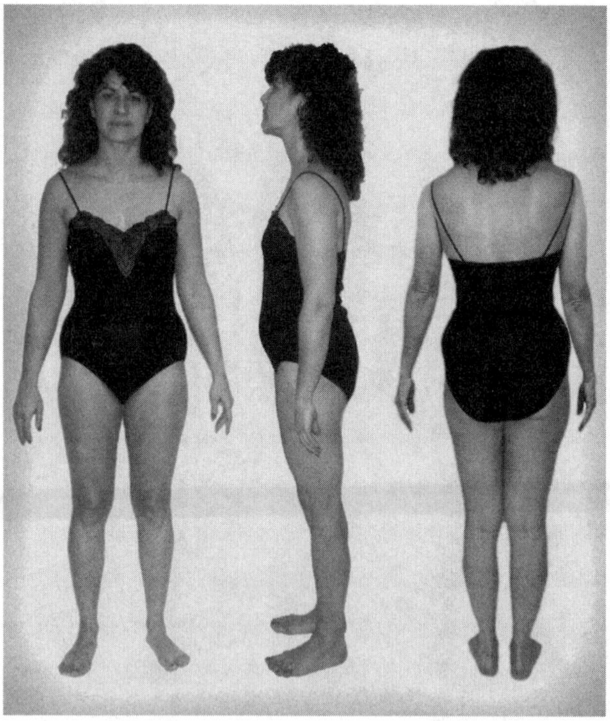

*Mild-mannered, even-tempered, sensitive, and caring with strong nurturing qualities. Naturally creative and artistic with a practical flair.

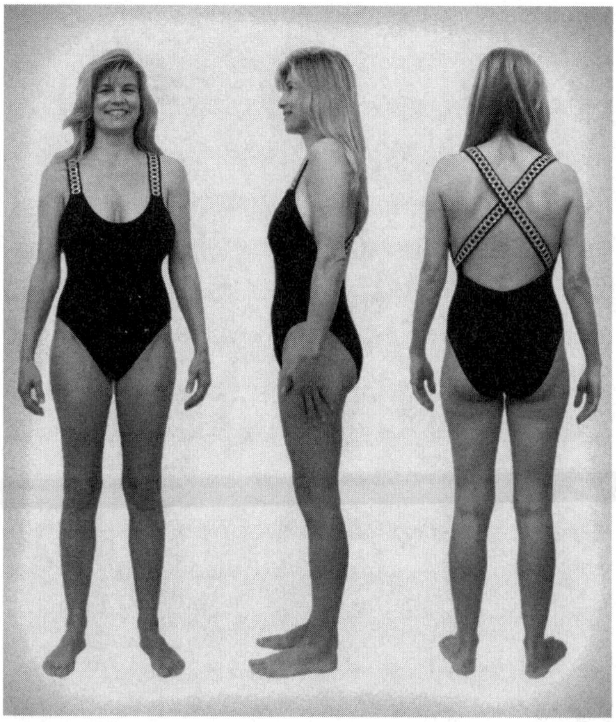

Emotionally expressive, they are known for making the most of the moment. Generally excel in music, dance, or some creative physical expression.

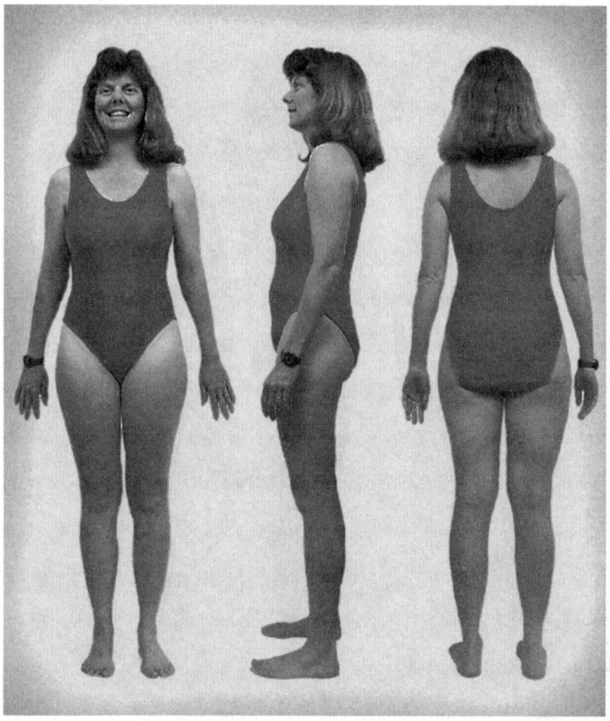

Low back curvature straight-to-average. Buttocks relatively flat-to-rounded. Height petite-to-average. Shoulders relatively even with hips.

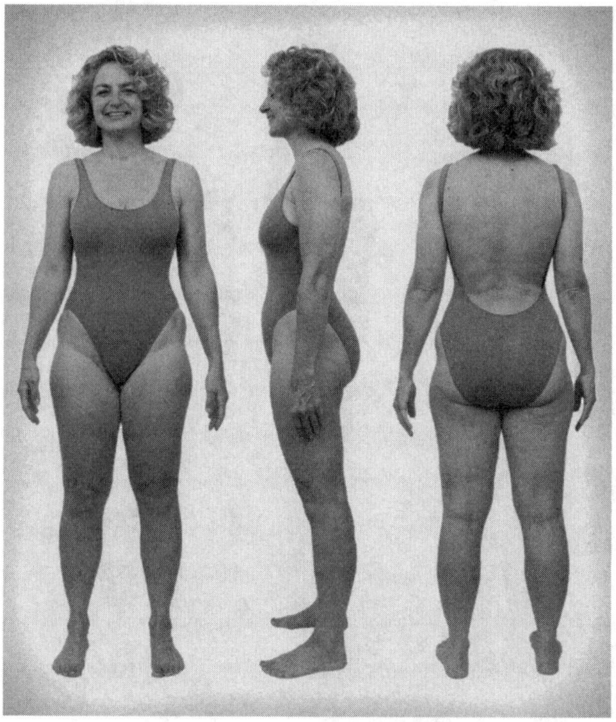

Average, elongated musculature. Bone structure small-to-medium. Hands average-to-slender, long, or delicate. Feet may be narrow.

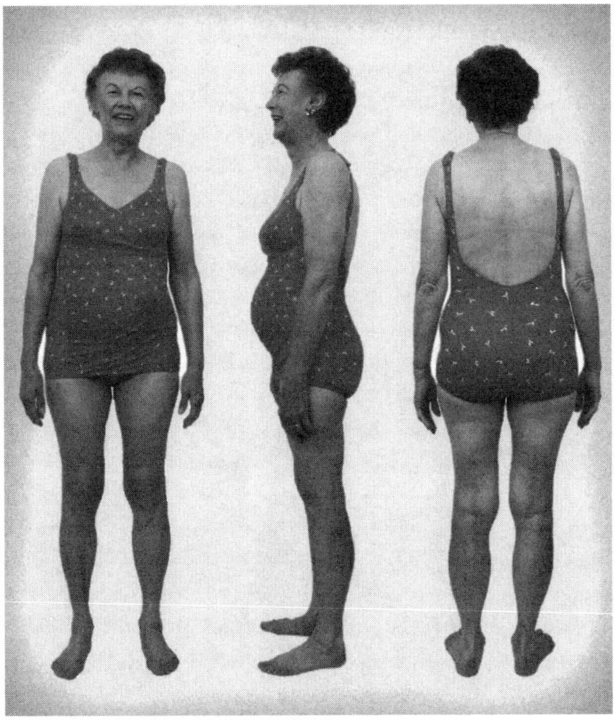

*Initial weight gain in lower abdomen, waist, and upper hips, with slight to no weight gain in thighs.

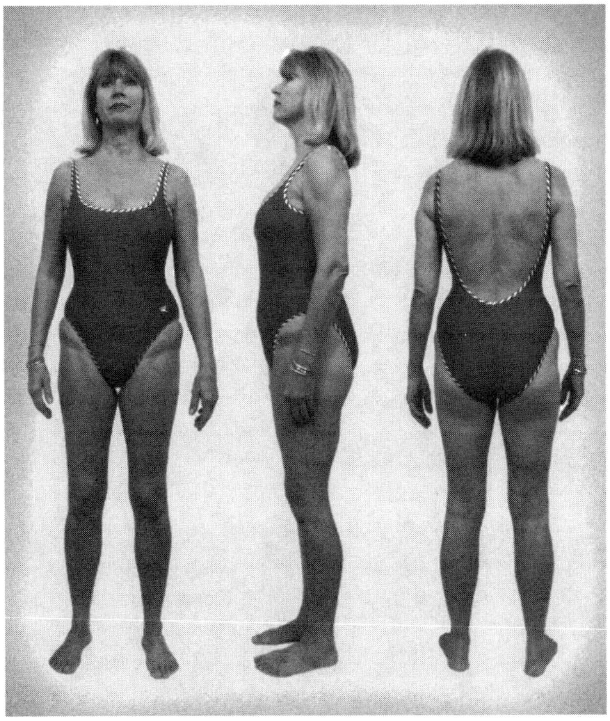

High cheek bones with square or V-shaped jaw, often with prominent chin or average oval or rectangular face.

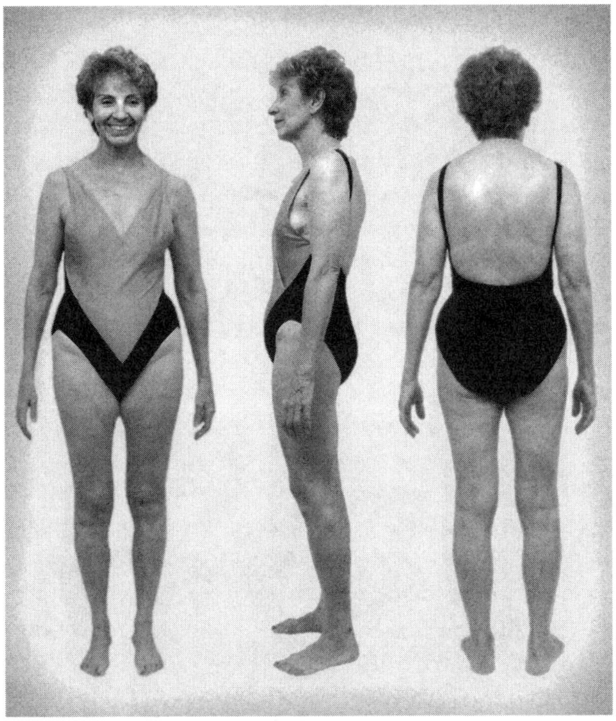

Body may be a full size smaller above the waist than below. Breasts small-to-average. Average torso with defined waist.

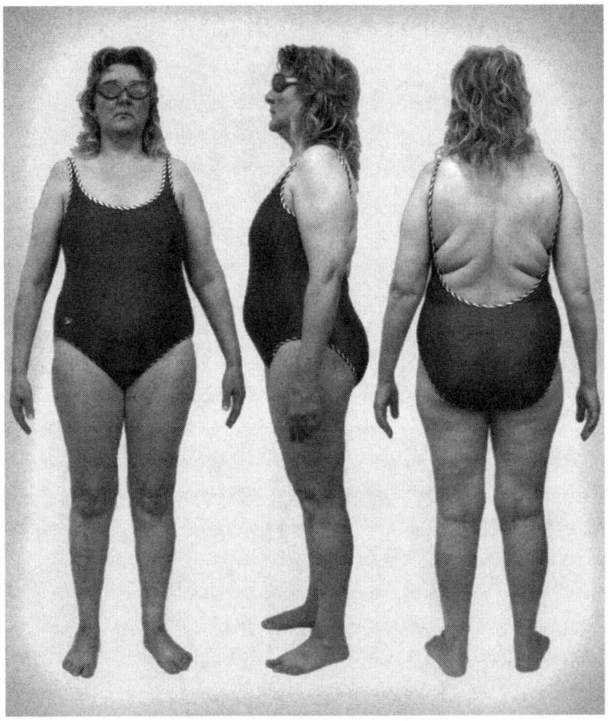

Secondary weight gain primarily in entire abdomen, middle-to-entire back, upper arms, possibly breasts, buttocks, face, under chin, and minimal gain in entire upper 2/3rds of thighs.

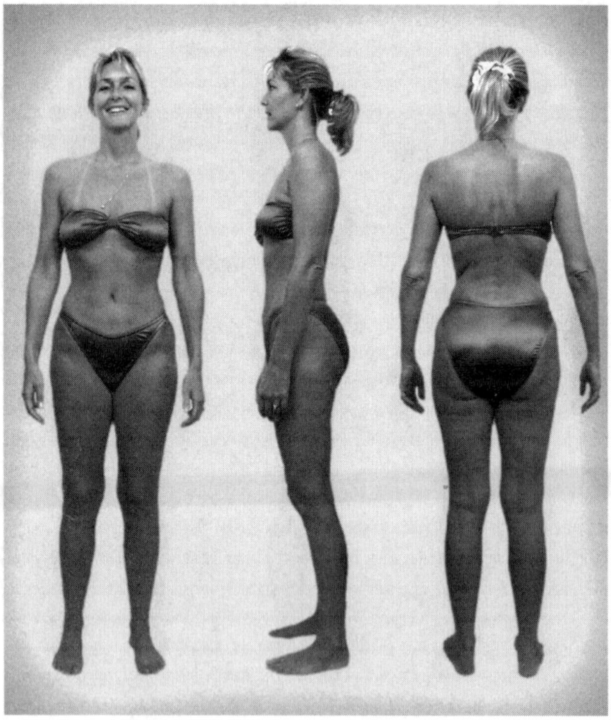

Physical exercise is essential. Usually athletic, with broad shoulders and well-proportioned, attractive face and body.

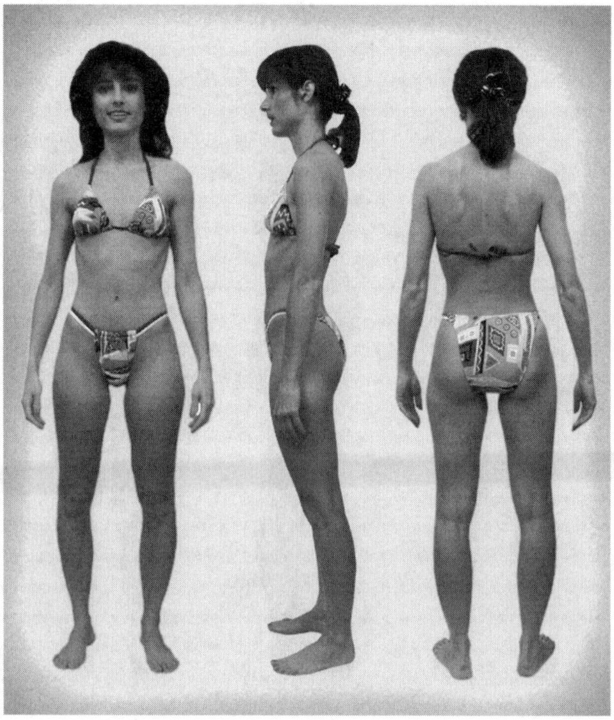

Height very petite to average. Low back curvature average-to-swayed. Buttocks rounded-to-prominent.

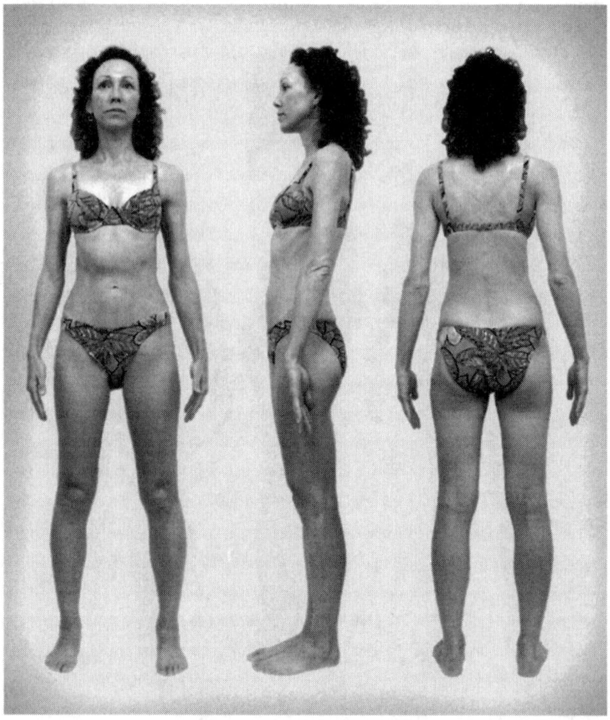

Head rectangular and proportionate to body, but may have long appearance. May have difficulty gaining or maintaining weight.

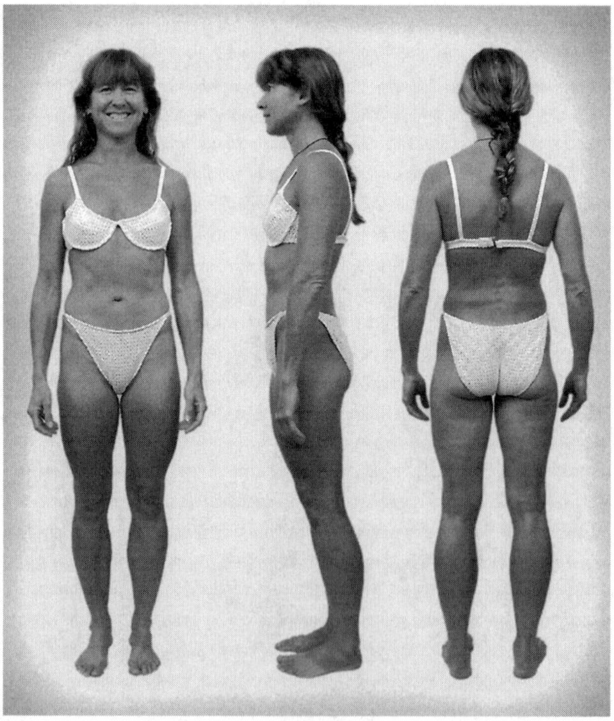

Generally playful, bright and quick-witted. They thrive on excitement. Strong abdominal muscles and thighs. Average, elongated musculature.

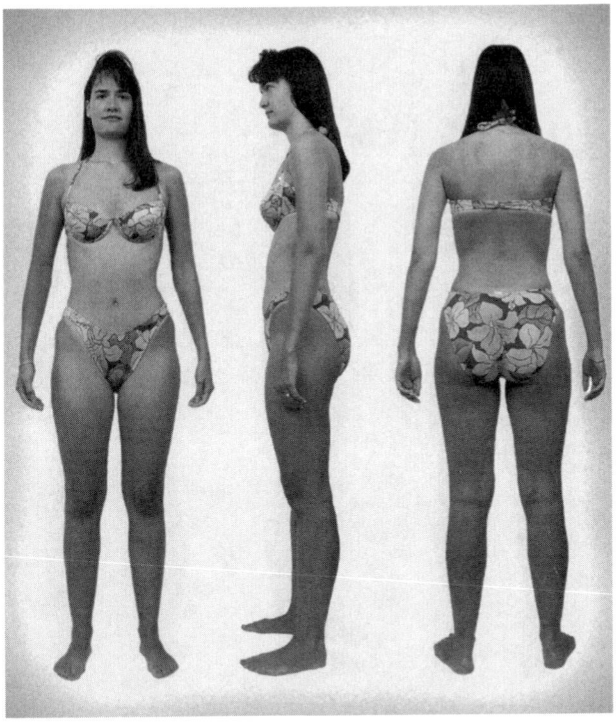

*Initial weight gain in entire upper 2/3rds of thighs including upper inner thighs, buttocks, and possibly upper hips.

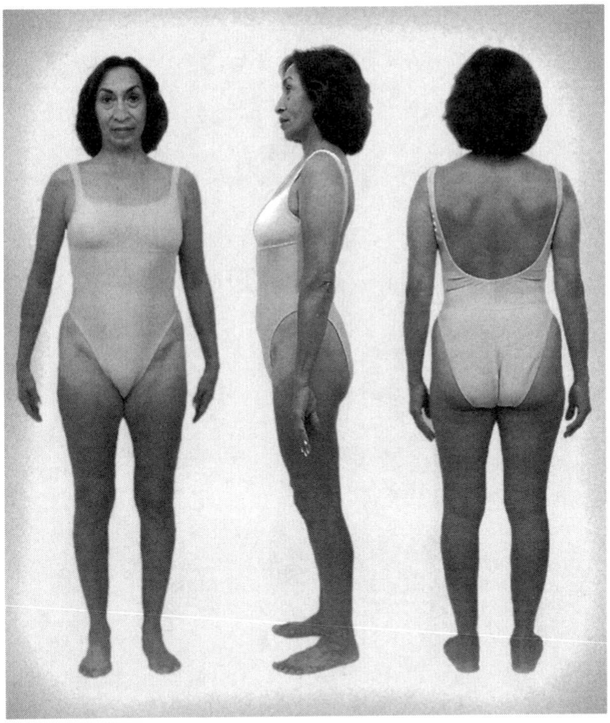

Shoulders relatively even with, to broader than, hips. Waist straight-to-defined. Average to long-waisted. Bone structure small-to-medium. Breasts small-to-average.

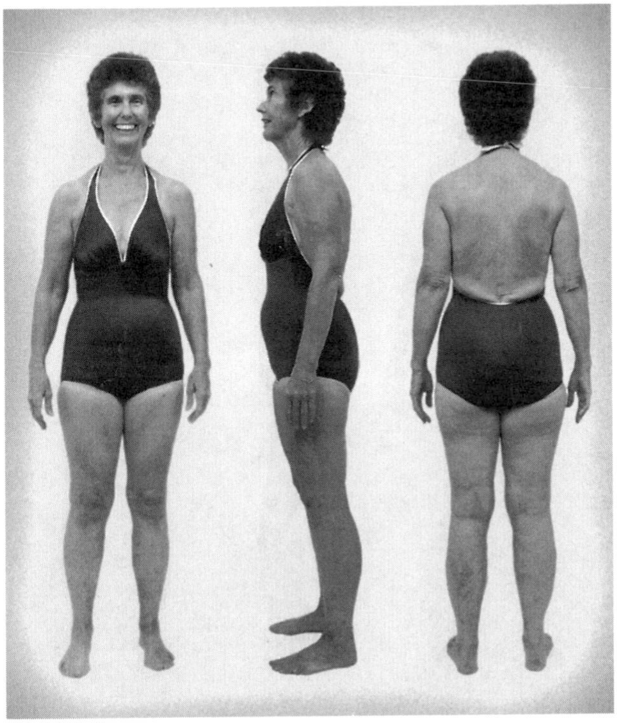

*To prevent stagnation, require regular physical or mental stimulation. Change, variety and movement keep them happy.

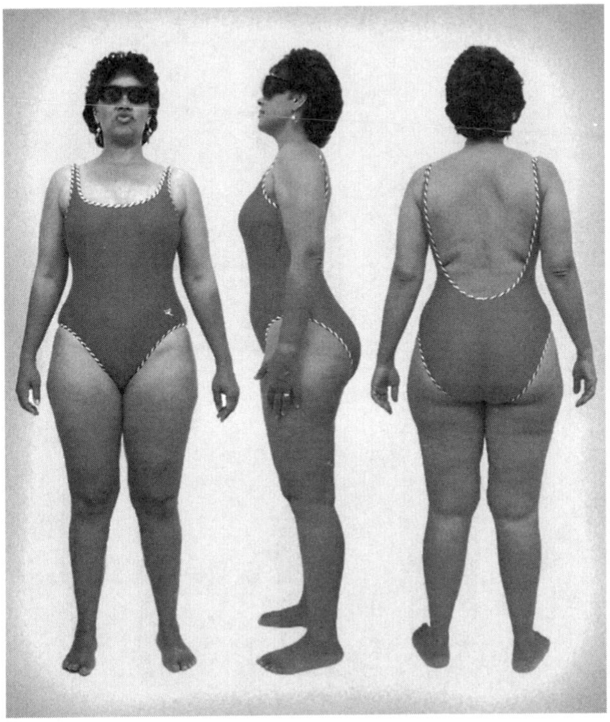

Secondary weight gain in lower abdomen, waist, hips (predominantly upper or lower), thighs extending to knees, middle back, and upper arms.

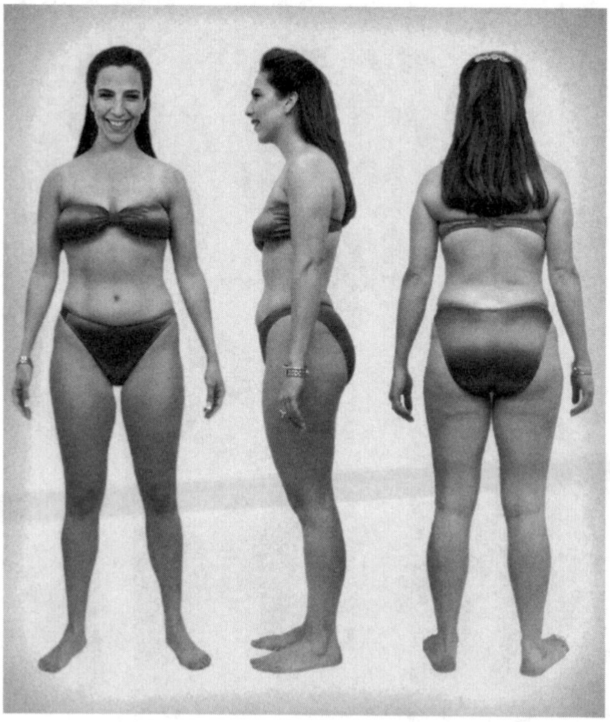

*Typically low forehead with heavy eyebrows, although can have high forehead. Character is generally steady, stable, and persistent.

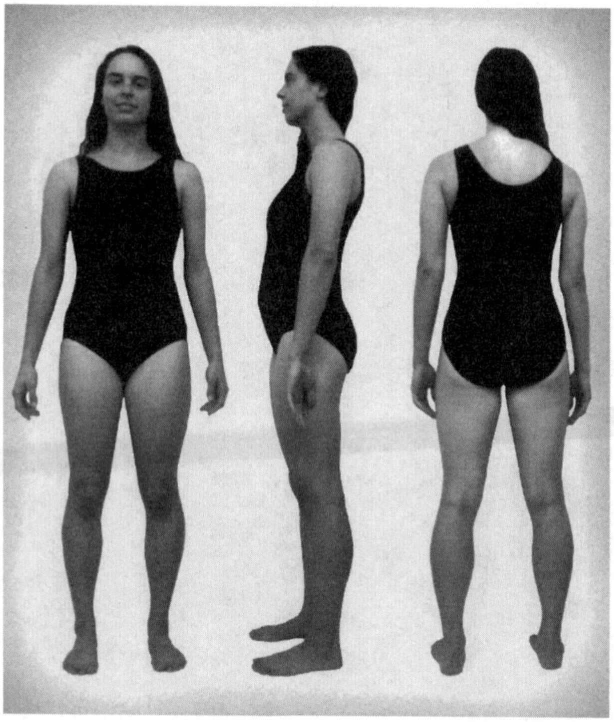

Average, elongated musculature. Easily build muscle mass with regular exercise, but require sustained exercise to lose weight.

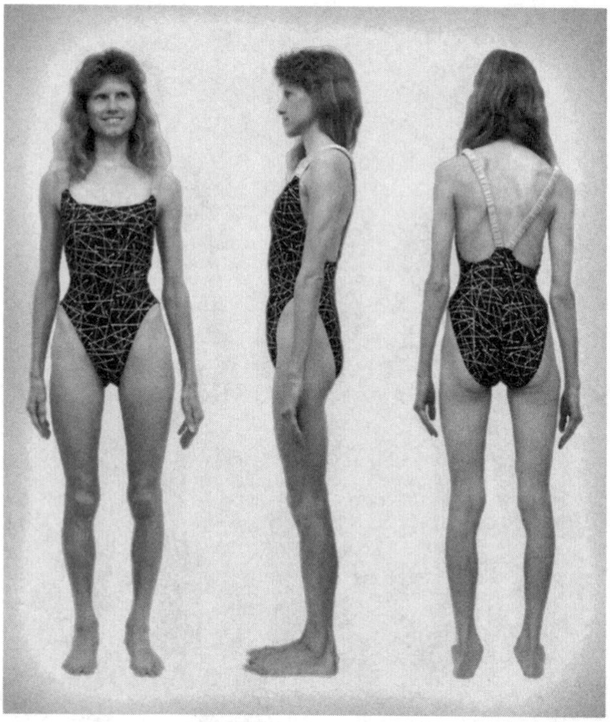

Low back curvature average. Buttocks relatively flat-to-rounded. Waist straight-to-defined. Average to long-waisted.

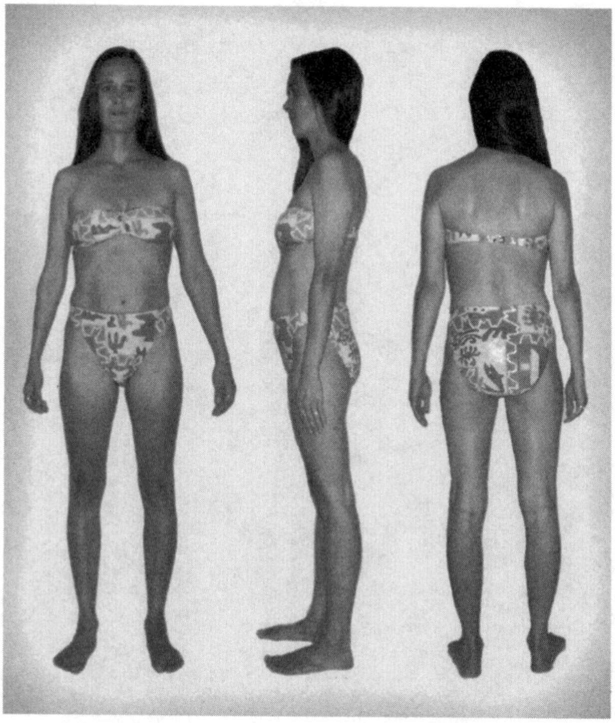

Face average oval, rectangular, or heart-shaped. Hair average-to-thick. Feet average-to-wide.

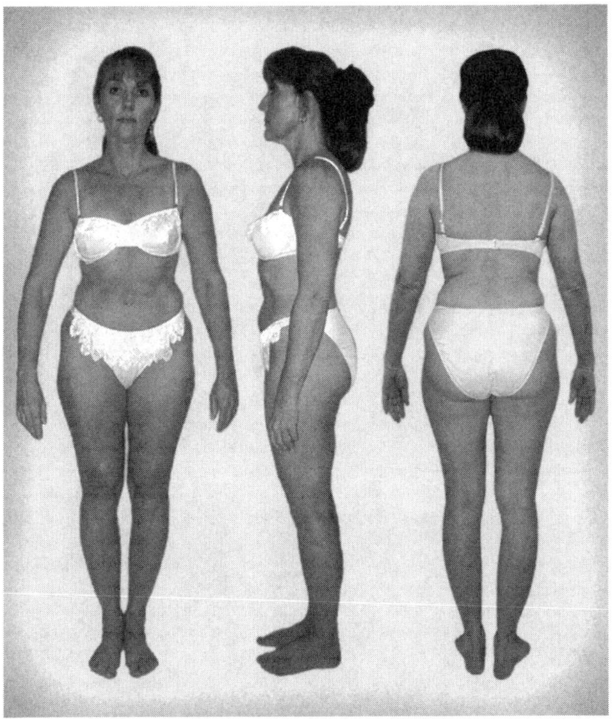

*Initial weight gain in lower abdomen, entire upper 2/3rds of thighs including upper inner thighs, upper hips, waist, and middle back.

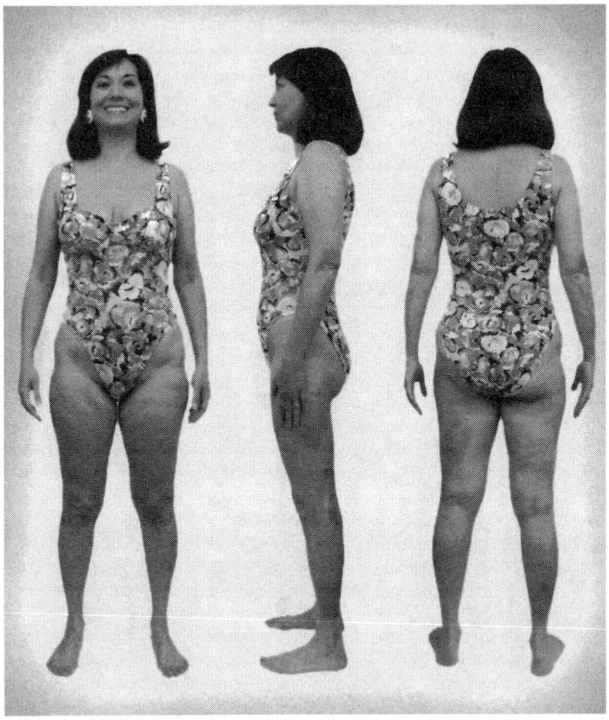

Shoulders relatively even with hips. Breasts average. Bone structure small-to-medium. Height average-to-tall.

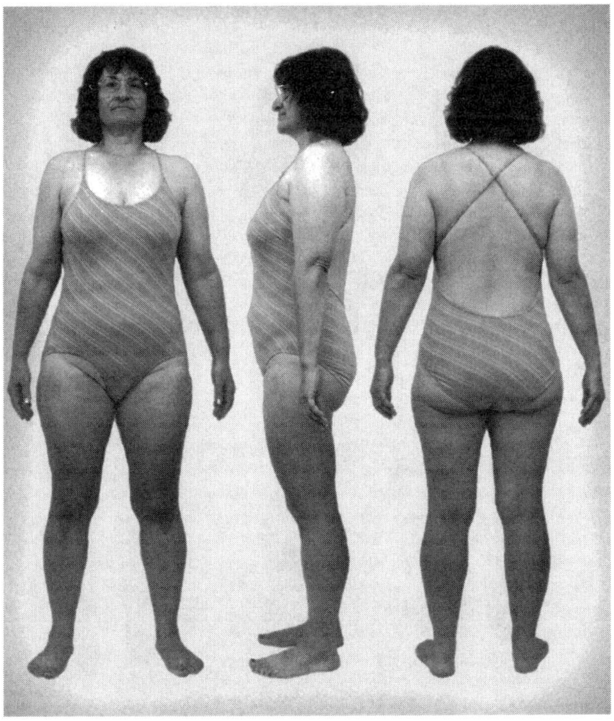

Hands may be large and broad, with rectangular or square palms and short, thick fingers, which sometimes have knobby knuckles.

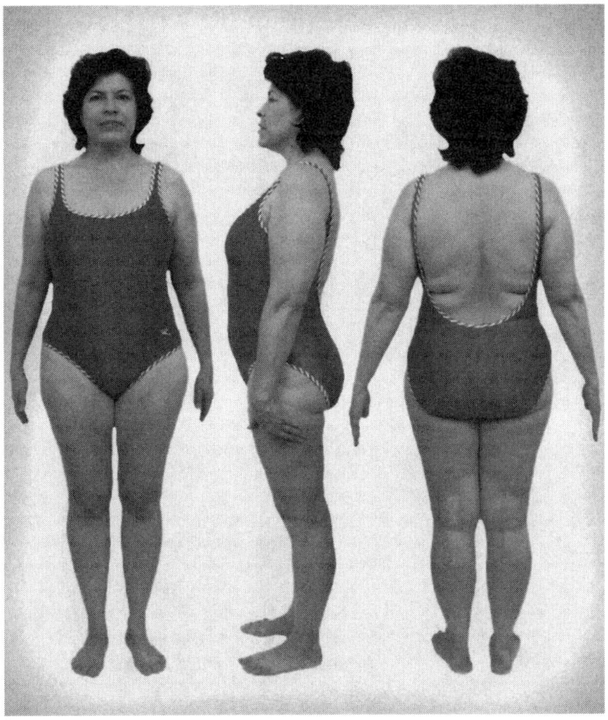

Secondary weight gain in waist, entire abdomen and back, buttocks, upper arms, and face. Weight loss occurs first in face, then lower back.

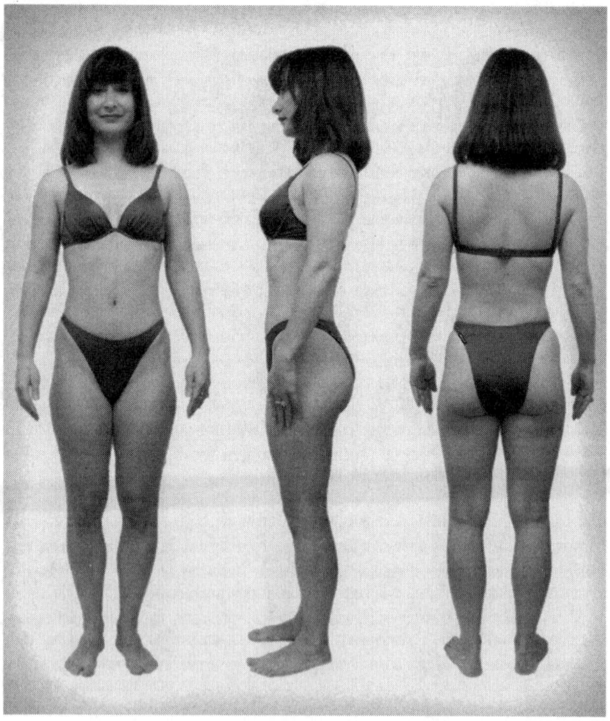

*Integrated, strong, solid body. Generally, quite verbal with good integration and common sense. Enjoy introducing and connecting people.

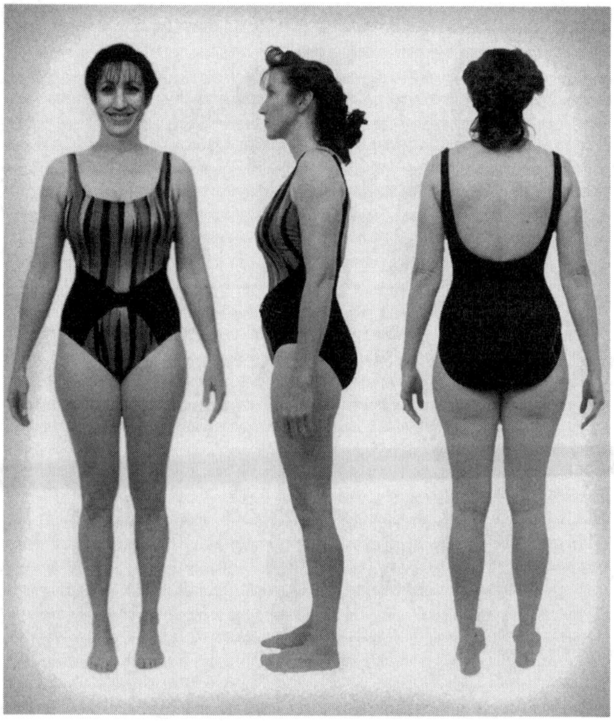

*High energy, excellent stamina and determination. Practical and efficient. Known for accomplishing what they set out to do.

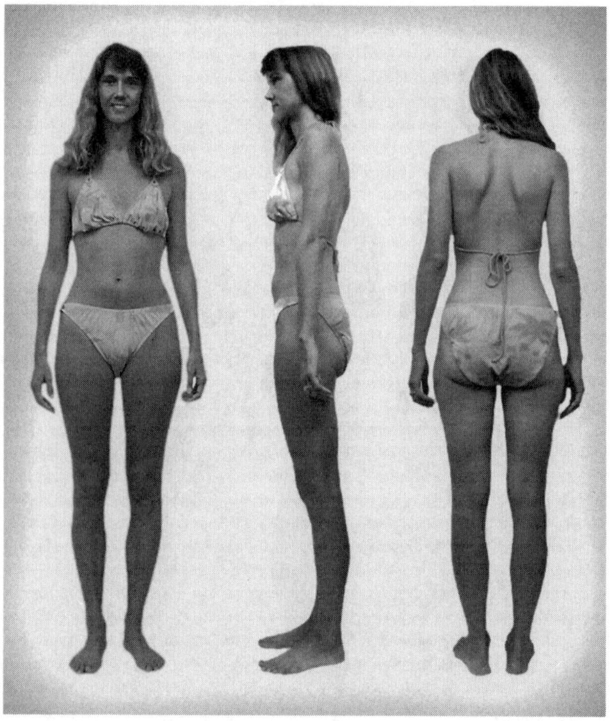

May have difficulty gaining weight. Buttocks relatively flat-to-rounded. Low back curvature average-to-swayed.

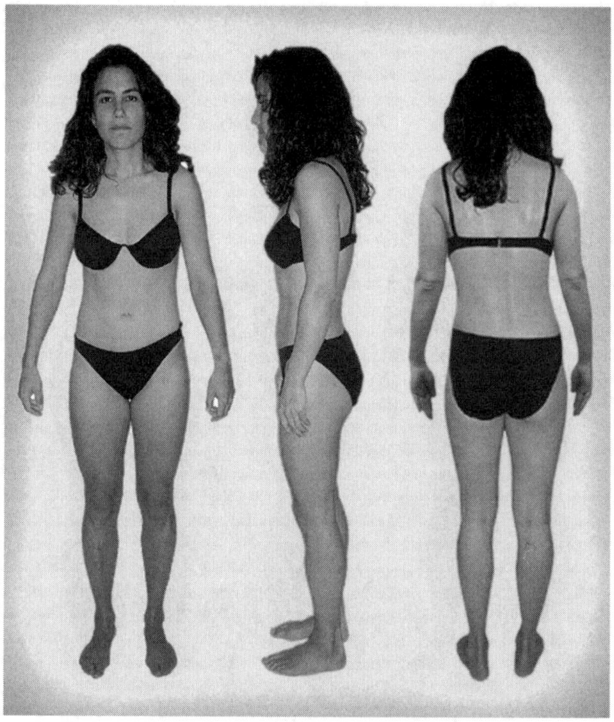

High forehead. Average-to-large head with long, oval, or rectangular face, which often comes forward at chin. Frequently have square or firm jaw, indicative of strong determination.

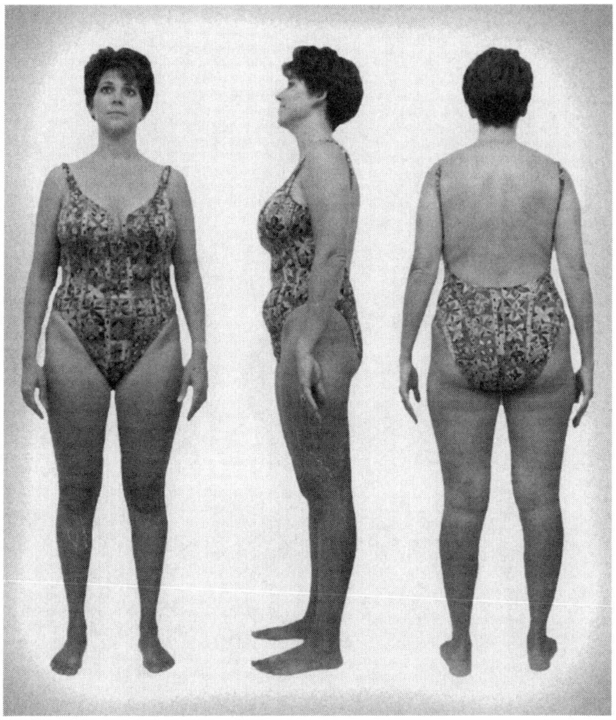

*Initial weight gain in lower abdomen, entire upper 2/3rds of thighs including upper inner thighs, upper hips, middle back and waist, or all over.

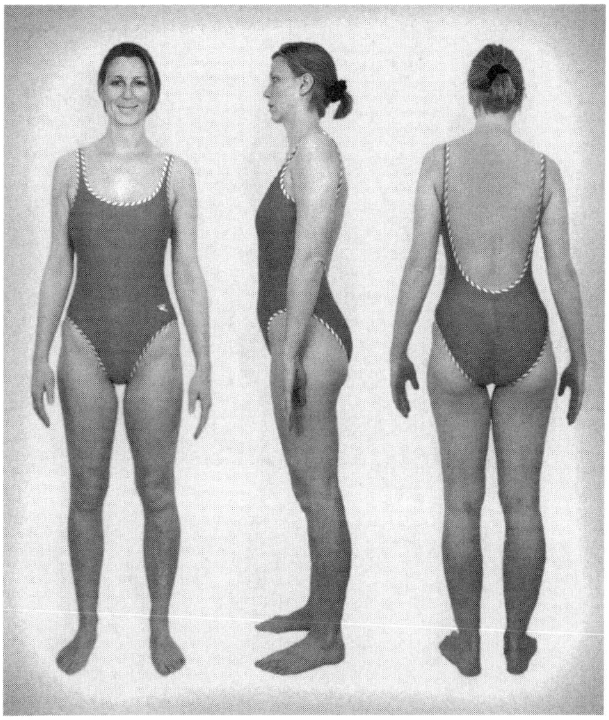

Height petite to very tall. Bone structure small-to-medium. Breasts average. Waist straight-to-defined. Average to long-waisted.

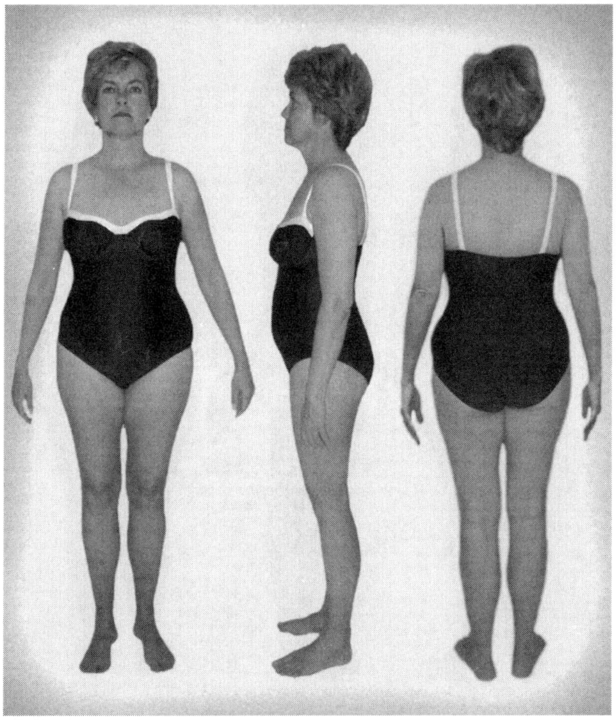

Shoulders relatively even with hips. Average, elongated musculature. Capable of putting on and losing large amounts of weight.

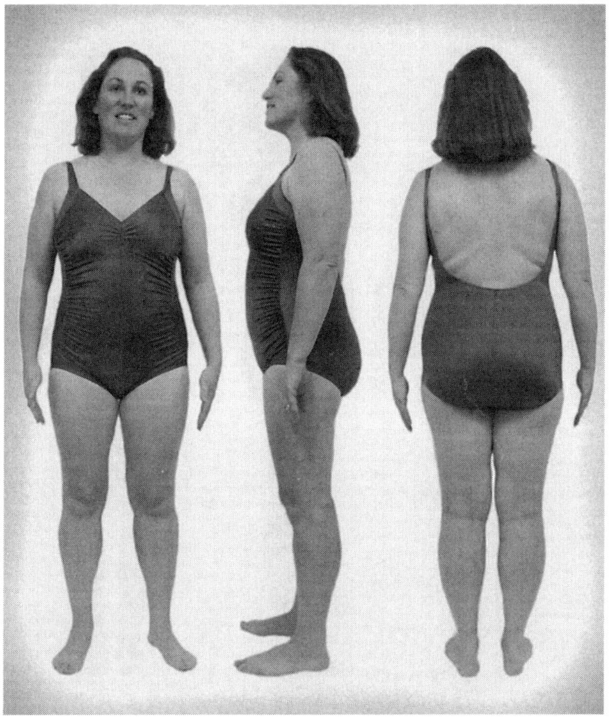

Secondary weight gain extending into entire abdomen, entire back, upper arms, buttocks, thighs, breasts, face, and under chin.

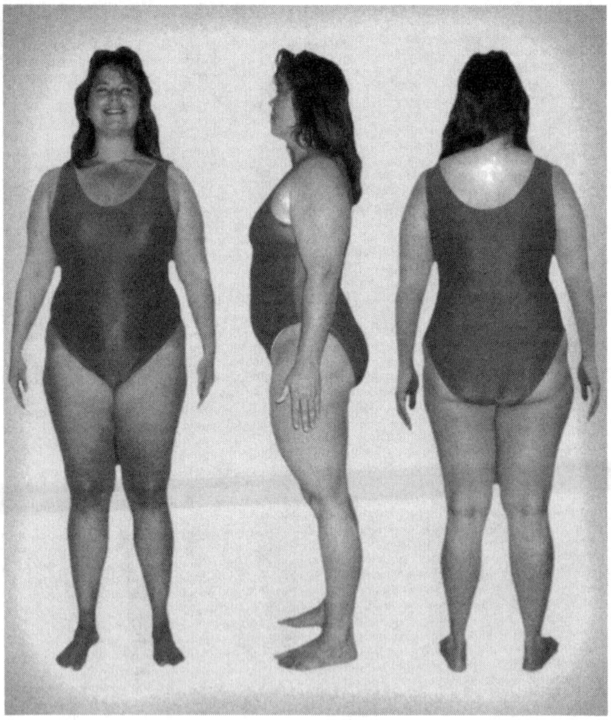

*Tendency toward "rut" eating – eating same food for 3 to 4 days in a row. Can put on large amounts of weight and have difficulty losing and keeping it off.

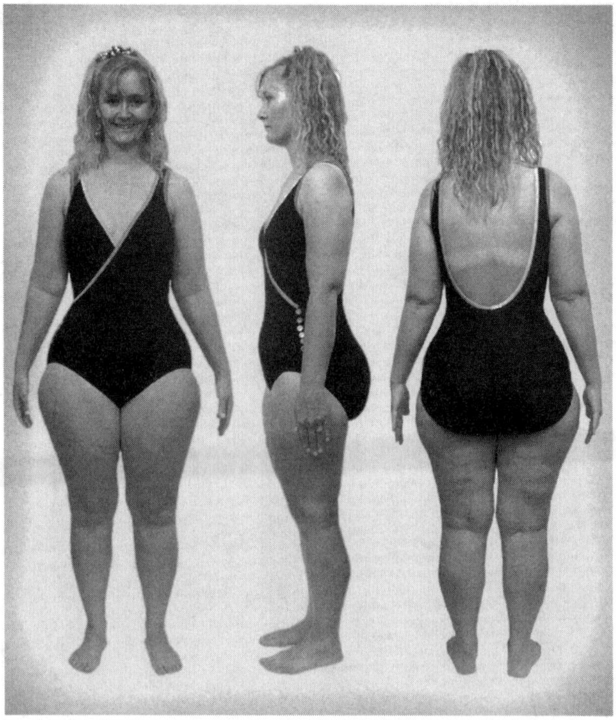

*Small hands and often small feet, with little weight gain from knees to feet or elbows to hands. Waist defined to well-defined. Hair frequently thin or fine.

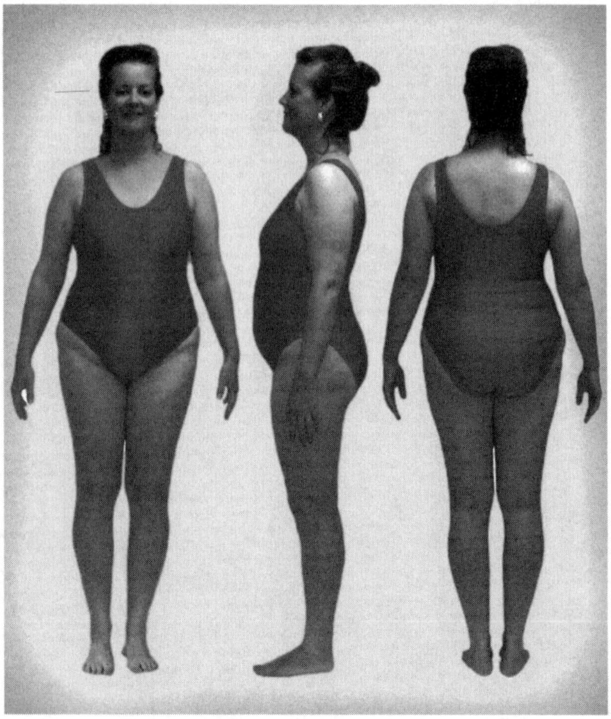

Long rectangular, or average-to-long oval-shaped face. Shoulders narrower than, to relatively even with, hips. Average, elongated musculature. Average to short-waisted.

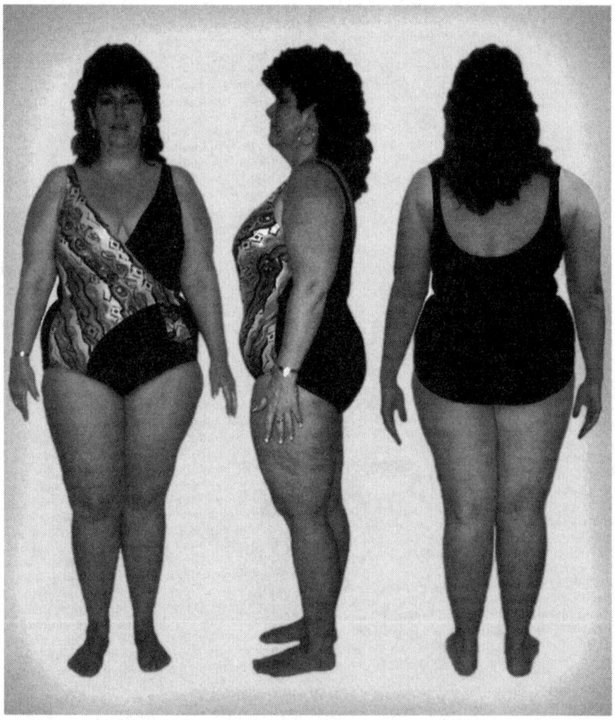

*Predominantly rounded in appearance, particularly noticeable from behind – in upper hips and buttocks. Height generally petite-to-average. Known for bringing joy.

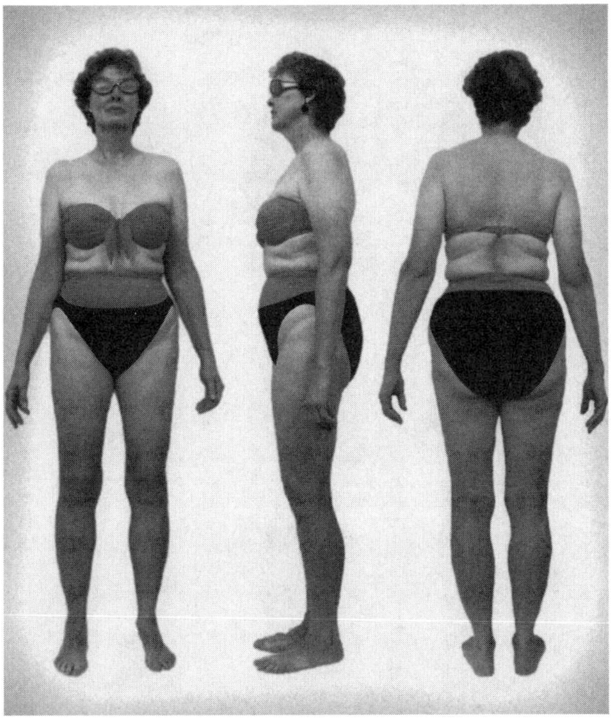

*Intial weight gain in lower abdomen, upper hips, upper inner thighs, inner knees, middle back, and waist in firm rolls. Excess fat initially firm, not flabby.

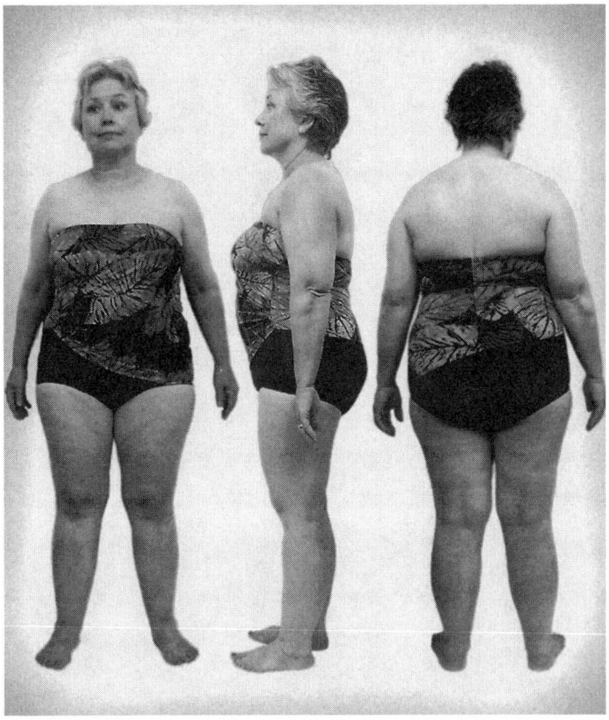

Secondary weight gain in entire abdomen, upper hips, entire back, upper arms, breasts, entire inner and possibly entire thighs extending to knees, buttocks, face, and under chin.

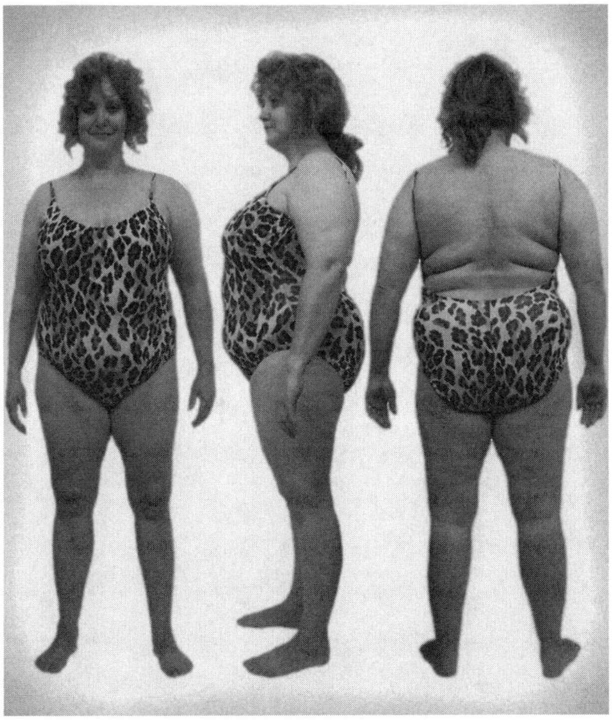

Bone structure small-to-medium. Breasts average-to-large. Low back curvature straight-to-average. Buttocks rounded, with rounded upper hips.

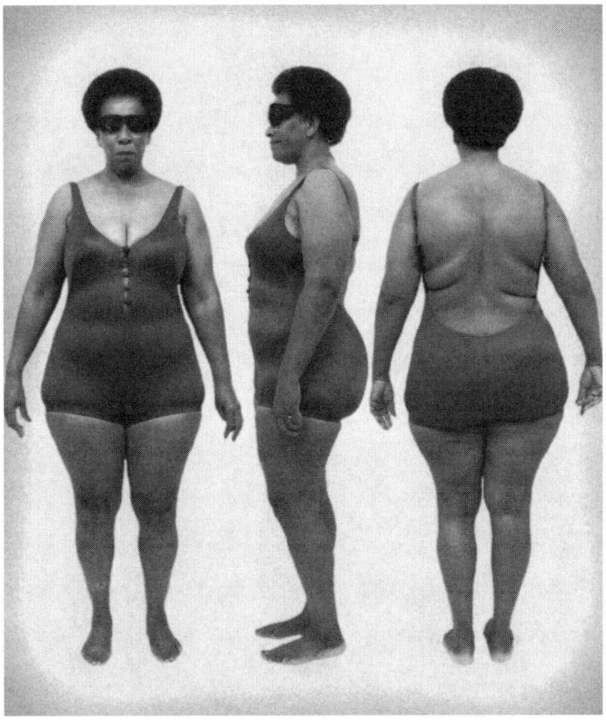

Alternative secondary weight-gain pattern: lower buttocks, lower hips, and entire upper 2/3rds of thighs, with cellulite predominantly on buttocks and thighs.

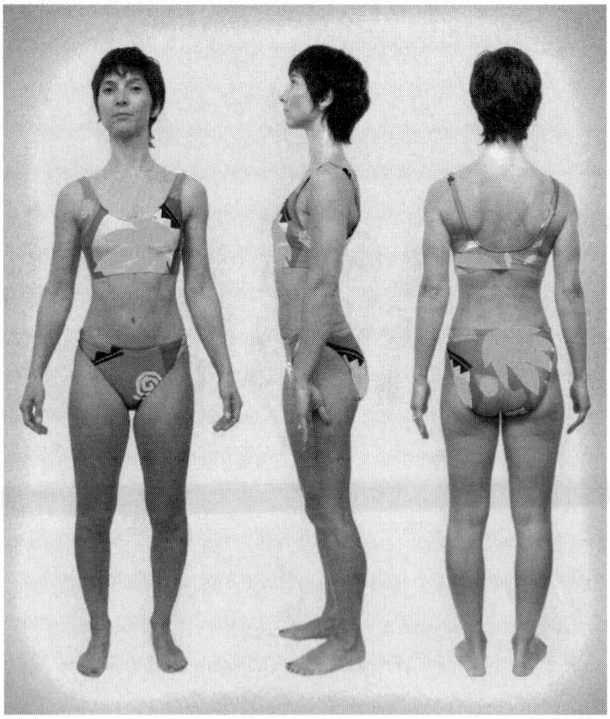

*Small head in relationship to body. Have physical need for sunlight. Prone to depression, mild to severe, when sunlight is unavailable. Known for talking to collect or focus thoughts.

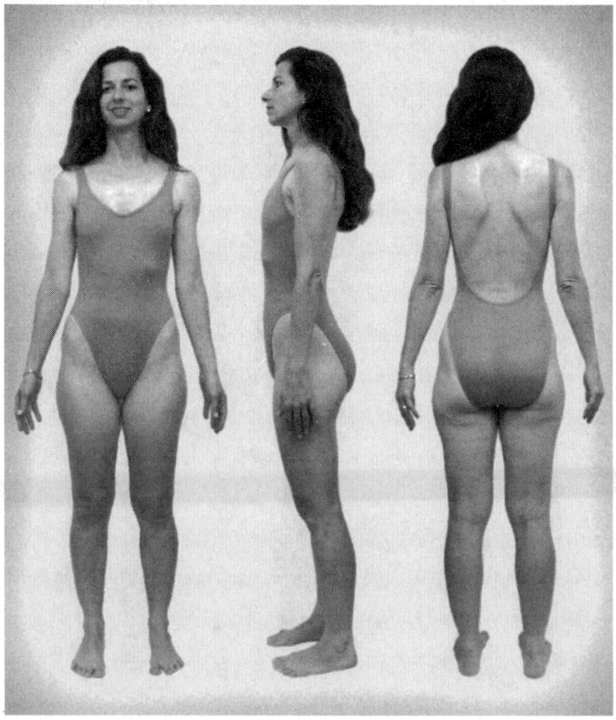

Buttocks relatively flat-to-prominent. Low back curvature average-to-swayed. Average, elongated musculature. Height ranges from petite-to-tall.

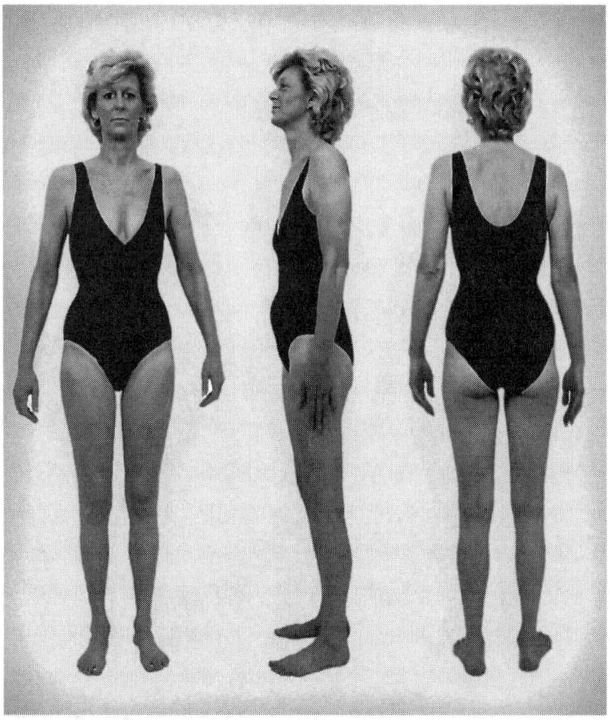

May be chronically underweight or have difficulty maintaining weight. Average-to-long oval or rectangular face with thin lips.

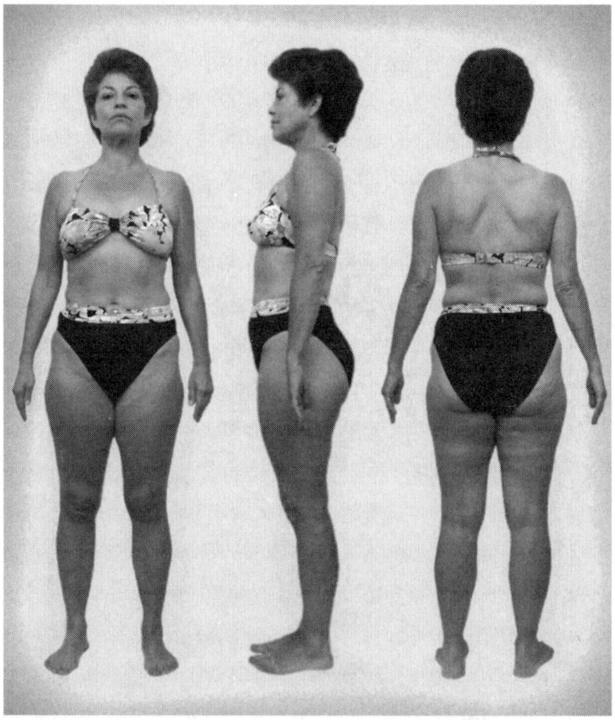

Long-waisted with small breasts or short-waisted with large breasts. Defined waist. Bone structure small-to-medium.

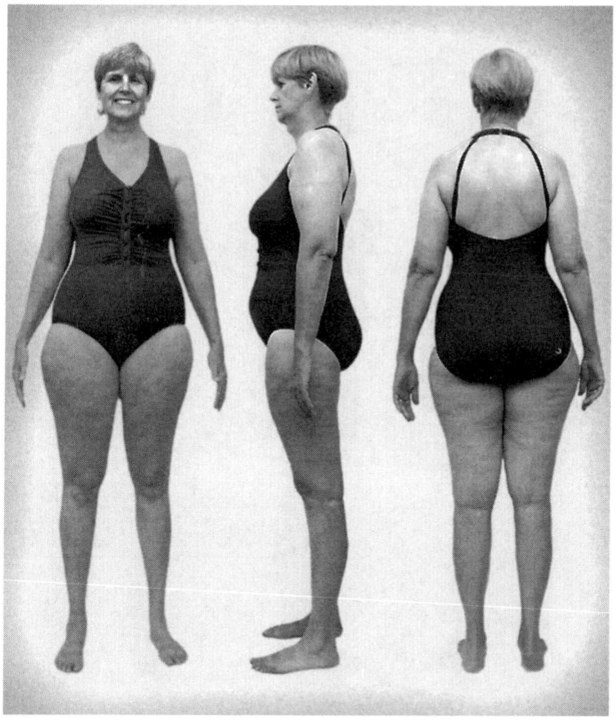

*Initial weight gain in lower abdomen, buttocks, waist, upper hips, and entire upper 2/3rds of thighs including upper inner thighs.

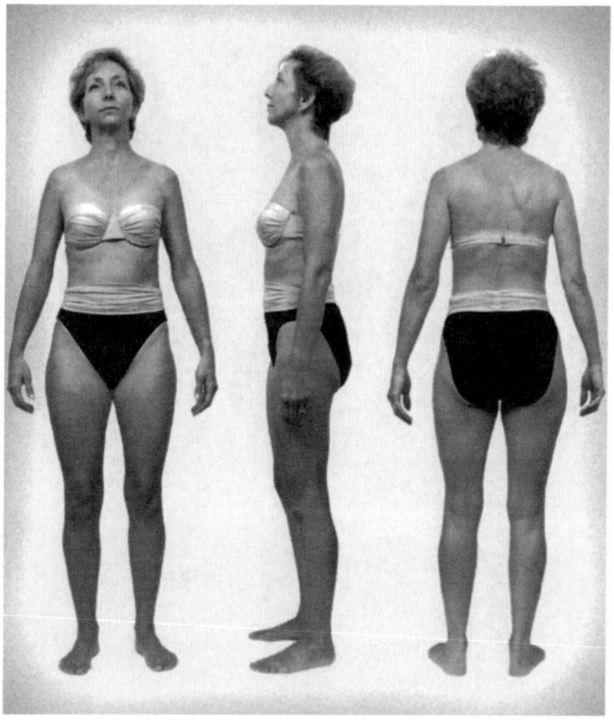

Alternative weight-gain pattern: lower hips, buttocks, and entire thighs. Cellulite below buttocks, possibly since childhood.

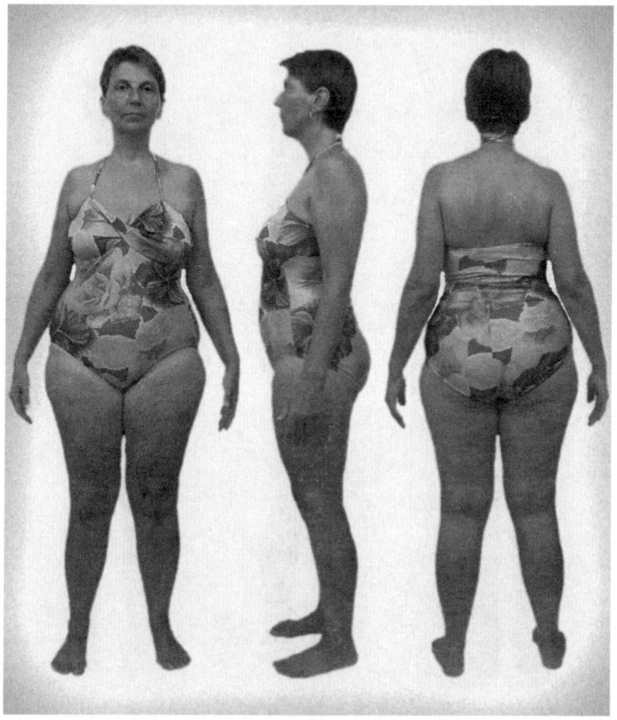

Upper body may be smaller than lower body. Shoulders narrower than, to relatively even with, hips. Alternative secondary weight gain in upper and lower hips.

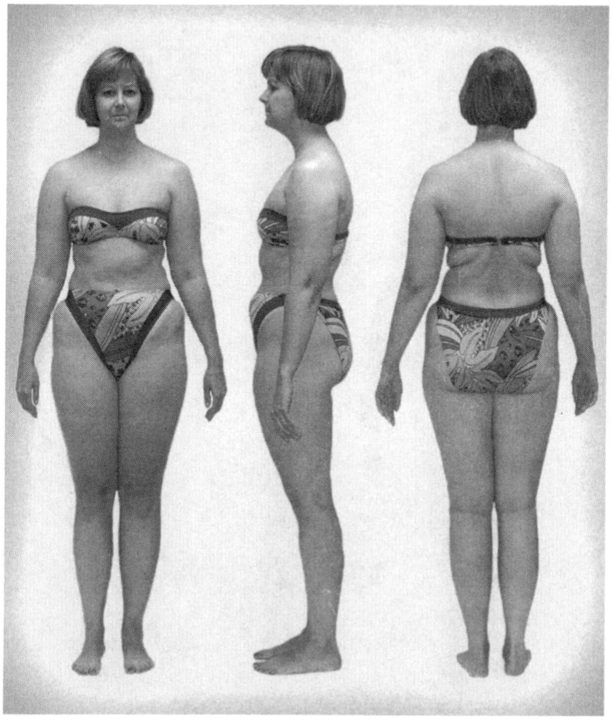

Secondary weight gain on upper arms, entire back, breasts, and eventually extending into entire abdomen, face, and under chin.

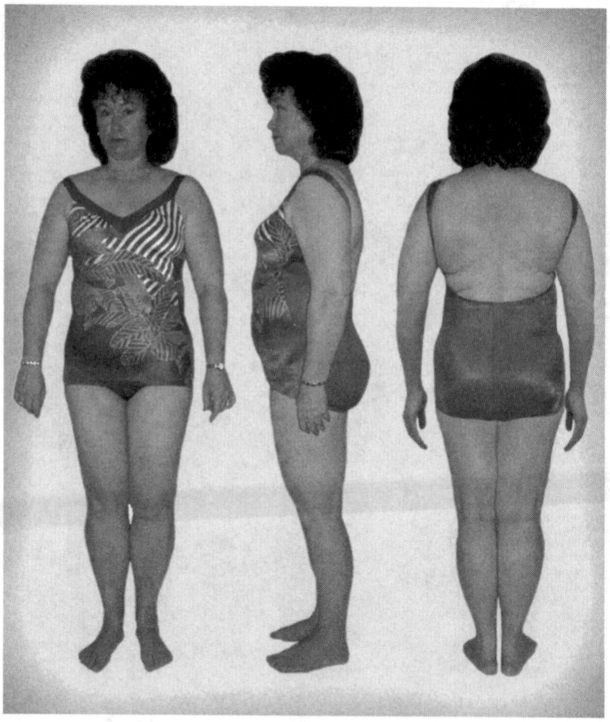

*Large head in proportion to rest of body and generally positioned in front of shoulders. Soft, child-like, underdeveloped look, often with rounded stomach.

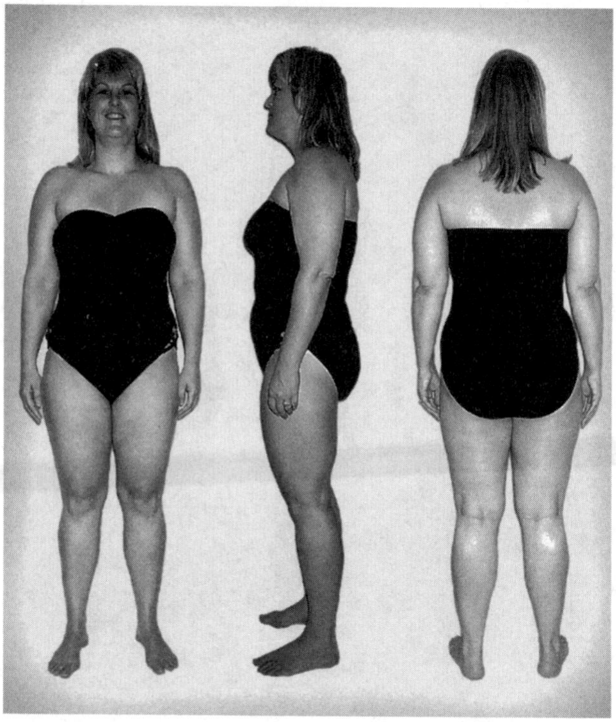

Weight gain all over (like baby fat), especially around knees, which tend to be pudgy. Generally retain baby fat over entire body throughout life. Tend to make life fun.

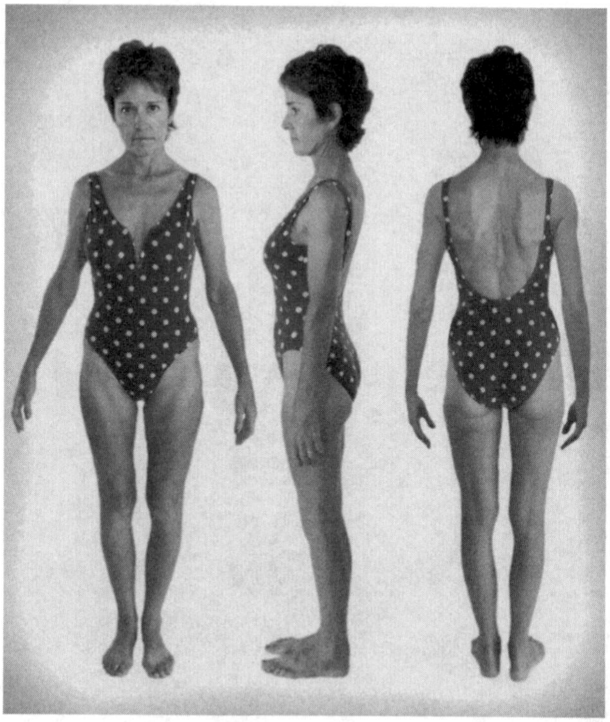

Often high forehead that is wider than cheekbones by 1/4 inch or more. Layer of softness covering muscles, or average, elongated musculature. Face round, oval or long oval.

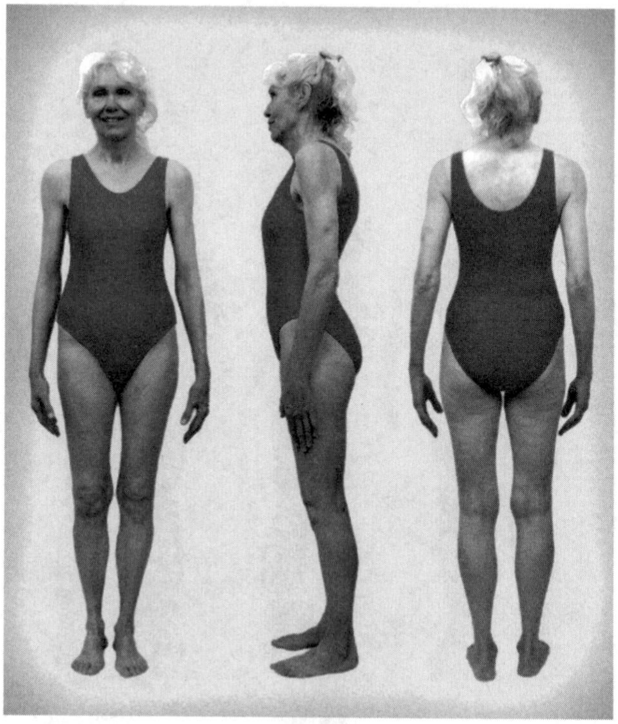

Occasionally have difficulty gaining weight. Height petite-to-tall. Bone structure medium-to-large. Prefer mental to physical activity. Breasts average-to-large.

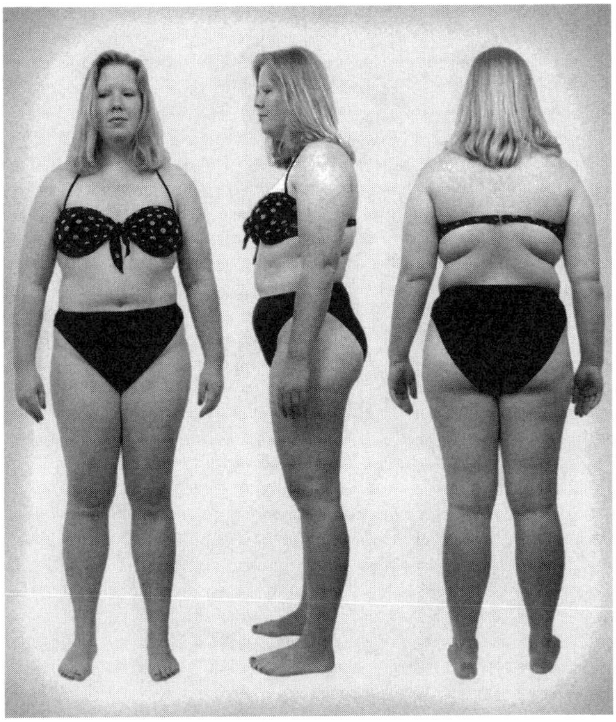

*Initial weight gain in lower abdomen, waist, upper hips, upper inner thighs or entire thighs, and inner knees. Generally gain evenly in soft rolls over entire body, including hands and feet.

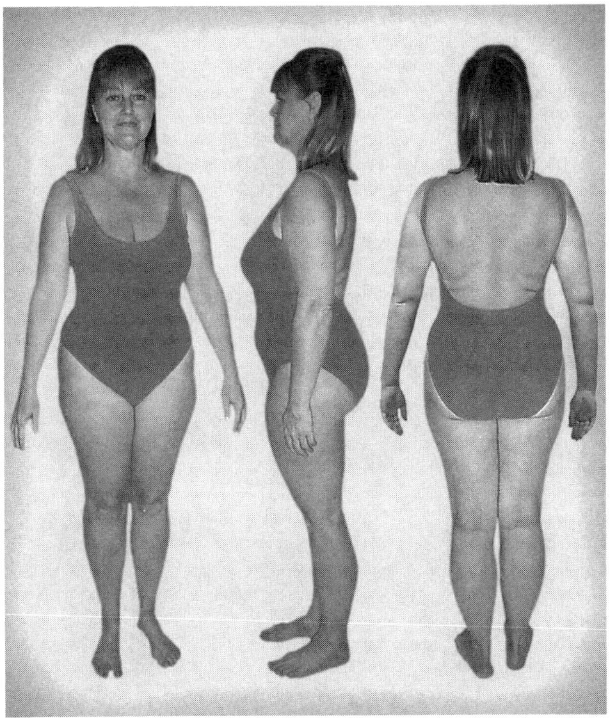

Buttocks relatively flat-to-prominent. Low back curvature straight-to-swayed. Shoulders relatively even with hips. Waist straight-to-defined. Average to short-waisted.

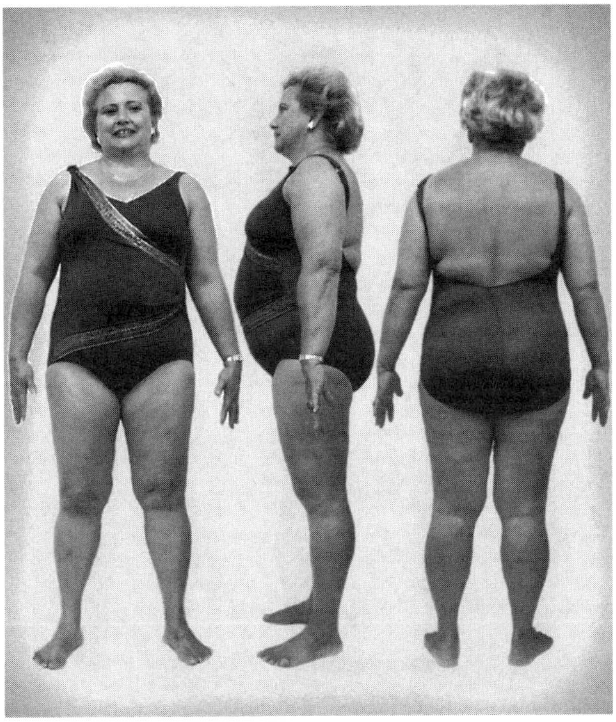

Even when short, general appearance is large. Alternative weight-gain pattern is predominantly in abdomen with small buttocks and little if any gain in thighs.

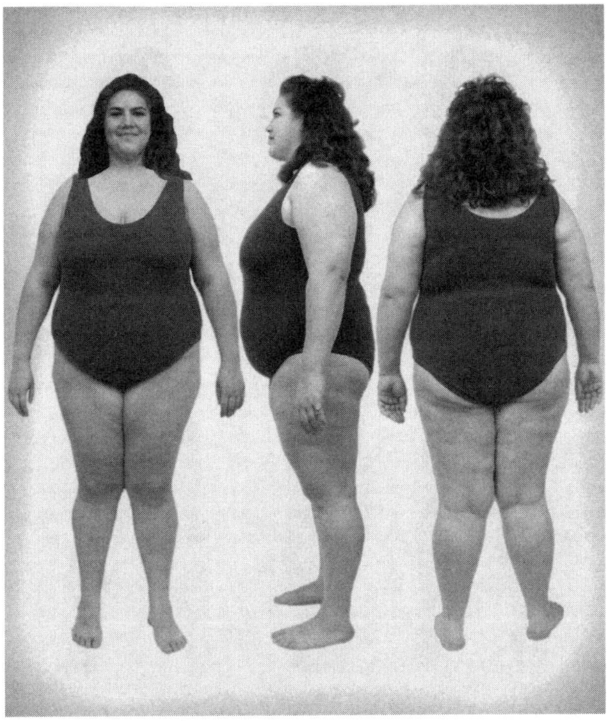

Secondary weight gain in entire abdomen, upper-to-entire back, upper arms, breasts, face, under chin, entire inner thighs or entire thighs to knees, and buttocks.

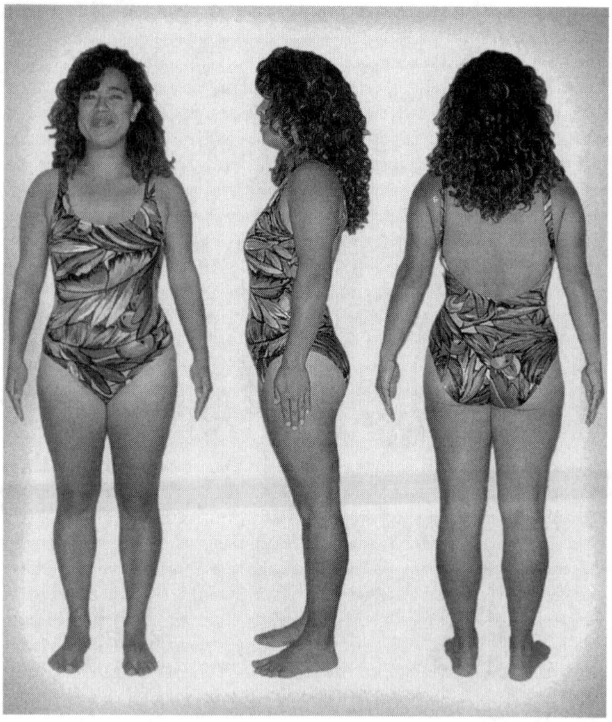

*Soft, gentle appearance. Full face, which gets fuller with weight gain. Average-to-long oval or round face. Communicate through feeling.

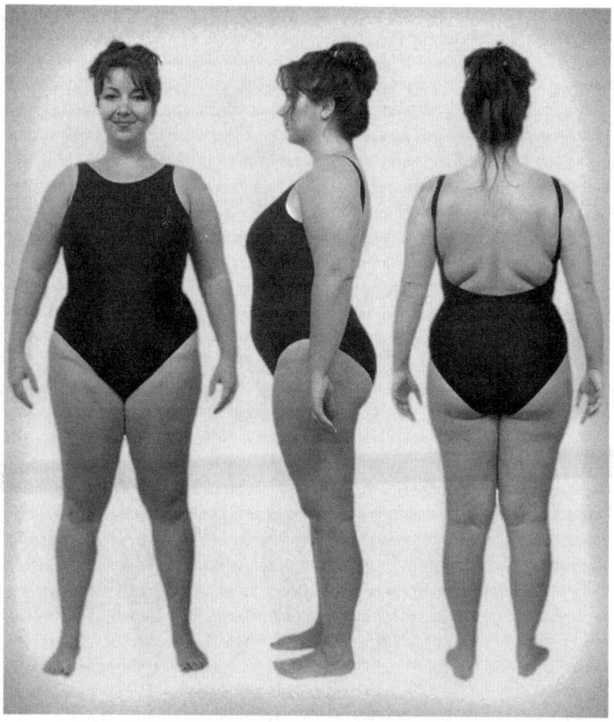

Rounded-to-prominent buttocks, generally firm and shapely, occasionally flat. Low back curvature straight-to-swayed. Breasts small-to-large. Height very petite (less than 5 ft.) to tall.

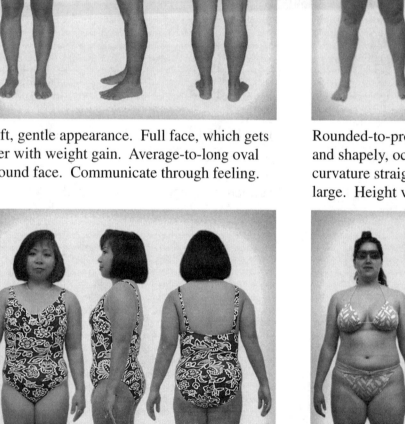

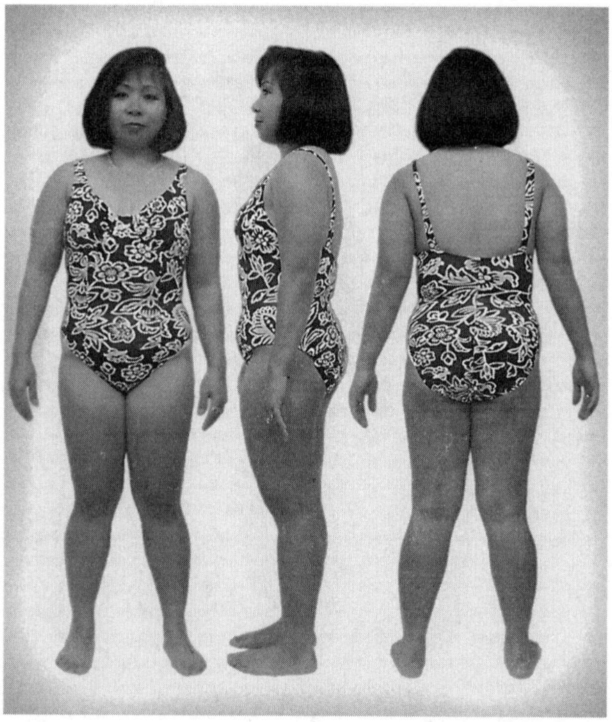

*Puffiness in hands and feet to extent that tendons in back of hands are not visible, even at ideal weight. Ring size goes up and down depending on weight gain or fluid retention.

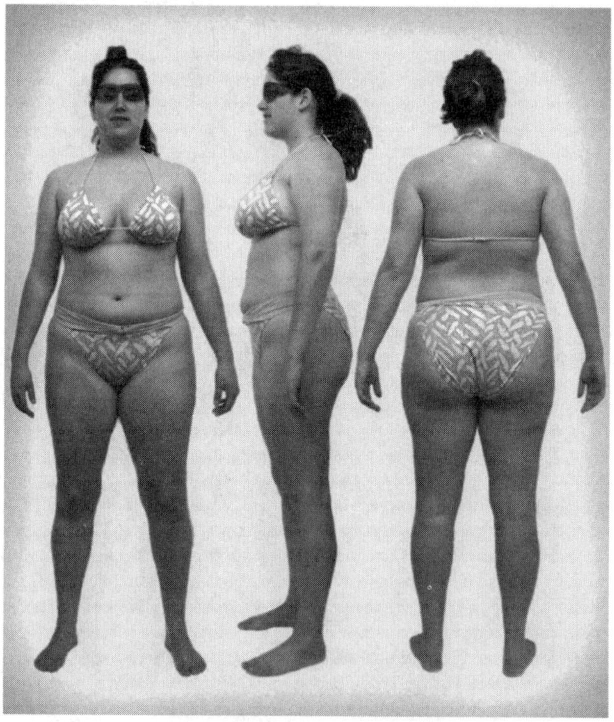

Square, flat upper back extending across shoulders and shoulder blades with relatively straight torso extending to waist. Shoulders relatively even with hips.

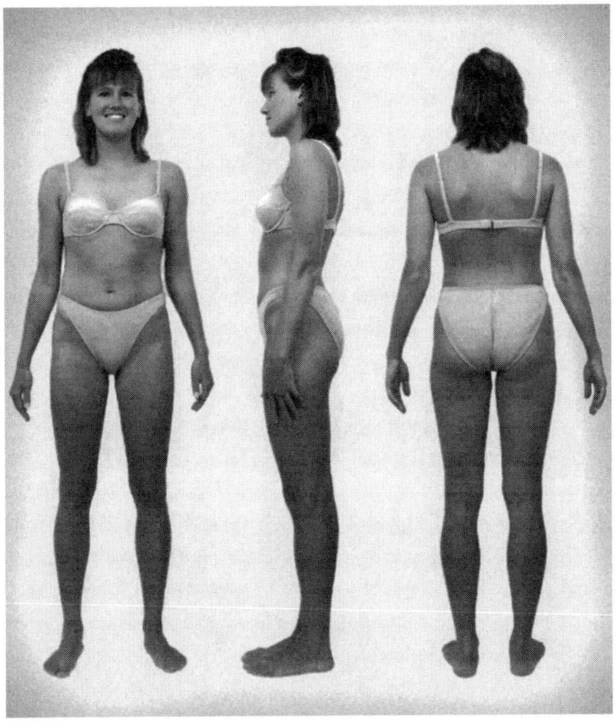

*Initial weight gain in lower abdomen, upper hips, waist, middle back, face, and entire upper 2/3rds of thighs including upper inner thighs. Straight-to-defined waist. Average to short-waisted.

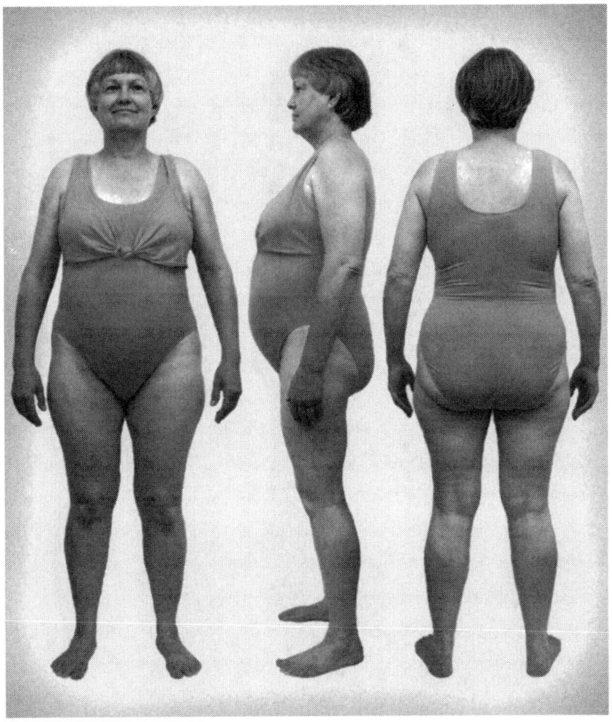

Alternative weight-gain pattern: entire abdomen, upper hips, waist, face, and inner thighs, with little, if any, on outer thighs.

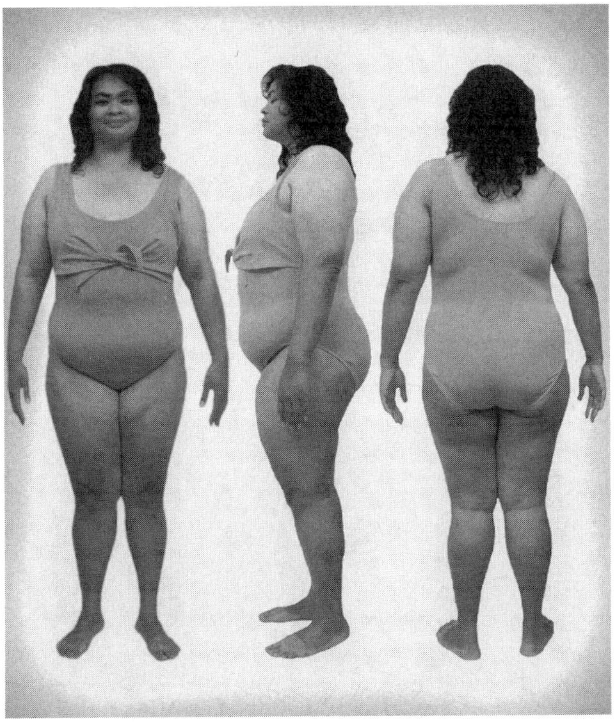

Secondary weight gain in buttocks, back, then all over – including upper arms, hands and feet. Usually medium-to-large bone structure, but with small-to-average hands and often wide feet.

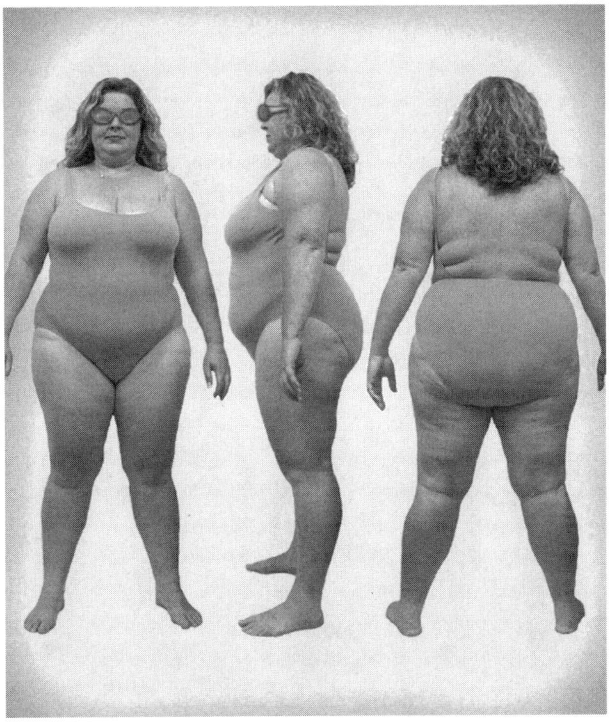

Majority of weight carried in torso – either in front of body or balanced between abdomen and buttocks. Layer of softness covering muscles or average, elongated musculature.

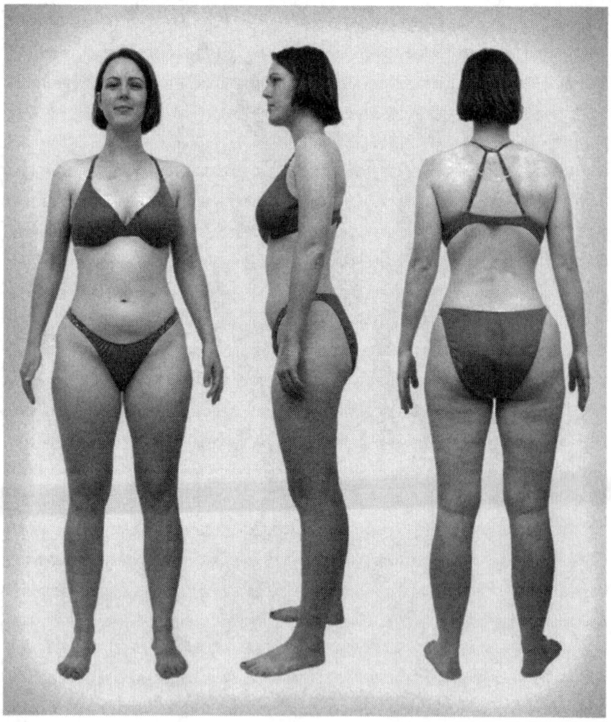

*Friendly, down-to-earth personality, and/or intense, tenacious, determined and strong-willed. Known for making things happen by disseminating energy.

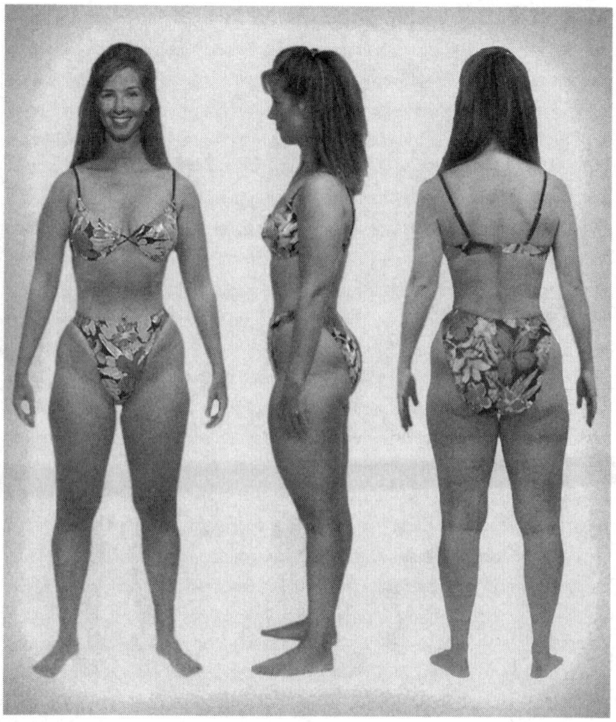

Buttocks rounded-to-prominent. Low back curvature straight-to-swayed. Defined to well-defined waist. Average torso. Solid body, with muscular or heavy/chunky legs.

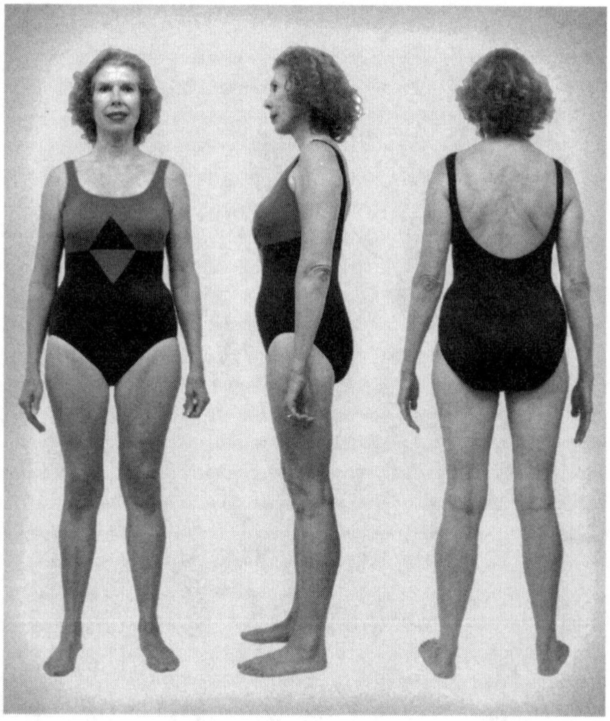

Shoulders narrower than, to relatively even with, hips. Height petite-to-tall. Bone structure medium. Hands small-to-average, often with short fingers.

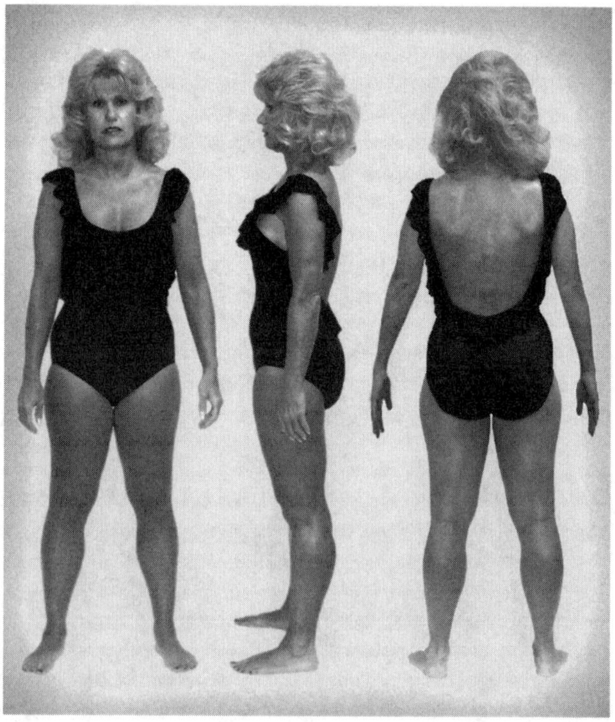

Average oval-shaped head which may be large for body size, although will appear small if much excess weight is gained. Average, elongated to dense, solid musculature.

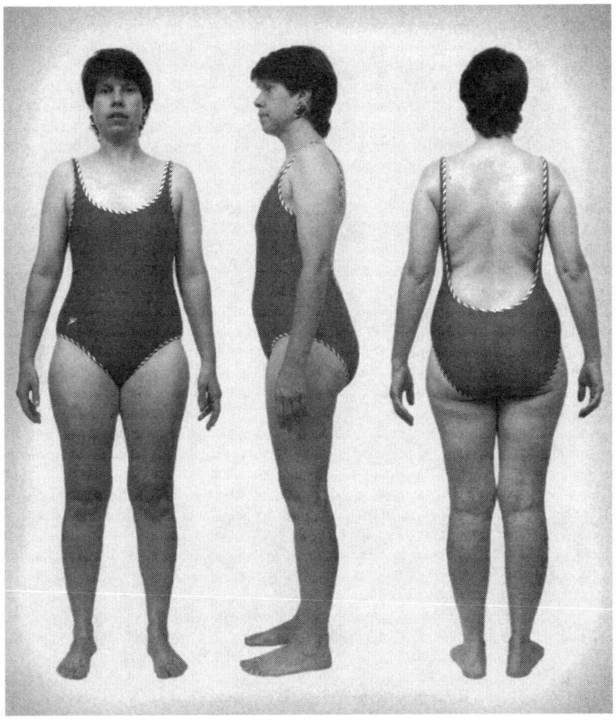

*Initial weight gain in lower abdomen, entire upper 2/3rds of thighs including upper inner thighs, buttocks, upper and lower hips, waist, and middle back.

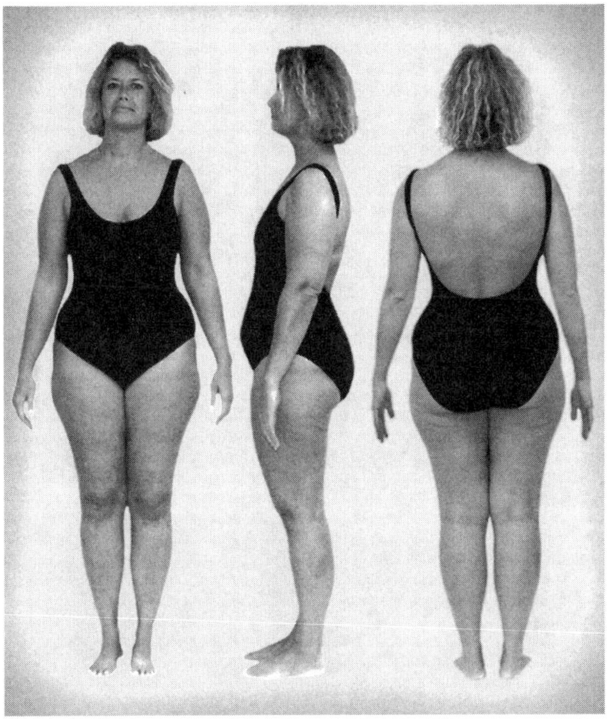

Often carry bulk of weight and cellulite in legs, which can then appear chunky. Thighs and calves often heavy with solid, dense appearance.

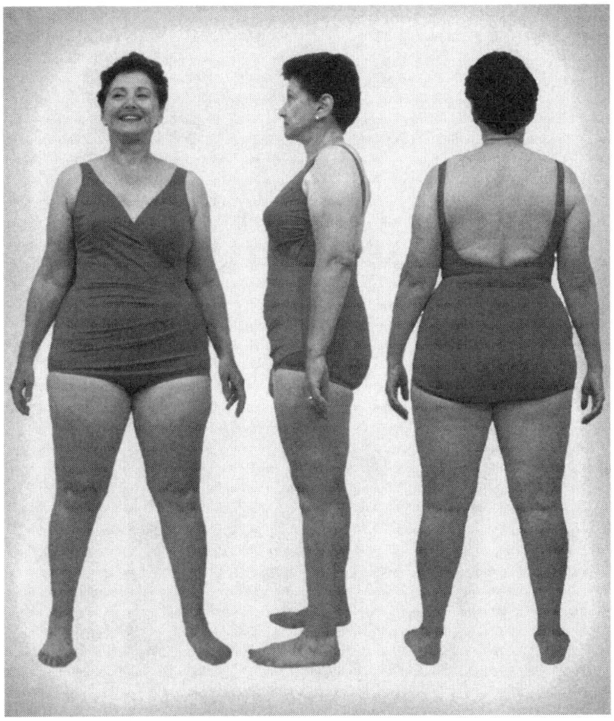

Lower body often at least full size larger than upper body, with hips generally more wide than thick. Breasts average.

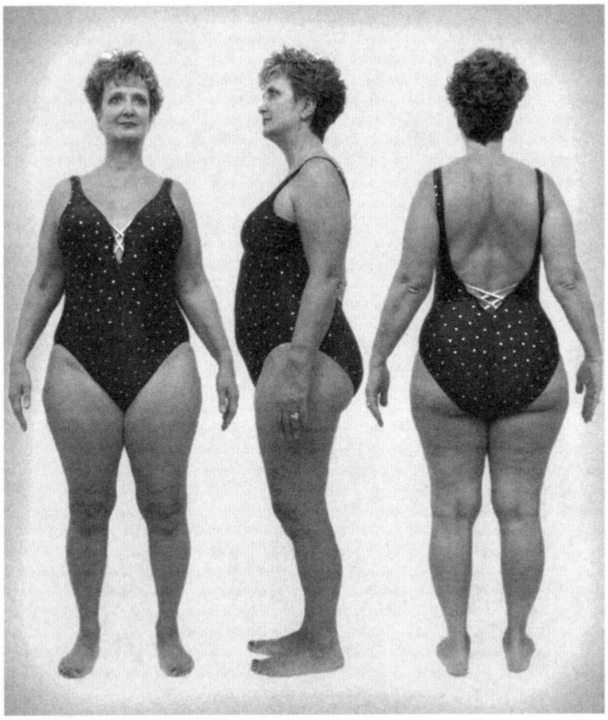

Secondary weight gain in entire abdomen, breasts, upper and entire back, entire inner thighs to knees, face, and upper arms. First place weight is lost is in face.

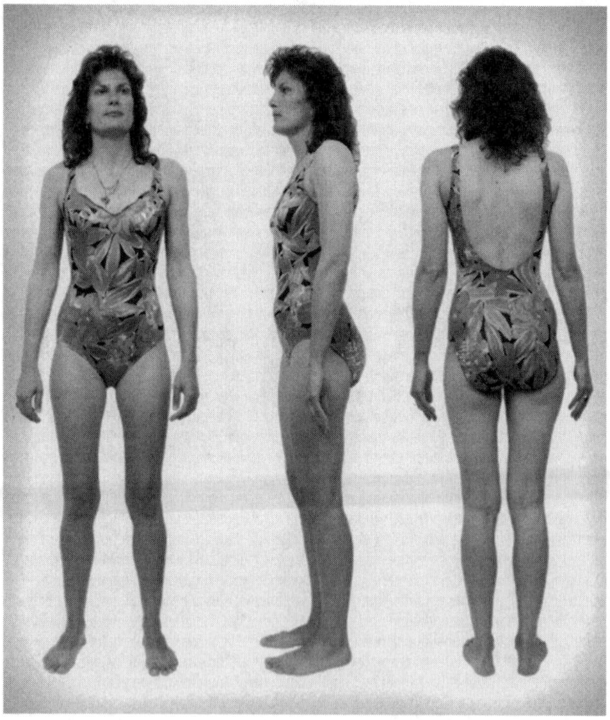

*Average-to-large, dominant, striking head and face with prominent chin. Characteristic head posture is lifting chin and tilting head backward.

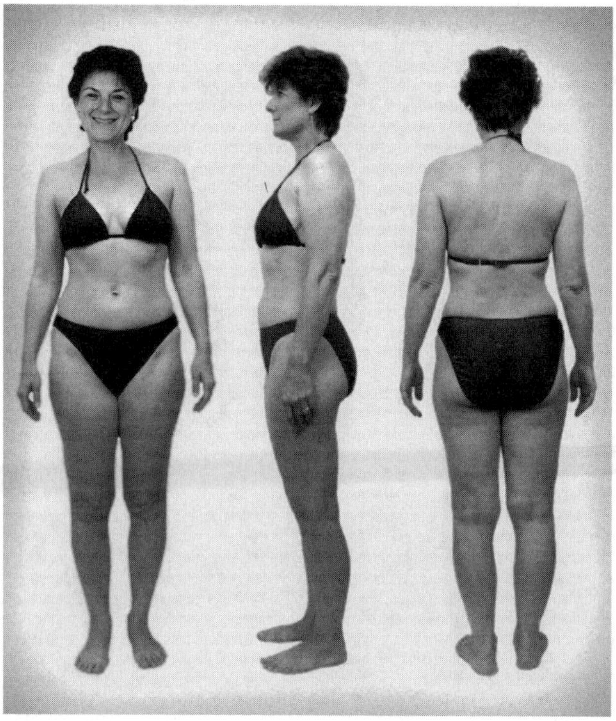

*Their passion, coupled with an intense mental focus, enables them to accomplish their goals. Exceptional ability to come in and take charge.

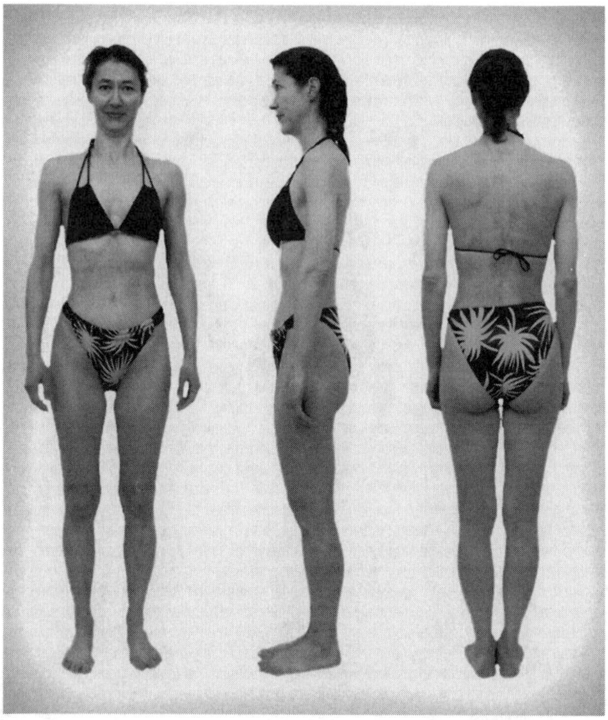

Shoulders relatively even with, to broader than, hips. Buttocks relatively flat-to-rounded. Low back curvature straight-to-average. Breasts average.

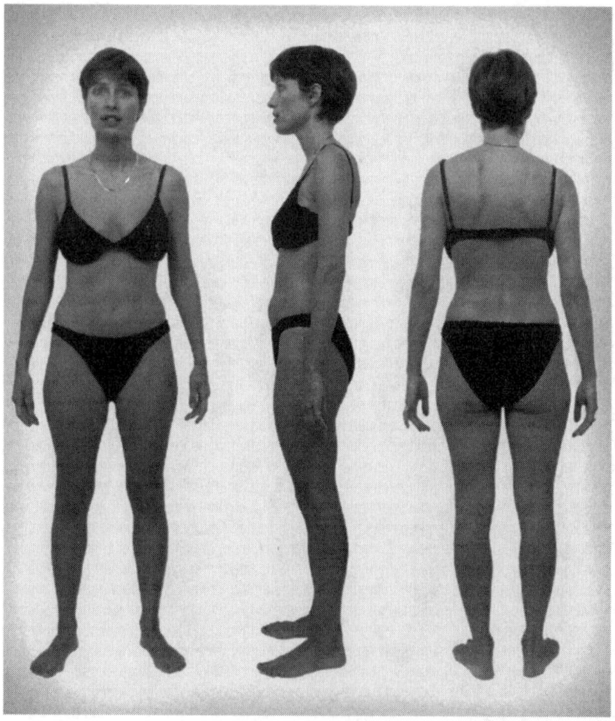

Strong body with good stamina. Average, elongated musculature. Waist straight-to-defined. Average to long-waisted.

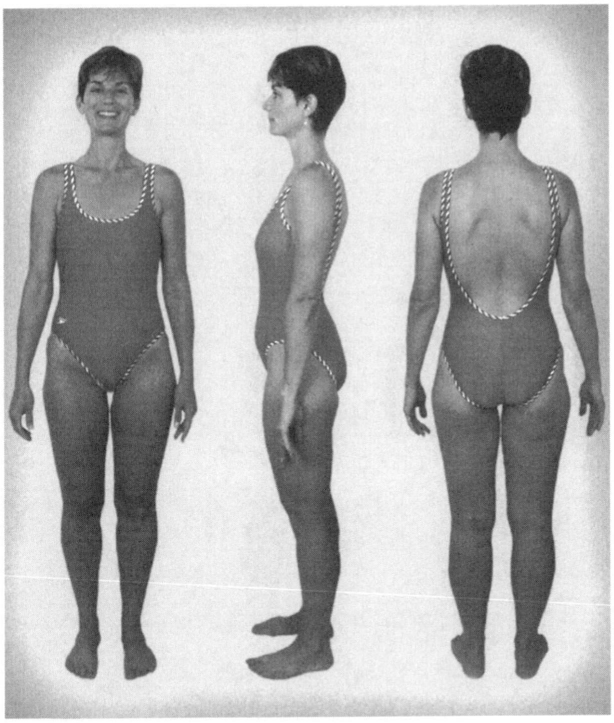

*Initial weight gain in lower abdomen, waist, upper hips, upper back under arms to middle back, and entire upper 2/3rds of thighs including upper inner thighs.

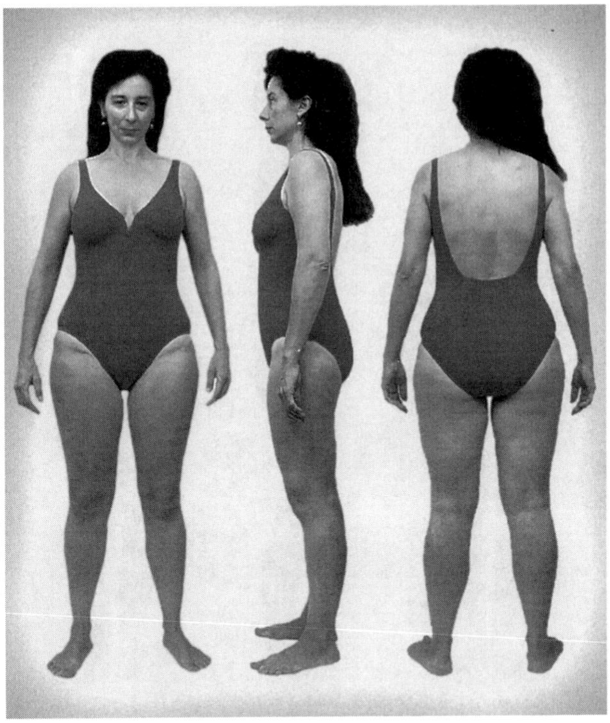

Height petite-to-tall. Bone structure small-to-medium. Square, strong jaw, often with thin-to-average upper lip or lips.

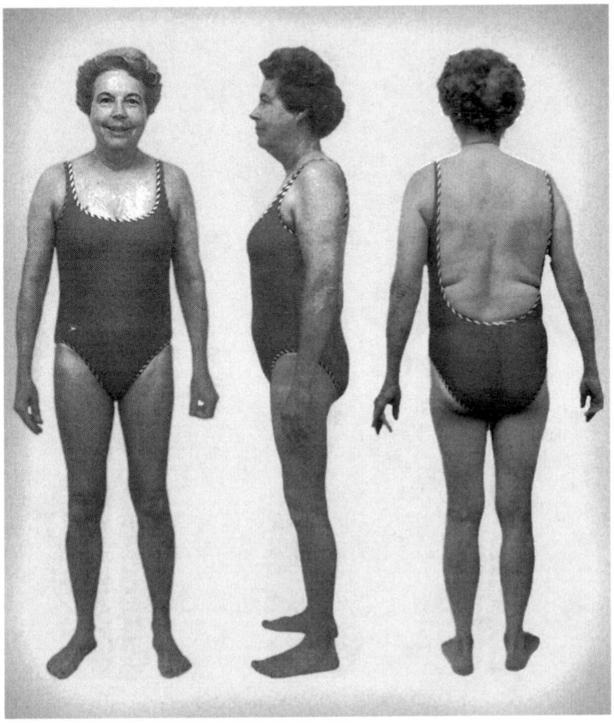

Alternative weight-gain pattern: upper-to-entire abdomen, upper hips, waist and possibly breasts. Body may be at least a full size larger above waist than below.

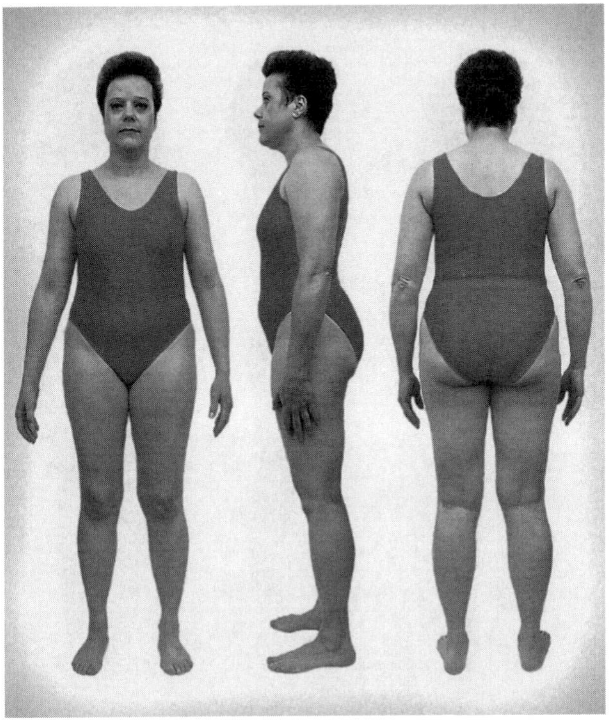

Secondary weight gain is fairly even over body including entire back, upper arms, breasts, thighs, face and under chin.

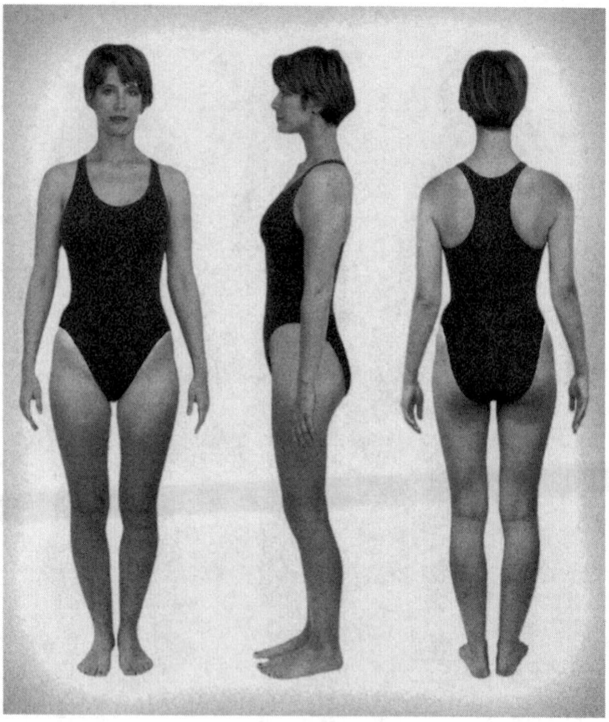

*High, wide and/or dominant forehead, with long, slender oval face or long-to-average rectangular face.

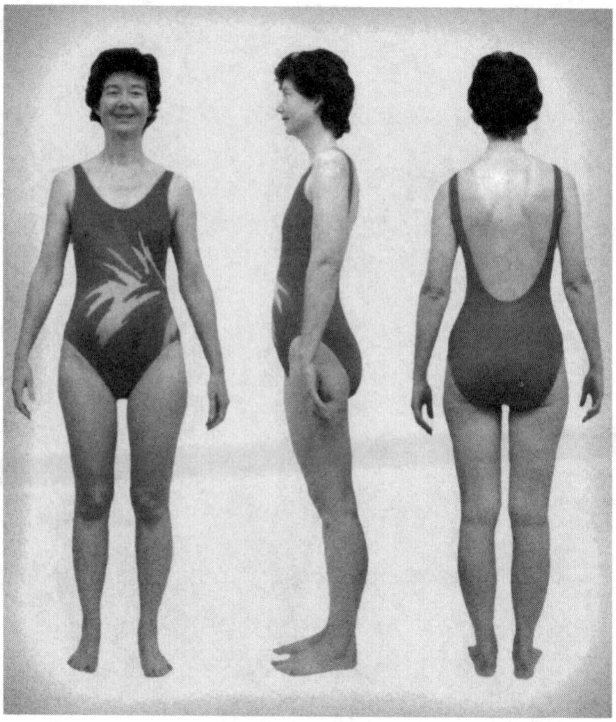

*Continuous arching abdominal musculature with lower abdominal protrusion. Typically slender, delicate appearance, even with weight gain.

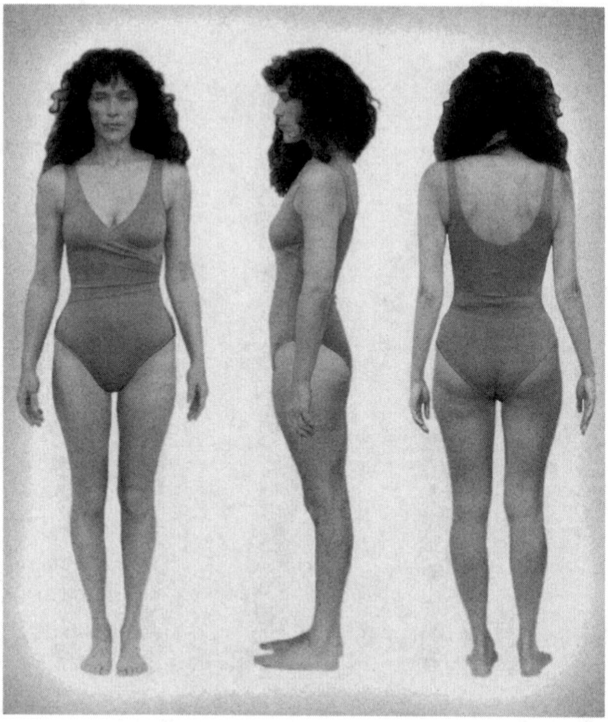

Height generally average-to-tall. Bone structure small-to-medium. Average to long, slender hands. May have difficulty gaining or maintaining weight.

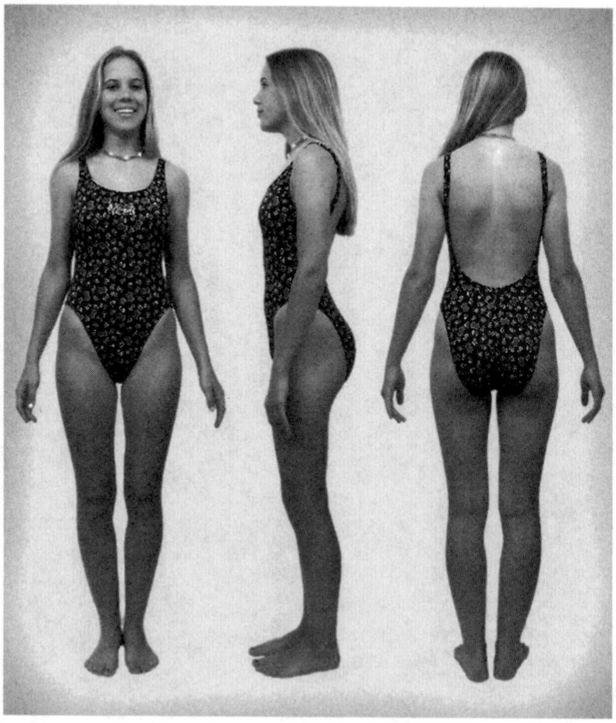

Energy focus is predominantly in head as they are noted for collecting and evaluating information that comes their way.

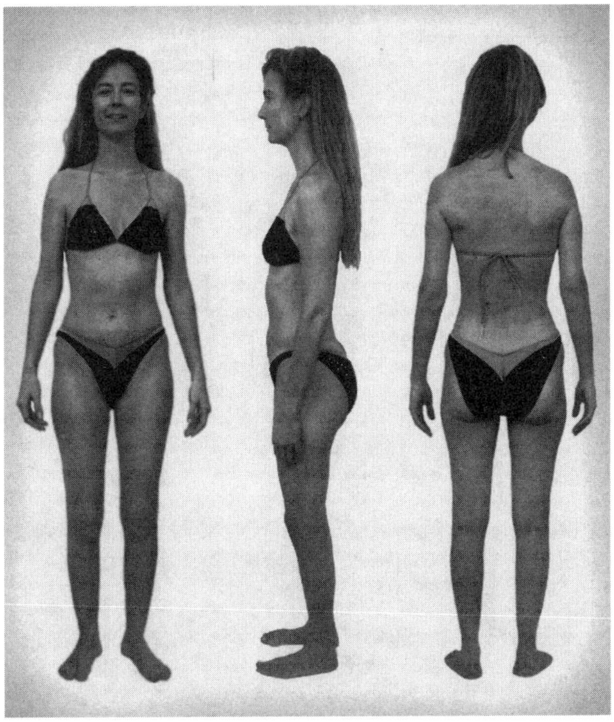

*Initial weight gain in lower abdomen, face, entire upper 2/3rds of thighs, including upper inner thighs, and upper hips.

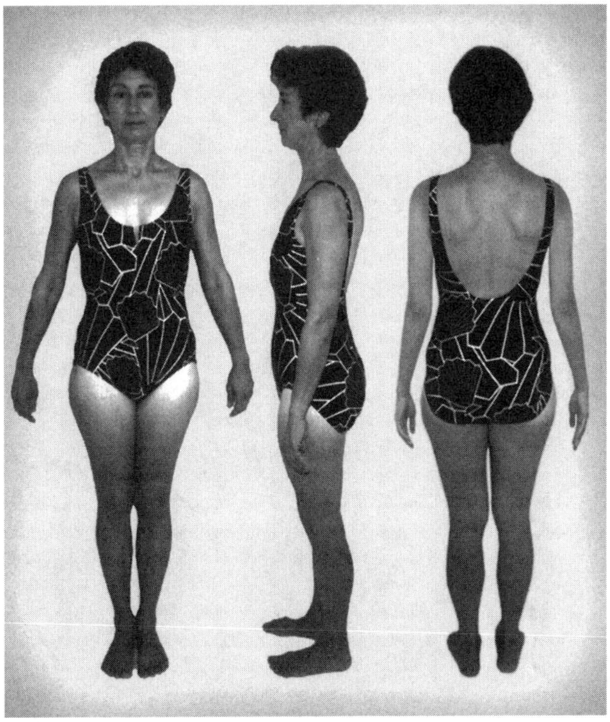

Buttocks relatively flat-to-rounded. Low back curvature average-to-swayed. Breasts small-to-average. Shoulders relatively even with hips.

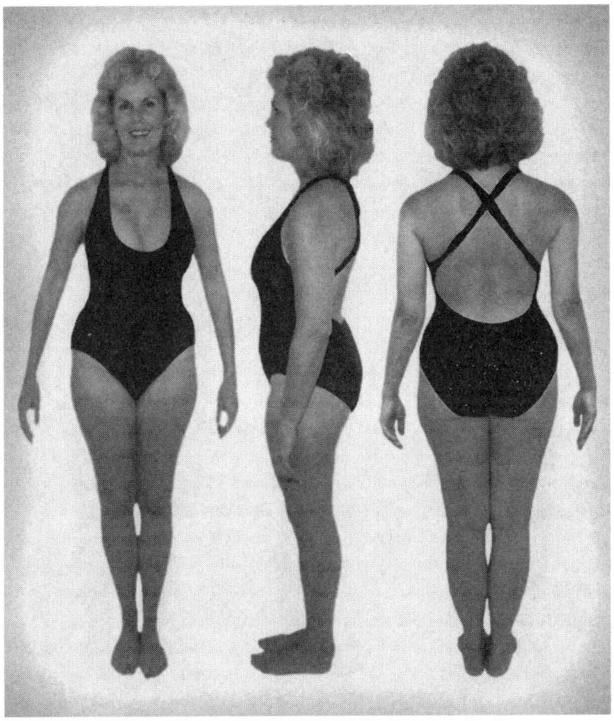

Defined waist. Average, elongated musculature. Average to long-waisted. Body often a full size smaller above waist than below.

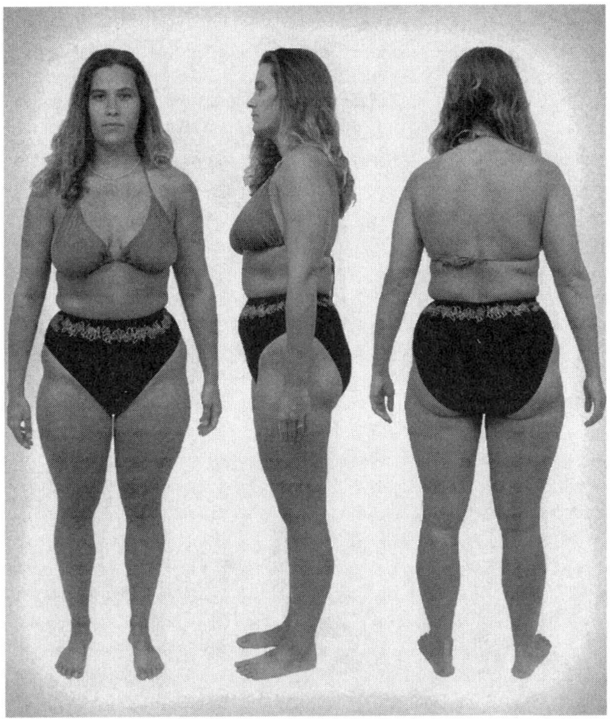

Secondary weight gain in waist, entire abdomen, middle-to-entire back, upper arms, buttocks, lower hips, thighs, calves, and breasts.

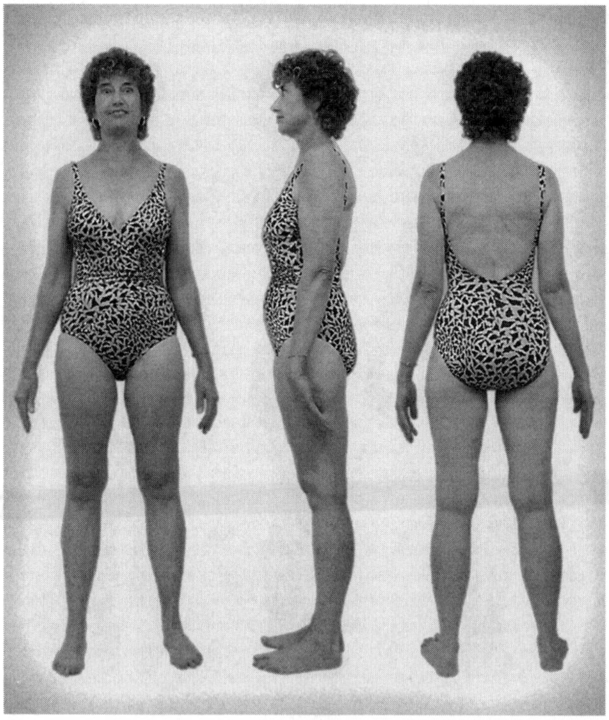

*Tall to very tall with long-limbed appearance. Well-meaning, take-charge demeanor which can be forceful, and sometimes perceived by others as controlling.

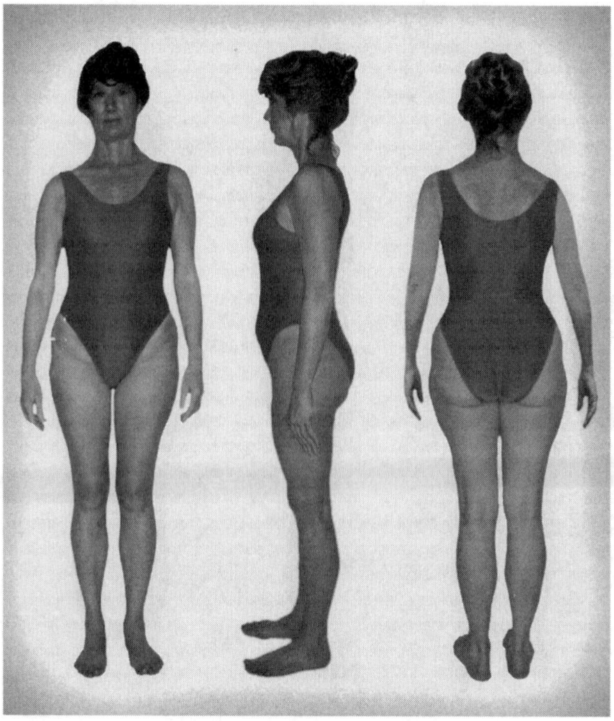

Their strong sense of responsibility and loyalty coupled with their forceful presence allows them to bring stability into their environment.

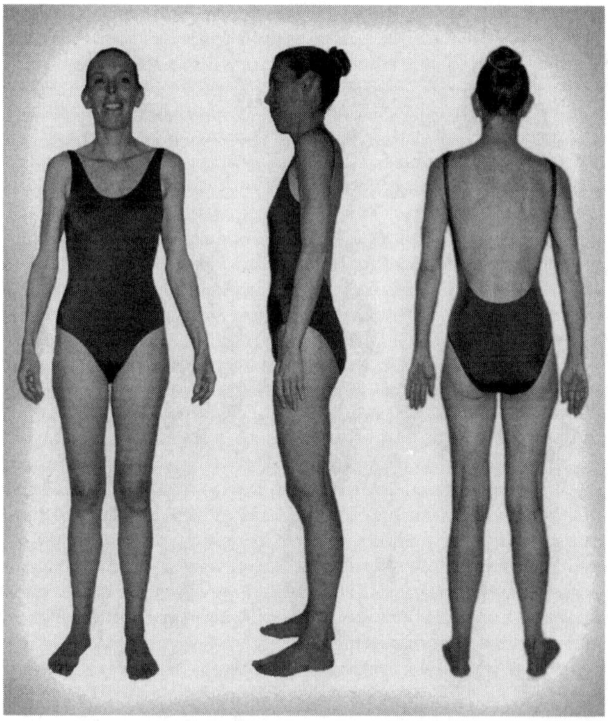

May have difficulty gaining or maintaining adequate weight. When at ideal weight, generally have stable weight pattern throughout life.

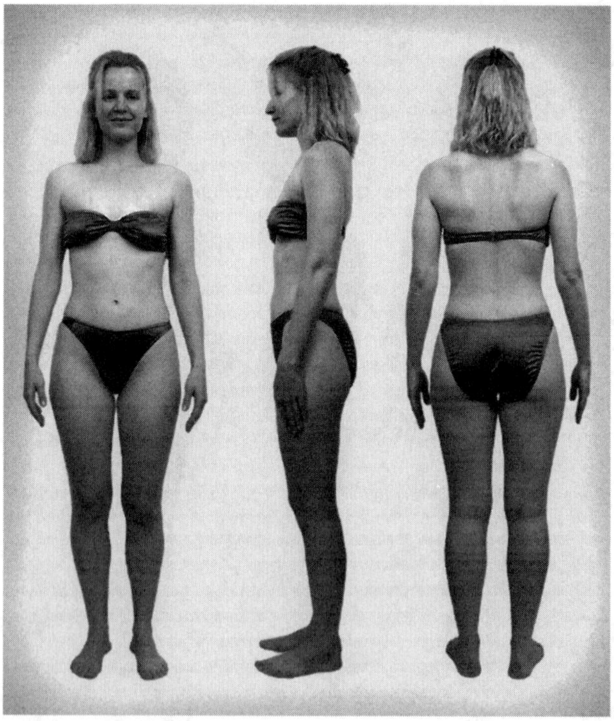

Shoulders relatively even with hips. Average, elongated musculature. Waist straight-to-defined. Average to long-waisted.

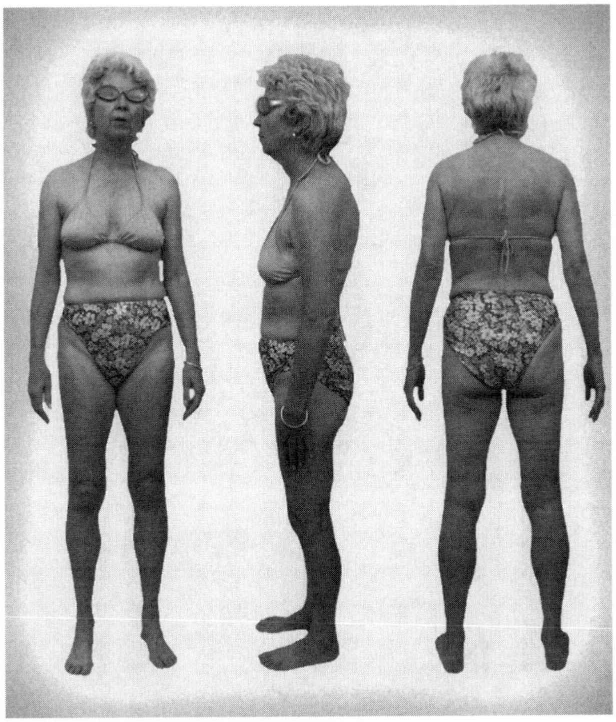

*Initial weight gain in lower abdomen, waist, possibly upper hips, and either entire upper 2/3rds of thighs or only upper inner thighs.

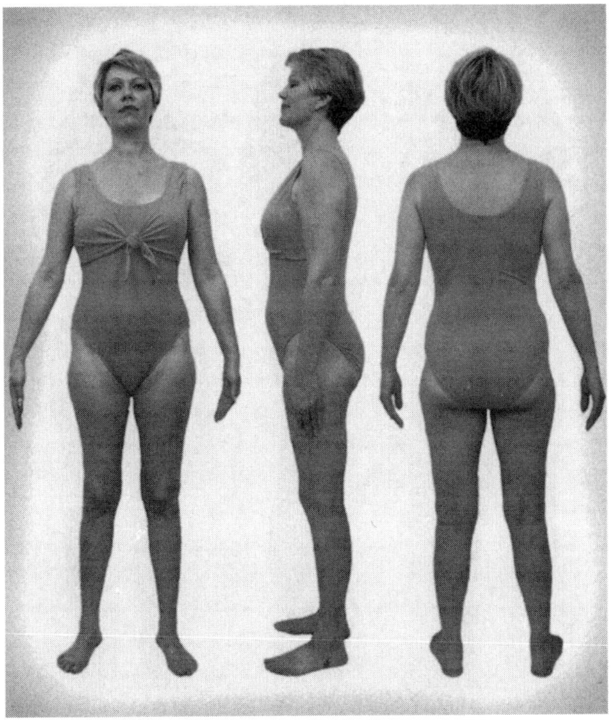

Buttocks relatively flat-to-rounded. Low back curvature straight-to-average. Bone structure medium. Breasts small-to-average. Height tall to very tall.

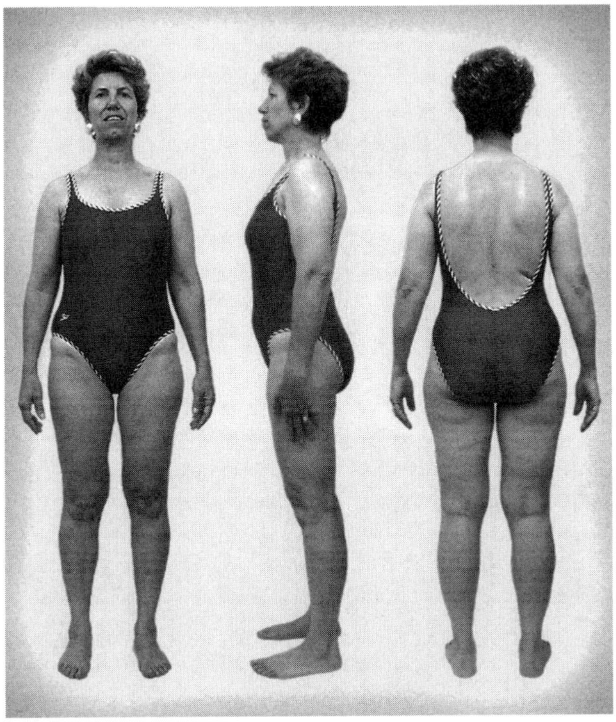

Average-to-long oval or long, rectangular face which often appears slender or small. Large, wide hands with long, slender fingers proportional to hands. Long arms.

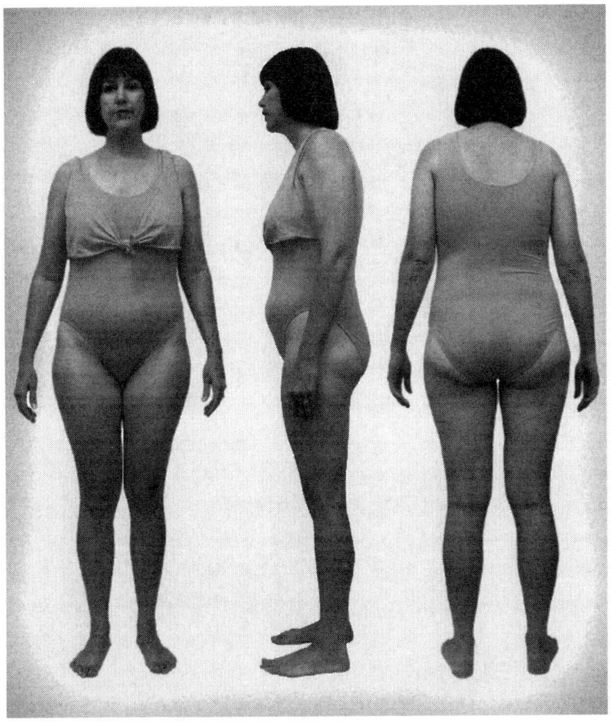

Secondary weight gain in thighs, buttocks, upper and/or lower hips, and middle back. Alternative weight gain pattern same except for minimal gain in thighs.

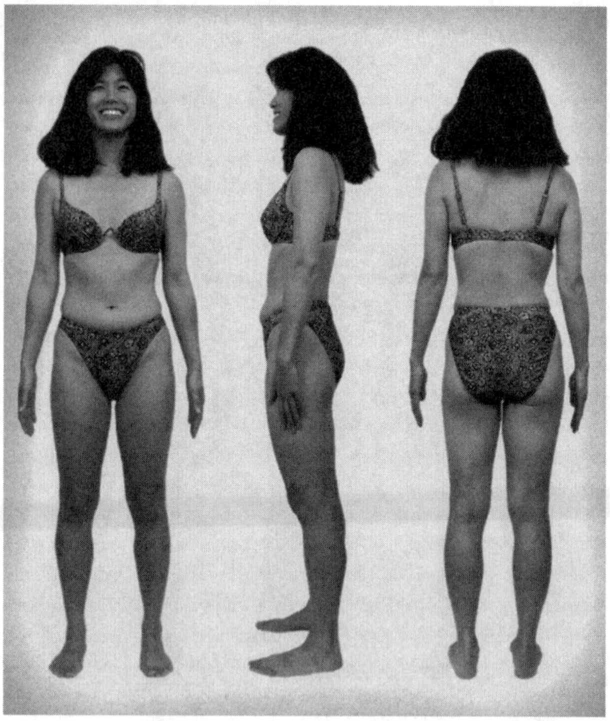

*Eyes reveal brightness and sensitivity. Known for being able to see what needs to be done and getting it done.

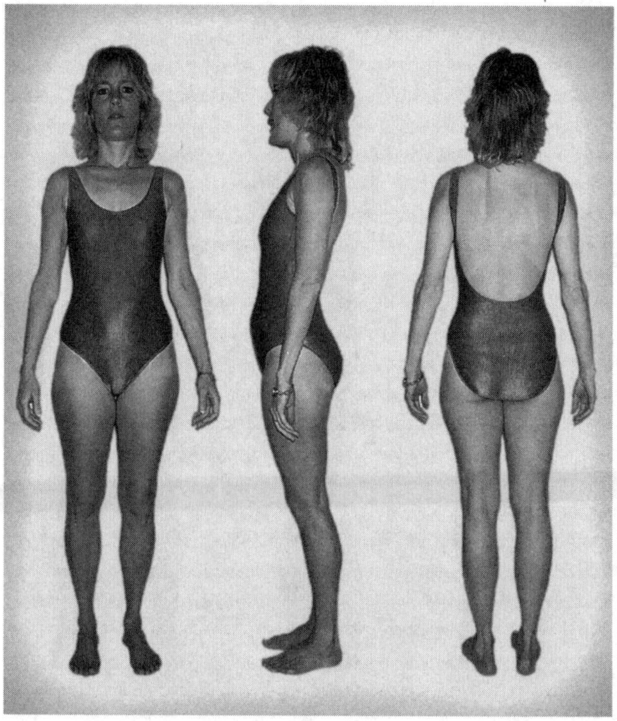

*Body well-proportioned, usually with delicate or slender hands; long, tapered fingers and narrow feet. Often with delicate appearance.

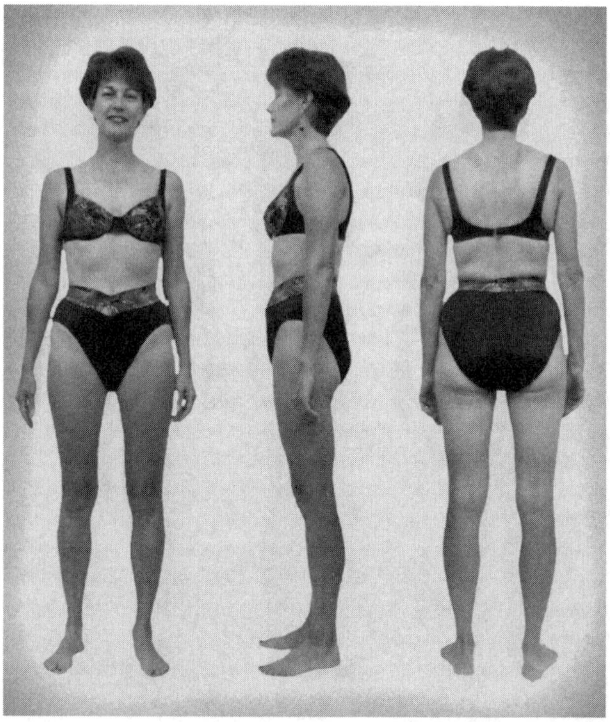

Low back curvature straight-to-average. Buttocks relatively flat-to-rounded. Shoulders relatively even with hips.

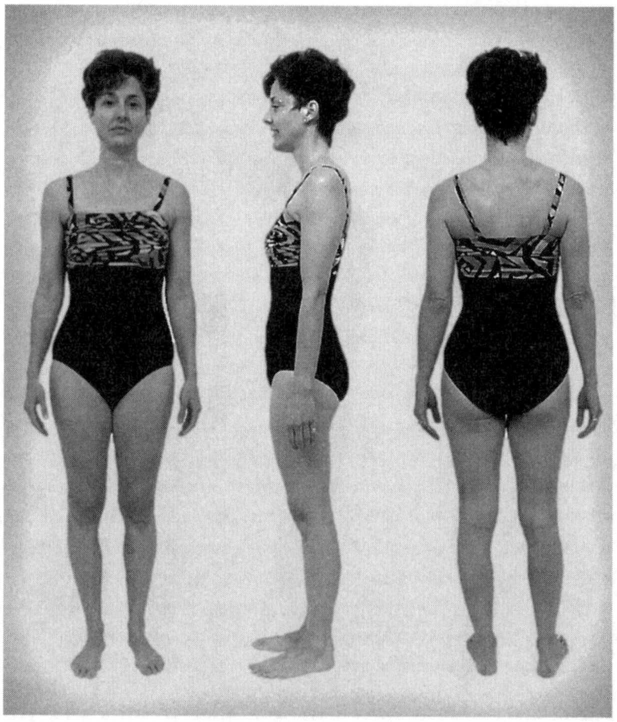

Hair generally thick-to-average, healthy and abundant. Defined to well-defined waist. Average to long-waisted.

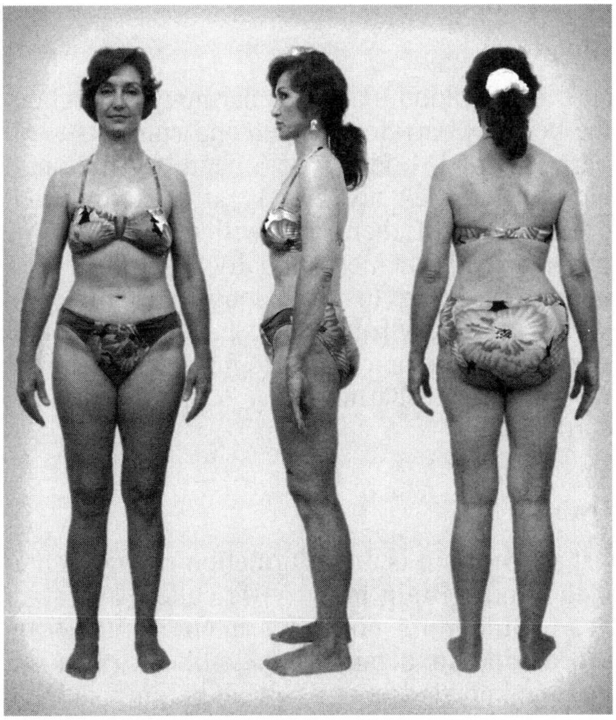

*Initial weight gain in lower abdomen, waist, upper hips, entire upper 2/3rds of thighs including upper inner thighs, inner knees, and middle back.

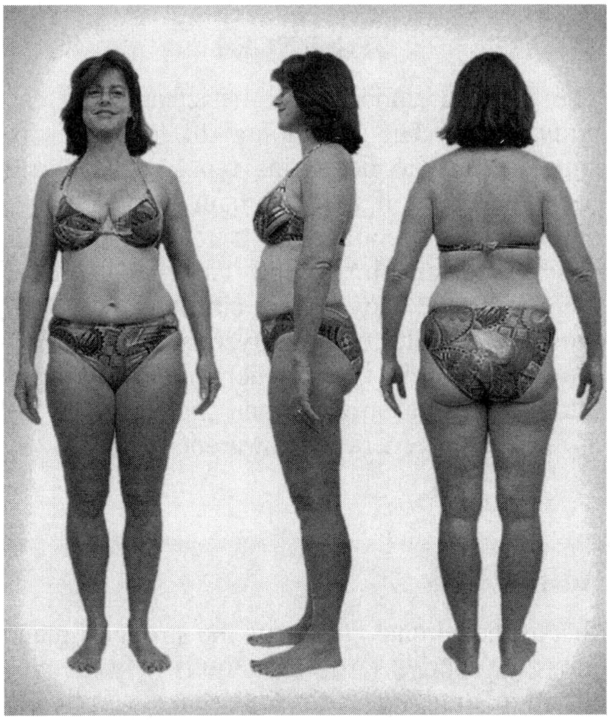

V-shaped jaw on either average oval or heart-shaped face. Shapely legs, with muscular, well-defined calves. Average, elongated musculature.

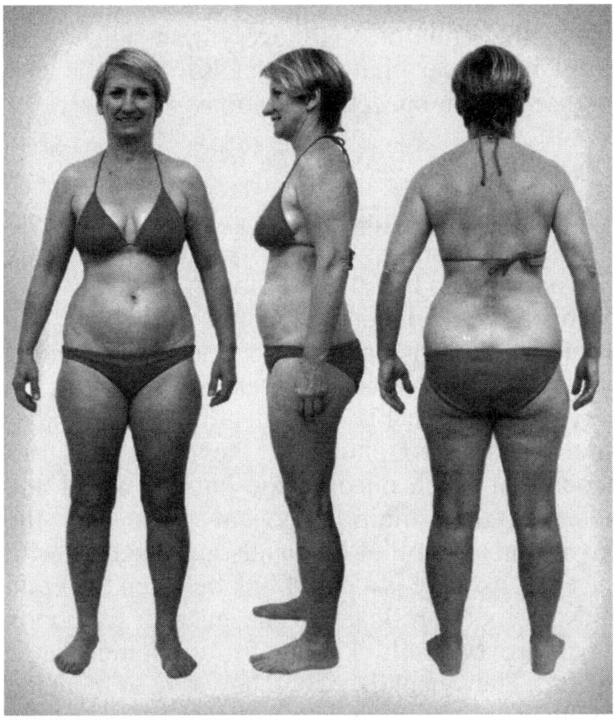

Height petite-to-tall. Bone structure small-to-medium. Breasts average; may increase with age and/or weight gain.

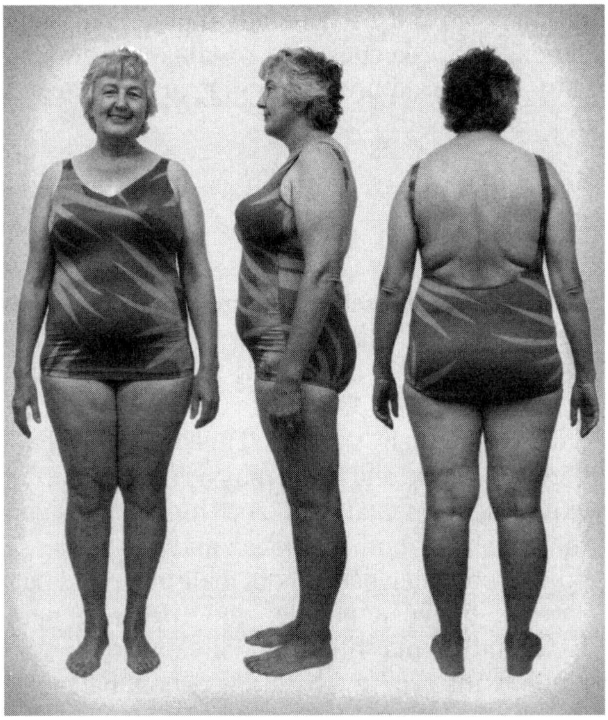

Secondary weight gain extends into entire abdomen, upper arms, entire back, thighs extending to knees, face, under chin, breasts, and buttocks.

ESSENCES

The Essence embodies the basic nature of each body type. The Psychological Profile is the simplest way to determine type, as supporting foods can shift if the dominant gland becomes depleted. Psychological traits are generally observed from birth and can be useful in identifying the body type of children. Becoming familiar with the personality characteristics and motivation for the type can help in gaining insight into the personal strengths and challenges, as well as expanding general self-awareness.

Adrenal

Just as the adrenal glands are the strongest glands in the body, Adrenal body types are distinguished by their high energy, physical strength, and endurance. This dominant physical energy is reflected in their heavy, solid musculature, commanding presence, and physical comfort in the world. Forceful and dynamic, they easily make themselves known as soon as they enter a room and are generally the first ones in an audience to ask questions or make comments. They are, by nature, outgoing, often charming and charismatic.

Balanced

Just as the Balanced body type is not controlled by any single gland, organ or system, but is dependent upon everything working together synergistically, Balanced body types need balance in their world. This means balance between work and play, physical and spiritual expression, mental and emotional states, and relationships, both personal and business. In other words, balance in both their inner and outer worlds, between people, and life in general. Essentially playful and adventurous, they embody the synergy that brings about balance.

Blood

Just as the blood maintains harmony throughout the body by carrying oxygen and nutrients to all parts, Blood body types need to maintain harmony. They are greatly affected by what others think of them and will readily become physically ill when emotionally upset. They are noted for going to great lengths to maintain social and environmental harmony. Their strength lies in their ability to make people aware of the effect disharmony has on people and the earth.

Brain

Just as the brain is the information storage center of the body, Brain body types collect and store data. Brains are noted for intensely gathering information in detail, as they like to have all possible knowledge on a subject before making a decision. Memory, logical thought, and control of voluntary muscle responses are the brain's primary duties. It's the brain that is responsible for moving the body safely through the world. Since so many of our routine daily activities are done by automatic muscle memory, the brain knows the value of doing everything right. This desire to do everything right leads them to be very precise in their speech and actions.

Eye

Just as our eyes link us to our outer world and environment, and provide a window to our soul, Eye body types link the world with themselves by connecting the inner and outer worlds through implementing visions. The world of the human body is connected and activated by the eyes, as they are responsible for integrating the body's intelligence throughout all the cells. It's our hands that reach out into the outside world and provide the main physical link to the environment. Use of the hands is connected with the eyes, as there is a direct link between the brain and the motor reflexes in the hands. Eye body types are typically known for implementing a vision. They visualize what they want to manifest and then set out to make it happen.

Gallbladder

Just as the gallbladder can be depended upon to store bile manufactured by the liver (which is essential for the breakdown of fats) and release it as needed, the Gallbladder body type is dependable. Known for being helpful, loyal and consistent, Gallbladder types create a steady, stable environment. They prefer to work behind the scenes, doing the jobs that are essential to keep a home or business running. Their quiet, steady strength is often expressed in what appears to be a timid or shy nature. They are exceptionally reliable and loyal, and feel most fulfilled when they are being useful.

Gonadal

Just as the gonads are a pleasure center, the nature of the Gonadal body type is to create pleasure and be playful. They bring a light, playful, spontaneous quality to their work, relationships, and to all aspects of their lives. Integration, balance, and enjoyment create genuine playfulness. Highly emotional, Gonadals are prone to being controlled by their emotions. Difficulty focusing or concentrating is typical when tired or stressed. To compensate, Gonadals will look for and do "no-brainer" jobs like shopping, gardening, or routine tasks. Playtime or time to completely relax is essential, as it allows them to re-connect with their essence.

Heart

Just as the heart beat regulates the flow of the blood throughout the body, Heart body types regulate the beat of their environment. Heart types can walk into a room and create either harmony or discord within a group, even causing conflict when they so desire. Their approach can be quite subtle, especially when they are in a new environment, first getting in step with what is going on, and then deciding whether to shift it. Being able to set the beat, they have the natural ability to influence the moods of those around them. Physically softer than most other types, they impress others as being sweet and lovable. Women are often round and heart-shaped, while men and boys are huggable like teddy bears. Like the heart, they bring their own rhythm or music to their environment.

Hypothalamus

Just as the hypothalamus gland is responsible for and in charge of the involuntary functions necessary for life, including regulating the heartbeat, body temperature, blood pressure, metabolism and blood-sugar levels, as well as directing the pituitary gland, Hypothalamus body types have an intense sense of responsibility for their behavior. They seem to be intuitively aware of the significance of their actions, and have a sense of responsibility for accuracy in all they do. Consequently, they approach life with a certain caution. They will generally gather all the necessary tools, study the directions, and formulate a plan before starting a project.

Intestinal

Just as the intestines openly accept everything that comes in and then discern between nutrients and waste material or what to keep and what to release, the Intestinal body type is discerning. They approach life with an openness, taking everything in, and then letting go of what isn't appropriate. This often leads to a thorough analysis of everything new and a prejudice ("pre-judge") against anything similar to something already analyzed in the past. While their initial response to life is emotional, they generally don't trust their emotions, so they gather as much information as possible to make a logical decision. New experiences are vital since expansion is essential, and if it doesn't occur mentally, emotionally, or spiritually, Intestinals will expand physically.

Kidney

Just as the kidneys regulate body fluid levels and are responsive to arterial pressure, Kidney body types rise to the occasion when under pressure. They respond and function best when they are needed, particularly if coupled with time or performance pressure. If sufficient outside pressure doesn't exist, they will create it, procrastinating until they get behind in their projects to the point of discomfort, which forces them to excel and move beyond their previous limits. Fearful by nature, successfully meeting challenges builds confidence and prepares them for their next experience, allowing them to move further than they had ever dreamed.

Liver

Just as the liver is in charge of converting substances into usable forms and filtering out what can't be used, the Liver body type unifies life. Livers are noted for putting pieces together and fitting them into the flow of the day or project. Placing a high priority on family, loyalty, and stability, they excel at helping with whatever needs to be done. By seeing something in the flow, they create the desire, that when coupled with their tremendous physical strength, results in accomplishment or manifestation. Teaching, often through leadership, is their way of insuring the unity of life, as the knowledge gained by one generation can flow to the next.

Lung

Just as the lungs supply the oxygen needed for life, the Lung body type takes in life. Nurturing and creative, Lungs give life to their world by expressing positive, supportive emotions. Their strength lies in being able to shift emotional energy, like changing hurt into creativity. This allows them to express the energy of negative emotions in a safe, constructive or positive manner. By using emotions as an indicator rather than a response, respecting emotions, and getting the essence from them, emotions can be used to move into a greater richness and fullness of life, which is what enables Lungs to excel at making the most of the moment.

Lymph

Just as the lymphatic system requires stimulation to move the waste away from the tissues, the Lymph body type needs continual stimulation in the form of movement and change. It's this constant movement that adds variety to life. Lymph types require a lot of variety through physical activity or mental stimulation to maintain mental clarity and a sense of vitality. They are happiest when they feel excitement. Fun loving and playful, activity allows them to feel vibrant and alive. Consequently, stimulation, either mental or physical, is essential.

Medulla

Just as the medulla or brain stem is responsible for controlling respiration and heart rate, functions that require steady perseverance, Medulla body types are known for their consistency and persistence. Undaunted by time or trends, Medulla types are unwavering in their activities and beliefs, staying with what they choose to be doing with unusual resolve. With an abundance of patience, Medullas possess an intense sense of responsibility and remain loyal indefinitely, especially when they have identified with the group or cause. It's their high sense of responsibility that makes them patient teachers, and the appreciation of their students, patients, or clients makes it all worthwhile.

Nervous System

Just as the nervous system connects all parts of the body and keeps the brain informed of what is happening, Nervous System body types connect all parts on all levels. They enjoy listening to others and connecting people according to their needs, desires, or interests. Practical and efficient, they are happiest when they are connecting people and ideas. Nervous System types tend to have an abundance of nervous energy, and manifest it through a myriad of activities. For the Nervous System, listening to others is an adventure.

Pancreas

Just as the pancreas, by breaking down carbohydrates or sugars, releases energy, Pancreas body types release energy, bringing joy. They love socializing, especially around food, and are usually the life of a party. Food, particularly sugar, produces energy. Likewise, Pancreases, in their exuberance, produce joy. Conscientious and reliable, when their energy is channeled into a particular area, Pancreases can be quite dynamic. They are the ones that continually release the energy that keeps an organization running. With their genuine concern for people and their ability to use laughter to burst out of the most uncomfortable situations, they are known for bringing joy to their environment.

Pineal

Just as the pineal is sensitive to light and regulates the sleep cycle, Pineal body types listen to their intuition. The pineal gland is derived from a third eye that begins to develop early in the embryo and later degenerates. Likewise, our intuition is present early in life and can be developed or suppressed. Pineals tend to retain their intuition longer and stronger than most types. Generally sensitive on all levels, their challenge is to learn to accurately listen to their intuition and balance it with their mental acuity. Being highly susceptible to a barrage of internal information, talking is a way of collecting or focusing, as well as a means of sorting out what is most appropriate.

Pituitary

Just as the pituitary gland controls growth hormones necessary for a child to grow, Pituitary body types manifest the childhood quality of making life fun. They approach life with a childlike openness and wide-eyed innocence that makes them fun to be around. As the master gland in charge of directing the entire body, the pituitary gland has to be extremely responsible. Likewise, Pituitaries are naturally capable, responsible people. Lighthearted and creative, Pituitaries are stimulated by new ideas and concepts which they use to bring happiness.

Skin

Just as the skin communicates with the outside world, Skin body types communicate through feeling. Feelings are used as a way of receiving information. While they are generally very open to others and their environment, when stressed, Skins will retreat by detaching, disassociating, or essentially closing down and turning their focus inward. Strongly attached to and affected by their environment, Skins have a strong connection with the earth, nature, and animals which allows them to naturally recharge. Highly visual, they generally see, remember and learn through pictures. Many are extremely sensitive, easily "picking up on" subtle energies and vibrations – including sounds and voice inflections.

Spleen

Just as the spleen stores blood and the spleen acupuncture point draws energy into the body to be disseminated through the blood as needed, Spleen body types disseminate energy. They have a strong ability to organize and delegate, making sure projects get done, many of which often involve food and social or group interaction. Noted for their tenacity, Spleens will stay with a subject until they get the results they want. They are most comfortable when they can solve a problem in a logical step-by-step fashion, and are noted for providing the sustaining energy needed to get a job done right.

Stomach

Just as the stomach focuses all its attention on the food it's digesting, Stomach body types focus on what's in front of them, allowing them to ignite their passion and truly live in the present moment. It's their focus, passion, and physical stamina that enables them to accomplish their goals. When dealing with a problem, they will often talk it out, either alone or with someone else, chewing the data until they have sufficiently digested it. They make their best decisions after they have thoroughly processed the material. Igniting their passion brings an aliveness to everything they undertake, which is especially apparent when expressed through music and dance.

Thalamus

Just as the thalamus collects information and files it for storage in the cerebral cortex or brain, Thalamus body types collect and evaluate information. They like to be effective and tend to be perfectionists. Hearing is often their dominant sense, making them extremely sensitive to vibrations, and easily stressed by noise. Conversely, music is essential to them and can be used to shift out of their strong mental focus into a relaxing, creative, or nurturing mode. This is because music provides a direct link to their emotions. Just as they readily take in information, they are just as willing to let it go as new data becomes available, making them open-minded and willing to change.

Thymus

Just as the thymus gland eliminates unknown protein – generally bacteria and viruses – to keep the body's internal environment safe, Thymus body types stabilize their environment. They are protective of their own and will go to great lengths to keep their environment constant, generally resisting change of any kind. Judging everything as good or bad, right or wrong, makes maintaining a constant, stable environment easier. Their initial response is usually negative as this eliminates the need for examining anything new further. Since being safe is generally associated with known situations, there is a deep seated fear of change. Their innate desire to protect and keep life constant gives rise to a sense of loyalty and responsibility that towers above most other types.

Thyroid

Just as the thyroid gland regulates the metabolism, ensuring the adequate release of energy into the body, Thyroid types are known for manifestation or getting things done. Extremely responsible, they will go to great lengths to fulfill their obligations, often at their own expense. Thyroids thrive on doing things that are worthwhile and are often idealistic, wanting to make a contribution to their world. With an affinity for both the theoretical and the practical, Thyroids are constantly formulating theories, then testing and refining them based on their practical application. Bridging the gap between the head and the body, or the mind and the emotions, Thyroids are able to see both sides of an issue, distill it, and communicate its essence.

CONFIRMING YOUR BODY TYPE

There are a number of different ways to accurately determine your type. Using several methods also provides a way of verifying, so you can feel confident you've identified your body type.

Photo Recognition

If you are visually aware or highly intuitive, look through the photos of the various body types and see if you can recognize yourself and others you know. A quick way to learn to identify body shapes for a specific type is to cover the heads and compare the bodies. The similarities will amaze you! You can also take a small photo of a person's head and place it on the various photos of the body types until you find the type that "looks" right, even with weight variations.

Photos & Essences

For a more detailed approach, evaluate the photos and note the types that are closest to your own set of photos. Once you have narrowed it down as much as you can, read the "Essences", choosing the one or ones that most accurately describe you. Read the complete "Psychological Profile" to make a final determination of your body type.

Weight Gain Pattern

Your first clue to determining your body type, or your dominant gland, is your weight-gain pattern. Where do you gain weight first? What area of your body poses the greatest challenge when you try to lose weight or maintain your figure? Your dominant gland corresponds with this particular area.

Physical Characteristics

Your general body build will also help identify your dominant gland. Height and bone structure, relative shoulder and hip width, the size and shape of your head and hands, are all considerations in determining your body type. Some types have particular identifying characteristics, such as head size in relation to body size, or thick, heavy eyebrows.

The key characteristics that are distinguishing factors for all body types include the degree of curvature of the lower back; the shape of the buttocks; and, most importantly, the areas of weight gain. There is a questionnaire available that uses these and other factors to help you identify your specific type.

Diet recognition

Look at the "Frequently" and "Rarely" foods for each of your considered types. Are the "Frequently" foods, for any one of these, the foods that you enjoy and eat often? Are the "Rarely" foods either those that you dislike or find don't agree with you?

Some people are so in tune with their bodies that they can identify their body type by finding the eating plan that they know best supports them. You may recognize your type simply by reading through the diets until you find the one that you know works for you. Most people who do this find that the diet validates what they intuitively knew, gives them menu suggestions, new ideas, and answers their nagging questions. In general, it fills in the missing gaps.

You may choose to simply experience different diets. This way you can follow a different diet until you find the one where you feel best. Even if you do select the wrong diet, you wouldn't be doing any more harm than you currently are if you don't know what is right for you or if you are trying one fad diet after another. If by any chance the diet you have chosen no longer feels appropriate, switch to another. Eventually, you'll find the right one.

Food Cravings

Another way to identify your dominant gland is to notice which foods you crave when your energy is low. Think about what you might want to eat if you were out shopping and stopped for a quick bite to eat. Would you choose sweets, such as ice cream or pastries? Or would you look for a fast food restaurant for something containing meat or salt?

Gonadal types, who crave fats, or Pituitaries, who like creamy foods, would probably choose the ice cream. Thyroid types would go for carbohydrates or sweets and would find a bakery where they could get a muffin or croissant. Adrenals, who are stimulated by salt and protein, would opt for the fast food restaurant where they could get a hamburger or a taco.

The Body's Response to Foods

Since certain foods stimulate, while others support or rebuild specific glands, the most accurate way of determining body type is by determining the body's response to particular foods. The easiest way to communicate directly with the body is through muscle testing, as this is a means of by-passing the conscious mind and all its beliefs and judgements. To distinguish body type, there are certain foods that types respond to differently, they are the "Key Indicator Foods By Type" and are found in the "*Muscle Testing*" booklet.

Psychological Profile

In addition to the physical characteristics, there are certain psychological tendencies, more pronounced in certain types, that will help you better define your body type. The "Essences" are the heart of the "Psychological Profile", and will give you a good idea of the basic nature of each type. You may wish to read through them until you find the one that fits. If you identify with several, read the entire "Psychological Profile".

Points of Connection

Points of Connection are your dominant traits. Do you rely most heavily on your mind or your emotions? Knowing whether a person's dominant sense is mental or emotional is invaluable in the job market, as it makes matching personalities with jobs much easier.

For example, Emotionals excel in jobs that require consistently meeting a lot of new people. Mentals are better suited for high stress jobs that require a lot of decision making.

Area of Attention

Another clue to determining body type is to notice the area of the body where your attention is immediately drawn. When you look at a person from a distance or in a full body photograph, do you focus on a specific area, such as the chest, lower abdomen, or head? If you're looking at a photo, you can cover one area at a time and observe where the energy is most noticeable. It may be in one region or, as in the case of the Lymph, Blood and Nervous System, all over. Once you've located an area, refer to the diagram on page 91 for the glands and organs found in that region. Investigate those types further, as the dominant gland, being the strongest, will emit the greatest amount of energy.

POINTS OF CONNECTION

A person's psychological profile is strongly influenced by the dominence of two out of four traits. Everyone has a stronger connection with either their mind – Mental, or feelings – Emotional as well as with either their Spiritual – intuitive or Physical aspects. The strongest ones seem the most real. The two dominant traits are referred to as "Points of Connection." All of the 25 types fall into one of these four categories. Identifying your strongest traits will go a long way in accurately determining your type.

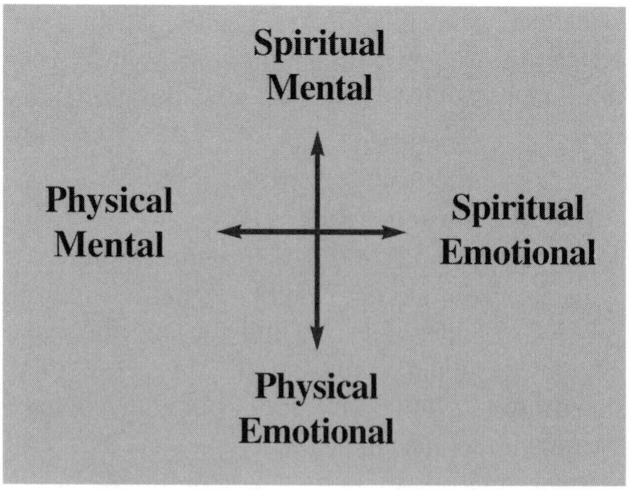

The first step is to identify your two dominant or connected traits. These "Points of Connection" are the areas you identify with most. One of our challenges in life is to connect with and integrate the other two points. The more you have done to develop the opposite trait, the harder it is to distinguish your strongest tendency. *If you have done this, remember back to a time before you made the decision to develop your complementary aspect.*

To determine your points of connection, honestly look at yourself. With both sets of statements, select the set that is most true for you. *Answer according to your feelings, not what you were taught.* Remember one is not better than another, it is just what you need for your life experience and it's absolutely perfect for you.

MENTAL *vs.* EMOTIONAL

What sense do you ultimately rely on most heavily, mental or emotional? This is often your first impulse, or your strongest influence. When faced with a difficult situation, do you rely most heavily on your ability to think it through logically (mental), or your feeling sense of how to handle the situation (emotional)?

Mental		Emotional
• My dominant sense is mental.	*vs.*	• My dominant sense is emotional.
• My initial response to things is to think first, feel later.	*vs.*	• My initial response to situations is to feel first, then think about it.
• At home, when someone wants me to do something, I respond best to suggestions or reasons why I would do it.	*vs.*	• At home, when asked to do something, I prefer people tell me what they want me to do.

PHYSICAL *vs.* SPIRITUAL

Do you relate or identify more with your body or your spirit? Are you a spirit with a body or a body with a spirit? If you identify most with your body, your reality is closely associated with your physical body, strength, or physical presence. If you identify most with your spirit, your reality is characterized by sensitivity, intuition, and a knowingness. People with a strong spiritual connection often approach unfamiliar situations and physical experiences with caution, while physicals will jump right in.

Physical		Spiritual
• I am a body with a spirit.	*vs.*	• I am a spirit with a body.
• I am much happier when life is not so complex.	*vs.*	• I prefer to accept life as it comes and adjust to it.
• I tend to look at new ideas and concepts after I've heard them 3 times.	*vs.*	• I tend to look at new ideas and concepts the first time I hear about them.

QUADRANTS

PHYSICAL/MENTAL

- **Adrenal**
- **Lymph**
- **Medulla**
- **Nervous System**
- **Spleen**
- **Stomach**
- **Thymus**

SPIRITUAL/MENTAL

- **Balanced**
- **Brain**
- **Eye**
- **Hypothalamus**
- **Pineal**
- **Pituitary**
- **Thalamus**
- **Thyroid**

PHYSICAL/EMOTIONAL

- **Blood**
- **Gallbladder**
- **Gonadal**
- **Kidney**
- **Liver**
- **Lung**
- **Pancreas**
- **Skin**

SPIRITUAL/EMOTIONAL

- **Heart**
- **Intestinal**

ICONS

The icons are *color-coded* according to the "Points of Connection". (See Centerfold.)

Red is Physical

Blue is Spiritual

Yellow is Mental

Rose is Emotional

Now read the "Essence" of the types in your selected quadrant. The one that rings most true is your type. As you read each "Essence," be aware that some will fit while others do not apply. One or two will ring very true for you.

Hint: To distinguish between the two or three types that are very close, highlight the phrases that are true with one color, the phrases that aren't as accurate with another, and those that don't describe you with a third color.

LOCATION OF THE 25 BODY TYPE GLANDS, ORGANS, OR SYSTEMS

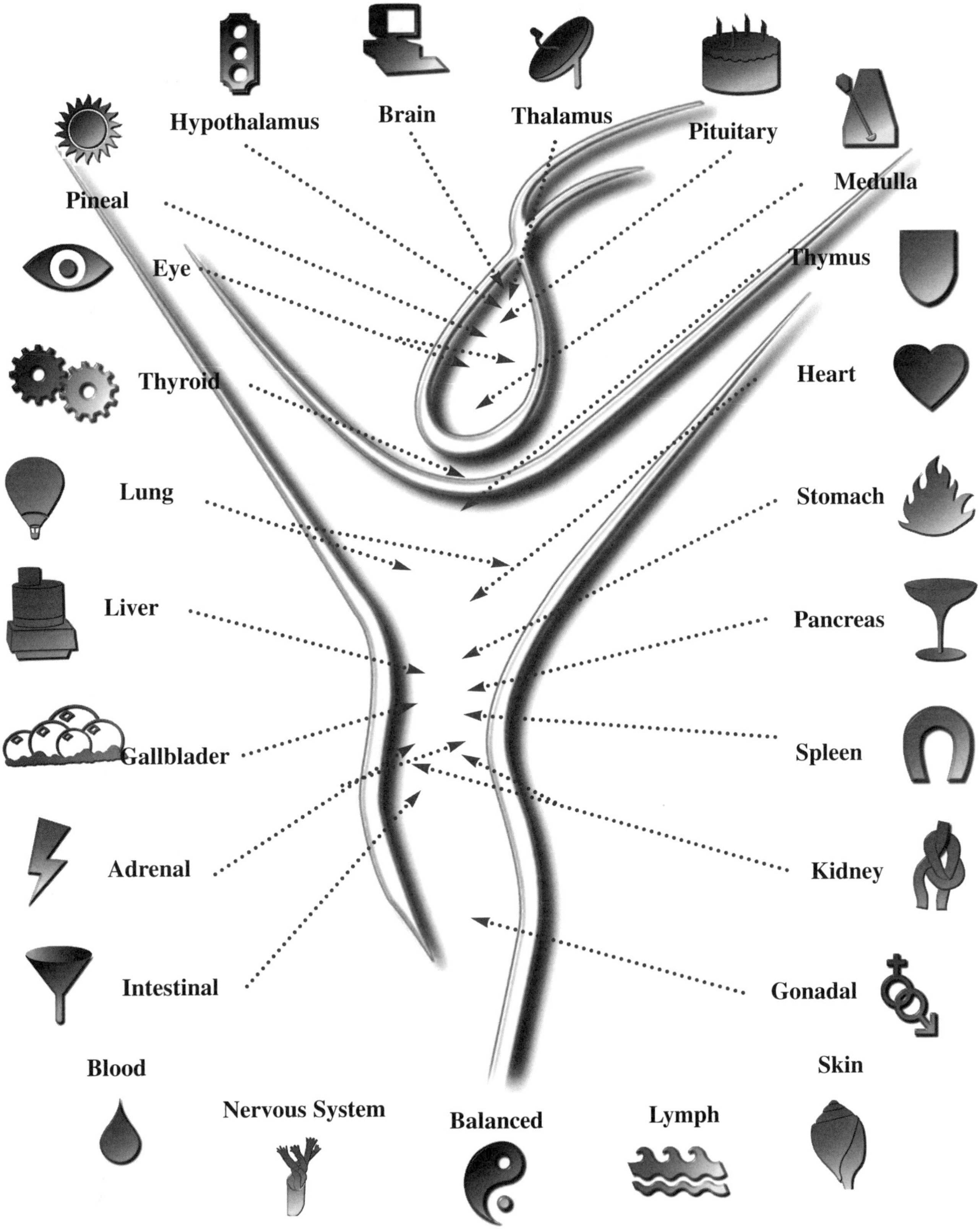

These organs or systems shown at the bottom of this page are located throughout the body.

AREA OF ATTENTION

A quick, visual way to narrow your choices of body types is to notice the area of the body where your attention is immediately drawn. When you look at a person from a distance or in a full body photograph, do you focus on a specific area, such as the chest, lower abdomen, or head?

If you're looking at a photo, you can cover one area at a time and observe where the energy is most noticeable. Since the dominant gland is the strongest, it will emit the greatest amount of energy. Consequently, the glands located in this area are the ones you will want to further investigate.

You may be drawn to one particular region or, as in the case of the Lymph, Skin, Blood and Nervous System, all over. Once you have located an area, refer to the diagram of the "Location of the Glands, Organs and Systems" (page 91).

Having identified the glands in your area of attention, go to the "Essences" (beginning on page 82), reading the ones you have selected until you find the one that fits. You've just identified your type!

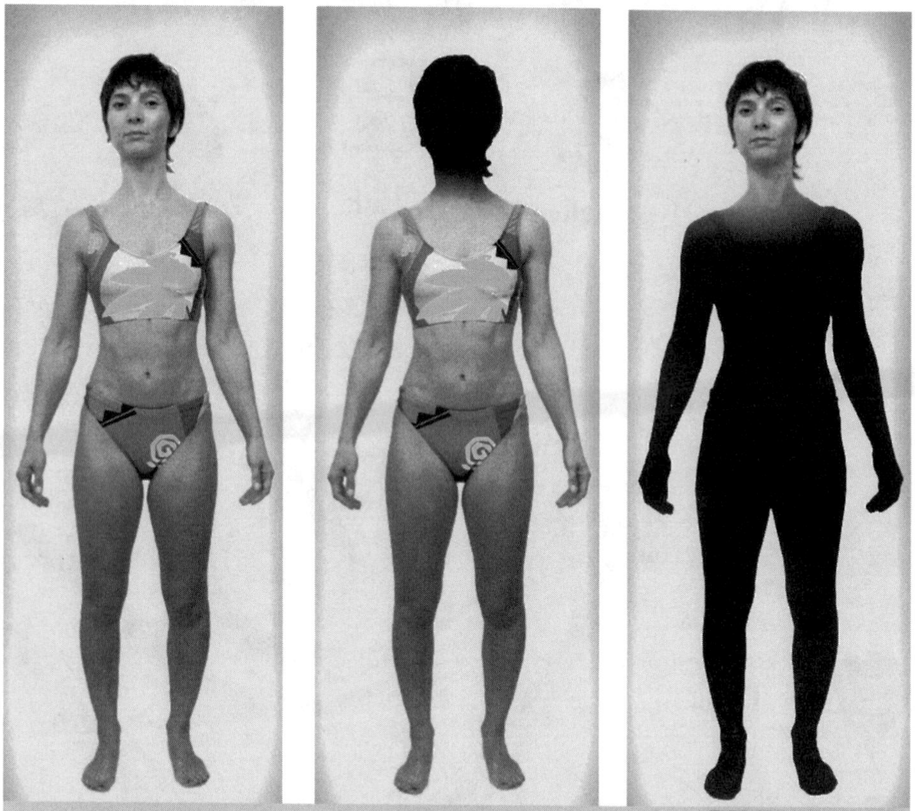

PINEAL

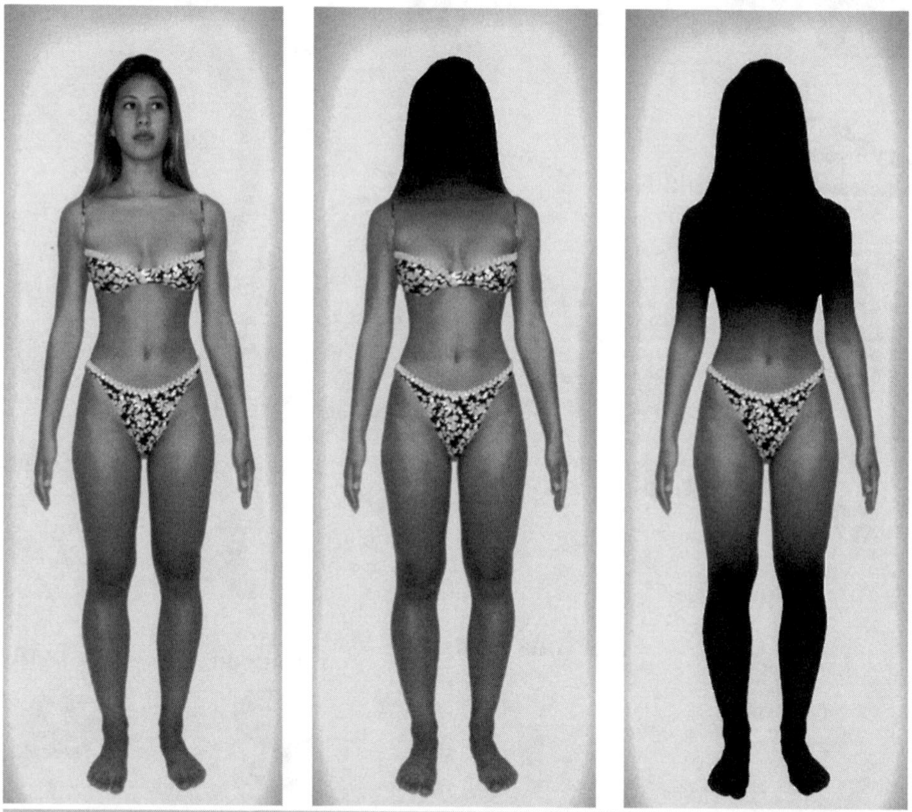

GONADAL

If you are not sure or would like further confirmation, refer to the "25 Body Type Photos" section. This will give you weight gain patterns and dominant characteristics.

DETERMINING THE AREA OF ATTENTION

• Look at the complete photo and notice where your attention is drawn.

• Look at the second photo. Is the person still there, or did they disappear?

• Look at the third photo. You will notice that Mr. Stomach disappeared but the other three are quite present.

• Take a photo of yourself and cover different areas. Notice when you disappear.

• Match the area of the body with the glands located in that area.

• Read the "Essences" for these glands. The one that fits you is your body type.

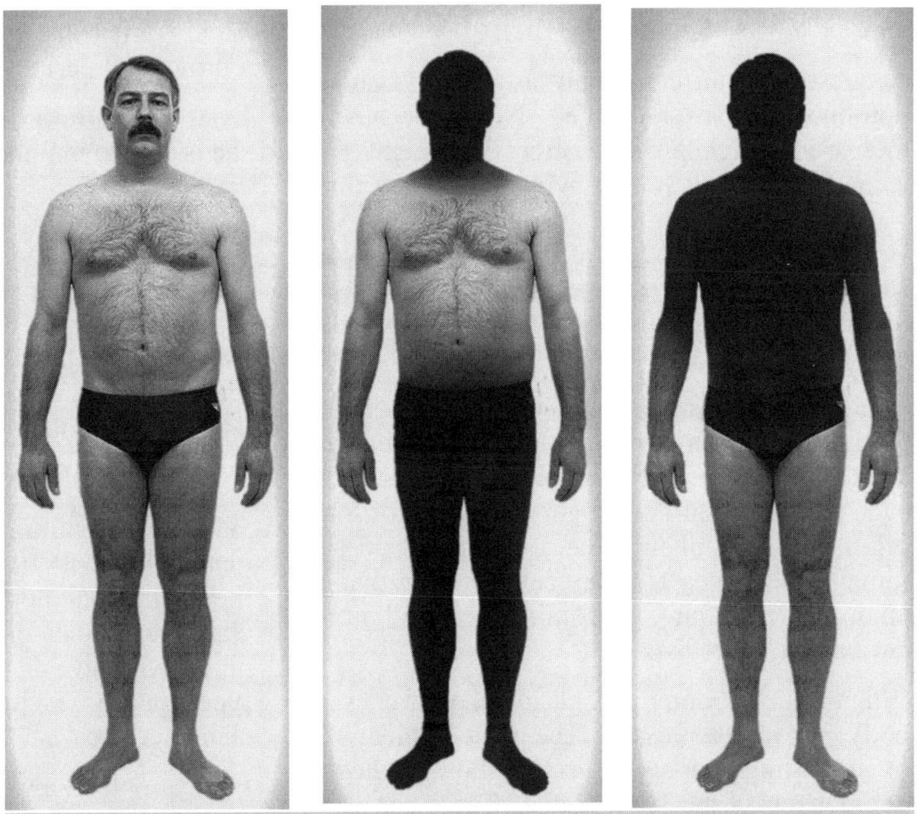

STOMACH

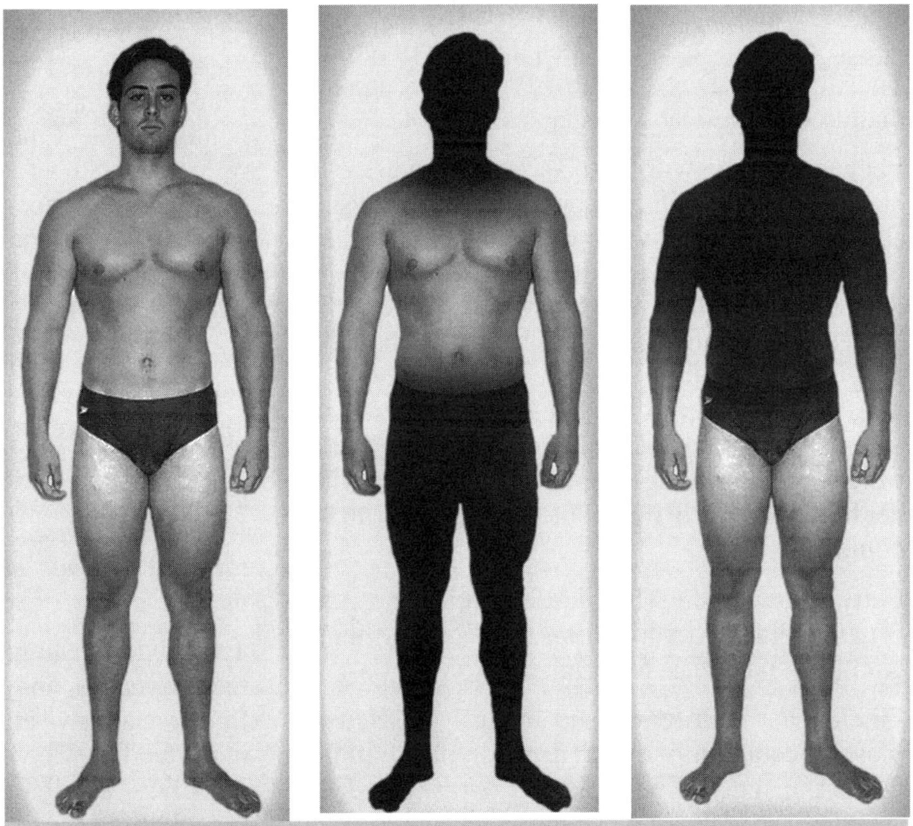

LYMPH

DOMINANT GLANDS: IMMUTABLE BUT EXHAUSTIBLE

A question I am commonly asked is, "Can my dominant gland ever change?" No, but because of increased weight gain, changes in weight gain areas, or different food cravings, you may think your dominant gland has changed. If you find yourself wanting different foods, your subdominant gland may be taking over. This is often an indication that your dominant gland is exhausted.

The dominant gland always stays the same, even though there can be major glandular changes, such as menopause. Redirection of life focus can even produce a shift in weight gain areas for some types. In spite of this, the dominant gland still remains the same. You can feel, however, that it's changed if your subdominant gland, also permanent, takes over.

When your subdominant gland takes over, your body is severely stressed. The most efficient way of supporting your system is by following the key components of the Thyroid diet. These consist of dense protein, a good variety of vegetables, and simple grains such as rice or oats. For some types, potatoes can be eaten instead of grains. The Sensitive Diet for most types is comprised mainly of protein and vegetables.

I began working with Betty, a woman in her mid-30's who had an obesity problem. Her physical characteristics were those of a Pancreas type, but through muscle testing I found that her body did not respond well to Pancreas foods. Betty did, however, respond well to Thyroid foods, so I suggested that she follow the Thyroid diet until those foods began to lose their appeal. Then she was to check the Pancreas foods to see if they were more appealing. This would indicate when her body was ready for the diet consistent with her dominant gland.

Betty followed the Thyroid diet until her system was strengthened enough to allow her dominant gland, the pancreas, to regain control.

Finally, her nutritional and dietary needs were those once again of the Pancreas type. Initially, when she ignored her diet and overstressed her system, she found she needed to eat more of the Thyroid foods to regain balance. Now, imbalance occurs only if her system is severely stressed over a prolonged period of time.

Even when Betty is remiss in her eating habits, she is able to maintain most of her weight loss and can easily return to her ideal diet. She is no longer susceptible to colds, has lost 30 pounds, and continues to lose her excess weight in a safe, comfortable manner. It is especially difficult for the Pancreas type to lose weight and keep it off. Betty's example shows that the correct body type diet can solve even the most difficult and stubborn weight loss problems.

VARIATIONS IN TYPE APPEARANCES

When determining someone's subdominant gland, you will find that it is most apparent in their physical appearance. Some people are classic examples of a particular body type, while others will have distinguishing features of another type along with their dominant gland characteristics.

For example, if a woman's dominant gland is 85% Pituitary and the subdominant is 15% Nervous System, she will look like a Pituitary with some minor Nervous System characteristics. If she is 55% Pineal and 45% Gonadal, she will have the prominent buttocks of the Gonadal and the small head of the Pineal. These details are also reflected in the foods and psychological profile for each body type. You may recognize your own subdominant gland more from the psychological profile for the type than from physical characteristics.

While it is interesting to learn what your subdominant gland is, it really isn't essential to know it. However, it can explain why people of the same body type, with the same dominant gland, appear so different. *Regardless of what your subdominant gland is, you will still follow the diet of your dominant gland, although you may be aware of some subdominant preferences.*

The subdominant gland provides the "coloring" for the grey areas in your body type determination. Since we all have all the glands, organs, and systems in our bodies, we will be able to recognize parts of ourselves in all of the body type descriptions, especially in the psychological profiles.

BASIC SIMILARITIES WITHIN TYPES

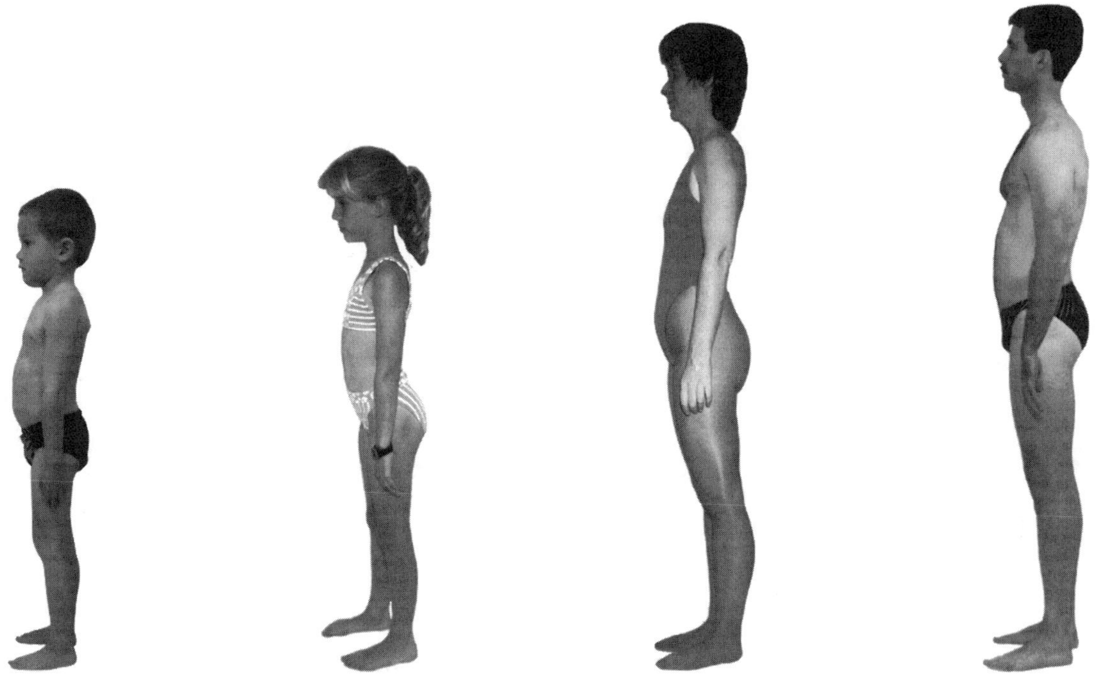

Slender appearance.
Average, elongated musculature.
Sway back.
Small buttocks.

Continuous abdominal arching
with slight protrusion
in lower abdomen.

THALAMUS BODY TYPE

Notice the similarity in body structure of the Thalamus body type. They all have a slender appearance, sway back, small buttocks, similar musculature of the thighs and calves, and a continuous abdominal arching, with a slight protrusion in the lower abdomen.

The basic body type characteristics are consistent within a type. These characteristics are apparent at an early age and are true for both men and women.

CONSISTENCY REGARDLESS OF AGE

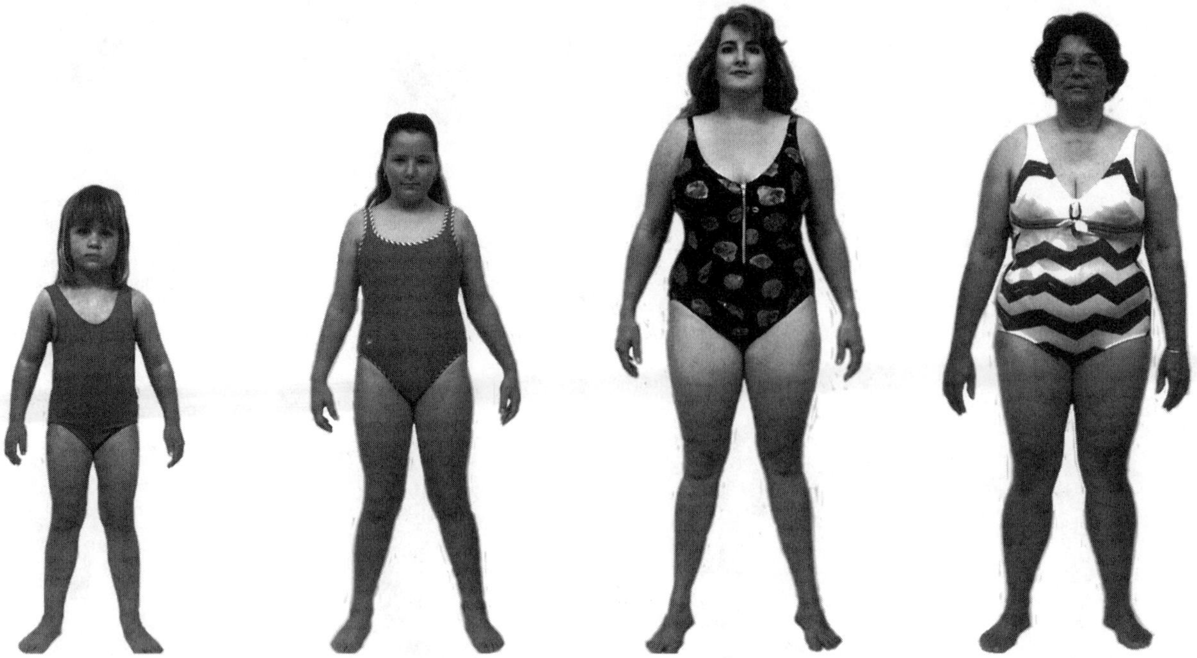

Wide sturdy grounded stance.
Strong, solid physical appearance.

Straight, poorly defined waistline.
Dense, solid musculature.
Short, thick neck.

ADRENAL BODY TYPE

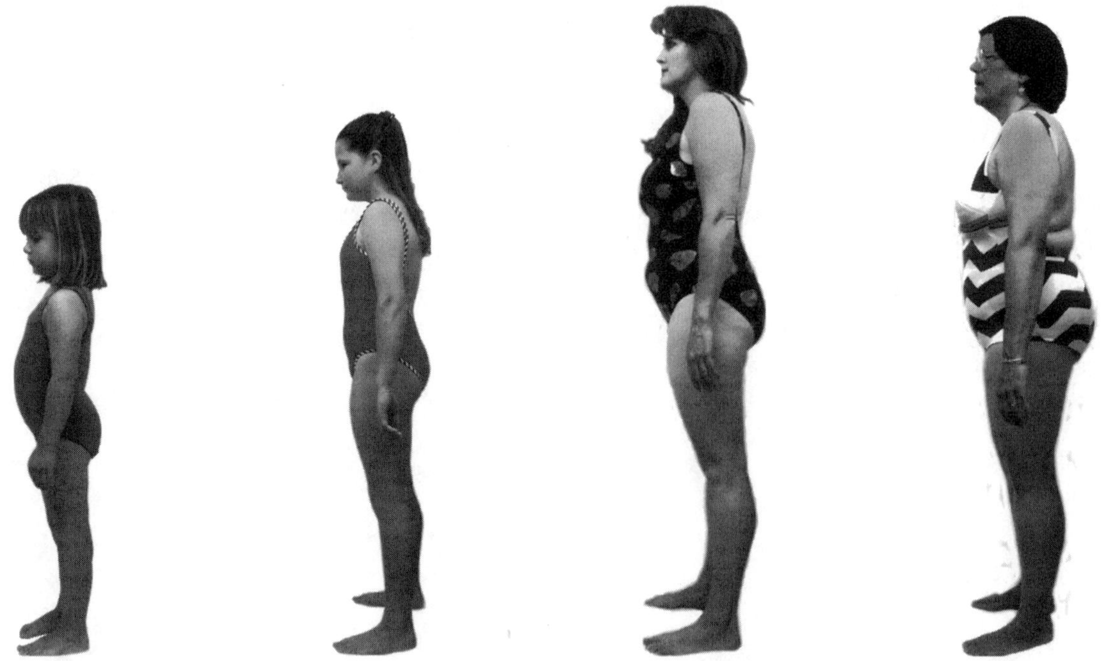

Small, rounded buttocks.
Average low back curvature.

Weight gain across upper back causing
"rounded" shoulders, thick torso.

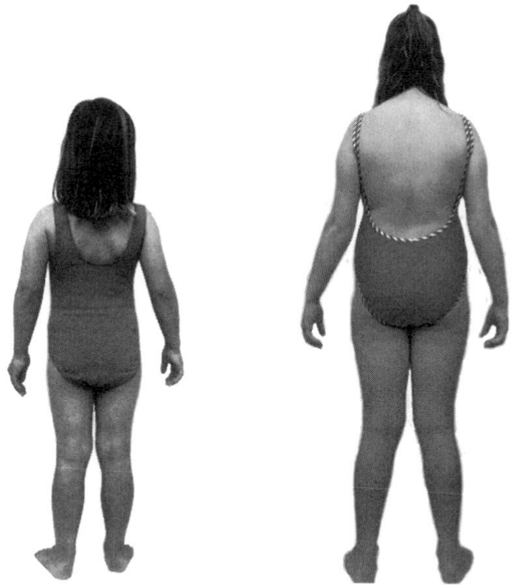

Relatively even hips and shoulders

Age is not a factor in identifying body type, nor is weight, as the relative proportions of the body will always remain the same. The size of the head, the shape of the face, back, and buttocks, the bone structure, definition of the waist, and relative width of the hips and shoulders will remain constant.

These Adrenals depict this consistency. There is also a similarity of stance, foot and leg placement, general posture, and the way the arms are held. Regardless of age, the width of the hips and shoulders are even, and the musculature in the torso, arms, and legs is dense and solid.

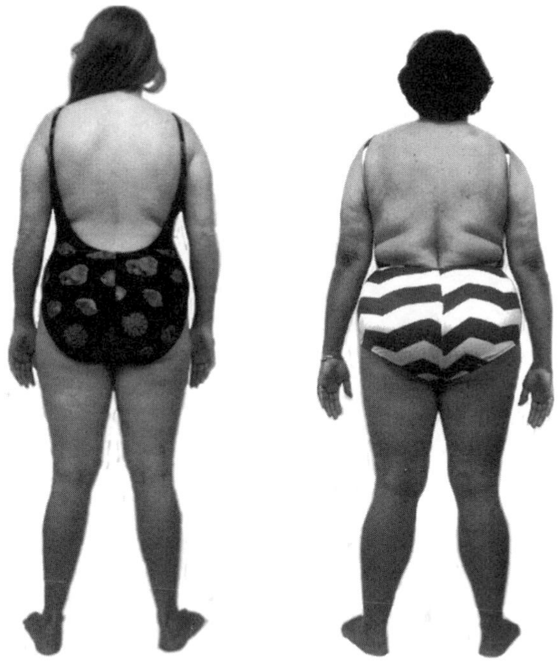

Weight gain in lower back, waist, and upper hips.

Whether you are looking at the 5 year-old or the 60 year-old, you will see the classic "boyish" Adrenal figure with the straight, poorly defined waistline. The feet are firmly planted on the ground, and the buttocks are small and rounded. You can see weight gain across the upper back (notice the "rounded" shoulders), lower back, waist, and upper hips. These are the types of characteristics that differentiate body types.

CHAPTER 3

THE FOUNDATION FOR DIETS

Debra first came to my office five years ago because she was interested in her diet. As a physical exercise instructor, she was very conscious of her weight and her overall health. As with many of us, she had accumulated a lot of conflicting dietary information over the years as to how and what she should eat. Because of the spiritual path she was following, she was on a vegetarian diet. While she was very conscientious about getting ample vegetable and dairy protein, she just was not feeling as well as she knew she should.

Debra was listening to "myths", "old wives' tales", and trying to make some sense of these in her own life. Because she lacked sufficient protein in her diet, she craved sweets. The fruits and vegetables she was consuming left her feeling like she needed "something more," but she didn't know what it could or should be. I told her that because of her body type she needed to eat more protein in the form of eggs, chicken, and fish. She was very reluctant to give up her well-engrained vegetarian habits, but she agreed to try it for two weeks.

Debra began to follow the Thyroid body type diet, and within the first week she noticed a marked improvement in her health. She lost her cravings for sweets and experienced more energy and a feeling of well-being. In spite of her dramatic success, old habits can be hard to break. So every so often, she'd slip back into them. Sometimes she'd just try different diets or get lax with her protein consumption, only to return to her body type diet when she felt her energy dropping or her body getting out of balance.

In health and diet, as with any subject, there are always "myths" that are prevalent and commonly accepted as fact. These are sometimes "old wives' tales" handed down through generations, or often simply new "fad" ideas that come into being and are accepted by a large number of people without scientific proof. The interesting thing about these myths is that they are so often repeated and widely believed without considering the effect they have on one's health.

NUTRITIONAL FACTS AND MYTHS

Myth #1 Cut Fats

Currently, the first, and perhaps most prevalent, dietary myth is, "The best way to lose weight is to cut the fats out of your diet." Actually, fat is essential in your diet, and its complete elimination, even for a short time, can damage your health and even cause weight gain. The key is knowing which kinds of fat and how much fat is best for your body type.

Myth #2 Margarine vs Butter

A second complementary myth is that vegetable fats are better than animal fats, which leads to "Margarine is better for you than butter." The problem is that we need essential fatty acids, of which butter is an excellent source, while margarine is not. Even worse, margarine contains molecules harmful to the body's cell structure, and its trans-fatty acid compounds (TFA's) have been directly linked to increased risk of coronary disease.

Myth #3 Raw Foods

A third misconception is, "If you eat only raw fruits and vegetables, you will lose weight." While this is true for some body types, such as the Adrenal, it is not true for everyone. For many other body types, this raw food diet can stress the body, causing it to produce excess hormones which are then deposited in weight gain areas.

Myth #4 Vegetarian Diets

A fourth assumption is, "Vegetarian diets are ideal for everyone." The truth is that only 13 of the 25 body types can get adequate nourishment from a vegetarian diet. This means that their bodies can obtain sufficient protein by eating only plant or dairy foods. However, when stressed, as is the case when they are carrying excess weight or fighting an illness, they need to include dense protein to make adequate protein absorption easier. Of the 13 types who would be able to stay healthy on a vegetarian diet, the percentage of dense protein (eggs, fish, chicken, beef, pork, etc.) that they might comfortably assimilate ranges from a low of zero to 10% for the Adrenal, Gonadal, and Pancreas, to a high of 30% for the Pituitary. The 12 body types who cannot get the protein they need from a vegetarian diet range from requiring a minimum 5-35% of dense protein for Blood types to a high of 10-40% for Eye types. The average range for most types is 10-30%.

Myth #5 Whole Wheat Bread

Another widely accepted myth is, "Whole wheat bread is an ideal source of complex carbohydrates." Of the 25 body types, only the Adrenal and Stomach can eat whole wheat bread more than twice a week without stressing their digestive systems. This stress is most commonly manifested as bloating and weight gain. Nine other body types should eliminate whole wheat bread completely or eat it no more than once a month. These are the Gallbladder, Gonadal, Heart, Kidney, Liver, Lung, Pancreas, Pituitary, and Thyroid. The remaining types fall somewhere between these extremes, with average consumption of once or twice a week.

Even the 7-grain, multi-grain, or 7-grain sprouted breads don't offer a better solution unless you are a Lung type. Most types have as much difficulty digesting them as they do the whole wheat breads. The Pancreas, Pineal, Pituitary, and Thyroid types should eat these breads only on a "rarely" basis.

The best sources of complex carbohydrates are whole grains, including oats, corn, pasta, and especially rice. Rice is the only grain that is not a "Rarely" food for any type. Many body types can eat oat bread, even though it contains wheat flour that is generally refined. Ideally, rice or oats should be eaten in the whole grain form. Breads, which consist of a combination of grain, yeast, and sweetener, often are difficult to assimilate. Since tortillas and pastas consist of simple grains, they are much easier to digest.

Myth #6 Sugar For Energy

Have you ever heard someone say, "I need some quick energy. I'll have a candy bar." A common misconception is that if you want to get a "boost" you should eat something that contains refined sugar. While sugar is essential for the body and the brain to function properly, it is glucose, the body's sugar, that is used for energy, muscle movement, and brain activity. Glucose is the end product of carbohydrate metabolism. Carbohydrates are sugars found in grains, vegetables, and fruits.

However, the simple sugars found in fruit are not the same as refined sugar. The difference is that natural sugars also provide nutrients that help digestion. Refined sugar may seem to boost energy but continual consumption can soon cause problems, as it will eventually exhaust the adrenal glands and deplete the body's mineral reserves. The problem is that refined sugar does not contain the minerals necessary for its digestion, so in the long run, refined sugar is a "downer."

Myth #7 Artificial Sweeteners

There is a common fallacy that "Artificial sweeteners are better for you than sugar." My own clinical experience suggests that each of the artificial sweeteners, including aspartame (NutraSweet®), are toxic to the liver and, in most cases, even more harmful than refined sugar.

Myth #8 Fruit Isn't Sugar

A misconception about fruit is, "Fruit is a safe substitute for sugar and since it's a natural food, it can be eaten anytime." The belief is that fruit doesn't count as sugar, which means that if a cookie is sweetened with fruit or fruit juice it moves out of the dessert and into the meal category. The reality is that fruit is still sugar. It just contains the necessary minerals to digest it. Unfortunately, fruit is not as easy for the body to utilize as you would think. For most types, there are one to two meals where it is best to avoid fruit, and while consistent within a type, this varies from type to type.

Fruit is a simple sugar, so it quickly gets into the bloodstream. It is more demanding on the body than complex sugars like grains, that require more steps to break down and take longer to move into the bloodstream. Because of the demand that regulating blood sugar places on the body, the best time to eat fruit is when your body has access to the greatest amount of energy. This generally corresponds to your high energy periods.

Myth #9 Liquids Are Water

Another incorrect assumption is about water. "In order to meet your body's need for water, you can drink any kind of liquid – coffee, tea, juice, soda, etc." It is a fact, that for optimal functioning of all bodily processes, especially elimination, an ample amount of plain drinking water is essential. When you drink other liquids, or even water that contains impurities, there is a reduced efficiency of your bodily systems that depend on clear water for proper functioning. The result of not drinking enough water is increased bodily stress. This doesn't mean that you shouldn't drink other liquids, but that you should always get plenty of plain water. To make sure you get the water your body requires, the basic rule is to drink a half gallon of water a day, that's 64 ounces, which equals eight 8-ounce glasses.

Myth #10 Microwave Cooking

Finally, the assumption that microwaved foods are as healthful as those cooked by conventional methods is false. Research continues to show that the molecular changes in food caused by microwave radiation make this food very stressful to the body. Read on for a more complete explanation.

MICROWAVE COOKING

When Ted came to me, he complained of a problem that he thought might indicate food allergies. Being nutritionally minded, he wanted to make sure he was eating right so he could eliminate the source of his discomfort. Ted had open sores, bright redness, and an extreme sensitivity in his mouth that had suddenly appeared. This could come from any one of a number of things, so I first questioned him about his eating habits. We went through what he was eating and then he told me that he cooked all his food in a microwave oven.

I checked his body's response to microwaved foods through muscle testing, and the response was a definite "no." I advised him to stop microwaving immediately and to notice if it had any affect on the redness in his mouth. One week later Ted came back to see me. The worst mouth sores I had ever seen were completely healed. He could eat anything without discomfort. Ted was a classic example of someone with a sensitive body type who was dramatically affected by microwaved foods. More often, I find people who notice increased colds and symptoms of a weakened immune system when using the microwave oven. There is enough evidence from controlled studies, as well as my personal observations, to support the premise that microwave ovens should not be used for cooking or even reheating foods.

In past years, microwave cooking has become an accepted method of cooking and heating foods. Only recently have we been warned of the dangers of radiation leakage in these appliances. It is well known that exposure to direct radiation from microwaves is definitely hazardous, and we have safety standards in place to minimize the risk. But there is another concern in using microwave ovens, and that is the harmful affects from eating irradiated food. Because these are indirect and not easily observed, there is little attention given to this aspect of microwave cooking.

It is assumed that microwaved food isn't affected in any way that makes it harmful to humans. The World Health Organization denies having information that microwaves adversely affect food. However, recent studies suggest that this information may be forthcoming.

A 1989 Microwave News report by University of Vienna researchers, first published in The Lancet, stated that milk heated in a microwave oven forms neurotoxic compounds (substances that have a toxic effect on nerve tissues) because of molecular changes in some of the amino acids.

Researchers at the Stanford University School of Medicine reported in the April, 1992 issue of Journal of Pediatrics that microwaving breast milk to warm it destroyed 98% of its immunoglobulin-A antibodies. These antibodies are necessary for the passive immunity breast milk gives the infant, as well as 96% of its lipsome activity, which inhibits bacterial growth. It was concluded that antibodies and proteins, which normally inhibit bacterial growth in breast milk, are broken down by microwave heating, reducing infection fighting properties of the milk and letting bacteria grow at a much higher rate than normal.

In a German study conducted in 1992, eight people ate a morning meal of either milk or lightly cooked vegetables, with some given food that had been microwaved. During the course of the two month study, each subject had blood drawn three times a day to test the nutrient and bacteria levels. Blood measurements of those who ate microwaved foods were especially disturbing, indicating food alterations which were impossible to measure before ingestion.

Among the findings:

1. A decline in various hemoglobin levels due to microwaving. This may signify anemia which can lead to rheumatism, fever, and thyroid insufficiency.

2. Those given microwaved vegetables showed the greatest drop in lymphocytes and the highest rise in leukocyte counts. This indicates the body responded to the food as if it were an infectious agent.

3. Both high density and low density level lipoproteins, measures of cholesterol, rose significantly after the vegetables were eaten.

4. The radiation levels of light emitting bacteria were highest in those who ate microwaved food, indicating the microwave energy may have been transferred from food to subject.

It is not surprising that microwaving food results in nutrient loss. This happens with all heating and cooking methods, but microwave cooking seems to produce the greatest loss of essential nutrients. What alarmed researchers most was that the blood of those who ate microwaved food showed pathological (disease related) changes in the body's cell structure. This was reported by Dr. Julian Whitaker in _Health and Healing: Tomorrow's Medicine Today_, 1993.

Swiss scientists Bernard H. Blanc and Hans U. Hertel conducted a study in 1989, using blood tests to determine effects of microwaved foods compared with those cooked in a conventional oven. Results showed that eating microwaved foods caused changes in blood chemistry similar to those present in the early stages of cancer. Eating microwaved foods increased the body's tendency toward anemia and caused elevated cholesterol values, which are known to increase when the body is exposed to stress causing factors like radiation and toxic substances.

Regarding microwaved food, the report explained that "atoms, molecules and cells hit hard by this electromagnetic radiation are forced to reverse polarity 1-100 billion times per second. There are no atoms, molecules and cells of any organic system which are able to withstand such violent, destructive power. Structures of molecules are torn apart, molecules are forcefully deformed, and thus become impaired in quality." This shows how direct microwave radiation alters the molecular structure of foods to form unnatural patterns. Eating these microwaved foods results in bodily stress because the elements are difficult to digest, assimilate or eliminate.

After testing hundreds of people for tolerance to microwaved foods, I have yet to find any food or drink that has been cooked or heated in a microwave oven to be nutritionally acceptable. In working with overweight patients, I found that many noticed weight problems soon after they began using a microwave to cook or heat their food.

It is possible that, because of molecular alteration, all or part of microwaved foods can't be digested and thus become toxic substances in the body. If the body does not have the necessary energy reserves to eliminate the toxins, they are stored in fat cells or suspended in extracellular fluid, resulting in weight gain due to fat accumulation and/or fluid retention.

Not all body types react to toxicity in the same way. Some experience weight loss, especially if it is hard to keep weight on. Those with very strong systems are often not aware of adverse affects as they are strong enough to absorb the energy drain without any obvious symptoms. But, regardless, the immune system suffers the most stress, so you should avoid using a microwave for any kind of food preparation, even defrosting foods and heating water. This is vitally important if you have a weight problem or trouble with your digestive or immune system. It may seem a hardship, but you will be healthier for it.

ALTERNATIVE COOKING METHODS

I'm always amazed when I tell patients to give up microwave cooking at how many of them will ask me, "If I don't use the microwave, how can I heat my food?"

Go back to cooking the way you did before microwaving food became popular.

- **Steaming is excellent**, and if you don't want the extra moisture, use a double boiler. If you're heating food that contains a lot of juices, put it in a dish inside the steamer; this way the juices will stay in the dish.
- When you're at work where you don't have a stove, **use a fifth burner.** You can even bring your food in a corning ware dish so you don't have to wash an extra pan.
- **Toaster ovens** are excellent for certain foods, as are convection ovens, especially if want to reduce cooking time.
- **Leftovers can be heated** in a skillet, frying pan, wok or by steaming.
- When you cook, package the leftovers into **individual serving sizes.** This is a good way get away from rut eating, because now when you're hungry you don't have to go to all the work of preparing a healthy meal. Simply take your food out of the freezer and put it in the steamer. This is usually what I do in the mornings for breakfast. I'll put something on, go take my shower, come back and it's ready.

THE SEVEN ESSENTIALS OF LIFE

Dietary Basics and Other Frequently Overlooked Facts

Judy came to me complaining of low energy, frequent infections, and a sensitivity to many foods. She had tried to eat "light" with meals of rice, legumes, and vegetables, but she was left feeling tired, irritable, and often bloated. When she resorted to eating just salads, she would lose weight, which was the last thing she needed as she was naturally thin. In determining Judy's body type, I found her to be a Pineal. Unfortunately, her eating habits were not supporting her type. By following the basic Pineal diet, she was able to meet all her dietary needs. Now she was able to support her body and keep her system in a good healthy balance.

In planning any dietary regimen, there are basic nutritional requirements that must be met. These basics, and your understanding of them, offer the foundation you need for your own eating plan.

Dietarily, the seven essentials of life are: protein, carbohydrates, fats, minerals, vitamins, water, and fiber.

The reasons for including all of these elements in your diet will become more clear as you understand their importance.

Protein

As protein is digested, it is broken down into amino acids. There are 22 different acids, all of which must be present for the body to make its own protein. However, only ten of these are essential for life, as they cannot be made by the body but must be supplied by what you eat. Amino acids, the building blocks for protein, are used in the structure of your body's tissues, hormones, enzymes, brain control substances, and antibodies. Your immune system is also heavily dependent upon protein which explains why chicken soup is such a good cold remedy.

Best Sources

The best sources of high quality protein, meaning protein that contains all the essential amino acids in abundance, are fish, chicken, turkey, animal meats, and eggs. The protein found in these foods is referred to as dense protein.

Small amounts of one or more essential amino acids can be found in beans, rice, grains, cereals, and soybeans. Consequently, these are not considered good sources of protein. Half the body types are able to obtain adequate protein from these foods, and therefore, are able to maintain a vegetarian diet when balanced and healthy. The other types require the previously mentioned, high quality, or dense protein.

Why we require protein

Protein is found more abundantly in the body than any other substance except water, and is crucial for good health. The deficiency of this substance can cause stunted physical growth, weakness, poor stamina, hormonal problems, brain dysfunction, depression, and learning difficulties. Lack of adequate protein can also cause poor immune system function, with a lowered resistance to disease, and a slower recovery from illness and injuries.

Essential amounts of protein will vary with individuals and the seasons, but adequate consumption of protein is extremely important for everyone. What you, in particular, may need will vary as your body goes through its natural cycles of building and cleansing.

Your body will need more protein during a "building" phase, such as after an illness or when you are under an extreme amount of stress. During a "cleansing" phase, your body will require less protein and you can eat more of either fruits or vegetables, depending on your body type. As your body goes through these different phases, you can learn to recognize its needs and eat accordingly.

Protein requirements vary with body type. Adrenals, for example, can generally get adequate protein from a vegetarian diet because of their inherently strong bodies. Thyroids, on the other hand, are more delicate and need highly concentrated protein, more than they are able to obtain from vegetable sources.

The best sources of protein for you will depend upon your body type. Eating protein unsuited to your type can lead to a protein deficiency and an imbalance in your system.

Protein Assimilation

A quick way to check for poor protein assimilation is to notice your body after you've eaten dairy products. If you have excess mucous in your throat, your protein is not being completely assimilated. Dairy protein is the easiest to digest and unless you have a dairy sensitivity, excess mucous indicates that you are not completely assimilating the other protein you are eating either.

Noni

The best product I have found to aid in protein assimilation, as well as enhance digestion in general, is Noni™. Noni is a fruit that has been used as a main healing agent in the Polynesian Islands, Hawaii, and parts of Australia for over 2000 years. Dr. Heinicke identified the active substance as a precursor to an alkaloid that he named xeronine. Xeronine is a substance the body produces in order to activate enzymes so they can function properly. It is basic to the functioning of proteins, so it energizes and regulates the body, and strengthens the immune system. The body must have it before it can do anything that requires protein, which includes manufacturing digestive enzymes, antibodies, hormones and doing any form of healing. Noni is probably the best source of proxeronine that we have today. It's available in a liquid form, and is best taken on an empty stomach. Noni can even be applied topically to problem areas. It's one of the few products I've found that benefits most people. Additional information is located in the back of this book.

Listen to and be aware of what your body is telling you. If you're still having problems, you may need to use a digestive aid or work with a professional to enhance your digestive system.

VEGETARIAN DIETS

We now know that protein requirements, as well as the protein sources most easily assimilated, vary with each body type. Certain types, such as the Adrenal, Pancreas, and Hypothalamus, are well suited for obtaining adequate protein from dairy, beans, seeds and nuts, as long as their systems are healthy. When fighting an illness, or even when wanting to lose weight, dense protein is usually a better choice.

Other types, particularly the Lymph and often Medulla, are able to assimilate high quality protein in its most basic form, that is algae, especially the blue/green variety. Still other types, the Thyroid and the Eye, for example, need to obtain their protein from higher sources such as fish, shellfish, and fowl.

In choosing which protein you are going to eat, the quantity as well as quality is important. Too small an intake will cause the problems we have already mentioned, and too much protein can stress your system. It is possible to overload your system with protein, and this can eventually produce problems that range from clogged arteries to excessive toxicity. Either of these can have life threatening implications.

When your system becomes overloaded, either with an excess or deficiency of protein, it will often manifest a distinct body odor. With protein toxicity your body is unable to adequately remove dangerous wastes. Your body type profile will help you choose the type and amount of protein you need so you can avoid these problems.

Studies of people with a history of cardiovascular problems are usually done on the Adrenal and Blood body types, as they are most prone to heart attacks and fat clogged arteries. These types need to minimize their intake of high cholesterol foods such as eggs and beef, and in some cases eliminate them entirely.

Adrenal types do exceptionally well on vegetarian diets, and when healthy, their systems are actually stressed when more than 10% of their calories come from dense protein sources. This is very little protein, as 10% of a 2000 calorie diet is equal to 5.5 ounces of chicken breast or 6 ounces of tuna. This constitutes the entire allowance for a whole day! The typical male Adrenal eats twice this amount of protein in one sitting, and will generally do this at least twice a day. It is no wonder that, in my experience, coronary heart disease among Adrenal body types is so common.

Blood body types, on the other hand, need a minimum of 5% dense protein in their daily diets, and they can assimilate up to a maximum of 35% protein. So, in comparing these two types, only the Adrenal type would benefit from a completely vegetarian diet.

Carbohydrates

Carbohydrates are the foundation of all healthy diets, and eating an insufficient amount of them can create numerous problems in the body. Some of these include poor growth, low energy levels, anemia, impaired wound healing, and learning difficulties. Inadequate carbohydrate consumption can also result in the breakdown of lean muscle mass and proteins, as the body attempts to get its "fuel" from other sources in your body.

Best Sources

The principal carbohydrates are sugars and starches. One of the best sources of simple carbohydrates, which the body immediately absorbs, is fruit. The best sources of complex carbohydrates, which take longer to break down, are whole grains, such as oats and rice, and starchy vegetables, like potatoes, yams, squash, and peas.

When you eat complex carbohydrates in the form of whole foods, the time it takes for the system to break down the elements insures that sugar can be released into the bloodstream at a controlled rate. All the nutrients for proper digestion and assimilation are present in these foods, along with the bulk essential for proper intestinal activity and good elimination.

Poor Sources

Refined or highly processed foods are very poor sources of complex carbohydrates. Processed foods such as white flour and polished rice lack the fiber that is present in whole foods. These refined foods are also low in vitamins and minerals. Even though a package states that the food is "enriched," it does not necessarily mean that all of the essential nutrients that were removed during processing have been replaced.

Some other poor sources of carbohydrates are white sugar, honey, and high yield fructose from corn. They are poor because of the negative effect they have on blood sugar levels, as well as their deficiency in vitamins, minerals, and enzymes. *If sweeteners must be used, those refined from natural sources are preferable to artificial sweeteners.*

In testing people for their tolerance to artificial sweeteners, including aspartame, which is known as NutraSweet® or Equal®, it was found that the effects of these products can be quite damaging to the system. These substances are known to be toxic to the liver and even more detrimental than refined sugar. If you must sweeten your food, or drink soda, use sugar or drink regular soda instead of the artificially sweetened products.

Rice

Rice is an excellent complex carbohydrate. The next question is which variety. There is a general belief that brown rice is the better choice over white. The truth is that not everyone can digest brown rice, and there is even a difference between the assimilation of short and long grain brown rice. Gonadal and Thyroid types fare much better with short grain brown rice than the long grain variety.

Of all the rices, white basmati is the easiest to assimilate and is a "Frequently" food for all body types except the Nervous System. There is also a brown basmati rice which is even easier to digest than short grain brown rice. White basmati rice smells like popcorn when cooked, and is naturally white in color.

The white polished rice that is commonly sold in the United States is simply brown rice with the outer brown skin removed. These outer skins, or rice polishings, are then sold as rice bran. Another product is rice bran syrup, which is high in B vitamins and is an excellent sweetener.

Blood Sugar and Refined Sugar

Refined sugar is very similar to the glucose found in the blood, which we refer to as blood sugar. This blood sugar is critical to the proper functioning of your body and must be carefully regulated by your system. If your blood sugar level gets too high, you could go into a diabetic coma. If your blood sugar level drops too low, the result is insulin shock

The "ups" and "downs" you feel in your energy level are due to variations in the level of blood sugar in your system. *Since your brain is the largest consumer of sugar in your body, the first indication of a low blood sugar level is "fogginess" or irritability.*

Your liver is the primary controller of your blood sugar level, and measures the amount of sugar in your blood. When the level needs an adjustment, the liver signals the pancreas to secrete insulin, or tells the adrenal glands to secrete adrenalin. Increased insulin causes your blood sugar level to drop, and adrenalin will cause it to rise.

Sugar Sources and Their Effects

The body is designed to derive most of its blood sugar from complex carbohydrates. It takes time for the body to reduce these complex sugars to simple ones that pass easily into the bloodstream. When sugar is released into the bloodstream at a relatively slow rate, the body is able to maintain a fairly constant blood sugar level. That is, only minor adjustments from the pancreas and adrenal glands are needed for the body to perform smoothly.

When you eat simple sugars, like refined sugar, it throws the body's regulating system into chaos as this sugar instantly goes into the bloodstream. This occurs because refined sugar is very similar to the glucose found in your blood.

When this happens, the blood sugar level will rise dramatically. Then the liver signals the pancreas to secrete more insulin to offset the increase. The pancreas asks, "How much?" and the liver responds with, "I don't know! Sugar is coming in so fast, there is no way to measure. Dump whatever you have!" As the pancreas releases all its insulin into your bloodstream, your sharply rising blood sugar level suddenly drops.

The liver, which is carefully monitoring this situation, now signals the adrenal glands that the blood sugar level is getting dangerously low and directs them to secrete adrenalin. Increased adrenalin causes the blood sugar level to rise once again, stabilizing the system and avoiding a crisis.

This process occurs each time you eat refined sugar, and over time this seesaw effect between the liver, pancreas, and adrenal glands puts an excessive strain on your system. If you do this often enough, it eventually leads to exhaustion. Usually, your adrenal glands are affected first and then your pancreas.

When your adrenal glands become exhausted, the result is low blood sugar, also known as **hypoglycemia.** This occurs when your adrenal glands can no longer bring your blood sugar level back up to normal. Pancreas exhaustion affects carbohydrate metabolism and insulin production. *When any gland or organ is exhausted, your system becomes unbalanced. This imbalance affects your overall health, energy level, and weight.*

Since refined sugar is in almost everything, what can you do? Sugar is not inherently bad, and most types can handle some refined sugar in moderation. While your body needs sugar, it prefers to get it from complex carbohydrates.

When you have an imbalance, it is usually best to eliminate refined sugar as much as possible until your system has recovered. Once your balance has been restored, you can use small amounts of refined sugar in conjunction with other foods as these other foods can help supply the missing minerals. For example, molasses is the by-product of the sugar refining process and still contains all of the minerals that were removed in that process. By mixing it with granulated sugar, you restore the minerals that aid in digestion and assimilation of sugar.

An occasional large dose of sugar from a soft drink or candy bar can usually be tolerated without any noticeable effects. However, to keep your system healthy and in balance, these should only be occasional treats, preferably no more than once a month.

Other Sweeteners

Unfortunately, **artificial sweeteners** are not the solution they were expected to be. They are very hard for your body to break down and should be avoided. While they don't cause extreme blood sugar fluctuations, they are toxic to the liver. Aspartame has even been linked to brain seizures, vision problems, and dry eye syndrome. If you are noticing confusion, memory loss, or difficulty wearing contact lenses due to decreased tears, stop your diet drinks and artificial sweeteners. Using these in place of sugar is just exchanging one problem for another.

Honey is not the answer either. It is difficult for most types to digest, unless you are a Spleen or a Lung type. For the rest of the types, honey is a "Moderately"" or "Rarely" food as indicated on the food lists.

Some types, like Thyroids, can even be sensitive to the sugars in **sweet fruits,** such as oranges and bananas. Fruit sugars can overstimulate the thyroid gland. Anyone with a blood sugar problem should reduce and possibly eliminate fruit. Frequency and best time of day to eat fruit varies from type to type, so consult your food list for what's best for you.

Tart fruits like cherries, apricots, blackberries, or cranberries can provide the sugar that is often helpful in digesting protein without over-stimulating the thyroid gland.

Fruit juices can also provide a viable option for the desire for something sweet, as can vegetable juices like fresh carrot juice. Just be aware that sugar is still sugar and use accordingly.

For the most part, fruit is the best sugar source when you are craving something sweet. Heart types digest their lunch better when they have fruit for dessert. Adrenals need the thyroid gland stimulation they receive from eating very sweet fruits like bananas and dates. So, again, check your individual profile to find what is best for your type.

Fats

Fats are an important part of your diet for several reasons. They are a more concentrated form of energy than carbohydrates, and are needed by your body's system to properly use certain vitamins and minerals. Fats contain fatty acids, which like some specific amino acids, are essential to good health. These fatty acids cannot be produced in your body and must be supplied through the foods you eat.

Essential Fatty Acids

When your body is low on essential fatty acids, you will experience low stamina. Stamina is defined as strength and endurance, rather than energy. A simple way to test your stamina is to repeatedly test or challenge a muscle.

While you can use any muscle in the body, I like to use the pectoralis major clavicular muscle, which is a muscle in the upper chest that is described in test #2 of the *Muscle Testing* booklet. Test #1 works equally well, as the purpose is to determine your level of muscle endurance.

When performing the muscle test, apply pressure to the muscle, then release it. Repeat this cycle at the rate of about one test per second. Ideally, you should be able to resist pressure on the muscle for a minimum of 25 repetitions. If the muscle weakens before 25, you are low in essential fatty acids. If you stayed strong throughout the test, you have good stamina and could continue testing for a while without weakening.

Sources

If you do require additional fatty acids in your diet, the next step is to determine which source will be best for your body. From a maintenance standpoint, the best source is butter. Add this to your diet if you tested strong at 25 or weakened in the 20's.

If the muscle test showed a weakening before 20 repetitions, you will need the added support of a nutritional supplement. Professionally, I use a concentrated source of essential fatty acids. The best one varies from individual to individual. Those from which I consistently get good results are by Standard Process, Inc: Chlorophyll Complex Perles, Cataplex F Perles, Sesame Seed Oil Perles, Linium B6, and Super EFF, or Biotics Research Corp.: Flax Seed Oil, or Bioctasol Forte, or Metagenics or Ethical Nutrients: Chlorotene. If you have questions regarding your particular needs for fatty acids, contact your health professional.

Fat Sources

The best sources of fats in your diet are fish, chicken, turkey, animal meats, butter, and egg yolks. Egg yolks, in some cases raw, have been found to be excellent in lowering cholesterol, which may seem contrary, since egg yolks contain large amounts of cholesterol.

The reason for the beneficial effect of eggs is that for many types they build the adrenal glands. Foods that support the body lower the overall stress on the system, and this in turn lowers cholesterol.

Cholesterol

Only 10-30% of your body's cholesterol comes from the foods you eat. The other 70-90% of your total cholesterol is manufactured internally. The liver senses the amount of dietary cholesterol present in your system at any given time. It then synthesizes what your body needs through an internal communication network that includes the intestinal cells and the adrenal cortex. *Cholesterol production is essential as it is needed for hormone production, as well as the manufacture of antibodies and enzymes.*

When your body is stressed, it's the adrenal glands that initiate the "fight or flight" response by pumping adrenalin into your system. Cholesterol is used to form the hormones secreted by the adrenal cortex. It is reasonable to say then that the adrenal cortex has the highest cholesterol synthesis rate of all cells. Adrenalin goes directly to your muscles, so you have a choice to "fight or flee" when faced with a stressful situation.

It is not often that your reaction will call for the "fight or flight" response that would effectively burn up this adrenalin. *So, when adrenalin is not used, it backs up in the body and is stored as fat.*

Since stress, whether it be physical, emotional, dietary or immune, is so much a part of daily life, the adrenal glands eventually become exhausted. Once this happens, the body will call on your dominant gland to produce whatever hormones are manufactured by that gland. Then, if these hormones are unable to solve the problem, they will be stored away as excess fat in the corresponding weight gain area.

Cholesterol is essential for the formation of hormones, enzymes and antibodies. If your cholesterol is high, it may be because your body is (1) producing an excessive amount of hormones due to system imbalance, or (2) it is forced to make large amounts of enzymes because of poor diet, or (3) the immune system is fighting an infection and needs to build antibodies.

When under stress, the body's cholesterol levels rise to enable it to produce what it needs. High cholesterol is a symptom of stress. The solution to correcting the condition is to identify and solve the problems that caused the stress.

Adrenal body types are the most susceptible to cholesterol problems because their strong adrenal glands represent their body's backup system. Their bodies will actively "prepare" for stress by maximizing cholesterol from everything they eat.

When Adrenals are stressed, they crave salt and red meat, which stimulate the adrenal glands and cause them to produce even more cholesterol. Since Adrenals are prone to heart attacks and strokes, the recommendations put out by the American Heart Association should be heeded by all Adrenal types. The suggestions are for regular physical exercise and strict limits on eating eggs, salt, and red meat as preventative measures. The best form of exercise for Adrenals is daily running, as this releases the excess adrenalin stored in their muscles.

While these guidelines are generally good, they don't completely apply to all types. The Thyroid body types, for example, need to eat more protein to strengthen and rebuild their adrenal glands. Chemically speaking, the lack of thyroid hormones in the system increases blood cholesterol concentration, while excess thyroid hormones decrease it.

The Adrenal body types need to stimulate the thyroid gland by eating more sugar, such as those found in sweet fruits, while the Thyroids need to minimize these sugars and eat more protein. Since eggs are the most complete protein source, as well as the greatest source of cholesterol, they are an ideal food for Thyroids who tend to be more predisposed to cancer than heart attacks and strokes.

Lowering the cholesterol in your diet is usually not sufficient by itself to bring a high cholesterol level down to normal. It can actually aggravate the problem if the change in diet puts additional stress on the system. For example, eggs are a supportive food for the Thymus type who actually thrives on four eggs a day, particularly for breakfast. Ideally, they should eat four eggs six times a week! Eliminating them would remove that support. While cholesterol in the diet is reduced, the increased stress on the system could actually result in higher cholesterol levels.

Eggs have just the opposite effect on Adrenal types because they are stimulating to their systems and will aggravate a cholesterol problem. Even though the actual cholesterol content of certain foods may be incidental, it is how the body responds to them that is important. In some cases, cholesterol-rich foods like eggs can cause major stress to the system, causing cholesterol levels to rise significantly. Eliminating these foods can reduce stress and effectively reduce cholesterol.

There is a great deal of negative emphasis on high cholesterol levels which often causes people to think it is healthy to have unusually low cholesterol levels. However, having a very low cholesterol level is a condition that can be even worse than having levels that are too high.

When cholesterol levels are high, it means the body is responding to a problem and its defense mechanisms are working. When the cholesterol levels drop below normal, it can mean that the body's system is just too exhausted to activate its defenses. A person with low cholesterol levels is apt to be extremely ill.

Inadequate Fats

In most diets you will find that there is an emphasis on the elimination of fats, as well as cholesterol. However, these diets rarely distinguish between fats that are beneficial and those that are harmful. Certain fats are necessary for good health, while others cause problems.

Sources

The obvious fats to reduce or eliminate in any diet are those that don't supply the body with essential fatty acids. These are lard, saturated oils like peanut and coconut, hydrogenated or partially hydrogenated oils, and polyunsaturated oils.

Hydrogenated polyunsaturated oils, which are found in many of our processed and prepared foods, are the primary ingredient in margarine.

Hydrogen is added to these oils to make them solid at room temperature. This causes the molecules to be twisted in such a way that, when eaten and taken into your cell membranes, they impede normal cell function. These are also difficult, if not impossible, to break down.

Effects

Some of the negative effects of these products are a weakened immune system, impaired growth, accelerated aging of the skin, and arterial damage including hardening of the arteries. Needless to say, these are not conditions that would be acceptable or attractive to any of us.

TFA's

In an article in American Journal of Public Health (1994) two Harvard scientists spoke out against the ingestion of margarine. They wrote that margarine contains compounds called "trans-fatty acids", which are by-products of the hydrogenation process that converts oil into a semi-solid spread to make it usable in cooking and eating. They discussed how these trans-fatty acids, or TFA's, can raise blood levels of bad cholesterol, LDL, while lowering levels of the good kind, HDL.

These scientists cautioned that the ingestion of TFA's could be much worse than eating saturated fats. They estimate these substances cause 30,000 deaths a year in the U.S. from heart disease. Reducing calories by using margarine instead of butter is not a valid reason for eating it. The calories in a tablespoon of butter and a tablespoon of margarine are just about the same. The increased risk to health by eating margarine instead of butter is far too high.

Fats In Weight Loss

When your body does not get a sufficient amount of fatty acids, you can suffer any one of a number of ailments. In women, a deficiency in these fats is directly related to hormonal imbalances that can cause menstrual problems, PMS, and the inability to become pregnant. Weight gain is also a common occurrence.

I once worked with Betty, a woman who was determined to lose weight. She started by lowering her fat consumption, which she assumed was a reasonable means of getting rid of her body fat. Unfortunately, the result of Betty's efforts was a weight increase of 25 pounds in the course of 5 years, because she wasn't getting enough fat.

Betty is a Gallbladder, a type that does not do well on low fat diets. Fats are essential for the digestion of carbohydrates. When Gallbladder types don't get enough fat, they gain weight in their lower abdomen due to poor carbohydrate digestion. They can assimilate bread and butter, but the bread alone is too hard to digest and results in weight gain. Other types, like the Stomach and Adrenal, need a very low fat diet if they are to lose weight.

Fat Deficiencies

Fat deficiencies can also result in poor growth and skin problems. Gonadal types will often have dry skin and very stiff hair on their arms if they don't get enough of the proper fats in their diet. With all types, the development of a callous around the heel of the foot is a symptom of poor fat assimilation.

While butter is an excellent general source of fatty acids, a few body types are better off eating other fats. Olive oil or walnut oil is a better choice for some. The best fat sources are consistent within types and are listed in the individual profiles.

My stressing the importance of adequate fat consumption does not mean that I advocate a high fat diet. The point I am making is that fats are an important dietary element and must be consumed from the proper sources in appropriate quantities. Either too much or too little can be detrimental. *Optimal health requires maintaining the correct balance of fat in the diet, and this varies according to the body type.*

Fats are essential because the body requires them to produce antibodies which are at the core of the immune system.

The Immune System

In order for you to maintain good health and live a long happy life, you must have a strong immune system. Your immune system is a structure of antibodies, blood cells and chemicals that protect you against illness and disease. These are the "soldiers" of your body, guarding you against bacteria and viruses. Keeping these "troops" in top condition is vital to staying healthy.

Chronic pain or weakness is often the result of inflammation caused by bacteria normally present in your body in small amounts. When your immune system is impaired, these bacteria multiply and cause pain in your joints, like arthritis, or weaknesses in various organs, such as the stomach, liver and bladder.

Eliminating all of the harmful bacteria from what you eat, while maintaining a nutritionally sound diet, would be an impossible task. But you can exercise cleanliness in the preparation of your food and avoid spoiled food or that which is past its "prime" eating time. These measures will help to minimize the bacteria, so they can be easily controlled by a healthy system.

The acids in your stomach usually destroy most of the bacteria in the foods you eat, and the healthy functioning of your immune system keeps the remainder under control. But, if your digestive organs are overstressed because of poor diet, that is, one that does not support your particular body type, then you may be opening yourself to bacterial infection.

This can occur when your stomach acids have become too weak to break down the bacteria, allowing a larger number than usual to get into your body. Now your immune system must get to work to eliminate the bacteria, but it is already overworked trying to remove all the undigested protein that got into your bloodstream because of a weakened digestive system. Imagine the chaos going on in your body!

Now the immune system is scrambling to get rid of the excess bacteria coming out of the stomach, and to eliminate the foreign protein molecules that were not properly digested. Needless to say, the eventual condition is that of immune system fatigue and illness. The bacteria have begun to win the battle and the effectiveness of the immune system is significantly diminished. Your "soldiers" are exhausted and your "troops" are retreating. Poor diet, which caused digestive weakness, in turn, is causing the immune system to fail.

Bacteria: Staph and Strep

Staph (staphococcus) and strep (streptococcus) are the most common bacteria found in the body. When the immune system is weakened, these bacteria multiply and attack weak areas. Strep goes after the blood vessels in a debilitated area.

Anyone who has a genetic tendency towards vascular weakness will be especially vulnerable to the damage that strep can do to the blood vessels. When the blood vessels are attacked, the body attempts to "patch them up" with cholesterol, which builds up on the vascular wall and eventually causes a constriction in the flow of blood and hardening of the veins and arteries.

When there is a build-up of cholesterol in the blood vessels, one can experience headaches (often after exercising), fatigue, low-grade fever, light-headedness and a general lack of energy. The buildup of cholesterol in the blood vessels is a symptom of the more serious issue of a weakened immune system.

Vascular problems, chronic pain and weakness are some of the ailments associated with a diminished immune system that can originate from a poor diet. The body has the ability to heal itself if given the support it needs including a proper diet on a continuing basis.

Minerals

There are numerous minerals in your body and skeletal structure, and the constant replenishment of them is important to staying healthy. Minerals are vital. If you don't get the ones you need in sufficient amounts, either in your diet or through supplements, or you're not absorbing them, you won't be able to absorb vitamins either.

The minerals most abundantly found in the body are sodium, potassium, calcium, chloride, magnesium, and phosphorous. Sodium and potassium are needed to control water balance in your tissues. Calcium is necessary for nerve conduction, and magnesium is vital to the vascular and cardiovascular systems.

Other minerals essential for your body are manganese, which benefits your ligaments and connective tissue, iron that enriches your red blood cells, and copper, which helps to utilize the iron. The body needs zinc for the prostate and immune system, iodine for the thyroid, and chromium for the pancreas to regulate blood sugar.

Selenium, in very small amounts, will help to prevent cancer and heart disease. Also needed is cobalt, an important element in Vitamin B12 which prevents and cures anemia, and the trace mineral, molybdenum. Additionally, there are about 35 other trace minerals that are needed in the diet in varying amounts.

The body needs these minerals for vital functions such as water balance, nerve conduction, enzyme regulation, bone formation, and muscle contraction. Mineral deficiencies can cause dysfunctions such as irregular heartbeats, breathing difficulties, water retention or edema, high blood pressure, a weak immune system, and poor bone growth.

Sources

It is understandable how your daily functioning could be extremely hampered with a severe deficiency in the proper amount of minerals in your diet. The best sources for minerals are fish, chicken, turkey, animal meats, nuts and seeds, green and yellow vegetables, and fruits.

Highly processed or refined foods, especially those with extra salt and other additives, may seem more appealing and tastier than the more "natural" foods. However, they are very poor sources since many of the essential minerals have been removed.

Calcium: Necessary Factors for Assimilation

One of the biggest health problems many older people face, particularly women, is inadequate calcium utilization and the resulting diseases. It is often assumed that one can simply take a calcium supplement and all will be well, but it is not quite that easy. Even when there is sufficient calcium, all too often it simply isn't being assimilated by the body because of deficiencies in other elements, especially magnesium.

Magnesium

While essential to the assimilation of calcium, magnesium is also needed for the flexibility of muscles and ligaments. Infants, who have a high flexibility factor, have a high magnesium-to-calcium ratio. Older people, however, who are stiff, inflexible, and arthritic, have this ratio reversed. Fortunately, this can be helped with proper diet and nutritional supplements.

Sources

As with any other element, it is possible to get too much magnesium. If this happens, you get diarrhea. Simply stop your magnesium until the diarrhea clears, then resume at a lower dosage. Excellent sources of both calcium and magnesium are fresh green vegetables, such as broccoli, and nuts, especially almonds. The best way to determine your mineral levels and ratios is through a mineral analysis using your hair as the tissue sample.

Assimilation

Insufficient amounts of Vitamin B6 can also cause improper calcium assimilation. Some good sources of this vitamin are meats and whole grains. Also, people who tend to be rather sedentary are at a greater risk of calcium deficiency than those who exercise regularly. Walking each day, especially in sunlight, can help improve your calcium assimilation.

There are some excellent nutritional formulas developed to prevent osteoporosis. Supplements are often necessary to correct any mineral deficiencies you may have, especially if your system is extremely out of balance. As you become healthier, the best way to get your minerals is from the food you eat. Eating a diet that contains the proper minerals ensures that they are found in combination with other elements needed for their digestion. Muscle testing is one of the best ways of determining whether you need supplementation, and if so, which products are best for you.

Chemical Balance

Acid/alkaline balance or sodium/potassium ratios are another way of determining your relative state of health. The key to health is balance. The challenge is to find what will bring you back into balance and keep you in a harmonious state.

This balance is often reflected first in your energy level. When your system is too acid, you will tend to be full of nervous energy, or "hyper", and find it very difficult to relax. On the other hand, when your system is too alkaline, you feel tired, sluggish, and generally fatigued.

Maintaining a good acid/alkaline balance is essential to good health. When your body is too acid, you can bring it back into balance by eating acid foods. While this sounds counterproductive, it is because in chemistry, adding acid foods to an acid environment produces alkalinity. The most acid food, and the one that acts most quickly on the system to restore alkalinity, is lemon.

If your system is too alkaline, it can be brought back into balance with acid forming foods. These are foods that form acid as they are digested, rather than foods that are acids themselves. The most acid forming foods are meats.

Acid forming foods include meats, fish, eggs, milk, cheese, and grains. Alkaline forming foods include fruits and vegetables. Vegetables can be primarily acid or alkaline, depending upon how you prepare them, as this will affect their sodium/potassium ratio. Sodium (salt) is acid while potassium is alkaline.

Raw vegetables have a high potassium-to-sodium ratio and are considered alkaline. However, when you cook the vegetables, you reverse the ratio. This is because potassium is lost in the cooking process, which consequently increases the relative sodium levels. So, your vegetables become acid when cooked.

Although sodium is an acid, the rule about adding one acid to another to produce an alkaline condition does not apply here. Adding sodium, or salt, to either an acid or alkaline environment will always increase acidity. You need potassium to neutralize the acidity caused by sodium. This is also true in the reverse; you need sodium to balance the alkalinity produced by potassium.

The two body types that are at the extreme ends of the acid/alkaline polarity are Adrenals and Thyroids; the other body types fall somewhere in between. Adrenals have the most acid systems, with an inherently high sodium level, while Thyroids are the most alkaline with high potassium levels. *One way to identify whether you tend more towards acidity or alkalinity is by considering your response to stress.* Adrenal glands are known to produce energy, so when Adrenal types are stressed, their body temperature increases causing them to get sweaty and "hyper." They will often turn up the air conditioner, start shedding their clothes, get louder, scattered, or more active.

Since this type is naturally high in sodium, and therefore highly acidic, they need additional potassium to balance their systems. Eating more salt, which is generally what they crave when they get like this, stimulates the adrenal glands even further, compounding the problem. *Exercise can be helpful to release stress while, dietarily, they can increase potassium levels by eating raw vegetables and drinking vegetable juices.*

On the other hand, the alkaline Thyroid reacts to stress in just the opposite way. Their body temperature drops and they tend to feel cold. When their energy levels plummet, they turn up the heat, eat, or want to retreat, going somewhere to curl up, get warm, or perhaps go to sleep. *Because of the excess of potassium in their systems, they should lightly steam most of their vegetables before eating them to increase their sodium-to-potassium ratio.*

Considering the reactions of these two types to stress, assess your own reactions and determine where you fall on the scale. Do you get "hyper"? Sweat a lot? Feel agitated? Or do you fall into a slump, want to go off by yourself, curl up and have a nap to escape the problem? Your reaction could be a clue to your sodium/potassium ratio or chemical balance.

If your system is too alkaline, adding more salt to your food usually is not the best answer to the problem. Regular table salt is an extreme acid and can throw sensitive systems way out of balance. Body types that tend to be alkaline generally have a more sensitive nature.

Eating salt stimulates your adrenal glands, making them more agitated. This is certainly not a viable option, particularly if your adrenals are *already* exhausted. Excess salt can also cause fluid retention, especially in the feet and ankles or around the eyes, increased thirst, and bloating.

Sodium Sources

There are other ways to get the sodium you need in your diet without these negative effects. Corrected Salt™ by Life Plus™ balances sodium with chloride, sulphur, and magnesium, or you can balance sea salt with kelp. For this formula, add one part powdered kelp or kelp flakes to four parts sea salt, and use as you would regular salt. Since kelp is high in iodine, which is the mineral that supports the thyroid gland, it can help keep sensitive systems in balance. Sodium can be very helpful in protein digestion. So cooking with some salt is beneficial. As in everything else, balance is essential.

Another way to get your sodium is from vegetables, with celery being one of the highest sources. *When cooking vegetables, steaming is a better method than boiling as it helps to increase sodium levels while keeping the loss of vitamins to a minimum.*

While Thyroids benefit from steaming most of their vegetables, this doesn't mean they shouldn't eat anything raw. Ideally, 30% of the vegetables in their diet should be fresh and raw. Adrenals, however, thrive on just the opposite ratio, eating most of their vegetables raw.

Body types that have their dominant gland in the head, that is the Pituitary, Pineal, Brain, Thalamus, Hypothalamus, Medulla, and even the Thymus will do best with Thyroid's ratio. Those types with dominant glands below the neck are like the Adrenal.

Determining PH

An easy way to determine your acid/alkaline balance is by using pH paper to check your saliva. You can get this paper at most drugstores. The best one to get registers a range of 6.0 to 8.0 in increments of .2 to .4. To use, tear off a strip, put one end of the paper in your mouth, and get it thoroughly wet with saliva, then check the resulting color against the graph on the dispenser. The ideal result is a pH between 6.8 and 7.0.

If you find that your level is less than 6.8, your system is too acid. Eating more raw vegetables and acid fruits like lemons, limes, and oranges, will usually increase your alkalinity. This is a typical example of two acids producing alkalinity.

If your reading is greater than 7.0, your system is too alkaline, and you'll need more acid-forming foods. These would include high protein foods like meats, grains, and steamed vegetables.

The most common imbalance is acidity. If you're getting enough fruits and vegetables and you're still too acid, it could be caused by one of several factors. Generally it means your immune system is stressed, like when you're fighting a cold, chronic illness, or toxic condition. Following a diet that does not provide enough essential fatty acids will also produce acidity. If your system does not respond by simply changing your diet, see your health care professional.

Vitamins

Vitamins are divided into two categories, fat soluble and water soluble.

Fat Soluble

Fat soluble vitamins are A, D, E, and K, and are used in the body's production of hormones, cell membranes, anti-oxidants, and anti-inflammatory agents. They are also important for healthy skin, proper growth, immune system function, blood clotting, and the regulation of the minerals in your system.

Sources

The best sources of vitamins A, D, E, and K are fish, particularly firm white meat as found in cod, roughy, sea bass, shark, and swordfish, animal products, algae, and vegetables. If supplements are used, vitamin A is best obtained as beta carotene, which is converted to vitamin A in the body.

Poor sources of fat soluble vitamins are processed foods, hydrogenated fats, consisting of vegetable shortenings and margarine, polyunsaturated oils, including corn, soy, and sunflower, and saturated fats, which usually come from animal sources.

Water Soluble

Water soluble vitamins include B1 (Thiamine), B2 (Riboflavin), B3 (Niacin), B6 (Pyroxidine), B12 (Cobalamin), Biotin, Choline, Folic Acid, Inositol, Pantothenic Acid, PABA (Para-aminobenzoic acid), Vitamin C, and the Bioflavinoids (Vitamin P), which make Vitamin C more effective.

Sources

The best sources of water soluble vitamins are all green and yellow vegetables, fruits, fish, chicken, turkey, animal meats, whole grains, and whole rices. Poor sources of these vitamins are all processed foods as well as "fast foods".

Deficiencies

Vitamin deficiencies can cause a wide array of health problems. Some of these are a poor immune response, hormonal imbalances, inflammatory diseases, mineral imbalances, blindness, and even death. It is certainly evident, based on these facts, that a good intake of all essential vitamins can help to prevent, if not cure, a number of undesirable conditions and ultimately prolong life.

Martha was complaining of irritability, fatigue, and depression. I discovered that she was suffering from a hormone imbalance caused by a deficiency of Vitamin D. Since her dominant gland was Pineal, and the pineal gland is activated by sunlight which supplies Vitamin D, adding a Vitamin D supplement to her diet produced dramatic results. Martha quickly reported a major improvement in her temperament and mood. Sometimes something as simple as one vitamin can make a world of difference.

Water

Even though our bodies contain many elements, they are made up of 90% water. Consequently, good health is dependent upon the quantity and quality of water we drink each day, since water helps to maintain body temperature and carry waste products out of the body. *It's important to drink water that is free of chlorine, added fluoride, bacteria, or other toxic residues and chemicals.*

Water Choice and Its Ramifications

The water that comes out of your tap generally comes from **surface sources** such as streams, rivers, and lakes. The original water usually contains at least a moderate amount of pollutants that have been carried into the water from the surrounding terrain or atmosphere. These pollutants often include pesticides, or fertilizers from agriculture, as well as elements that come from the air, such as factory and automobile exhaust residues. There may have also been bacterial pollution in the natural waters of the rivers and lakes.

When the water comes into the filtration facilities for cities and towns, it is treated to remove these pollutants. To accomplish this, various chemicals including chlorine, fluorine, phosphates, sodium aluminates, and other chemical elements are added to the water.

While some of these chemicals have been implicated as cancer-causing agents, they continue to be widely used in municipal water systems. If present in your drinking water, they, as well as various other chemicals, are stressful to your body. This is because the body identifies them as foreign elements and must work harder to eliminate them, thus putting additional stress on your system.

Obtaining an analysis of your city water supply through your municipal water company may be worthwhile, as knowing what kind of chemicals you are ingesting can help you determine the best way to have clean drinking water.

Tap water that comes from **deep wells** is often much cleaner than surface waters, but it can also contain pollutants from the surface ground, especially if it is a rural agricultural area. The grazing of animals on the land and fertilizers and other chemicals used in farming can work down into the aquifer and pollute the water.

Also there is always the possibility of an excess of certain minerals in well water, depending upon the chemical nature of the soil. The best well water will contain a moderate amount of minerals and be free of toxic residues and bacteria.

Whether your water comes from a city system or a well, a water filtration or purifying system can be very useful in purifying the water you drink. While there are many good systems available, the ideal system varies depending on what residues your water contains. I have found that **reverse osmosis** systems remove so much of the minerals that the water is unsuitable for most people.

Minerals are the body's foundation. If a food or even water does not contain the necessary minerals to be assimilated, minerals are leached out of the body. This is a problem I have found with distilled water, as well as reverse osmosis systems.

In certain parts of the country, like southern California, buying **bottled drinking water** is often the best alternative. It's important to select a water that contains a moderate amount of minerals in balanced quantities.

Distilled water contains no minerals and usually should be avoided. If you choose to drink this water, it will tend to leach out the mineral stores from the body to supply what your system needs. Distilled water can be beneficial when your system needs to be flushed, but under normal conditions you need the minerals normally found in drinking water. Distilled water is often advised when large quantities of minerals are taken, as in the case of certain cancer treatments.

If you buy **drinking water in soft plastic containers**, such as the gallon jugs found in the supermarket, you may detect a "plastic" taste. You can pour this water into glass containers and let it sit in the sun for a day to get rid of the taste. **Hard plastic containers,** like the ones the bottled water companies use to deliver water, usually do not affect the taste, so no treatment is needed.

Your best indication of the best water for you is taste. If you don't like the taste of a particular water, it usually isn't the best one for you. It's easy to drink water when you like the taste. Muscle testing is a simple, effective tool that can be used to help you determine whether a particular water source is suitable for you.

Improving Water

If you have a water that is close, but not quite right, there are several options that will often upgrade a water, making it acceptable. There are devices available that can be used to polarize water, such as the Harmonizer by Rainbow Crossings or polarizer wands or pillows by Spring Life Polarity. Both will neutralize chemicals and bacteria, and consequently improve the taste.

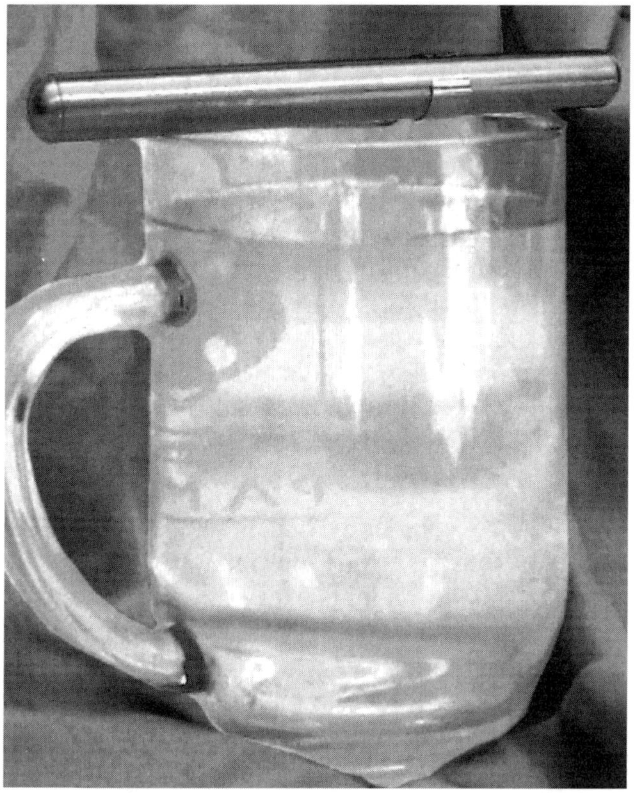

A polarizer being used to treat water.

Here is a simple test that you can do to determine the effect these devices have on your water: Take 2 glasses of tap water and place a polarizer wand on the top of the glass. It will initially rock and roll back and forth, then it will stop. When it stops, remove it and taste the water. Then taste the water in the untreated glass and compare the difference. The polarizer removes the chlorine taste, improving the quality of the water. You can also use muscle testing to determine your body's response to the water.

Another way to upgrade your water is to add a small amount of juice, such as lemon, lime, apple, or grape. Sometimes this is enough to balance its mineral content and improve taste. When you are eating in restaurants or traveling and must drink water from an unknown source, adding a few drops of lemon juice will help improve taste and neutralize chlorine or any other toxic substance.

Sparkling Water

Sparkling water is an alternative for people who experience regular water as being "heavy". Some types, like Liver, Pancreas, and Pineal, tend to prefer water with carbonation, and still others prefer the added fruit flavor. The "bubbly" content does tend to make it taste "lighter" and feel lighter in the stomach. Some people prefer to drink only sparkling water while others find it helpful only during an illness, like a cold or flu.

How Much Water?

Most people should drink at least a half gallon of water each day. While this sounds like a lot, in reality it is only eight 8-ounce glasses or four 16 ounce glasses. The Kidney body type often does well with a little less than this amount, but most other types can require between 1 1/2 quarts and 3/4 gallon of water daily. If you live in a hot, dry climate or are especially active during the day, you may require even more.

Benefits of Water

To get the maximum benefit possible from your intake of water, it should be in as pure a form as possible. Other liquids like coffee, fruit juice, soft drinks, soups, etc., are "registered" by your body as food. So if you are drinking anything other than plain water, even though it contains water, the body doesn't use it to cleanse your system.

Substituting other liquids for plain water adds stress and a potential for increased toxicity and sluggishness to your system. Your body requires plain water to regulate digestion, aid assimilation and elimination, and carry nutrients throughout your system. *Without sufficient water, you can actually gain weight as the body will suspend accumulated toxins in the extracellular fluids.*

The lymphatic system eliminates waste products and infections. It is activated by water and physical activity like walking, stretching, or muscle movement of any kind. Waste material is eliminated through several systems, depending on its form. The largest source of elimination is the kidneys, ideally moving 50% of all the waste. The skin is the second largest elimination organ, moving 28%, the lungs are responsible for 20% which consists of carbon dioxide. The remaining 2% is eliminated through the bowels in the form of solid material.

This gives you an idea of how much waste material the body has to process. If the kidneys are not able to fully eliminate their share, the load falls on the skin, causing it to break out. The lungs aren't equipped to help the kidneys, and the bowels can only carry a small percentage of total waste. Consequently, the kidneys need all the support they can get. They're just one of the systems that require water.

The bowels need water for proper lubrication and elimination, and the waste particles expelled from your lungs are suspended in water. Perspiration is the result of your skin eliminating waste through the pores. If you don't drink enough pure water, these systems can't function properly and your body quickly becomes toxic.

Ken, one of my Thymus type patients, suffered from lower back pain. Upon examination, I discovered it was directly related to his overloaded kidneys. While there was some structural involvement, the problem was primarily dietary. Even though his total intake of liquids through various sources was adequate, his body wasn't satisfied. He didn't like water and thought since it was included in the liquids he was drinking, it should be enough. Once he followed my recommendation to drink at least 1/2 gallon of plain water a day, his back pain completely disappeared.

Water will also curb your appetite. Many people eat not because they are really hungry, but because they are dehydrated. *In addition to flushing the toxins out of the body, water can help burn calories.*

Edema or Fluid Retention

Fluid retention, or edema, is a problem that confuses many people. It would seem reasonable to assume, that if your body is retaining water, you have too much, so you should drink less. The reality is that just the opposite is true. *Edema is a symptom of toxicity.* The body is suspending the toxic elements in fluid between the cells. If you do not drink enough water, the body is unable to flush the toxins out of your system. Rather than putting the toxins into the cells, it retains as much fluid as possible to keep them suspended until they can be eliminated.

Bloating is common before your period because this is when you have the greatest amount of toxins in your system. When your period starts and you get rid of the toxins, the bloating disappears. Chronic bloating occurs when the body is unable to eliminate the toxins. Drinking a lot of water for 2 or 3 days and then slacking off doesn't work. *The body needs water on a consistent basis and needs to know that it can trust you to drink it.*

To convince your body that it will always have enough water for proper elimination, you need to drink sufficient amounts every day. If you drink plenty of water one day, and then very little for the next several days, you will probably have a problem with fluid retention. *The solution is simply to be consistent, making sure you drink all the water you need every day.*

Depending on how toxic your system is and how long it has been abused, it may take from two days to two weeks of drinking enough water before your body returns to normal. The average time required is a week to 10 days. Some body types, particularly Pancreases, are more prone to fluid retention than others.

Edema is not always due to lack of sufficient water in the system. Kidney or heart problems, for instance, can cause fluid retention. The real cause of the problem is a system that is out of balance. Sufficient water, along with the correct diet, can do a lot to restore that balance.

Additional Dietary Support

If you know that you're having trouble with a particular organ or system, look at the list of "Frequently" foods for the body type that has that organ as its dominant gland. Select those foods that are also included on your "Frequently" or "Moderately" list and add them to your diet.

For example, if you have a problem with weak kidneys, look at the "Frequently" foods for the Kidney type. You'll see that foods like cranberries and asparagus are particularly supportive. Eating these foods will help strengthen the kidneys, so including them in your diet may help correct your problem.

When to Drink Water and How Much

Do you put water on the table with your meals? Have you ever wondered if you should drink water along with your food? There are different opinions on whether or not this is good for you. Some believe that drinking water with a meal interferes with the digestion by diluting the gastric juices. Others believe that water with food will aid the digestive process.

In my experience, most body types can drink water without any digestive upset immediately before and immediately after, but not with meals. A few can safely drink water or other liquids while eating, but some types are so sensitive that they should wait 15 to 30 minutes after eating to drink anything. Their delicate digestive systems need to separate foods from liquids.

Joan, a Thalamus type patient, complained of bloating and an upset stomach. I asked her about her eating habits and found that she drank water with all her meals. My recommendation was that she restrict her water to before and after eating. Sure enough, on her return visit, she reported that this simple change totally eliminated her digestive distress.

Finally, it should be noted that anything to excess, including drinking water, can be harmful to the body. Drinking too much water can leach out the mineral stores in your system and result in vitamin and mineral deficiencies.

Once again, the goal with everything is moderation, neither too much or too little. We want to achieve balance. If you're not sure about how much water you need, or to confirm what you drink at present is adequate, having someone muscle test you will help you to determine what is best for you.

Fiber

It is essential to have an adequate supply of fiber in your meals to keep your digestive system working properly. While fiber contains no nutrients, the proper absorption of sugars and the regulation of fats in the bloodstream depends on your fiber consumption.

Bowel diseases, such as cancer and colitis, have been attributed to insufficient fiber in the diet. Ideally, you should eat at least 30 grams a day, which is two to three times the average consumption of 10 to 15 grams.

Sources

The best sources of fiber include all green and yellow vegetables, fruits, whole grains, and whole grain cereals. Poor sources are processed and fast foods.

Benefits

Fiber keeps the bowels moving, helps to detoxify the body, and lowers cholesterol levels, and even provides an even blood sugar level so you are not constantly hungry.

CHAPTER 4

WEIGHT CONTROL CHALLENGES

Most weight loss diets are some form of starvation. This is why you gain back not only what you have lost, but extra, each time you go on a diet. Inadequate food intake tends to further deplete the body's resources and eventually causes problems. This is why the primary focus of this book is not on weight loss or how to lose 30 pounds in 30 days, but in creating an eating plan that is right for your body type.

When you follow an eating plan that benefits your entire body and builds its reserves, you eliminate cravings, imbalances, and excess weight in a way that actually supports and rebuilds your system.

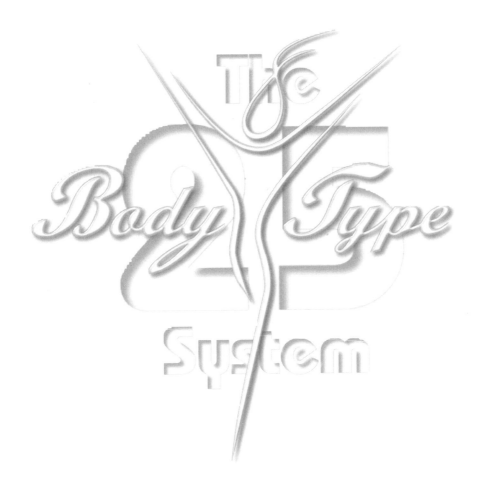

Weight Control

Too Skinny?

A healthy diet works for those who need to gain weight as well as those who desire to lose unwanted excess pounds. If an underweight person has a dietary imbalance, simply adding calories by increasing their food consumption will have only minimal, or unsatisfactory benefits.

Proper nutrition is essential for good body balance. When one of my patients was in high school, she decided that if she could only gain weight, her breasts would fill out. Unfortunately, in her effort to gain weight in her breasts, she put on 50 pounds, all in her hips, abdomen, and thighs. She then spent the next 20 years struggling to lose the excess weight in ways that would return her body to its natural proportions.

Simply adding calories to your diet does not insure that the weight gained will be exactly where you want it. Often, pounds are put on in places that give a disproportionate appearance, and then are difficult to take off. Whether you want to gain or lose weight, the key to success lies in eating the foods that are supportive of your particular body type.

Too Fat?

Linda, a nurse, is a Skin type who, like most Skins, puts on weight easily and had spent a lifetime struggling to lose it. When Skins do lose weight, the odds are against them keeping it off. As is so classic of this type, Linda had been overweight since childhood. She had tried countless weight loss programs, but had not been able to lose her excess weight and keep from gaining more. As an overweight child, she was put on doctor prescribed amphetamines to help her lose weight when she was only ten years old.

Over the years, Linda tried every kind of diet imaginable – vegetarian diets, liquid diets, Weight Watchers, Jenny Craig, Overeaters Anonymous, and several others. In her ceaseless effort to control her weight, she had done almost everything including radical fasting.

Linda came to me with her overweight problem. The first thing I did was determine her body type. From this point we planned a diet that would help her lose excess pounds and eventually maintain her proper weight. With this plan, she gradually began to lose weight, and at the end of six months, Linda had lost thirty pounds.

Linda's weight loss was not accomplished by dieting alone, but also by making important changes in her eating habits. The purpose of the body type diet is to identify and address the specific needs of the individual. What is amazing is the consistency within the types, so once your body type is identified, proper nutrition can begin. In many cases, a dieter's efforts fail because basic needs aren't being met.

Linda's body came with its own blueprint for gaining and losing weight and for staying healthy, of which she, like most people, was unaware. All the diets she had previously tried were not right for her body and consequently failed for various reasons. On some diets, she lost muscle rather than fat, while the deprivation on others caused her to return to her old eating habits. Then she gained back not only what she had lost, but added extra. Also the liquid diets she had been using included too many artificial sweeteners for her sensitive Skin system.

Since most Skins crave sweets, I soon discovered that the Skin body type has an extreme sensitivity to refined sugar, so Linda's source of sugar was mostly fruit. We worked on food combinations, which are vitally important for Skin types, especially regarding the mixing of food groups. We paid particular attention to not combining protein and grain and keeping fruit separate, as the chemistry of poor combinations would overload her system and throw it out of balance.

For instance, Linda could have chicken and green beans, which she digested very easily. But, if we added rice to the protein, her body would be stressed trying to produce the many kinds of enzymes needed to digest the starch along with the protein. The imbalance created would cause her to gain weight instead of lose it.

Timing of Linda's meals was also an important factor. She felt best when she ate her largest meal at noon and a light, early dinner. This way her body got the nutrients it needed at the times when it could best assimilate them, meaning it could digest the food instead of storing it, eventually as fat. She started drinking more water, enabling her system to flush out toxins. Fluid retention is generally due to toxins that can't get out of the body. Her weight gain was really a result of poor digestion and elimination, as well as improper eating patterns.

Many of the diets that Linda tried left her feeling unsatisfied after eating. Since the Skin diet nutritionally supported her system, she felt better than ever. She now has a renewed enthusiasm and no longer suffers from fatigue, headaches, or the restlessness that resulted from eating refined sugar. And with her system in balance, she no longer has a craving for sweets.

As a Skin type, Linda's physical system is sensitive, and so is her psychological makeup. Skins are one of the most sensitive types. They relate to the world through feelings, easily sensing the emotional needs of others, and responding to them.

Linda's compassion made her go beyond what was required of her as a nurse and the demands of her job, plus her tendencies to be overly giving were causing her stress and burnout. Once she understood the basis of her frustrations, she set more realistic limits on what others could expect of her.

LONG TERM EFFECTS OF WEIGHT LOSS DIETS

Weight loss diets that are designed to starve the body into burning up its fat reserves often do more harm than good, especially if they focus on completely eliminating one of the food groups – whether it be fats, carbohydrates, or proteins. The body needs all of these nutrients to function properly and cannot maintain good health for long without them.

Excess weight is a symptom of imbalance and depletion of the body's essential reserves. Going on a starvation diet only further reduces the already inadequate supply of nutrients and throws the system into even greater imbalance.

While you may initially lose weight with a radical diet, you ultimately do more harm than good, since you are throwing your body even farther out of balance. When you go off the diet, your body quickly puts the weight back on, and often adds more pounds than you were able to take off.

Additional weight gain occurs because reducing your food intake slows down the body's metabolic rate, meaning the speed at which calories are used. When normal eating is resumed, the body begins to store excess weight as a means of preparing for future food deprivation.

The body's interpretation of deprivation is that adequate food is no longer available and a "famine" exists. So, when food is plentiful again, the body's normal response is to store some away for that next inevitable "famine". This process is then repeated over and over again as you try one diet after another, a process which deprives your body of the nutrients essential to maintaining a healthy system.

When excess fat is a problem, it might seem that the reduction of fat in the diet would be a good way to get the body to use up its own fat reserves. Unfortunately, body fat is not the first thing to go when you eat a fat free diet.

The process that occurs when you begin to starve yourself is rather complex. First, the body uses its glycogen stores. Glycogen is produced in the tissues, especially the liver and muscles, and is changed into simple sugar when the body needs it for energy.

When the glycogen supply is depleted, your body gets energy by breaking down quality protein in the muscle cells. The reason people often feel so good when they are fasting is that they are getting good quality protein – their own. The body literally begins to consume itself, but once the fasting is over, it is very difficult to rebuild the "cannibalized" muscle.

Fat cells are the last to be tapped for the energy the body needs because they are the repositories for toxins and excess hormones. Being filled primarily with debris waiting to be dumped, and since house cleaning takes a lot of energy, fat cells make very poor fuel sources.

In order to burn fat you must consume a diet adequate for your body to perform normal day-to-day functions before it can tackle the job of cleansing the fat cells. These fat cells are used as "storage bins" for bodily refuse, and the body can only eliminate the fat and clean out the toxins when all of the other immediate needs of the body are met. So, proper nutrition is essential for the reduction of fat cells.

If you are on a starvation diet, and your body has reached the point of beginning to "burn" the fat cells, it will only take from them what it can, leaving the rest to be cleaned out later. If balance is not restored to your system, you will never get adequate energy reserves to complete the cleansing process. Binging on sweets and high fat foods adds more "refuse" to your fat cells, compounding the original problem and making weight loss even more difficult.

The key to permanent weight loss is to restore the body's balance. Once this is accomplished, the body can begin to clean up and deplete toxic fat cells.

Repeated dieting to lose weight is extremely stressful to the system and can cause severe physical damage. It is a well known fact that dieters tend to have more heart problems than those who consistently maintain a steady weight.

Dieting while under physical or emotional stress only magnifies health problems. It is important to stay with a permanent dietary plan that is appropriate for your body type because this is what will adequately support your system on a long term basis.

Staying with an eating regimen that is right for your body will minimize disease and illness, increase your energy, and stabilize your weight at a level that is right for you. Making the best food choices for your body type will pay off in terms of good health.

BODY BALANCE AND THE PROBLEMS OF WEIGHT MANAGEMENT

When you gain weight, it is often an indication that your system is unable to balance what you have eaten with what your body really needs. This is usually the result of one or all of the following problems:

- poor food choices which lead to depletion of minerals and/or enzymes,
- overloading the body with excess food, or
- an unbalanced condition within the body and consequent production of excess hormones.

Poor Food Choices

Karen was a candy eater – any kind, as long as it was sweet. Her body was a testament to the many years that she had craved sugar as a way to soothe her nerves, boost her energy, or give herself a treat. She celebrated every holiday with sweets, such as Valentine chocolates, Easter eggs, Christmas candy canes, and then treated herself many days in between. But she had now come to the realization that this refined sugar "comfort" she loved so much was also her downfall. If she were to lose any weight, she was going to have to banish this sugary treat from her life.

Refined Sugar

One of the simplest ways to get rid of unwanted pounds is to quit eating refined sugar. Often foods high in sugar are high in fat. Substituting artificial sweeteners for refined sugar doesn't solve the problem, however, as these are usually even more detrimental to your system.

It is possible, by following the dietary guidelines for your body type, to obtain ample simple sugars from the foods you eat. These can be safely supplied by fruits and complex carbohydrates. This way you can maintain a consistent blood sugar level and not add unwanted pounds.

Inclusion of Sweets

You don't even have to totally eliminate all sweets. The Pancreas type, for example, can lose weight while eating sweets as a bedtime snack, as long as the choice of sweets is rotated. Sometimes the body needs minerals, such as magnesium and copper, and they are present in chocolate. Women often become deficient in these minerals just before their periods and experience a craving for chocolate, so there are times when chocolate can actually be beneficial.

For some types, including the Thyroid, digestion is aided by eating some fruit after consuming protein, as long as the fruit is not too sweet. Tart fruits like cherries, apricots, or mangos provide plenty of sugar without stimulating the thyroid gland. The Adrenal, on the other hand, will benefit from stimulation of the thyroid gland with some very sweet fruits like bananas and dates. Again, this shows the need for you to know your particular body type and what kind of sugar you need in your diet.

The problem for most types is not so much with sugar consumption but in eating excessive amounts in the refined form. Whole foods are usually the best choices for getting natural sugars as these also provide all the vitamins and minerals necessary for proper digestion, which refined sugar does not.

For Karen it wasn't necessary to eliminate all sweets from her diet to lose weight, only refined sugar. Moderation is also important. She learned that eating the right kind of sweets only when her body was able to digest them was the sensible plan of action. Knowing how much sugar is right for you also means understanding what is right for your body type, and this will help you make the right choices in the kinds of sweets you eat.

Refined Foods

Poor food choices usually include too many refined foods. The problem with refined sugar is that all the minerals needed to digest it have been removed in the refining process. As a result, the body is forced to supply these minerals from its own reserves. When these reserves are used up, the sugar cannot be digested and is stored as fat. This same process occurs with other refined foods resulting in undesirable weight gain.

When the body's mineral reserves are depleted, the body must "borrow" what it needs for digestion from vital areas. This creates a weakness or dysfunction in those parts of the body that are affected. So, it's important to include unrefined, or whole foods in your diet, since all whole foods usually contain all the minerals necessary for their digestion.

Enzymes and Raw Foods

Enzymes are also necessary for good digestion as they act as catalysts to break down the foods you eat. Raw foods contain enzymes. Since enzymes are heat sensitive, they are destroyed at 110 degrees, so most cooking methods kill them. These enzymes can be preserved by cooking very slowly over low heat or by light steaming. Overcooking, using high heat, or even reheating foods, destroys enzymes as well as other nutrients.

When your food does not contain essential enzymes, your body must manufacture them. If the demand exceeds your body's ability to supply them, your digestion is inhibited. Consequently, the undigested food is stored as fat and you eventually notice weight gain.

Knowing this about enzymes, it might seem that the best diet would consist of eating only raw foods. However, totally raw diets put too much stress on the digestive systems of most body types. Balance again is the key. Certain vegetables, like broccoli for Thyroids, are easier to digest when steamed rather than eaten raw, while carrots may be eaten either cooked or raw. So, the solution is to eat some raw foods, with the amount dependent upon your body type and current state of health.

Generally, everyone's diet should contain both whole and raw foods. *How to make the best choices about which foods are right for you requires becoming aware of your personal needs. Your body intuitively knows what it wants and your challenge is to tune into its wisdom.* By paying attention to the subtle messages you continually receive from your body, you can make the food choices best suited for you.

Overeating

If you eat more than your body needs, you will gain weight! Overeating is the most common cause of weight gain in a healthy system even if you are eating all the right foods. Learning to listen to your body when it signals that it has had enough will aid greatly in keeping your weight at the proper level.

Do you remember when you were growing up, how you were encouraged to "clean your plate"! Were you told about starving children somewhere? And did you have to stay at the table until your plate was clean – under threat of terrible punishment? Do you realize that this may have set a definite pattern in your young mind that could stay with you forever?

Are you still listening to those old "messages" and responding to childhood programming in your adult life? Do you feel guilty if you don't finish everything on your plate – or the table, for that matter? Quit eating when your body tells you it doesn't need any more food. Pay attention! Listen to your body! It knows instinctively what it needs, and what it doesn't need.

Need for Chewing

Another problem many people have is that they don't chew their food properly. You probably remember your parents' admonishment of "Chew your food!" (Was it 28 times per mouthful?) They were right though, because chewing is an important part of the digestive process. When your food is not sufficiently chewed, you will often tend to eat more than necessary to satisfy the need to chew.

I was amazed to discover how strong the desire to chew actually is and how it is connected with the satiety (full) reflex. I found if I ate some raw foods, like carrots, or seeds or nuts, that required a definite amount of chewing, I would feel satisfied. When I ate soft foods that required little chewing, I noticed I needed to eat a lot more to get the same sense of fullness.

The need to chew provides yet another reason for including raw food in your diet, as these foods require much more chewing than those that are cooked. On occasion, when you are preoccupied with other activities, such as talking or watching TV, or even reading as you eat, you can forget to chew properly.

When your attention is focused elsewhere, it is easy to overlook the chewing process. Taking a mouthful of food and then only half chewing is a result of inattention to what you are eating. When this happens, you are also likely to miss the "I'm full" signal that your body sends. Paying full attention to the eating process obviously aids your digestion. This is a principle that is heavily stressed in both Chinese and Ayurvedic medicine.

Emotional Gratification

Janet was an attractive woman who would have been much more so with the elimination of her extra pounds. She knew she had a weight problem, and she had a good idea of what caused it. But Janet confessed to being powerless over the insatiable craving for foods like pasta, baked potatoes, and hot homemade breads. She said she just didn't feel "right" if she couldn't have some of these foods every day, and often at more than one meal.

When I body typed Janet, I found that she was a Stomach type, which explained her thickened waistline and upper abdominal weight gain. She had a sturdy, solid appearance with a medium bone structure. She was obviously carrying too much weight in the wrong places for her body. To help her solve her problem, I had to find out why Janet was craving the foods she wanted, so we explored that part of the problem first.

Janet had four children, all under the age of six. She told me she often felt she only "talked to children" as she kept so busy being a mother she didn't seem to have time for anything else. At the end of the day, when she was ready for conversation and stimulation, her husband came home tired and ready to relax in front of the TV.

So she found her challenges and pleasure in cooking, baking, and eating. Janet's problem is not unique. Many types see food as an ally, or constant friend, for a variety of reasons.

Many of us are inclined, at times, to eat as a result of emotional stress. We attempt to deal with anxiety, anger, loneliness, etc., by "treating" our egos with something tasty. We nurture ourselves with food, especially if we had a mother who used food as a reward or a way of showing her love. Instead of addressing the real problem, we cover it up with unnecessary eating and the risk of potential weight gain.

Whatever the reason, the problem of overeating can be solved, or at least moderated, by paying attention to what we are doing. Becoming aware of why we eat, what we do as we eat, and concentrating on the effects our food choices have on our bodies are the first steps in solving the problem. Responding properly to your body's actual needs requires paying careful attention to the messages it's sending you.

System Imbalance

Some people find themselves in the frustrating position of making good food choices, eating appropriate amounts, and still gaining weight. These weight increases generally occur when the internal functions of the body aren't operating properly. While the hormonal system ultimately causes the weight problem, it's not the only weak system. But it's one that relates to your dominant gland which, when stressed, produces excess hormones. Some dominant glands produce hormones that the body more readily stores as fat.

Consequently, certain body types are prone to putting on excess weight, while others tend to be slender or even lose weight in the same situation. Regardless, if you have a serious weight problem, it is likely that you have other physical problems as well. To provide some guidance and direction, I'll describe several areas that routinely cause problems.

Digestive Weakness

The initial stress that leads to a system imbalance is usually digestive. A problem that is basically universal is the ileocecal valve syndrome, as it is one of the greatest causes of poor assimilation. This is a condition where the valve between the small and large intestines does not close completely. The purpose of the ileocecal valve is to keep waste material that has moved into the large intestine from returning to the small intestine.

When this valve does not completely close, toxins are forced back into the small intestine, often as a fine mist. The problem is that the majority of food assimilation takes place at this very site, the end of the small intestine. Not only does this interfere with the absorption of nutrients, but instead of the toxins passing through as they were intended, they are absorbed. The first site of elimination for these toxins is the sinuses. This is why sinus problems are so prevalent. Dark circles under the eyes are often the result the absorption of ileocecal toxins, as are digestive problems, poor nutrient assimilation, constipation or diarrhea, abdominal bloating, gas and chronic pain in the right side around the appendix.

Correction involves establishing continuous nerve innervation to the area, and synchronizing the ileocecal valve with the movement of the small and large intestines. It is affected by diet, particularly improper food combinations, food additives, and too much refined sugar, as well as your emotional state.

Umbilical Hernia

Most people who suffer from chronic digestive problems do so as a result of an injury that commonly occurs shortly after birth. This injury, known as an umbilical hernia, is caused by excessive pulling on the umbilical cord or from the cord being cut too short right after birth.

You'd think that once you're born, you'd be done with the umbilical veins and arteries – not true.

They then become supportive ligaments. The process of becoming a ligament requires drying and results in shortening the veins and arteries. If the cord is cut too short, it will tear at the origin and insertion, resulting in an umbilical hernia. An umbilical hernia disrupts the energy flow in the abdomen and weakens the digestive system. This is why some people have always been aware of digestive weaknesses while others have excellent digestion.

Intestinal Parasites

Intestinal parasites are another common cause of digestive weakness. When the umbilical hernia is present, the stomach is not as strong as it normally would be so it isn't able to break down the bacteria that comes in. This results in low levels of botulism and salmonella frequently setting up permanent residency in the intestines. The resulting digestive weakness, commonly known as leaky gut syndrome, allows undigested protein molecules to enter the bloodstream. The immune system then identifies these molecules as foreign protein, and attacks them just as it does bacteria and viruses.

Immune System

When there are too many undigested protein molecules present, the overworked immune system becomes exhausted. It is then no longer able to effectively eradicate the bacteria and viruses already present nor defend against new invaders.

The bacteria and viruses are now free to take up residence in the body, creating chronic low-grade infection sites, as well as a serious energy drain. Chronic fatigue, recurrent sinus infections, swollen arthritic joints, and vascular weakness are just a few examples of possible problems.

Hormonal System

When the digestive and immune systems become overloaded, the hormonal system compensates by producing more hormones. Unfortunately, this doesn't solve the problem of bacterial or viral attack. Digestive or immune system problems are not the only cause of excess hormone production. Other types of stress (physical, mental, or emotional), can cause an abundance of hormones, particularly adrenalin.

As Hans Selye discovered in his research about forty years ago, the "fight or flight" response releases adrenalin into the system. When the response needs to be more civilized, the adrenalin isn't used by the muscles and becomes excessive in the body, as does any hormone that can't be used for its intended purpose.

As the stress continues, the body increases its hormone production, resulting in an excess of hormones. This excess, when it can't be released, is then stored as fat, just like it was during adolescence when the secondary sex characteristics were being formed. It's hormones that give us breasts, curvy hips and thighs, and unfortunately result in undesirable weight gain once we've reached a certain excessive level.

You may think you are handling the stress in your life, but if you are gaining weight for no apparent reason, your body is being overloaded. If you suspect that excessive hormone production or any of the other problems described are causing your weight problem, you should consult your healthcare professional. And if continual over-eating is your problem, perhaps the real cause could be psychological.

PSYCHOLOGICAL OBSTACLES TO CONTROLLING WEIGHT

If you have a weight problem, ask yourself, "Is my weight unconsciously serving some purpose?" Psychological factors can often be major obstacles to effective weight management and the power to gain or lose weight.

Imagine, if you can, what it would be like if you reached your desired weight. Think about this in great detail, envisioning yourself at that weight, and the image you create in your own mind, as well as how you think others will think of you.

Is it possible that weight loss or gain could lead to fear, discomfort, or conflict in your life? How would your life change? Would any of those changes be less than desirable, or actually hazardous? Honestly consider all of the changes that the loss or gain of body weight could bring about in your life.

It's a known fact that some people use excess weight as a psychological buffer or barrier that serves as a protection against perceived threats to their person. Losing that excess weight might open doors to new opportunities or experiences that may seem frightening or hostile.

Do you have a feeling that your weight serves to protect you from something, either real or perceived? Is it robbing you of the quality of life you desire? Is it inhibiting your personal growth and diminishing your self-esteem? If you can answer "yes" to these questions, you may need to seek professional counseling to overcome the problem.

Early Experiences

Your present weight may serve no useful purpose now, but could be the result of early programming that once was necessary. This could have been caused by sexual abuse or other experiences that created low self-esteem. If you recognize this in yourself, you can begin to consciously see how this is no longer appropriate or necessary in your current lifestyle. By facing the problem, you can begin to change and move out of the dilemma.

I have an Adrenal friend, Al, who was about 90 pounds overweight. As a child, his mother told him, "Eat all your food so you'll grow up big and strong like Uncle Jim." (Sound familiar?) Uncle Jim was a man who stood over 6' and carried his weight easily on his large frame. Al adored Uncle Jim and wanted to be "big and strong" just like him. His mother, in an attempt to get her little boy to eat, had unknowingly programmed Al to associate his uncle's size with strong, which meant eating a lot of food so he could be big and strong.

Al never grew any taller than 5'7" so the only way he could get bigger was to become "big around". Still, he unconsciously heeded his mother's "message", eating everything on his plate. When, through hypnosis, he finally recognized what he was doing, he was able to release that programming and shed his excess weight. He realized he didn't have to be big to be strong. Understanding the basic causes of our weight problems is often the very first step toward solving them.

Typical Dietary Challenges

FOOD CRAVINGS

Why is it that you sometimes have this awful, insatiable desire for a certain food at a particular time? Lemon meringue pie after a big meal or soda pop in the middle of the afternoon or dill pickles when you are pregnant. What causes a craving? And how should you deal with it?

Food cravings usually involve your dominant gland, and the need to stimulate that gland. In order to overcome the craving, you need to understand what your body is really wanting. The urge to eat certain foods could be caused by emotional stress, or the need for specific nutrients that you aren't getting in your diet.

For example, the Thyroid type craves sweets and carbohydrates because these are the foods that best stimulate the thyroid gland. When the body is stressed, the dominant gland, in this case, the thyroid, comes to the rescue and will continue to do so until exhausted and unable to respond. Once exhausted, symptoms of thyroid problems appear. In the meantime, the body craves foods which it knows will provide the greatest stimulation and the quickest energy lift. This is the basis of food cravings.

The answer is not to immediately start taking thyroid medication, but to give the thyroid gland a rest by eliminating sweets and simple carbohydrates. But, if the thyroid doesn't supply the energy, who will? The adrenal glands are designed to provide energy for the body. Unfortunately, because of the amount of stress we are routinely subjected to, most of us suffer from some degree of adrenal exhaustion. So, the adrenals need to be built up, and this is done by eating dense protein. By supplying the adrenal glands with the fuel they need, the thyroid gland won't have to come to the rescue. This means, that if you eat enough dense protein, your sweet cravings will disappear.

Giving in to your food cravings will eventually cause you to overload your dominant gland, and put undue stress on your system. The way out of this dilemma is to understand why you crave a certain food and what your body is really saying with the craving.

When you can determine what your system really needs, you can respond to this need in a way that supports your dominant gland as well as your body. Once you begin choosing the right foods in place of those that only stimulate, you are well on your way to achieving a healthy balance in your system.

SWEET CRAVINGS

There are several reasons for craving sweets. Have you ever noticed a particularly strong urge immediately following a large meal? Sugar is necessary to transport protein across the blood-brain barrier. The brain has a protective barrier that restricts protein from entering. This is designed to keep unwanted protein, such as bacteria, out. Consequently, if the good protein is going to get in, it needs a carrier to take it across, and that carrier is glucose or sugar.

Sugar stimulates the thyroid gland, which regulates metabolism. Overeating can overload the system, demanding an increase in metabolism, and requiring the thyroid to work harder. So, you crave sweets to boost the thyroid.

The need for fats is another reason for craving sweets. Sweets generally contain fats, and fats are necessary for digestion. Fats stimulate the gallbladder to release bile which acts like soap in the small intestines. If you don't digest fats, you won't digest protein or carbohydrates either.

COMMON EATING HABITS

Lack of Dietary Rotation

Food rotation is an essential part of any diet regimen, even when you are eating foods that are appropriate for your body type. Good nutrition and the achievement of balance depends upon variety.

A typical diet could consist of orange juice, dry cereal with milk, and coffee for breakfast; vegetable soup and a turkey sandwich for lunch; then chicken, potatoes, green beans and a tossed salad for dinner. Let's say that this is a nicely balanced combination of foods that you enjoy, and that it happens to be right for your body type.

However, if you eat these same meals all week, day in and day out, you will find that these foods gradually become less appealing. You may think that this is due simply to boredom from the repetition. Actually, this combination of foods, while beneficial in the beginning, can begin to strain your body.

As mentioned before, the digestion of food requires enzymes, that are depleted when the demands for them are excessive. In order to digest a particular selection of foods, a specific combination of enzymes is needed.

So, each time you repeat the same menu, especially at the same time of day, it puts greater stress on the pancreas to produce the same enzymes, over and over again. If you continue to eat this same combination of foods without change, the pancreas will temporarily exhaust its ability to produce the necessary enzymes.

When the body can no longer digest its food properly, it has to store it until the right enzymes can again be produced. Over time this accumulated stored food becomes unwanted fat and excess weight gain.

Rut Eating

The body types that tend to get into the habit of eating the same food for 3 to 4 days in a row, and then move to another food are Pancreas, Spleen

Stomach, Liver, and Brain. Many of the other types will eat the same thing for one meal, often breakfast. "Rut eating" is defined as eating the same food for 3 to 4 days in a row or eating the same food at the same meal day after day.

The problem with "rut eating" is that it initially stimulates and then exhausts the pancreas gland by depleting the enzymes necessary for digesting that particular food.

The type that excels at "rut eating" is the Pancreas. The main function of the pancreas gland is to break down carbohydrates or sugars which provide the main fuel source for the body. Likewise the Pancreas body type is the most efficient when it comes to food, utilizing every single morsel; and what it can't burn it stores as fat. Pancreases like food, and not just one type, but everything. So they don't crave any one food, plus they like things to be easy and convenient. When their bodies get stressed and their dominant gland demands stimulation, they simply eat what's available, which is often the same food they had earlier.

To give you an idea of what this does to the body, lets's say that you had some limburger cheese and that you really liked it. The first time you ate it, it would taste delicious and your pancreas would evaluate it and secrete the appropriate enzymes. If you ate it again for your next meal, it would still taste good and the pancreas would check its stores of enzymes and release the appropriate amount. By the third meal, the cheese doesn't look as good to you and the pancreas is getting worried since it's running out of some of the necessary enzymes. By the fourth meal, you're getting tired of it mainly because the pancreas goes into a panic since it's out of the necessary enzymes. So the limburger cheese has to be stored for later digestion when the pancreas has had a chance to recover.

It generally takes four days for a food to completely leave the digestive system. In order to give the pancreas gland sufficient time to replenish the enzymes for any one food, it should not be eaten again for four days. To go back to our illustration, you probably won't want any more limburger cheese for at least a week.

Sometimes this kind of rotation is just not practical, particularly for basic foods, so there is a modified rotation that can be used. It involves varying the time of day that the food is eaten. For example, ideally, if a Pancreas type eats turkey for dinner on Monday, turkey should not be eaten again until Friday. The modification would allow them to eat turkey again at lunch on Wednesday. Varying the time relieves the pressure, especially when given a day's rest.

Other body types are usually not as sensitive in their need for rotation. Nor are they as abusive to the pancreas gland. However, many people eat the same food for breakfast every day. So, to maintain a healthy pancreas, a four-day meal rotation is a good habit to get into. The easiest way to do this is to select four breakfast meals from the menus and rotate them.

Excess Sugar Consumption

Many health problems are a direct result of poor response to the body's needs. For example, when blood sugar levels drop, energy declines, and something sweet is often craved to provide an energy boost. If refined sugar is selected, the energy level comes back quickly, but drops again just as rapidly.

The immediate impulse is to eat more sugar to get the energy high again. *Repeated consumption of sugar produces a whiplash effect, so energy goes up and then down. The result is adrenal exhaustion and an imbalance in the system.* It also makes maintaining a good energy level and ideal weight difficult.

Eating sugar to get a quick energy "fix" often happens when the foods eaten at breakfast and lunch don't provide the fuel to maintain proper energy throughout the day. So, something sweet is used to get an energy boost to make it to the next meal.

Those who get into this kind of eating habit invariably are famished at the end of the day. They sit down and eat a very large evening meal, often containing even more sugar. This overloads the digestive system and causes the body to work harder at a time when it is tired and needs rest.

As a rule, eating a heavy meal late in the day is not a good idea for most body types. The exceptions to this are the Adrenals, Gonadals, Livers, Lymphs, and Stomachs. These types usually do well consuming a moderate to large meal in the evening, and eating light to moderately at breakfast and lunch. Eyes and Thyroids may also do this as they have more flexibility. Most body types function best eating their larger meals earlier in the day, with a small to moderate meal for dinner.

Skipping Meals

Meal skipping is not a good idea for anyone. The body needs periodic "refueling" in order to maintain a constant energy level. Eating only one meal a day, and then trying to make up what wasn't eaten the rest of the day, or what would normally be consumed in three meals, puts undue strain on the digestive system.

When meals are skipped the body interprets this as starvation, so it responds by lowering the metabolic rate and storing extra fat. If you are trying to lose weight, it is obvious that you should eat regular meals. When the body is confident that food will be provided on a regular basis, it will not attempt to accumulate surplus fat.

Time Between Meals

The time span required between meals varies with different body types. For some there should be four hours between breakfast and lunch, and five to six hours between lunch and dinner. This allows the body time for digestion and a chance to burn fat.

The Liver type, especially, needs to stay on a good eating schedule for any weight loss program to be effective. Other types need equal time between breakfast, lunch, and dinner, and some do well with frequent small meals spaced through the day rather than three large meals.

It isn't necessary for everyone to stick to rigid meal schedules as some types are more flexible. The important thing is to eat regularly, as it helps to maintain a good energy level and regulate fat storage. Regular eating also reduces stress on the digestive system, especially the stomach, allowing it to function more efficiently. A routine meal schedule will be less stressful than an unpredictable one and reduces the potential for overeating.

Overeating

When you wait too long between meals, or skip meals, there is a tendency to "wolf" your food when you finally sit down to a meal. When this happens, you eat more than you need, don't chew properly, and overload your digestive system. The obvious result is weight gain.

It's important that you take time to eat more slowly and chew your food thoroughly so that it is well combined with saliva, which aids digestion. Eating slowly also makes it more likely that you will get the "I'm full!" signal when your body has had enough. Including raw foods in your diet provides a way to slow down your eating, since these foods require time to chew.

When to Consume Liquids

Liquids that are consumed before or after a meal can act as a digestive aid. However, liquids during a meal should be minimized because they dilute the digestive juices and inhibit good digestion. The need to avoid the amount of liquids with meals will vary with different individuals, so it is important to be aware of your own body's needs. *Remember, if for any reason you are not properly digesting your food, your body is apt to store it as fat.*

CHAPTER 5

IMPLEMENTING YOUR DIET

Finally, you have reached the end of the search for the ideal diet. Now that you know your body type, you can start using food to truly support your body. Your body type diet gives you the guidance you need to develop the perfect diet for you. Knowing which foods truly support you, enables you to listen to your body and understand what it really needs. This allows for flexibility and variety within a supportive structure.

Becoming in tune with your body is a process. The most important thing to remember is to set the pace that is comfortable for you. The most effective way to change a pattern is to focus on one aspect long enough to incorporate it into your lifestyle. Once you've mastered that one, add another one.

Goals are achieved one step at a time. So, regardless of whether your goal is to gain, lose, or maintain your weight, or simply to feel vibrant, healthy and fully alive, your goal is within reach. You've taken the first step.

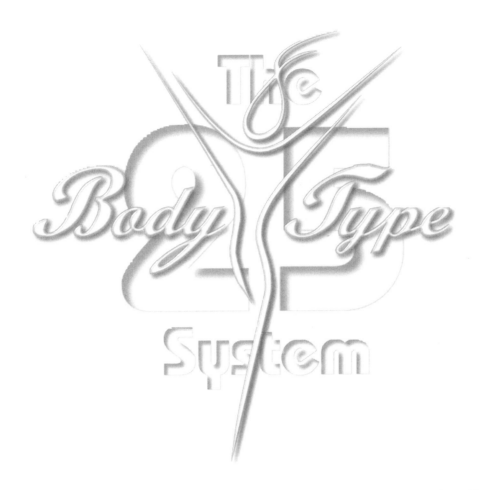

FOOD LISTS AND MENUS

FREQUENCY FOOD CATEGORIES

The food lists are divided into 3 categories: "Frequently," "Moderately," and "Rarely."

"**Frequently**" foods are those that best support your particular body type and can be eaten most often, which means they can be included in 3 to 7 meals per week. When you are hungry and can't think of anything that you especially want to eat, look on your "Frequently" list for ideas. Just make sure you get variety from these foods, rather than relying exclusively on the same ones over and over again.

"**Moderately**" foods offer variety in your diet. These are the foods you would eat 1 to 2 times a week. Frequency of foods refers to the individual foods rather than the entire group. For example, under grains you may eat semolina pasta twice a week, corn once as corn tortillas and once again as corn bread, and rye once as rye crackers and later as rye bread. This way you have your grains and variety. The lists are designed to be as complete as possible, so don't let unfamiliar foods scare you. You don't have to eat it just because it's listed. However, since no one food contains all the vitamins, minerals, and amino acids, and every food contains some of them, variety is essential. *By adding the nutrients from different foods to your diet, you will provide your body with more complete nutrition than you would with a diet that has limited food selections.*

"**Rarely**" foods are those that you should eat no more than once a month. While these foods aren't the best for you, it isn't the foods that you seldom eat that cause problems, but those that you eat 80 percent of the time. So, being able to eat these "Rarely" foods once in a while eliminates the feeling of deprivation, especially if something you love happens to be on this list.

What happens if you frequently eat "Rarely" foods? They tax your body by taking more energy away than they provide. This is usually done through excessive stimulation of your dominant gland or overloading your digestive system. You may not experience an immediate stomachache or headache after eating a stressful food. You could get a delayed reaction, ranging from mild to severe, that could include queasiness, upset stomach, mouth sores, lethargy, fatigue, constipation, diarrhea, dry or burning lips, dry skin, immune system weakness, nervousness, hyperactivity, or a craving for sweets. Symptoms may also be vague or hard to associate with a given food. Weight gain is often the result of eating too many of the "Rarely" foods since the body will often store what it can't assimilate.

By paying attention to what you are eating, you will eventually get to the point where you will be in tune with what your body needs. This is when you have a good sense of what is best for you to eat or avoid at any given time.

As a small child you had an intuitive sense of what was right for you, as long as you had reasonable choices. At times, such as after a cleansing diet, you probably found it was easier to be aware of which foods you needed and which ones you shouldn't eat. Ideally, we want to recapture our childhood intuition and awareness of our body.

Since the body controls its own metabolic processes, it knows what it needs and will be your best guide when it comes to what to eat. Your challenge is to correctly interpret the messages your body sends you. Generally, if you don't like a certain food, neither does your body.

HEALTHY VS. SENSITIVE FOOD LISTS

Select foods from the Healthy Food List when you feel strong and healthy. Select foods from the Sensitive Food List if you have digestive problems or when you are stressed.

The **Healthy** and **Sensitive Food Lists** constitute two perimeters. Most people fall somewhere between them rather than being completely in one or the other. If you are basically healthy, start with the Healthy Food List. As you look through it, you will probably find some foods you don't like or don't digest well. If these foods are in the "Frequently" or "Moderately" category on the Healthy List, they will probably be in the "Moderately" or "Rarely" category on the Sensitive Food List. Use the lists as a guide, being aware that the foods can change categories as your health and awarenesses change.

The foods, food combinations, and menus are recommendations, suggestions designed to give you a place to start. Ultimately, you want to be aware of and *listen to your body.*

MENUS: HOW TO SELECT AND USE

Most of the menu selections in diet books include foods that don't work for many people. They either overload the system by containing too many foods or the foods are inappropriate for the body type, leaving the person with a dull headache, mildly upset stomach, or lack of mental clarity. Also, these menus often take too much preparation time.

Cooking methods should be simple and uncomplicated, cutting down on preparation time by steaming, sauteing, or baking. Instead of rich sauces, season with herbs, combinations of herbs, or small amounts of salt and butter.

Keeping in mind the busy lifestyles most of us have, the focus is on menus that are practical. More importantly, once you have learned which foods are right for your body type, you can instantly evaluate any recipe as to how it is likely to affect you.

A wide range of menus is included. So if a food, or food combination, isn't something you would eat, you can simply cross it off and continue down the list. You are not limited to these combinations, and as you work with your diet, you'll develop your own favorites.

Quite often there are differences in food choices between types. What one person finds delicious may be downright inedible to another.

Each one of these menus has been "pre-tested" for each particular body type. *"Pre-tested" means that these specific food combinations are supportive for that particular type.*

Food combinations are important in that what is good for one type may not be for another. It's not enough to simply eat protein with any vegetable. You need to know the right combination if you want to optimize your diet. For example, some types can combine almost any vegetable with chicken, while others need to be far more selective. Skin types can add broccoli, cauliflower, carrots, green beans, zucchini, asparagus, chard, mushrooms, or celery, using any one or several simultaneously. Thyroids, on the other hand, can combine broccoli and/or carrots, green beans, or asparagus with chicken, but not all of these at the same time.

Combinations can be responsible for how well you digest certain foods. Putting together the wrong foods can cause symptoms ranging from mild indigestion, a heavy or sluggish feeling, nausea, bloating, fatigue, irritability, and weight gain to stomachaches and allergic reactions. While not every combination is listed, these menus will provide a starting point.

Muscle testing with another person or self-testing is also valuable in determining supportive food combinations. It enables you to determine what your body, rather than your head, needs. Combinations can change test results, so if there is a food you feel your body really needs, keep asking until you find the combination that will support you. *Please remember, too, that what your body wants today may be different from what it needs tomorrow.*

DIETARY CATEGORIES

There are several categories within the menus for each type: "Healthy", "Weight Loss", "Weight Gain", and "Sensitive". You may use different ones as your dietary requirements change.

"**Healthy**" includes all the menus and is the one most commonly selected. Use this for general body maintenance and when you are feeling well. As the ideal diet for your type, it shows you how to get the best nutrition as well as how to combine foods that are especially appropriate for you. Different foods have been combined to complement each other. The criteria are:

1) a strong muscle response when testing them, or
2) a positive physical effect after eating them.

Within a particular menu selection you will find food choices in parentheses. This designation means "with or without": that these foods are optional and can be safely deleted from the combination.

"Weight Loss" menus are designed to be low fat and low calorie, paying particular attention to specific body type requirements. They often revolve around foods that help to detoxify the body and include protein that is easily assimilated for rebuilding.

"Weight Gain" is for that neglected portion of the population rarely acknowledged as having a problem, specifically those who have difficulty maintaining adequate weight. People in this group are generally sensitive or have health problems interfering with assimilation. Also included here are athletes wanting to build muscle mass and people recovering from illness.

"**Sensitive**" menus are planned around the Sensitive Food List. These foods provide the greatest support and are the most easily digested. Originally developed for people who had severely depleted their bodies or were extremely sensitive, this menu is to be used when you don't feel well, are recovering from an illness, or are under a lot of stress. If you find yourself in the "sensitive" category, realize that as your system gets stronger, your foods will expand into the "Healthy" list.

If your body is extremely sensitive, as occurs when it has been severely stressed, usually from a chronic illness, prolonged fatigue, sleep deprivation, poor digestion or assimilation, hypoglycemia or low blood sugar, or obesity, the sensitive diet is often warranted. The basic sensitive diet, common to all the types, consists mostly of protein and vegetables. At times it will involve cutting down or eliminating sugars, including fruits, carbohydrates, and possibly reducing the grains down to only basmati rice. When the pancreas needs a rest, often the case with Pancreas and Skin types, limiting carbohydrate and sugar consumption to a period of less than one hour, once a day, will allow the pancreas to secrete insulin only once, thus reducing stress on the body. Some menus include "Very Sensitive" for types with extremely sensitive digestive systems.

VARIATIONS WITHIN THE DIET

The diets provided for the various body types are meant as a guide and can be modified to best suit your needs and desires. While your body is constantly adapting to changing conditions, the kind and quantity of food you choose to eat will vary with your activities.

The foods required to support your body during physical activity will differ from what is needed to support your brain during mental activity. Also, the amount of food you need at a particular time depends on what you are doing. If you are vigorously exercising, you will need to eat more than if you are sitting at a desk. The quantity of food eaten at meals will vary, as well as the choice of foods.

Example: *Thyroid types can eat from almost any of the food groups during the day and in varying amounts, depending on how active they are. Those who expend a lot of mental energy during the day do best with a moderate breakfast of protein with a vegetable or grain, possibly followed by fruit juice.*

A mid-afternoon snack is common if dinner is late. Also, the size and time of the evening meal often determines how heavy breakfast will be the next morning.

Regardless of the body type, it is important to change your diet appropriately when you are healing any part of your body or when you are under stress. This is also true when your level of activity or your environment changes.

WEIGHT LOSS TIPS

Since gaining weight is the first symptom of an imbalance in the body, the initial step to losing weight is to rebalance your body. The "Healthy" and "Sensitive" diets are designed to accomplish this goal. Occasionally, as individuals begin eating the foods they have deprived themselves of (sometimes for years), they experience weight gain. It is not uncommon to experience an increase in appetite for a short period before the system stabilizes.

There are a couple of pitfalls I'd like to caution you about. Some types have a strong *tendency to go overboard* on certain foods, especially if they have been depriving themselves of them. If the foods happen to be high fat or high calorie, weight gain can result, particularly if the diet is not adjusted accordingly.

The next common problem is *quantity of food.* The amount you eat is left to your discretion as it will vary according to your activities and diet earlier in the day or week. Naturally, if you have been eating large meals, you may be ready for less food. However, if your food consumption has been low, your body may be needing more fuel.

Another cause of weight gain relates to *body rebuilding.* When adequate nutrients are not available, muscle is cannibalized and often replaced with fat stores. This muscle must be rebuilt and fat eliminated. Since muscle weighs more than fat, body size may decrease (most often recognized when clothes begin to feel looser), while body weight actually increases.

Generally speaking, two weeks on the "Healthy" diet is sufficient to provide the nutrients that may have been missing and adequately support complementary systems so the body can rebuild. Then the actual dieting can begin, employing the weight loss menus.

FOOD ASSIMILATION AND WEIGHT MANAGEMENT

In order for a food to be considered a food it has to contain fat, protein, and carbohydrates, even if the quantity is too small to appear on package labels. If any component is missing, the body doesn't register the substance as a food and won't assimilate it. When foods are classified, they are put in categories of fat, protein, or carbohydrate, based on the dominant component. So meat is a protein, butter is a fat, and fruits and grains are carbohydrates.

The assimilation of these foods, however, still depends upon the presence of all three components of fat, protein, and carbohydrates. Without the three elements, digestion and assimilation are incomplete, which, of course, leads to a system imbalance.

Anything consumed that your body can't identify as a food is considered toxic and treated accordingly. Too much of a toxic substance will overload the liver and may trigger a migraine headache or cause headaches in general. Sometimes the body will keep the toxic substance in fluid suspension, resulting in bloating or fluid retention. Sometimes it will be stored in fat cells.

Carbohydrates, which break down into sugar, are necessary for protein assimilation. This became quite evident when I began testing a product called Re-Vita®.

Re-Vita®

Re-Vita® is a complete protein and contains all 22 amino acids. Initially, reading the ingredients, I was rather skeptical of its value since the first ingredient listed was fructose (a sugar), and the main component was spirulina, an algae that few people are able to assimilate. Another ingredient was ginseng, an herb which is beneficial for men, but not necessarily for women.

I was pleasantly surprised when I discovered that 70-80% of my patients, most of whom were very sensitive nutritionally, responded well to the Re-Vita®. I later learned that sugar was an essential factor in making this product easy to assimilate. Sugar enables protein to pass through a membrane between the bloodstream and the brain cells known as the blood/brain barrier. It also allows the same process to occur in other cells.

So, Re-Vita® duplicates what is naturally found in nature by using the fructose (sugar) to assimilate the protein (amino acids). This is also true for other sources of protein. It explains why carbohydrates are found in combination with protein in whole foods and why we desire something sweet after a high protein meal.

Proper assimilation of food also requires the presence of vitamins and minerals, which are often deficient in processed foods. A vitamin and mineral supplement sometimes helps provide these essentials but knowing which supplements to take requires an understanding of the body's needs. Muscle testing is helpful in making the right selection.

Most vitamin companies manufacture a multiple vitamin/mineral supplement, but in more than 20 years of testing I hadn't found one that was right for most people until I found Re-Vita®. In addition to protein, Re-Vita® contains minerals and trace elements in a form that is easy to assimilate.

Most minerals are simply mined from the earth and put into capsules. Unfortunately, our bodies aren't designed to assimilate them in this form.

Plants can convert minerals from the ground, but we can't. We can absorb them after the plants have converted them or from animals who have eaten the plants. If the plants don't get the minerals, they can't pass them on to us. This is why the algae is fed the minerals and why we assimilate minerals best from food sources.

Re-Vita® is different in that the assimilation is made possible by feeding the minerals to spirulina rather than simply adding them to the formula. The algae then processes the minerals into a form easily absorbed by the human body.

Food activates the digestive process. If vitamin pills are just swallowed the stomach has no way of knowing what's there. This is why the majority of nutritional supplements are most effective when taken with food. Consequently, mixing Re-Vita® with food maximizes its effectiveness. Some of the most popular ways to use Re-Vita® are with:

Grains as a

- sweetener on cereal like oatmeal, cream of rye or rice, and puffed corn or rice along with milk;
- syrup on pancakes, waffles, or French toast;
- flavoring for popcorn or in trail mix;
- "cookie" by melting butter, mixing oat flour, salt to taste, and Re-Vita® – then adding fine cut raw oatmeal. Proportions vary depending on quantity and the consistency you prefer for your "cookie". To make it stick together to form a flat patty or ball requires more butter. If you'd rather have it crumbly and eat it with a spoon or use it as a topping over fruit or yogurt, use less butter;

Fruit as a

- juice – use (Hain™) unsweetened cranberry concentrate, add berry Re-Vita®, and water;
- sweetener over cherries, rhubarb, or any other tart fruit. (May also be used as the sweetener in fruit desserts);

Dairy as a

- sweetener and flavor for yogurt, kefir, or milk;

Vegetables

- use over squash or pumpkin.

Basically use Re-Vita® as a sweetener or anything else that appeals to you.

HOW MUCH FAT AND PROTEIN

The consensus of most diet books is that weight loss is directly related to the consumption of fats. They say that an ideal diet should consist of no more than 25% fat for effective weight loss.

Example: If a 140 pound woman, consuming 1680 calories a day with no more than 47 grams of fat, wanted to lose weight, she would have to reduce the fat in her diet in proportion to her target weight. That is, if her goal was to weigh 120 pounds, she would need to reduce her fat intake from 47 to 40 grams. If she exercised vigorously, she might consume perhaps an additional 3 grams for every 100 calories burned. As metabolism slows, exercise should be increased and fat reduced.

The following table shows the number of calories and grams of fat based on percentage of calories from fats and the total number of calories consumed. Also included is a table for protein and

TOTAL PERCENTAGE OF FAT GRAMS AND CALORIES PER DAY

Total Calories	10%		15%		20%		25%		30%	
per Day	Grams	Calories	Grams	Calories	Grams	Calories	Grams	Calories	Grams	Calories
1000	11	100	16	150	22	200	27	250	33	300
1200	13	120	20	180	27	240	33	300	40	360
1500	16	150	25	225	33	300	41	375	50	400
1800	20	180	30	270	40	360	50	450	60	540
2000	22	200	33	300	44	400	56	500	67	600

TOTAL PERCENTAGE OF PROTEIN GRAMS AND CALORIES PER DAY

Total Calories per Day	10% Grams	10% Calories	15% Grams	15% Calories	20% Grams	20% Calories	25% Grams	25% Calories	30% Grams	30% Calories
1000	25	100	37	150	50	200	62	250	75	300
1200	30	120	45	180	60	240	75	300	90	360
1500	37	150	56	225	75	300	93	375	112	450
1800	45	180	67	270	90	360	112	450	135	540
2000	50	200	75	300	100	400	125	500	150	600

EXAMPLES

FATS	Fat Grams	Protein Grams	Cal.	PROTEIN	Fat Grams	Protein Grams	Cal.
1 tsp. butter	4	0	35	4 oz. chicken, light	4	35	187
1 tbs. oil (olive, safflower)	14	0	120	4 oz. turkey, light	3.3	34	175
1 tbs. blue cheese dressing	8	7	77	4 oz. chicken, dark	12.3	29	237
1 tbs. peanut butter	7	4	90	4 oz. turkey, dark	7.9	33	210
1 oz. Cheddar cheese	9	7	114	4 oz. tuna (water packed)	2	24	100
4 oz. cottage cheese, 2%	2	14	100	4 oz. shrimp	1.2	24	112
17 large almonds, roasted	14	9	180	4 oz. porterhouse steak	12.2	32	247
1 oz. sunflower seeds	14	6.5	162	2 oz. 1 beef frankfurter	17	7	181
1/2 cup avocado	19.9	2.4	204	1 egg, large	4.59	6	70

Source: *The Corinne Netzer Encyclopedia of Food Values*, Corinne T. Netzer, N.Y.: Dell Books, 1992.

food examples with their gram and calorie content.

In working with members of all 25 body types, I found that a diet with 25% fat is, overall, a good average. However, some types, such as the Stomach, need to reduce fat to 10-15% to lose weight. Conversely, types like Gallbladder and Eye gain weight if fat intake falls below 30%. Weight loss requirements can be quite specific, since not all fat sources are the same, and each body type has its specific sources from which to derive fat. This specific information is included in the profile under "Dietary Emphasis."

Even though your diet may call for 25% of your total calories from protein, the amount of protein per day may vary. For example, you may be really hungry one day and eat more protein, maybe even 50%, then feel like only eating vegetables the next day. The recommended percentage is designed to give you a realistic guideline to be used as a dietary average. This gives you flexibility and allows you the freedom to ultimately learn to listen to your body.

PROTEIN ASSIMILATION

A quick way to check for poor protein assimilation is to notice your body after you've eaten dairy products. If you have excess mucous in your throat, your protein is not being completely assimilated. Dairy protein is the easiest to digest, and unless you have a dairy sensitivity, excess mucous indicates that you are not completely assimilating the other protein you are eating either.

The best product I have found to aid in protein assimilation, as well as enhance digestion in general, is Noni™. Noni is a fruit that has been used as a main healing agent in the Polynesian Islands, Hawaii, and parts of Australia for over 2000 years. Dr. Heinicke identified the active substance as a precursor to an alkaloid that he named xeronine. Xeronine is a substance the body produces in order to activate enzymes so they can function properly. It is basic to the functioning of proteins, so it energizes and regulates the body and strengthens the immune system. The body must have it before it can do anything that requires protein, which includes manufacturing digestive enzymes, antibodies, hormones, and doing any form of healing. Noni™ is probably the best source of proxeronine that we have today. It's available in a liquid form and is best taken on an empty stomach. Noni™ can even be applied topically to problem areas. It's one of the few products I've found that benefits most people. Additional information is provided in "Resources".

Listen to and be aware of what your body is telling you. If you're still having problems, you may need to use a digestive aid or work with a professional to enhance your digestive system.

WATER

Our bodies are made up primarily of water. Consequently, the right kind of water in adequate quantities is essential. Approximately one-half gallon of water per day is ideal for most people. This sounds like a lot but it is only eight 8-ounce or four 16-ounce glasses. The Kidney body type often requires a little less, but most types need between 1-1/2 quarts and 3/4 gallons of water daily. If you live in a hot, dry climate or are especially active during the day, your requirements may increase.

Drinking water will curb your appetite. Many people eat, not because they are really hungry, but because they are dehydrated. In addition to flushing the toxins out of the body, water can help burn calories.

Many people think that because a beverage contains water it counts as water. Unfortunately, that's not true. The body registers liquids like coffee, fruit juice, soft drinks, soups, etc., as food. So, if you are drinking anything other than plain water, even though it contains water, the body can't use it as water.

The kind of water you drink will determine how easy it is for you to drink enough water. Heavily chlorinated water from the tap not only doesn't taste good but adds toxic substances to your body. Since the main reason to drink water is to cleanse your system, drinking anything other than pure water is counter-productive. The best waters contain some minerals. This is why drinking water from a fresh mountain stream can taste so good. Distilled water leaches minerals, as can water filtered through reverse osmosis.

One way to upgrade water is to add a small amount of juice such as lemon, lime, apple, or grape. Sometimes this is enough to balance its mineral content and improve the taste. When you are dining in restaurants or traveling and must drink water from an unknown source, adding a few drops of lemon juice will help improve the taste and neutralize the chlorine, as well as other toxic substances.

The best indicator of a good water for you is taste. If you don't like the taste of a particular water, it usually isn't the one that's right for you. It's easy to drink water when you like the taste. Muscle testing can also be used to determine your best water source.

POLARIZATION

There is a procedure that offers protection from toxins in food, water, and air called Polarization. Polarizing your food makes it easier to digest and neutralizes harmful bacteria.

I had an opportunity in Egypt to test the validity of one of these polarizers. Cholera is extremely common in the Middle East, so everyone is warned not to drink the water or eat any vegetables with a high water content. There were five of us within a larger tour group. During lunch, cabbage rolls were served. One woman took a bite, realized it contained lamb and stopped. Another woman ate one, which consisted of two bites. Rebecca ate two, and my roommate had three. I thought they were good and ate four. Prior to eating, my roommate and I used the "Harmonizer" to polarize our meal, while the other three women did not.

When we got back to the hotel, I received a phone call, "Rebecca is sick, and it was lunch." Lunch, I thought, I'm fine, my roommate is fine, what's going on here? I went next door, and Rebecca was so sick. Not only did she have cholera, but she had other intestinal bacteria as well. The other two women also had cholera, but when they realized they were getting sick, they immediately stimulated acupuncture points and were able to control the symptoms. My roommate and I were fine. The only thing we did differently was to momentarily hold the polarizer over our food before we ate it.

Polarization works by amplifying positive energy. In the northern hemisphere, everything that is positive spins in a clockwise manner, while everything with a negative polarity spins counter-clockwise. When an atom loses an electron, it loses it's positive spin and spins counter-clockwise. When an apple is bruised, the atoms in the bruised area lose an electron. They look for their missing electron and pull energy from the rest of the apple. This eventually causes the rest of the apple to go bad. And, this is how "one rotten apple can spoil the entire barrel."

Polarization supplies the missing electron by bringing in positive energy or electrons, thereby neutralizing the negative effects of the bacteria. I have made it a habit to polarize my food before I eat it since bacteria is so prevalent, and it also makes the food easier to digest.

Polarization is also good for general first aid. When an area has been traumatized like a cut or sunburn, the energy is disrupted or scattered. Polarizing the area allows the energy to be re-aligned, allowing healing to occur much quicker.

COMPATIBILITY BETWEEN TYPES

Laura consulted me because she was concerned about the eating habits of her entire family. It seems that they all wanted to eat different kinds of foods and she was going crazy trying to please them. She was buying food for meals and snacks that she thought would please everyone, but it just wasn't working out that way.

Laura couldn't understand why her husband, son, and daughter all wanted different things to eat and, to make it even more difficult, they wanted to eat at different times. In an attempt to please them all she had begun to think that she was the one with the problem.

Once I determined the body types of the entire family, it was easy to see why they were having such varied tastes. Even though they all seemed to look very much alike, with similar shapes and builds, they were an assortment of types. Laura was a Gonadal, her husband and son were Adrenals, and her daughter was a Kidney type.

In spite of the differences, there was a great deal of compatibility. After checking the menu suggestions and food lists for each type, we found that everyone in the family could eat bananas, apples, or oranges for breakfast, as well as oatmeal with raisins and oat bran toast. Laura and her daughter could have eggs, while her husband and son did better with cottage cheese and pineapple.

For lunch they could all include protein, vegetables, and grain. For example, a good meal might be chicken, potatoes, and broccoli, or they might like a tuna and lettuce sandwich on sourdough bread.

An ideal dinner for everyone would be pasta and vegetables. Laura, her husband, and son could have protein, such as fish or other meat, but her daughter, being a Kidney type, would utilize the protein much better at lunchtime or even for breakfast.

When we reviewed the dietary requirements for their different types, Laura began to see why she had been so confused. She had been trying to please everyone's desires without knowing their actual body type needs. Now, with this new plan, she has found enough similarities in the foods on each diet list to allow her to prepare meals and snacks that please everyone. The result is not only a happier family, but a healthier one.

It is a rare instance when every member of a family is the same body type. Couples are often complementary types, sometimes opposites, and on occasion, the same. Among children, perhaps none, or several, will be the same type as one of their parents.

Body types within a family will often be similar and generally compatible. This means that the types with dominant glands in their heads, such as the Pineal, are often attracted to similar types, such as a Thyroid. They can also be drawn to a type like a Lymph, Blood, or Nervous System, whose dominant system encompasses the entire body. In Laura's family, they all had their dominant glands in the lower portion of the body.

Opposite Diets

So, what happens if the food choices for a certain meal are not compatible for all family members? The Pituitary type, for example, needs protein for breakfast and lunch with only vegetables and/or fruit for dinner. Stomachs eat lighter in the morning, and heavier for lunch and dinner. So, if a Pituitary woman is married to a Stomach man, she can prepare chicken for dinner, along with vegetables and baked potatoes. Since dinner is a moderate to heavy meal for him and light to moderate for her, she can eat her potato and vegetables for dinner and save her portion of chicken for breakfast the next morning.

This way, everyone gets the foods they need at the time when their bodies can best utilize them, without having to cook two separate meals. The problem occurs if there is a strong family belief that everyone should eat some of everything on the table. The solution is to change this mindset to accommodate the needs of the individuals.

To determine which meals are compatible for all family members, check the food groups under "Scheduling Meals" in each body type diet for similarity. You are looking for protein, grains, vegetables, fruits, nuts, seeds, and dairy. Then compare the "Rarely" foods listed for each type and eliminate them from your choices. With the pared down list, you will be able to plan your meals to please everyone, adding other foods as needed for each individual family member.

HOW TO USE ADDITIONAL BODY TYPE INFORMATION

Since I only have one dominant gland, why should I bother to learn about the other body types? Why do I need the information on the other types?

The human body contains all of the glands, organs and systems. Your dominant gland is simply the strongest, meaning the one that exerts the strongest influence. If you have any health challenges, or are going through a healing process, you'll want to be aware of how to support the organ that is weak. For example, if you've been under a lot of stress and have exhausted your adrenal glands, you can refer to the healthy Adrenal food list.

Look at the foods under the "Frequently" category and compare them to the food list for your type. You'll probably find most of them in your "Frequently" and "Moderately" categories. Mark these foods and see which ones you feel like including in your diet for the next week or so. You can include the ones that are on your "Moderately" list twice a week, and those on your "Frequently" list can be eaten three to seven times. This is how you can focus on rebuilding your adrenal glands while still keeping your body in balance by following your diet.

DIETARY CHANGES: "TAKE IT SLOW"

"Listening to your body" is being sensitive to your body's reactions to the foods you eat. This is important in making changes in your diet and also in starting special diets. Sudden changes in what you eat, even when you go from a poor diet to a healthful one, can produce negative effects in your system. If the body's immediate needs are not met and those needs depend on the body's present condition, too radical a change can cause problems.

For example, when a person's system has deteriorated, whole, unrefined foods are usually indigestible. The body simply cannot tolerate a sudden change to a more healthful diet. A system used to highly refined "junk food" needs the fats and sugars that are easily metabolized for quick energy. These are stimulants that keep the system going but, at the same time, destroy health.

If an individual is eating "junk food", especially a child or a teenager, reducing this in their diet should be done gradually. The body must be given time to adjust to new foods and eating patterns and to rebuild the weakened systems.

When foods can't be assimilated by an unbalanced system, switching to a healthful diet can leave the person devoid of energy. This alone could encourage one to abandon the diet and go back to unhealthy eating, which at least will supply the energy necessary to function.

So, before making any serious dietary changes it is important to carefully consider what you are presently eating. Major changes usually need to be made in small steps, and care should be taken to eat those foods that will restore the depleted system.

"IF I FOLLOW THE DIET, WHAT CAN I EXPECT?"

Stand before a full length mirror in your underwear or a bathing suit. Turn and observe yourself from all angles, front, back, and side views. Take a careful look. Where do you appear to have excess weight? Is there a look of disproportion, a heaviness in some areas while others seem just right? Or you might need to put on a little weight in certain parts of your body.

The weight you carry on your body is a good reflection of how your system uses the food you eat. Eating the foods that are right for your particular body type, and also observing the times of the day when these are most effective for your system, will enable you to give your body just what it needs.

This "conscious" eating will cause your body to lose unnecessary weight so that your system can function properly without the mental and physical stress of "dieting". And if you want to gain weight, it will be much easier as you will know what to eat as well as the times of the day when your system will get the best results from the foods you eat.

Eating for your body type is different from the usual weight loss diets, since you are now supplying your system with foods which are supportive of it. Weight loss diets usually stress deprivation of some kind, which often causes a "rebound" effect when you go off the diet. Eating the right foods for your body type allows you to reach and then maintain your correct body weight. This, in itself, is a big step towards optimal health.

Without regard to weight loss or gain, there are other comments I hear from patients who have begun to follow the special diets for their body types. Most often I hear "I feel better!" Many tell me that they have a higher energy level, and that they no longer feel hungry between meals. Some are better able to avoid the sweets and caffeine that they were dependent on for that little "boost" that got them through the day. Often they are able to accomplish much more because of better endurance, and have more energy at the end of the day.

What it really comes down to is this: if you follow the eating regimen tailored to your particular body type, you will be using food the way nature, or your special nature, meant you to. When you support your body with a diet plan best suited for it, you can achieve an optimal state of physical health and well-being.

You must eat in order to live, so why not eat those foods that "enliven" you, unlocking the stores of energy and vitality that you may never have known before. And, with it, you can maintain that energy flow as it constantly replenishes and rebuilds your system.

MAINTAINING YOUR DIET

These diets are neither fads nor instant cures. It's about making permanent, long-term change. This lifetime eating program is based on sound dietary practices and what is individually right for each body type.

To get the greatest value out of your specific eating program, you'll need to change your eating patterns to the ways that truly support your body. In this process you will become more aware of when changes are necessary. Once you experience what it's like to feel really healthy, you will also know when your body is out of balance as well as how to regain that balance.

Long-term change rarely happens overnight, yet changing your eating habits can bring you better health and a more fulfilling lifestyle. Here's how some of my patients began to incorporate this program into their lifestyles:

"I looked at the diet, familiarized myself with what was ideal for me, and then compared it to what I was currently doing. I incorporated the parts that were easy for me, adding a single item I was attracted to, and put the diet away until I was ready for more."

""I worked on one part at a time, first the foods, then the meals. The foods meant adding or deleting certain foods. Meals involved using new menus, mainly at breakfast."

"I changed a pattern of eating sweets, like ice cream, cookies, candy, or pastries, from anytime during the day to only when my body could easily handle them. Now I save the sweets for later and if I still want them, eat them as an evening or bedtime snack."

"I shifted the time of day that I ate my largest meal from dinner to lunch time. It dramatically changed my energy level." (Pineal, Medulla, Skin, Pancreas, and Gallbladder types will definitely relate to this.)

"I followed the diet for 2 or 3 weeks and noted how I felt. Then I went back to the old way and noted the difference. I am convinced that it is definitely worth the effort to establish new patterns.

"I added 'balancing' foods. As a Medulla type, I found I could comfortably eat pepperoni pizza if I drank pineapple/coconut juice after it."

"I started keeping a diary of what I ate and how I felt after each meal. I read my diary while I'm riding my stationary bicycle. This motivates me to stay with my diet and keeps me from sliding back into my old habits. When I first started following my diet a year ago, I felt great. Then I felt I was invincible and could eat anything. It worked for a while, but then I gradually started slipping back into my old habits. My headaches returned, my energy was down, and I became irritable and short-tempered. I went back on my diet and felt dramatically better. That's when I realized I needed to keep a diary to keep reminding me that I can feel great and what it takes to do it."

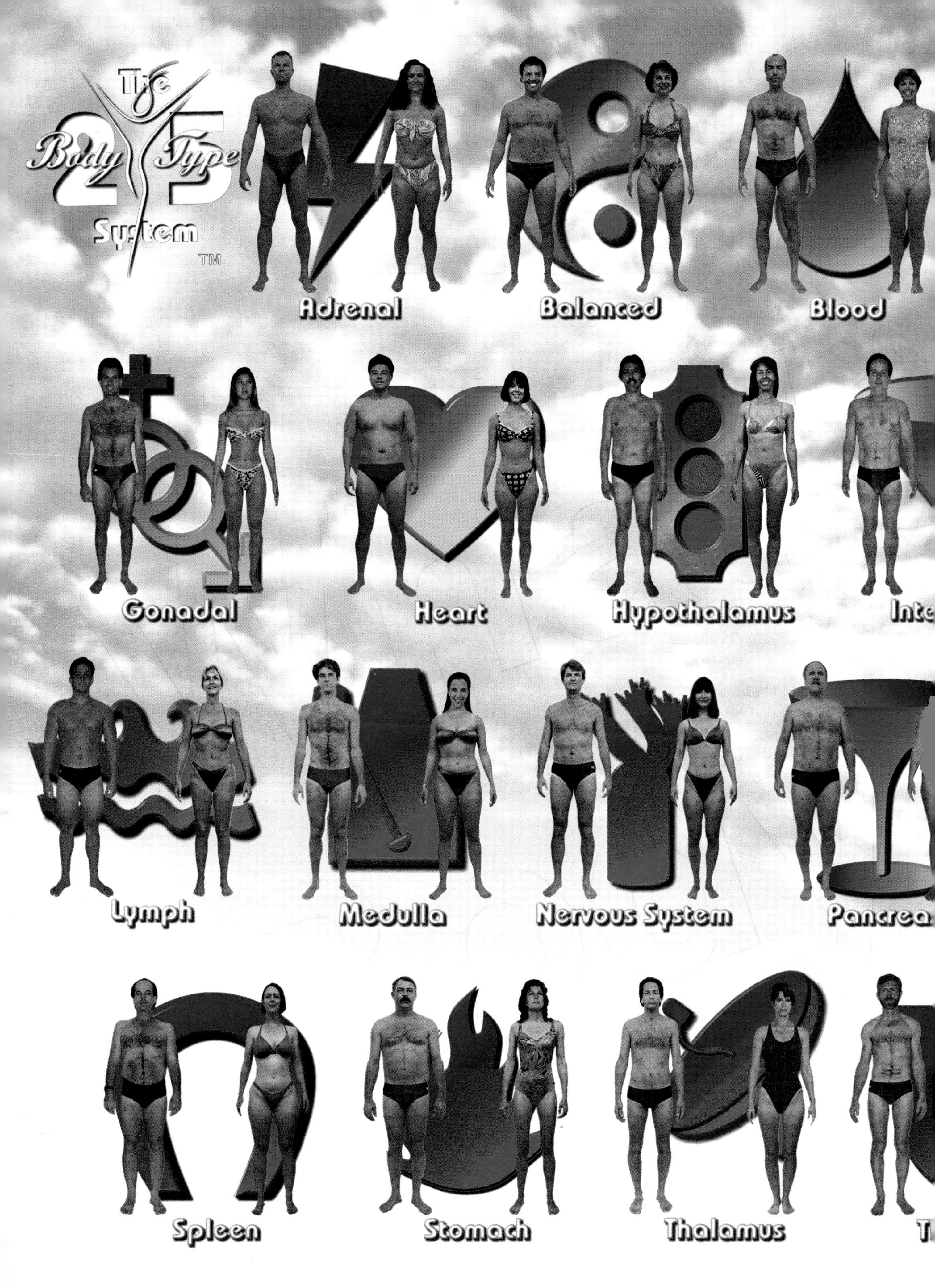

The Body Type 25 System
TM
Adrenal
Balanced
Blood
Gonadal
Heart
Hypothalamus
Lymph
Medulla
Nervous System
Spleen
Stomach
Thalamus

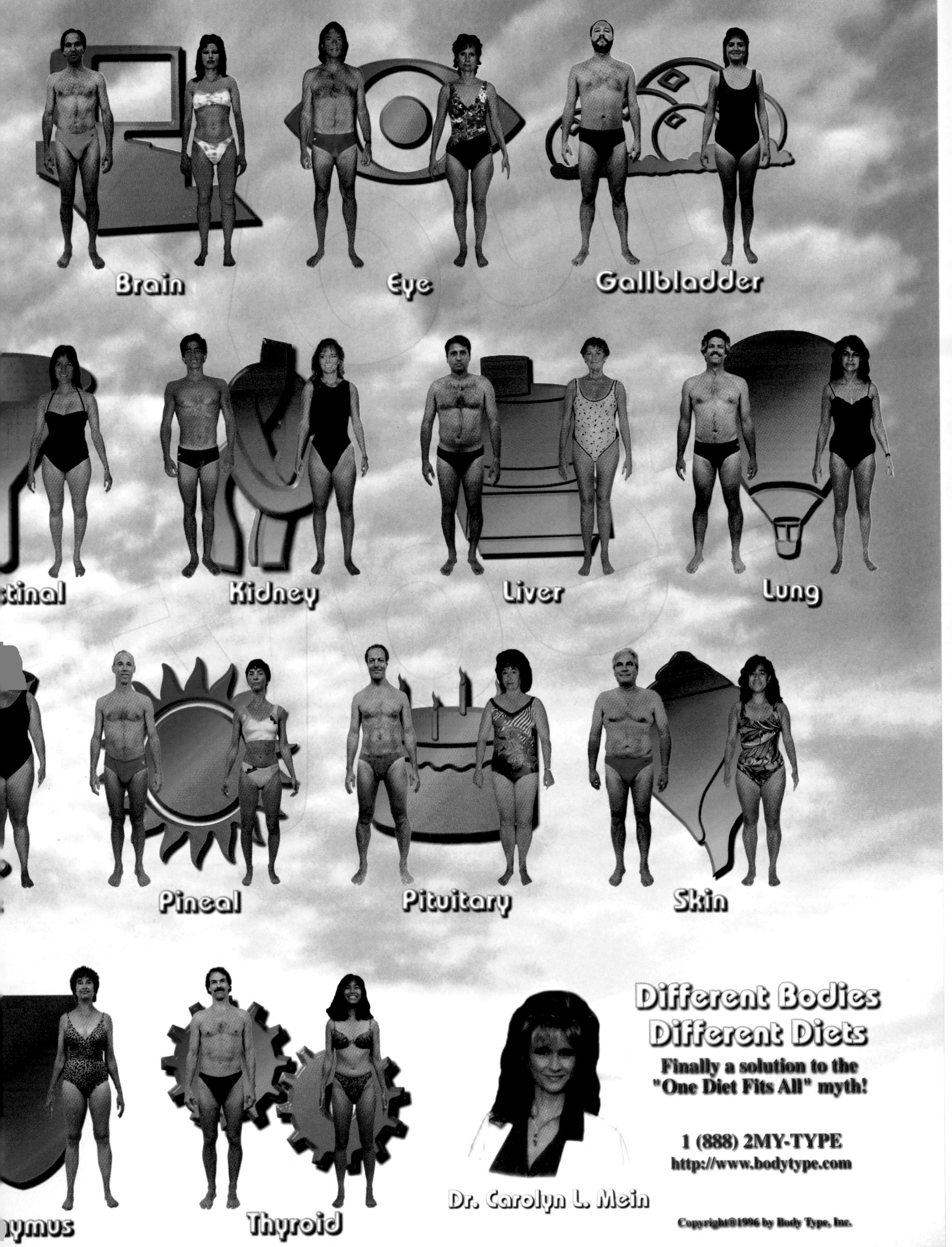
Brain
Eye
Gallbladder
stinal
Kidney
Liver
Lung
Pineal
Pituitary
Skin
ymus
Thyroid
Dr. Carolyn L. Mein
Different Bodies
Different Diets
Finally a solution to the
"One Diet Fits All" myth!
1 (888) 2MY-TYPE
http://www.bodytype.com
Copyright©1996 by Body Type, Inc.

PROFILES & DIETS

Each one of the 25 types is unique. No type is better than another. Each one has it's own specific strengths and challenges, and achievable potential. Every type, when they are able to consistently come from their "At Best", is awesome.

To be your best, you need to feel your best, and the diets are the easiest place to start. You'll learn to be in tune with your body, and from there your mind and emotions.

The basis of "The 25 Body Type System" is self-empowerment. The "Profiles and Diets" provide you with an owners' manual for your body – your unique guide to self-awareness.

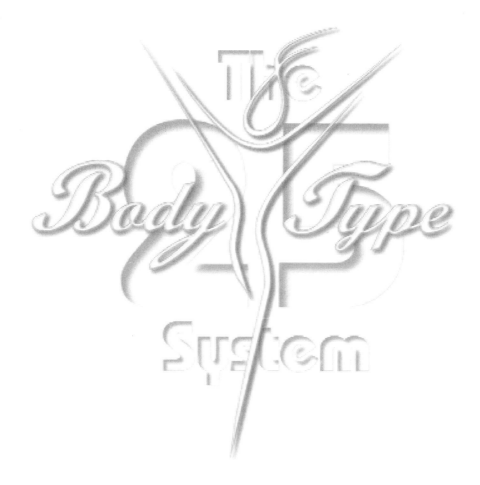

BRIEF EXPLANATION OF TERMS AND FORMAT

LOCATION & FUNCTION	Provides the location and function of the gland, organ, or system associated with each type. The location is where, when healthy, the majority of the body's energy resides and, when depleted, where the body is most vulnerable.
POTENTIAL HEALTH PROBLEMS	Identification of the problems your type is prone to develop when your dominant gland becomes exhausted, including early warning signs.
RECOMMENDED EXERCISE	Exercise is essential for some types as it activates the immune system. But, surprisingly, this isn't true for all types. For the majority exercise is helpful because of its affect on the emotions. It's an effective way to release stress, clear or calm the mind, and get energy moving in the body. From here it can have other emotional benefits or spillovers positively affecting the physical body. For others, whether you exercise or not doesn't make that much difference, making it optional. It's not that it doesn't have positive effects, because it does, it's just that exercise is a low priority for the body. The exercises listed are the ones that your type generally benefits from most. Excess weight accumulates in the weakest area of the body, in other words, the area where the energy flow is blocked or sluggish. For most of the 25 types this area is the lower abdomen. Exercise gets energy moving and tones muscles. With the demands I had on my time, I found it difficult to spend hours in the gym or work-out studio. So I began searching for the exercises that would be the most effective, particularly those that would specifically flatten and strengthen my lower abdomen. These exercise programs are the ones I have found to be the most effective and universally beneficial to all the 25 types. "Blisswork" developed by Juawayne Hope is by far the most effective and efficient way of strengthening and toning the body. Cathie Murakami of SynergySystems™ has developed a program based on the work of Joseph H. Pilates to strengthen the core muscles of the low back, pelvis and abdomen; it's available on video. The simplest and easiest way to incorporate exercise into your lifestyle is by using the Fitness Ball, a large exercise ball, as a chair. It gently forces you to use your lower abdominals and strengthens your core. Besides, it's fun.
DISTINGUISHING FEATURES	These features alone can often be sufficient to differentiate one type from another. However, while often present, not every member of a type necessarily has them, or has them to the degree that they are strongly evident.
ADDITIONAL PHYSICAL CHARACTERISTICS	Supplementary characteristics that are useful for comparing and contrasting different types. Since physical characteristics reflect ethnic and familial heritage as well as dominant and subdominant gland characteristics, they can vary considerably. I've described the characteristics that are most commonly seen within each type and noted the ones that tend to run the entire range. For example, height in Liver types can vary from very petite to very tall, even though the majority are of average height. So, don't rule out a type simply because one or two characteristics don't apply to you.

BRIEF EXPLANATION OF TERMS AND FORMAT

WEIGHT GAIN AREAS	The initial weight gain pattern is the most important, and is often the simplest and most obvious criterion for determining type in women. Secondary gain refers to over 15 pounds.
SCHEDULING MEALS	A quick guide for choosing which foods to eat for breakfast, lunch, and dinner and when to eat them. "Healthy" is when you feel strong and healthy with plenty of energy available to digest your food. "Sensitive" is when your body is under stress (physical, mental or emotional) so energy is directed elsewhere and less is available for digestion.
DIETARY EMPHASIS	Recommendations for weight loss or gain. Fat and protein requirements with best sources. Fats derived from other sources will not necessarily supply the essential fatty acids, so these fats would add to the total fat calories consumed, but not qualify to be included in the minimum fat requirement.
KEY SUPPORTS FOR SYSTEM	Suggested foods and/or activities to optimally strengthen or support your particular type.
COMPLEMENTARY GLANDULAR SUPPORT	Identifies the two glands needing to be rebuilt or supported in order to give your dominant gland a rest and suggests how this is best accomplished.
FOODS CRAVED	*(When Energy is Low)* The foods that, by stimulating the body's dominant gland, provide the greatest immediate but temporary energy lift.
FOODS TO AVOID	Foods that are particularly difficult for your body to assimilate or ones that cause excessive stress.
RECOMMENDED CUISINE	The cuisine most supportive to your system – particularly useful when dining out and needing to select the most appropriate restaurant. Also included are the foods best suited to your type on a daily basis.
PSYCHOLOGICAL PROFILE	The "Essence" embodies the basic nature of each body type. The profile is often the deciding factor in type identification as supporting foods can shift when the dominant gland becomes depleted. Psychological characteristics are often observed from birth and can be useful in identifying the body type of children. Becoming familiar with the personality parameters of the various body types can help you gain insight into your own personal strengths and challenges, as well as expanding your self-awareness. Additionally, aside from better understanding your own basic nature, increasing your knowledge about the psychological dimensions of the other body types can enhance your understanding and, hopefully, acceptance of others different from you. *Ultimately, you want to learn to be aware of your body and pay attention to it. Listening to your body is essential in knowing what foods to eat to feel and look your best, as well as understanding and accepting yourself.*

ADRENAL

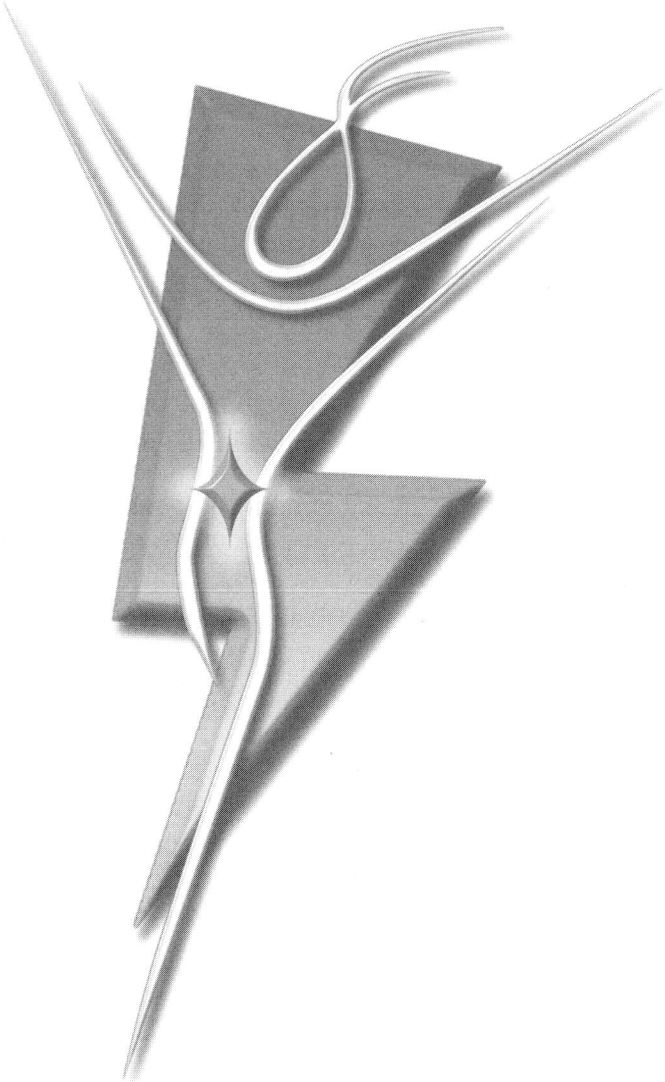

The "Adrenal Body Type"
is symbolized by the lightning bolt.
Forceful and dynamic, Adrenals are
characterized by their high energy,
physical strength, and endurance.
Charming and charismatic,
they readily make their
presence known.

Adrenal

BODY TYPE PROFILE

LOCATION	Situated on top of each kidney in lower back, at level of lower ribs.
FUNCTION	As strongest glands in body, produce hormones (including adrenaline) secreted under stress to prepare for "fight or flight" response.
POTENTIAL HEALTH PROBLEMS	Exercise is essential as it activates the immune system. To keep it continuously active requires exercising a minimum of 40 minutes daily, preferably after 3 p.m. Exercise is beneficial in all areas, including stress release, and is essential in losing and maintaining ideal weight. Running is excellent as are walk/run combinations and non-stationary activities, as they usually have a calming effect. Exercises such as Life Cycle or other stationary activities tend to build up energy in the body. Weight lifting is beneficial if you enjoy it. Activities such as swimming, tennis, and Tai Chi encourage hand/eye co-ordination, cardiovascular stimulation, and flexibility.
RECOMMENDED EXERCISE	Dense, solid musculature throughout torso, arms, thighs, and calves. "Boyish" figure with straight, poorly defined waist. Inherently high energy, strength, and endurance. Excess weight easy to gain. Strong, masculine energy, as reflected both by their muscle mass and forceful presence, which, when "feminized," becomes gregarious and vivacious, outgoing, and charming. The more masculine is direct and strong-willed, with a forceful presence.

WOMEN'S CHARACTERISTICS

DISTINGUISHING FEATURES	Very healthy and strong with consistently high energy and stamina throughout youth. Excess weight often problem as can easily put on weight by eating too much, failing to get sufficient strenuous exercise, and even from experiencing too much emotional stress. Conversely, can also lose weight easily, so known as "star dieters" – but also as "queens" of yo-yo dieting. Most diets are, in fact, designed for Adrenals, particularly those emphasizing raw fruits and vegetables, yogurt, and cottage cheese. Become confused and/or "hyper" when under stress and may have difficulty calming down. Classic disease patterns include sudden onset of high blood pressure, hypertension, arteriosclerosis, and cardiovascular disease.
ADDITIONAL PHYSICAL CHARACTERISTICS	Buttocks relatively flat-to-rounded. Low back curvature straight-to-average. Breasts average-to-large, depending on weight distribution. Shoulders and hips relatively even. Torso short-waisted to average. Wide, sturdy, grounded stance. Height generally average, but can range from very petite to tall. Bone structure medium-to-large. Dense, solid musculature throughout torso, arms, thighs, and calves. Hands often large and/or wide with strong, thick muscle at

Adrenal

base of thumb. Feet may be wide. Hair average to very thick and heavy. Typically square or rectangular face with strong jaw, or average-to-long oval face.

WEIGHT GAIN AREAS

Upper, lower or entire body with initial gain in upper, lower or entire abdomen; marked in waist; upper, middle, and entire back; upper hips; upper arms; breasts; entire thighs (consisting of front, back, inner and outer) covering upper 2/3rds or extending to knees including upper inner thighs; and face. Alternative weight gain pattern limits gain in thighs to upper inner, with predominant gain in upper body. If more masculine, weight gain in torso; if more feminine, in thighs. Area of gain can vary with life circumstances. Secondary gain all over, including under chin, with large amounts of weight accumulating mainly in entire abdomen, waist, and upper hips. Weight often fluctuates according to emotional state.

DIETARY GUIDELINES

SCHEDULING MEALS:

"HEALTHY"

Breakfast: Light, with fruit, dairy, vegetables, and/or grain.

Lunch: Moderate. May be heavy if dinner is moderate, with vegetables, grain, legumes, nuts, seeds, dairy, protein, and/or fruit.

Dinner: Heavy, or moderate if lunch was heavy, with grain, vegetables, protein, dairy, legumes, nuts, seeds, and/or fruit.

"SENSITIVE"

Breakfast: Light, with fruit.

Lunch: Moderate, with vegetables, grain, dairy, and/or legumes.

Dinner: Heavy, with protein, dairy, nuts, seeds, legumes, vegetables, and/or grain.

DIETARY EMPHASIS

- Yogurt, cottage cheese, and fruit.
- For weight loss, reduce food quantity, especially carbohydrates (including breads, rice, pasta, and potatoes), and, if tolerated, may use appetite suppressants. If adrenals are exhausted, include up to 20% dense protein (fish, turkey, and/or chicken). Ideal diet consists of raw fruits and vegetables, salads, protein, and soups. Best not to snack, but if cannot avoid, eat raw vegetables or fruit or about 1/2 cup of yogurt. Limit fats to 25% of total calories (if below 20% won't lose weight).
- For weight gain, increase food quantity. Include dense protein up to 30% of calories.

Adrenal

DIETARY EMPHASIS	• Vegetarian diet recommended when healthy and at ideal weight, particularly when dairy products are included. Normally, up to 10% of total calories, up to 30% when rebuilding, may be from fish, turkey, or chicken to balance body weight when under stress. • Fats, 20-25% of total daily calories, should be derived from almonds and dairy (yogurt, cottage cheese, cheese). If intolerant of dairy, include chicken and fish.
KEY SUPPORTS FOR SYSTEM	When healthy, eat more raw than cooked vegetables, while sensitive require more cooked than raw; whole grains; fruit (up to 40% of diet); protein, mainly from poultry or fish; and low fat dairy. Drinking mineral water and/or parsley tea can help reduce appetite and cleanse body.
COMPLEMENTARY GLANDULAR SUPPORT	Pituitary, through dietary stimulation with dairy, specifically yogurt and cottage cheese; thyroid stimulation with sugar, especially fruit; caffeine in moderation (1 to 1-1/2 cups/day) may be beneficial unless sensitive, as helps thyroid establish steady energy flow.
FOODS CRAVED	*(When energy is low)* Sweets, especially candy, chocolate, or ice cream. Salty foods like nuts (particularly peanuts), chips, and french fries. Protein such as eggs, chicken, and beef (typically steak or hamburger), particularly in evening. Energy lull around 5 p.m. (i.e., cocktail hour), at which time crave salty foods, sweets, and/or cocktails.
FOODS TO AVOID	Because salt and beef stimulate adrenals, best to stay away from both salty foods and hamburgers.
RECOMMENDED CUISINE	Mexican, Italian, Chinese, Sushi, Soup and Salad (Best daily fare: vegetables and rice noodles, salads, and soups).

Adrenal

PSYCHOLOGICAL PROFILE

ESSENCE

Just as the adrenal glands are the strongest glands in the body, Adrenal body types are distinguished by their high energy, physical strength, and endurance. This dominant physical energy is reflected in their heavy, solid musculature, commanding presence, and physical comfort in the world. Forceful and dynamic, they easily make themselves known as soon as they enter a room and are generally the first ones in an audience to ask questions or make comments. They are, by nature, outgoing, often charming and charismatic.

CHARACTERISTIC TRAITS

Adrenals thrive on excitement and obvious success. They possess a quick, powerful energy and approach life with a see, touch, get–in, get–out attitude. With their commanding presence, strong will, and being vocally uninhibited, they make themselves heard when they enter a room, and people listen. Consequently, they can easily control and lead a crowd, making them dynamic leaders. Highly competitive, they often gravitate toward sales and contact sports.

With inquiring, investigative minds, Adrenal types like to examine things from alternative perspectives. They are good at surveying the facts, and are geared to practical, down-to-earth solutions. Predominantly visually oriented, they readily examine, access, and see solutions to physical problems. Easily bored, Adrenals prefer to move on to something else once a task becomes routine. Mentally quick and alert, they don't like to stay with a task too long, making them appear to have a relatively short attention span. They prefer to see what needs to be done, delegate the tasks, then oversee the work.

Independent minded and prone to act, Adrenals like to be in total control of a task or situation so they alone can determine the outcome. With their quick, strong initiating energy, they are the first to dive into a project, even when not really sure how to do it. Competitive and hard driving, when uncertain how to proceed, their immediate impulse is to "power" through it anyway.

For Adrenals, stress is generally reflected by an "adrenaline rush." This excess hormone production can lead to scattered hyperactivity, or the inability to channel energy productively, resulting in "running around in circles." While prone to these "nervous highs," when their energy is exhausted, Adrenals are just as likely to feel low or depressed.

MOTIVATION

Adrenals tend to be unaware of their emotions or that something is bothering them until their feelings have become strongly aroused. When the internal pressure builds up to a certain point, they are likely to undergo a sudden emotional discharge that may include bursts of anger, tears, or outbreaks of excitement. Verbally uninhibited, Adrenals think nothing of asking questions or making comments that would embarrass other types. Likewise, when stressed, they will readily "blow off steam." The angry outburst will end as

Adrenal

MOTIVATION (Continued)

suddenly as it began and without any lingering hard feelings. For once Adrenals are able to express their feelings and get rid of the bottled up energy, they're prepared to forgive just about anything and to resume the relationship as though nothing at all had happened.

There is a basic fear of rejection that manifests as their having difficulty saying "no" for fear of being left out. They tend to be "people pleasers" because they are dependent upon others' responses to them, so they will generally strive to make a good impression. Consequently, they will often commit to an activity and fail to follow through. As they gain more emotional maturity, their fear of rejection becomes less of a motivation.

Recognition and approval from others is often closely linked to self–esteem. Being externally directed, career success and validation from outside themselves are crucial for a sense of well–being . Self–worth can hinge on doing well in their chosen line of work, and women Adrenals often experience a need to prove themselves in "a man's world." Especially sensitive to rejection, Adrenals are strongly motivated to make a good impression, making them extremely concerned about their image and how well they're accepted by others.

Blessed with resilient, robust bodies, and strong digestive systems, Adrenals initially seem to be able to eat anything. They can eat large quantities of food in an unconscious effort to numb themselves against distressful feelings with no significant side effects other than weight gain. When they're experiencing anxiety or emotional discomfort, Adrenals often experience a strong compulsion to eat. For Adrenal types, weight loss is directly related to quantity of food consumed and exercise, so most diets initially work. Since, with Adrenals, weight is actually regulated by their stress level, and because exercise relieves the stress produced by excess adrenaline, exercise is essential. However, unresolved emotional turmoil can result in weight gain or the inability to lose even though they are exercising and following their ideal diet.

"AT WORST"

When under stress, Adrenals experience an "adrenaline rush," often gradually, that disturbs their ability to channel their energy productively. They get scattered, hyperactive, or depressed. The tendency is to overeat to soothe their emotions, which can easily culminate in a food addiction or turning to alcohol or drugs. Strenuous physical movement moves the adrenaline out of the muscles, which reduces stress buildup and emotional blowups. Depression or exhaustion can bring out their tendency to be lazy.

When their energy is high and the excess energy is not dissipated through exercise, Adrenals experience mood swings and emotional volatility. Sensitive to rejection, when they don't get the approval they are seeking and their self–esteem is threatened, Adrenals will defend themselves through verbal attacks or blaming someone or something. Thriving on excitement and immediate success, they can easily become addicted to thrill-seeking and

Adrenal

adrenaline rushes. Feeling physically indestructible, they often go through a period in their lives where they live on the wild side and push their bodies to the limit.

With their inherent strength, Adrenals can easily become overpowering, controlling, tactless, and pushy. They may become physically aggressive, particularly when their fear of rejection has been numbed through drugs or alcohol. Verbally, they are often too forceful at the expense of the feelings and opinions of others. They can become overly analytical and critical, demanding that things be done their way, refusing advice or assistance from others. When the going gets rough, they hit a snag, or their success is not readily assured, Adrenals tend to lose patience with themselves, others, or with a task. This often results in their lack of follow-through on the project at hand. The tendency is to try to quickly power through the problem, and if that doesn't work, delegate or ignore it.

"Nothing breeds success like success" and "to be successful you have to look successful," are basic Adrenal philosophies. Their nature is to emphasize the physical expression and appearance of success. They use money to impress, often insisting on picking up the check even when they can't afford it. Their attitude is one of here today and gone tomorrow: High rolling and gambling, easy come, easy go, and living only for the moment results in money issues, particularly since there never seems to be enough to sustain all their wants and impulses.

"AT BEST"

When Adrenals redefine success by placing the real value on qualities and attributes, they begin to manifest true success. Success is then measured by their personal growth, emotional maturity, and caring for others. It's based on the development of their connection with their own inner guidance or intuition.

Once they have developed their intuition through their spiritual connection, life really works for them. They are then able to get off the emotional roller coaster and easily focus their attention so that productivity increases and social situations are more harmonious. Life takes on a new meaning with a richness, joy, and excitement unattainable through thrill seeking and adrenaline rushes.

Validating themselves from within, their self-esteem is no longer dependent upon others' responses and reactions to them. Their spiritual connection is what provides the inner peace that creates a stable inner environment. This is when Adrenals become balanced and can live with harmony and self–esteem. Emotional maturity comes through self-knowledge and insight.

Learning to flow with life, rather than forcing or trying to control it, allows Adrenals to effectively channel their high energy. The key is learning to connect and stay connected with Spirit. Being innately connected with the Universe. Once they learn to let go of thinking they are in charge, they step into the Universal flow, allowing them to experience manifestation, abundance, and prosperity in the physical world.

Adrenal

FOOD LISTS

HEALTHY FOOD LIST

FREQUENTLY FOODS	3-7 meals per week – refers to each food, rather than category.
DENSE PROTEIN	Chicken, chicken broth, chicken livers, turkey, cornish hen; anchovy, bass, bonita, catfish, cod, haddock, halibut, herring, mackerel, mahi-mahi, perch, roughy, sardines in tomato sauce, shark, red snapper, swordfish, tuna; calamari (squid)
DAIRY	Milk (whole, 2%, raw, goat), sour cream, yogurt (regular, low fat, nonfat, plain, or flavored), butter
CHEESE	Cream, feta, Jack, Muenster, Parmesan, ricotta, Romano, Swiss
NUTS and SEEDS	Almonds (raw, roasted), almond butter, filberts, macadamias (raw, roasted), macadamia butter, sesame seeds (raw, roasted), sesame seed butter
LEGUMES	Pinto beans
GRAINS	Amaranth, buckwheat, corn, corn grits, corn bread, corn tortillas, hominy, millet, quinoa, rice (white or brown basmati, short grain brown, Japanese, white, wild), cream of rice, rice cakes, brown rice bread, Chinese rice noodles
VEGETABLES	Asparagus, avocados, bamboo shoots, green beans, lima beans, bok choy, broccoli, cabbage (green, napa, red), carrots, cauliflower, swiss chard, celery, cilantro, corn, garlic, greens (beet, collard, mustard, turnip), kale, kohlrabi, romaine lettuce, okra, black olives, parsley, parsnips, peas, snow pea pods, bell peppers (green, red, yellow), potatoes (red, white rose, russet, Yukon gold), pumpkin, radish, sprouts (alfalfa, mung bean, radish), squash (acorn, banana, butternut, yellow [summer], spaghetti), tomatoes (canned, hot-house, vine-ripened), turnips
FRUITS	Apricots, bananas, blueberries, strawberries, cherries, grapes (black, green, red), lemons, limes, oranges, peaches, pears, dates
CONDIMENTS	Ginger, Vege-Sal®
SALAD DRESSINGS	Creamy Italian
SWEETENERS	Re-Vita®, stevia
MODERATELY FOODS	1-2 meals per week – refers to each food, rather than category.
DENSE PROTEIN	Beef broth, buffalo, calf's liver, lamb, pork, ham, bacon, sausage, veal, venison, organ meats (heart, brain); duck; flounder, salmon, sardines, sole, trout; abalone, clams, eel, lobster, mussels, octopus, oysters; eggs
DAIRY	Nonfat milk, half & half, sweet cream, buttermilk, kefir, frozen yogurt, ice cream (Alta Dena®, Breyers®, Ben & Jerry's®, Dreyer's, Haagen Dazs®, Swensen's®, Baskin-Robbins™ 31 Flavors)

Adrenal

CHEESE	American, blue, brie, Camembert, Cheddar, Colby, low fat cottage, Edam, goat, Gouda, kefir, Limburger, Mozzarella
NUTS and SEEDS	Brazils, water chestnuts, coconuts, hazelnuts, peanuts (raw, roasted), peanut butter, pecans, pine nuts (raw, roasted), walnuts (black, English), seeds (pumpkin, sunflower, raw or roasted caraway), sunflower seed butter
LEGUMES	Beans (adzuki, black, butter [lima], garbanzo, kidney, great northern, kidney, red, soy), lentils, black-eyed peas, split peas, soy milk, tofu, hummus, miso
GRAINS	Barley, oats, popcorn, long grain brown rice, rice bran, unsalted rice cakes, rye, triticale, whole wheat, wheat bran, wheat germ, refined wheat flour, flour tortillas, breads (French, garlic, Italian, sourdough, 7-grain, multi-grain, oat, corn, corn/rye, rye, sprouted grain, white, whole wheat), croissants, plain bagels, English muffins, Rye Krisp®, pasta (plain, artichoke, vegetable), couscous, udon noodles, cream of rye, cream of wheat
VEGETABLES	Artichokes, arugula, yellow wax beans, beets, broccoflower, brussels sprouts, eggplant, jicama, leeks, lettuce (butter, endive, iceberg, red leaf), mushrooms, green olives, onions (chives, green, brown, red, white, yellow, vidalia), chili peppers, pimentos, daikon radishes, rutabaga, sauerkraut, sea vegetables (arame, dulse, kelp, nori, wakame), shallots, spinach, sprouts (clover, sunflower), sweet potatoes, watercress, yams, zucchini
VEGETABLE JUICES	Celery, carrot, carrot/celery, parsley, spinach, tomato, V8®
FRUITS	Apples (Golden or Red Delicious, Granny Smith, Jonathan, McIntosh, Pippin, Rome Beauty), blackberries, boysenberries, cranberries, gooseberries, raspberries, grapefruits (white, red), guavas, kiwi, kumquats, loquats, mangos, melons (cantaloupe, casaba, crenshaw, honeydew, watermelon), nectarines, papayas, persimmons, plums (black, purple, red), pineapples, pomegranates, rhubarb, tangelos, tangerines, figs (fresh, dried), prunes, raisins
FRUIT JUICES	Apple, apple cider, apple/apricot, apricot, black cherry, cherry, cranapple, cranberry, grape (purple, red, white), grapefruit, guava, lemon, orange, papaya, pear, pineapple, pineapple/coconut, prune, tangerine
VEGETABLE OILS	All-blend, almond, avocado, canola, coconut, corn, peanut, flaxseed, olive, safflower, sesame, soy, sunflower
SWEETENERS	Fructose, honey, molasses, sorghum, brown sugar, date sugar, raw sugar, refined cane sugar, maple syrup, brown rice syrup, barley malt syrup, corn syrup, succonant
CONDIMENTS	Catsup, mustard, mayonnaise, horseradish, soy sauce, barbecue sauce, pesto sauce, salsa, tahini, margarine, vinegar, sea salt
SALAD DRESSINGS	Blue cheese, French, ranch, creamy avocado, oil and vinegar, lemon and oil, thousand island
DESSERTS	Custard, tapioca, chocolate, desserts containing chocolate, raspberry sherbet, orange sherbet

Adrenal

CHIPS	Bean, corn (blue, white, yellow), potato
BEVERAGES	Coffee, coffee with Re-Vita®; herbal tea, black tea, green tea, Japanese tea, Chinese oolong tea; mineral water, sparkling water; lemonade; wine (red, white), sherry, sake, beer, barley malt liquor, champagne, liqueur, gin, Scotch, vodka, whiskey; root beer, regular sodas
RARELY FOODS	No more than once a month
DENSE PROTEIN	Beef, beef liver; crab, scallops, shrimp
DAIRY	Most ice creams
NUTS	Cashews (raw, roasted), cashew butter, pistachios
GRAINS	Crackers (saltines, wheat, oat)
VEGETABLES	Cucumbers
SWEETENERS	Saccharin, aspertame, Equal®, NutraSweet®, Sweet'n' Low®
CONDIMENTS	Salt, MSG
BEVERAGES	Diet sodas

SENSITIVE FOOD LIST

FREQUENTLY FOODS	3-7 meals per week – refers to each food, rather than category.
DENSE PROTEIN	Calamari (squid)
GRAINS	Oats, brown basmati rice, rice milk
VEGETABLES	Avocados, green beans, lima beans, broccoli, celery, romaine lettuce, parsley, squash (acorn, banana, spaghetti), sweet potatoes, turnips
FRUITS	Strawberries, cherries, red grapes, peaches, pears
CONDIMENTS	Vege-Sal®
MODERATELY FOODS	1-2 meals per week – refers to each food, rather than category.
DENSE PROTEIN	Beef broth, buffalo, lamb, veal, venison, organ meats (heart, brain); turkey, chicken, chicken livers, chicken broth, cornish hen, duck; bass, bonita, cod, flounder, haddock, halibut, herring, mackerel, mahi-mahi, perch, orange roughy, salmon, sardines, shark, red snapper, sole, swordfish, trout, tuna; abalone, clams, eel, lobster, mussels, octopus, oysters

Adrenal

DAIRY	Milk (raw, goat), half & half, sweet cream, sour cream, buttermilk, kefir, plain or flavored regular yogurt, low fat or nonfat yogurt
CHEESE	American, blue, brie, Camembert, Cheddar, Colby, low fat cottage, cream, Edam, feta, goat, Gouda, Jack, kefir, Limburger, mozzarella, Muenster, Parmesan, ricotta, Romano, Swiss
NUTS and SEEDS	Almonds (raw, roasted), almond butter, Brazils, water chestnuts, coconuts, filberts, hazelnuts, macadamias (raw, roasted), macadamia nut butter, peanuts (raw, roasted), peanut butter, pecans, pine nuts (raw, roasted), walnuts (black, English), seeds (raw or roasted caraway, pumpkin, sesame), sesame seed butter
LEGUMES	Beans (adzuki, black, garbanzo, kidney, lima [butter], great northern, pinto,red), lentils, black-eyed peas, split peas, hummus, miso
GRAINS	Amaranth, barley, buckwheat, corn bread, corn grits, hominy grits, millet, popcorn, quinoa, rice (long grain brown, Japanese, wild), rice bran, unsalted rice cakes, rye, Rye Krisp®, triticale, wheat bran, wheat germ, refined wheat flour, breads (French, Italian, sourdough, oat, corn, corn/rye, rye, sprouted grain, white, garlic), croissants, plain bagels, English muffins, artichoke pasta, vegetable pasta, couscous, udon noodles, Chinese rice noodles, cream of rice, cream of rye
VEGETABLES	Artichoke, asparagus, bamboo shoots, yellow wax beans, beets, bok choy, broccoflower, brussels sprouts, cabbage (green, napa, red), carrots, cauliflower, Swiss chard, cilantro, corn, eggplant, garlic, greens (beet, collard, mustard, turnip), jicama, kale, kohlrabi, leeks, lettuce (butter, endive), mushrooms, okra, olives (green, ripe), onions (chives, green, brown, red, white, vidalia, yellow), parsnips, peas, snow pea pods, peppers (green, red, yellow), chili peppers, pimentos, potatoes (red, russet, Yukon gold, purple), pumpkin, radishes, daikon radish, rutabaga, sauerkraut, sea vegetables (arame, dulse, nori, kelp, wakame), shallots, spinach, sprouts (alfalfa, clover, mung bean, radish), squash (butternut, yellow [summer], zucchini), turnips
VEGETABLE JUICES	Celery, parsley, spinach, V8®
FRUITS	Apricots, bananas, blueberries, cranberries, gooseberries, red plums
FRUIT JUICES	Black cherry, cherry, cranapple, cranberry, red grape
VEGETABLE OILS	All–blend, avocado, coconut
SWEETENERS	Rice bran syrup, barley malt syrup, Re-Vita®, stevia
CONDIMENTS	Salsa, tahini, vinegar
SALAD DRESSINGS	Oil and vinegar, lemon and oil
BEVERAGES	Coffee with Re-Vita®; herbal tea, green tea, Japanese tea, Chinese oolong tea; mineral water, sparkling water

Adrenal

RARELY FOODS	No more than once a month
DENSE PROTEIN	Beef, beef liver, pork, ham, bacon, sausage; anchovy, catfish; crab, scallops, shrimp; eggs
DAIRY	Milk (whole, 2%, nonfat), ice cream, frozen yogurt, butter
NUTS and SEEDS	Cashews (raw, roasted), cashew butter, cashew milk, pistachios, sunflower seeds, sunflower seed butter
LEGUMES	Soy beans, soy milk, tofu
GRAINS	Corn, white basmati rice, short grain brown rice, whole wheat, corn tortillas, flour tortillas, breads (brown rice, 7-grain, multi-grain, whole wheat), cream of wheat, pasta, crackers (saltines, wheat, oat, rye)
VEGETABLES	Arugula, cucumbers, lettuce (iceberg, red leaf), white rose potatoes, sunflower seed sprouts, tomatoes (canned, hot-house, vine-ripened), watercress, yams
VEGETABLE JUICES	Tomato, carrot, carrot/celery
FRUITS	Apples (Golden or Red Delicious, Granny Smith, Jonathan, McIntosh, Pippin, Rome Beauty), blackberries, boysenberries, raspberries, grapes (black, green), grapefruits (white, red), guavas, kiwi, kumquats, lemons, limes, loquats, mangos, melons (cantaloupe, casaba, crenshaw, honeydew, watermelon), nectarines, oranges, papayas, persimmons, pineapples, plums (black, purple), pomegranates, rhubarb, tangelos, tangerines, dates, figs (fresh, dried), prunes, raisins
FRUIT JUICES	Apple, apple cider, apple/apricot, apricot, grape (purple, white), grapefruit, guava, lemon, orange, papaya, pear, pineapple, pineapple/coconut, prune, tangerine
VEGETABLE OILS	Almond, canola, corn, peanut, flaxseed, olive, safflower, sesame, soy, sunflower
SWEETENERS	Honey, molasses, sorghum, brown sugar, date sugar, raw sugar, refined cane sugar, maple syrup, corn syrup, fructose, saccharin, succonant, aspertame, Equal®, NutraSweet®, Sweet'n' Low®
CONDIMENTS	Catsup, mustard, mayonnaise, horseradish, soy sauce, barbecue sauce, pesto sauce, margarine, salt, MSG
SALAD DRESSINGS	French, creamy Italian, creamy avocado, thousand island, blue cheese, ranch
DESSERTS	Custard, tapioca, chocolate, desserts containing chocolate, raspberry sherbet, orange sherbet
CHIPS	Bean, corn (blue, white, yellow), potato
BEVERAGES	Coffee; black tea; wine (red, white), sake, beer, barley malt liquor, champagne, gin, Scotch, vodka, whiskey; root beer, regular sodas, diet sodas

Adrenal

MENUS

DIETARY EMPHASIS:

- Yogurt, cottage cheese, and fruit.
- When healthy, more raw vegetables than cooked (sensitive require more cooked); whole grains; fruit (up to 40% of diet); protein, mainly from poultry or fish; and low fat dairy.
- Drinking mineral water and/or parsley tea can help reduce appetite and cleanse body.

WEIGHT LOSS: (tips in order of priority)

- Reduce food quantity, especially carbohydrates (including breads, rice, pasta, and potatoes).
- May, if tolerated, use appetite suppressants (muscle test for tolerance).
- Include up to 30% dense protein, particularly fish, turkey, and chicken to rebuild the adrenals. Dense protein necessary when there is excess weight gain (over 20 lbs.), fatigue, and/or general feeling of being stressed.
- The ideal diet consists of raw fruits and vegetables, salads, protein, and soups.
- Best not to snack, but if cannot avoid, eat raw vegetables or fruit, or 1/2 cup of yogurt.
- Limit fats to 25% of total calories, but be aware that if intake drops below 20%, you will not lose weight (see fats).
- Exercise at least 40 minutes daily.

WEIGHT GAIN:

- Increase food quantity. Include dense protein up to 20%, possibly 30% of calories.

VEGETARIAN DIET:

- Recommended when healthy and at ideal weight, particularly a lacto-vegetarian diet which includes dairy products.
- Normally, up to 10% of total calories, up to 30% when rebuilding, may be from fish, turkey, chicken. Dense protein is often required to balance body weight when under stress.

FATS:

- 20-25% of total daily calories.
- Best sources are almonds and dairy (yogurt, cottage cheese, cheese).
- If intolerant of dairy, include chicken and fish.

SENSITIVE:

- Eat dense protein for dinner.
- Eat fruit only in the morning.
- Limit breakfast to fruit.

KEY

—all menus may be used by healthy persons
( ) around foods means that they're optional
L denotes weight loss menus
S denotes sensitive menus
G denotes weight gain menus

BREAKFAST:
6-8 a.m. Light, with fruit, dairy, vegetables, and/or grain.

SENSITIVE: Light, with fruit.

L S	Fruit, such as strawberries, peaches, pears, cherries, or red grapes
L	Pineapple, oranges, tangerines, or grapefruit
L S	Bananas, blueberries, or red plums
L	Fruit juice and fruit
L	Cantaloupe or watermelon
L	Plain yogurt w/banana or other fruit (carrot juice)
	Flavored yogurt
L	Low fat cottage cheese
	Cottage cheese (pineapple)
	Spinach quiche
	Cream of wheat w/milk and Re-Vita® or fruit
	Cream of rice (milk)

Adrenal

	G	Rice or rye w/milk and Re-Vita®
	G	Brown basmati rice w/vegetables, vary each day
		Unsalted rice cakes and Jack cheese
		Grape nuts® or bran cereal w/low fat milk
		Shredded wheat cereal and raisins or banana w/2% milk (carrot juice)
		Oatmeal (butter)
		Oatmeal w/raisins or strawberries and milk
	G	Toasted bagel w/cream cheese and fruit, such as banana, apple, or grapes
		Toasted bread (butter) (jam)
L		Miso soup
		Potato (cheese)
L		Celery
		Carrot juice
		Parsley tea
		Decaffeinated tea (honey)

MID-MORNING SNACK:
(Optional) Vegetables, fruit, grain, dairy.

L	S	Celery
L	S	V8® juice, unsalted
	S	Carrot/celery (parsley, spinach) juice
L	S	Peach, pear, apple, or strawberries
L	S	Raisins
L		Low fat vanilla yogurt
	S	Herbal tea

LUNCH:
12-2 p.m. Moderate, may be heavy if dinner is moderate, with vegetables, grain, legumes, nuts, seeds, dairy, protein, and/or fruit. Lunch and dinner menus are interchangeable.

SENSITIVE: Moderate, with vegetables, grain, dairy, and/or legumes.

	S	G	Brown rice and broccoli
			Brown rice, brussels sprouts, and salad w/cottage cheese
	S	G	Potato and zucchini
	S		Oatmeal
			Oatmeal and prunes
L			Low fat cottage cheese and fruit, such as banana, apricot, or avocado
L			Caesar salad
		G	Caesar salad (chicken w/croutons) and cornbread
L	S		Salad: romaine lettuce, tomato, onion, broccoli, cheese, and avocado salad (Italian or ranch dressing, or vinegar and oil)
L			Chicken pita sandwich w/lettuce (sorbet)
		G	Chicken or ham and Swiss cheese croissant or sandwich
L			Chicken or bean burrito
		G	Sesame bagel w/tuna (lettuce)
			Fresh tuna and tomato
		G	Lobster bisque, tuna sandwich, and green salad
			Taco salad
L			Chicken taco (cole slaw)
L			Sushi

MID-AFTERNOON SNACK:
(Optional) Vegetables, fruit, grain, dairy, protein, nuts.

		Almonds (garlic and onions or seasoning)
	G	Peanut butter (celery, apple, or bread)
	G	Guacamole and chips
L		Plain nonfat or low fat yogurt (fruit)
		Cottage cheese and pineapple
		Sherbet
		Frozen fruit, such as cherries, grapes, or peaches
		Banana or pear

LUNCH or DINNER:

	G	Grilled cheese sandwich w/sourdough or rye bread and white cheese such as Jack, mozzarella, or Swiss.
	G	Gyro sandwich in pita bread and Greek salad

Adrenal

- L — Turkey and salad: romaine lettuce, tomato, onion or scallion, and broccoli (cheese and/or avocado)
- G — Chicken, garlic, red and green bell peppers, and potatoes
- G — Garlic or orange chicken and rice
- L — Tuna salad w/fresh tuna and tomato (pickles)
- G — Mahi-mahi and rice (tomato sauce, or raw or stuffed baked tomato)
- G — Sole, halibut, or orange roughy, rice, broccoli and carrots, or salad
- G — Clams and linguini (red or white sauce and peas) (salad)
- L — Greek salad: celery, tomato, black olives, and feta cheese
- L — Romaine lettuce salad and cheese
- Salad, corn bread, and beans
- G — Baked potato w/yogurt or Cheddar cheese
- G — Potatoes and garlic
- G — Jack cheese, avocado, tomato, and sprouts on pita bread
- Unsalted rice cakes and Jack cheese
- Mozzarella cheese melted on wild rice, mushrooms, and broccoli
- Baked eggplant w/ginger and any rice (soy sauce)
- L S — Wild rice, mushrooms, and broccoli
- L S — Baked eggplant – plain
- Brown rice, nori seaweed, and ume boshi plum
- S — White and brown rice w/succotash
- S — Rice and beans (salsa)
- L S — Stir-fry vegetables and rice
- S — Black beans and rice w/celery and onions
- L — Black beans w/garlic and Parmesan cheese
- G — Refried beans, corn or flour tortilla, and salsa
- Bean and cheese relleno (salsa)
- G — Bean burrito
- Hummus, pita bread, and cheese or salsa
- Meatless chili (on potato)
- L S — Vegetable soup or stew
- Chicken noodle soup
- L — Spaghetti w/meatless tomato sauce, Parmesan cheese, or garlic pesto sauce
- G — Cheese ravioli and tomato sauce (salad)
- G — Vegetable lasagna (tomato sauce)
- G — Pasta w/vegetables or tomato sauce
- G — Pasta w/white or cream sauce (vegetable or salad)

DINNER:
7-9 p.m. Heavy, may be moderate if lunch was heavy, with grain, vegetables, protein, dairy, legumes, nuts, seeds, and/or fruit.

SENSITIVE: Heavy, with protein, dairy, nuts, seeds, legumes, vegetables, and/or grain.

- S G — Lamb, red potatoes, snow pea pods, and carrots
- L — Ground turkey, vegetable pasta, and garlic
- S G — Turkey, rice, snow pea pods, and carrots
- L S — Turkey, vegetable rotellis, and leeks
- S — Chicken, brown basmati rice, and zucchini
- S G — Chicken, potato, and spinach or cole slaw
- G — Chicken teriyaki, miso, and rice
- S — Chicken teriyaki and rice
- S — Chicken and rice curry
- L S — Cornish game hen, celery, carrots, and onions
- L S — Sushi (soy sauce and/or green mustard)
- L S — Tuna, avocado, and romaine lettuce
- S — Tuna, brown rice, and broccoli
- S — Swordfish and broccoli (rice)
- S — Salmon and rice (broccoli, and/or squash)
- S — Bass, brown basmati rice, and spinach or green beans
- L S — Mahi-mahi and zucchini
- L S — Caesar salad (chicken, turkey, or fish)
- G — Chicken Caesar salad and sourdough bread

Adrenal

Chicken burrito and cabbage salad

L Chicken fajita and salad

Broccoli w/cheese, white rose potatoes, and cottage cheese

Fettuccini w/tomato sauce, and salad

Fish w/almonds, garlic, and onions (rice and/or zucchini w/tomatoes)

G Chili rellenos, Spanish rice, and refried beans

L Soup and salad

S Miso soup and sushi (California roll)

L S Chicken soup

Turkey stew w/tomatoes, zucchini, kidney beans, and pasta

Note: Use vegetable cooking water to cook rice, potatoes, pasta, or use as soup base.

EVENING SNACK:
(Optional) 10 p.m.-2 a.m. Fruit, vegetables, grain, protein, dairy, nuts, sweets. Rotate foods.

Brown rice w/vegetables

L Sushi

L Fruit

L Watermelon

Frozen cherries, grapes, or peaches

Frozen fruit smoothie

G Chocolate chip cookies

Sherbet or sorbet

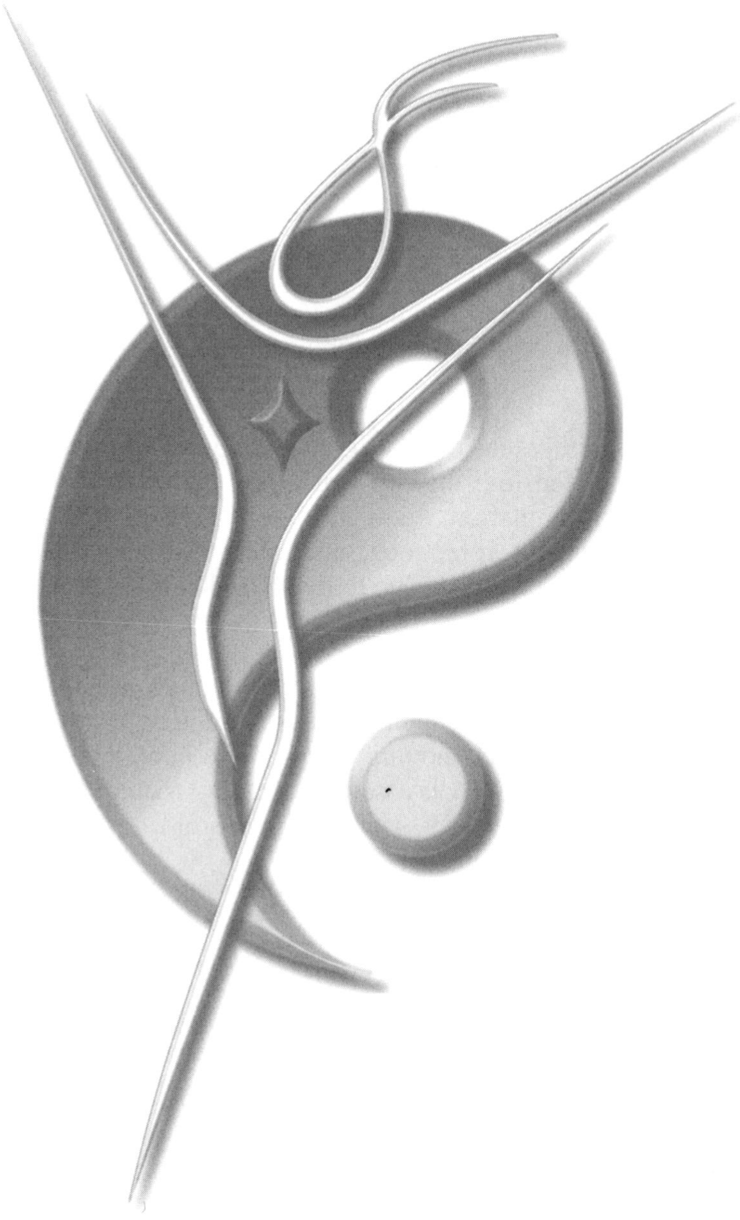

The "Balanced Body Type" is symbolized by the Yin/Yang symbol. Dependent upon everything working together synergistically, Balanced body types need balance between work and play, as well as all other aspects of life. Essentially playful and adventurous, they embody the synergy that brings about balance.

BALANCED

Balanced

BODY TYPE PROFILE

LOCATION	All over, since no one gland is in charge.
FUNCTION	With Balanced types, all glands, organs, and systems must work together harmoniously for optimal functioning.
POTENTIAL HEALTH PROBLEMS	Headaches, either tension or migraine (frequently relieved by caffeine); neck and shoulder tension; digestive distress, such as indigestion, constipation, intestinal inflammation; food allergies (may be hidden); hypoglycemia; kidney or bladder infections; and menstrual distress. May experience weakness or hyperactivity due to low blood sugar if meals are skipped.
RECOMMENDED EXERCISE	Exercise is helpful. Its benefit is initially emotional. It gets energy moving, lifts spirits, adds variety to daily activities, and activates the physical body by getting the lymphatics moving. Sunlight is beneficial. Being around water often important. Variety is essential and may include Callanetics™, dancing, walking, hiking, bicycling, swimming, weight lifting, baseball, or tennis.

WOMEN'S CHARACTERISTICS

DISTINGUISHING FEATURES	Buttocks somewhat flat, due to blending into upper and outer thighs, creating a rather droopy appearance. Bright, sparkling eyes – especially when smiling. Essentially playful and adventurous, they embody the synergy that brings about balance.
ADDITIONAL PHYSICAL CHARACTERISTICS	Rounded-to-prominent buttocks that appear flat. Low back curvature average-to-swayed. Breasts small-to-average. Shoulders relatively even with, to broader than, hips. Defined waist. Long-waisted with short-to-average legs, or short-waisted with long legs. Height generally average, but can range from petite to tall. Bone structure small-to-medium. Average, elongated musculature. Hands average-to-broad, square palm with square or short fingers, characterized by wide reach. Good joint flexibility. May have had long arms as child, sometimes also as adult. Average oval or rectangular face with high forehead, or heart-shaped, pixie-like face with V-shaped chin.
WEIGHT GAIN AREAS	Lower body with initial gain in entire upper 2/3rds of thighs extending into lower buttocks, upper inner thighs, lower abdomen, minimally in waist, upper and/or lower hips. Secondary gain in entire thighs, eventually extending into entire abdomen, middle back, upper arms, and upper hips.

Balanced

DIETARY GUIDELINES

SCHEDULING MEALS	Breakfast: Light-to-moderate, with grain and/or fruit, vegetables, dairy, nuts, and/or seeds. Emphasize carbohydrates, with moderate fats. Lunch: Moderate, with protein, grain, vegetables, and/or dairy. Emphasize protein. Dinner: Moderate, with grain, vegetables, legumes, protein, and/or dairy. Emphasize grain and vegetables.
DIETARY EMPHASIS	• Balance raw and cooked vegetables. • For weight loss, avoid caffeine, stimulants (including Ma Haung and alcohol), and sugar; derive no more than 25-30% of caloric intake from fats (caution: if fats fall below 20%, weight will stabilize); limit portion size; eat light dinner, consuming majority of calories at breakfast and lunch; eat fruit only for breakfast; avoid snacking after dinner; delete starches (especially breads and grains with wheat) at dinner; reduce dairy; and rotate foods. Emphasize protein and vegetables with 15% of caloric intake from dense protein. To keep weight off, especially important to lose it slowly. • For weight gain, increase protein when underweight; if at ideal weight or above, sugar, including dried fruit and honey, and dairy, especially ice cream and milk, will add extra pounds. • Vegetarian diets inadequate, since require 10-30% of calories from dense protein. • Fats, 20-30% of caloric intake, should be derived from butter and dense protein (chicken, turkey, eggs, fish, beef).
COMPLEMENTARY GLANDULAR SUPPORT	Thyroid, through consuming two oz. of dense protein (chicken, turkey, eggs, or fish) with grain, such as rice or pasta, five times weekly; and pancreas, through rotating foods.
FOODS CRAVED	*(When energy is low)* Sweets (pastries, cookies, chocolate – especially Reese's™ peanut butter cups); fruit (strawberries as child); carbohydrates (popcorn, white and wheat breads, hoagie sandwich, pizza); fats; or salty foods like chips, processed meats; drinks with caffeine.
KEY SUPPORTS FOR SYSTEM	Rotation essential – ideally, allow four days before repeating food. Balance choices from all food groups.

Balanced

FOODS TO AVOID

Any food that is a problem for you. Some of the more common ones are: raw onions, because they can cause indigestion; chocolate, because it can raise blood pressure; cookies, because they can raise body heat excessively, even to point of facial flushing; sugar, because it can cause fatigue or sleep disturbances; wheat or yeast, because they can cause sleepiness or loss of mental focus. Leg pain may result from certain food combinations, such as carrot/celery/beet juice. In general, search out food sensitivities (which can come from any food group) and eliminate.

RECOMMENDED CUISINE

Chinese, Thai, Sushi, Japanese, Moroccan, Mexican, French, Indian. Foods moderately seasoned, protein and grain combinations.

PSYCHOLOGICAL PROFILE

ESSENCE

Just as the Balanced body type is not controlled by any single gland, organ or system, but is dependent upon everything working together synergistically, Balanced body types need balance in their world. This means balance between work and play, physical and spiritual expression, mental and emotional states, and relationships, both personal and business. In other words, balance in both their inner and outer worlds, between people and life in general. Essentially playful and adventurous, they embody the synergy that brings about balance.

CHARACTERISTIC TRAITS

Sensitive by nature, Balanced types have a fragile equilibrium and will go to great lengths to maintain their delicate balance. On the outside, they are often light, playful, personable and entertaining, while being reserved on the inside, reluctant to share their true feelings. Generally quite social, people are readily attracted to them but rarely allowed to get very close emotionally until they've proven that they can be trusted.

Balanced body types have a strong sense of adventure and like to travel or move frequently, giving them the opportunity to meet new people and try new things. They love performing or being the center of attention, and since they are typically in their glory when interacting with people, will often be the life of the party. They mix well with others and can be quite good at making favorable impressions. They are basically easy-going, forgiving, optimistic, and open- minded individuals, with a positive attitude toward life.

Adventure is what creates an aliveness and a love of life that is often expressed as new ideas, concepts and designs. Imaginative and creative, with a strong attraction to the Arts, Balanced types have a need for order and structure that allows them to be extremely precise in their music, dance or creative expression. Sensitive and artistic, they are also practical, logical, and

Balanced

CHARACTERISTIC TRAITS

technically adept. Their acute sense of sight, hearing and touch is balanced with a natural sense of rhythm and timing which they often use to discover their inner sense of stability and balance.

MOTIVATION

Because of their extreme sensitivity to imbalances, Balanced types have a heightened need for security and stability, causing them to go to great lengths to control their environment. They need to work in situations that ensure maximum predictability and harmony. They often find it difficult to delegate tasks or supervise others and feel that it's faster and more effective to do a job personally. Consequently, they prefer to work alone, taking full responsibility for the outcome and offering their personal guarantee that the job will be done right. By working alone they also avoid the unpleasant task of criticizing or correcting co-workers.

Despite the care they take in projecting a positive image, Balanced types are known to undermine their own efforts. For example, by placing such a high value on honesty, truthfulness can override diplomacy and result in tactless comments. There is a tendency to speak without censoring words. They have difficulty keeping secrets and don't like others to be secretive, often becoming very impatient when others withhold information.

Being intuitively aware of the dangers relationships pose, and taking commitments seriously, they are cautious about making them. Consequently, as a protective mechanism, they may have a fear of intimacy, which compels them to distance themselves from others and limit close friends to a select few. They need to develop relationships slowly and to know others well, before they are willing to reveal their innermost thoughts and feelings.

"AT WORST"

Balanced types can become extremely impatient both with themselves and others when things go wrong and their need for order and balance isn't satisfied. Unless they've developed considerable self-control, they may display anger or even rage, and then regret it later. They can overreact with rigidity and intolerance or retreat from problems through compulsive/addictive behavior in the form of an activity, a relationship, or substance abuse.

If they haven't developed an inner sense of stability, Balanced types will typically look to others to provide it. Since relationships can never fulfill what can only come from within, expecting to gain stability from outer relationships makes them prone to disillusionment, or settling for relationships that are detrimental to their personal growth and inner peace.

Motivated by the need for acceptance by others, Balanced types will often suppress or even deny their feelings, causing them to appear distant, detached, or preoccupied. Their fear of rejection can cause them to keep their feelings hidden to avoid upsetting themselves or others. These suppressed emotions generally surface as physical complaints, like

Balanced

"AT WORST"

headaches or digestive problems. Balanced types use play and adventurous activities to release stored-up emotional energy. When out of balance, they can get so caught up in their play and fantasies that they lose sight of reality.

"AT BEST"

Balanced types are persistent, goal-oriented self-starters who like to be in control of their work, gladly accepting responsibility for the completion of a task. They are good at seeing to the heart of a matter, focusing more on the big picture or the main objective than on technicalities, so as not to be distracted by surface appearances. While they are not primarily detail-oriented, they'll make sure the details are correct before finally releasing a project. Conscientious and competent, they can be depended upon to fulfill their promises and are often found working late into the night to finish a project.

Engaging in adventurous activities and daring pursuits that capture the imagination and challenge their problem solving abilities allows Balanced types to get rid of pent-up stress and revitalize themselves through play. They find the balance between work and play by finding their passion and making work and play synonymous. Balancing work with play helps them find the harmony they need for a sense of well-being. This in turn helps them maintain an optimistic, open-minded, positive attitude toward life enabling them to bounce back from adversity.

Having developed their intuitive nature, they are guided by their deep sense of stability and balance, causing them to create positive experiences in relationships and in life overall. By solidly connecting with their spiritual center and developing their own stability, they are able to establish a nurturing relationship with themselves, and break free from their fears and self-imposed restrictions. By discovering their deeper truths and movements, they are able to live more from the potential that each day and each moment offers.

Balanced types are self-contained and at peace within themselves. Having developed an inner sense of harmony and balance, they have an easygoing, forgiving, and humorous nature that brings a lightness and balance into the lives of those they touch.

Balanced

FOOD LISTS

HEALTHY FOOD LIST

FREQUENTLY FOODS	3-7 meals per week – refers to each food, rather than category.
DENSE PROTEIN	Chicken (white), turkey (white), cornish hen; anchovy, tuna; octopus
DAIRY	Whole milk, raw milk, nonfat plain yogurt, butter
CHEESE	Cheddar, cream, feta, mozzarella, Muenster, Parmesan, ricotta, Swiss
NUTS and SEEDS	Almonds (raw, roasted), almond butter, water chestnuts, coconuts, sunflower seeds (raw, roasted), sunflower seed butter, pumpkin seeds (roasted)
GRAINS	Oats, oatmeal, rice (long or short grain brown, brown or white basmati, Japanese), cream of rice, breads (corn, oat, 7-grain), bagels, pasta, vegetable pasta
VEGETABLES	Avocados, green beans, carrots, eggplant, jicama, bell peppers (green, red, yellow), sweet potatoes, mung bean sprouts, yams
FRUITS	Cherries, nectarines, Fuju persimmons, pineapples, pomegranates, cantaloupes, dates, Mission figs (soaked)
SWEETENERS	ReVita®, stevia
BEVERAGES	Coffee with cream (morning), decaf coffee with ReVita® (morning or evening), cafe' au lait, espresso
MODERATELY FOODS	1-2 meals per week – refers to each food, rather than category.
DENSE PROTEIN	Beef, beef broth, beef liver, veal, buffalo, pork, organ meats (heart, brain); turkey (dark), chicken (dark, broth, livers); bonita, catfish, cod, flounder, haddock, halibut, herring, mackerel, mahi-mahi, perch, orange roughy, salmon, sardines, shark, red snapper, sole, swordfish; abalone, calamari (squid), crab, clams, eel, lobster, mussels, oysters, scallops, shrimp; eggs
DAIRY	Nonfat or low fat milk, half & half, sweet cream, sour cream, buttermilk, kefir, regular or low fat yogurt (plain, black cherry, raspberry, boysenberry, lemon, strawberry, cinnamon apple, apricot, pineapple/coconut), frozen yogurt, ice cream (Breyers®, Ben & Jerry's®, Dreyer's)
CHEESE	American, blue, brie, Camembert, Colby, cottage, Edam, goat, Gouda, Jack, kefir, Limburger, low fat mozzarella, Romano
NUTS and SEEDS	Brazils, raw cashews, filberts, hazelnuts, macadamias (raw, roasted), macadamia butter, peanuts (raw, roasted), pecans, pine nuts (raw, roasted), pistachios, walnuts (black, English), pumpkin seeds (raw), sesame seeds (raw, roasted), caraway seeds (raw, roasted)
LEGUMES	Beans (adzuki, black, butter [lima], garbanzo, kidney, great northern, pinto, red, soy), lentils, black-eyed peas, split peas, hummus, miso, soy milk, tofu

Balanced

GRAINS	Amaranth, buckwheat, corn, corn bread, corn grits, corn tortillas, hominy grits, popcorn, quinoa, wild rice, rice bran, rice cakes, rye, triticale, refined white flour, flour tortillas, whole wheat, wheat bran, wheat germ, breads (French, Italian, garlic, multi-grain, corn, corn/rye, rye, rice, sourdough, sprouted grain, white), English muffins, croissants, crackers (oat, rye, saltines), couscous, udon noodles, Chinese rice noodles, cream of rye, cream of wheat
VEGETABLES	Artichokes, arugula, asparagus, bamboo shoots, lima beans, yellow wax beans, beets, bok choy, broccoli, brussels sprouts, broccoflower, raw cabbage (green, napa, red), cauliflower, celery, chard, cilantro, corn, cucumber, garlic, greens (beet, collard, mustard, turnip), kale, kohlrabi, leeks, lettuce (Boston, butter, endive, iceberg, red leaf, romaine), mushrooms, okra, olives (green, ripe), cooked onions (chives, green, brown, red, white, vidalia, yellow), parsley, parsnips, green peas, snow pea pods, chili peppers, pimentos, potatoes (red, white rose, russet, yukon gold, purple), pumpkin, radish, daikon radish, rutabaga, sauerkraut, sea vegetables (arame, dulse, kelp, nori, wakame), shallots, sprouts (alfalfa, clover, radish, sunflower), spinach, squash (acorn, banana, butternut, spaghetti, yellow [summer], zucchini), cooked or raw tomatoes (canned, hot-house, vine-ripened), turnips, watercress
VEGETABLE JUICES	Carrot, celery, carrot/celery, carrot/celery/parsley, parsley, spinach, tomato, V-8®, green juice
FRUITS	Apples (Golden or Red Delicious, Granny Smith, Jonathan, McIntosh, Pippin, Rome Beauty), apricots, bananas, blackberries, blueberries, boysenberries, cranberries, gooseberries, raspberries, guavas, kiwi, kumquats, lemons, limes, loquats, mangos, melons (casaba, crenshaw, honeydew, watermelon), papayas, peaches, pears, Hychia persimmons, rhubarb, tangelos, tangerines, figs (fresh, dried), prunes, raisins
FRUIT JUICES	Apple, apple cider, apple/apricot, apricot, black cherry, cherry, cranapple, cranberry, grapefruit, guava, lemon, orange/mango, papaya, pear, pineapple, pineapple/coconut, prune, tangerine, watermelon
VEGETABLE OILS	All-blend, almond, avocado, canola, coconut, corn, flaxseed, olive, safflower, sesame, soy, sunflower
SWEETENERS	Honey, molasses, sorghum, brown sugar, date sugar, raw sugar, refined cane sugar, maple syrup, brown rice syrup, barley malt syrup, corn syrup, fructose, succonant
CONDIMENTS	Catsup, mustard, horseradish, barbecue sauce, soy sauce, pesto sauce, salsa, tahini, vinegar, salt, sea salt, Vege-Sal®
SALAD DRESSINGS	Blue cheese, French, ranch, creamy Italian, creamy avocado, thousand island, vinegar and oil, lemon juice and oil
DESSERTS	Custards, tapioca, puddings, pies, cakes, raspberry sherbet, orange sherbet
CHIPS	Bean, corn (blue, white, yellow), potato
BEVERAGES	Coffee, coffee with ReVita®; herbal tea, black tea, Chinese oolong tea, green tea, Japanese tea; mineral water, sparkling water; wine (white, red); root beer, diet soda, regular soda

Balanced

RARELY FOODS	No more than once a month
DENSE PROTEIN	Lamb, ham, bacon, sausage, venison; duck; sea bass, trout (with cornmeal, moderately)
DAIRY	2% milk, goat milk, nonfat yogurt (mandarin orange, strawberry/banana), regular or low fat yogurt (vanilla), most ice creams
NUTS and SEEDS	Roasted cashews, cashew butter, peanut butter, sesame seed butter
GRAINS	Barley, millet, polished rice, wheat crackers, breads (7-grain, whole wheat)
VEGETABLES	Cooked cabbage, raw onions
VEGETABLE JUICE	Beet
FRUITS	Grapefruits (red, white), grapes (black, green, red), oranges, plums (black, purple, red), strawberries
FRUIT JUICES	Grape (purple, red, white), orange (with grapefruit and tangerine)
VEGETABLE OIL	Peanut
SWEETENERS	Saccharin, aspertame, Equal®, Sweet'n Low®, NutraSweet®
CONDIMENTS	Mayonnaise, margarine
DESSERTS	Chocolate, desserts containing chocolate
BEVERAGES	Sake, beer, barley malt liquor, margaritas, champagne, gin, Scotch, vodka, whiskey; regular Pepsi®, diet Pepsi®, diet Coke®

SENSITIVE FOOD LIST

FREQUENTLY FOODS	3-7 meals per week – refers to each food, rather than category.
DENSE PROTEIN	Tuna
NUTS and SEEDS	Coconuts, sunflower seeds (raw, roasted), sunflower seed butter
GRAINS	Oats, oatmeal, Japanese rice, cream of rice
VEGETABLES	Green beans, carrots, jicama, sweet potatoes, bean sprouts, yams
FRUITS	Cantaloupes, cherries, nectarines, pineapples, pomegranates, dates, figs (fresh, dried)
MODERATELY FOODS	1-2 meals per week – refers to each food, rather than category.
DENSE PROTEIN	Beef, veal, organ meats (heart, brain); anchovy, bonita, catfish, cod, flounder, haddock, halibut, herring, mackerel, mahi-mahi, perch, orange roughy, salmon, sardines, shark, red snapper, sole, swordfish; abalone, clams, crab, eel, mussels, octopus, oysters; eggs
DAIRY	Raw nonfat milk, half & half, sweet cream, sour cream, plain yogurt, butter

Balanced

CHEESE	American, blue, brie, Camembert, Cheddar, Colby, low fat cottage, cream, Edam, feta, goat, Gouda, Jack, kefir, Limburger, mozzarella, Muenster, Parmesan, ricotta, Romano, Swiss
NUTS and SEEDS	Almonds (roasted), almond butter, Brazils, cashews (raw), hazelnuts, pistachios, caraway seeds (raw, roasted)
LEGUMES	Beans (kidney, pinto), lentils, soy milk, tofu, hummus, miso
GRAINS	Corn, corn bread, corn grits, corn tortillas, popcorn, brown or white basmati rice, wild rice, rice bran, rice cakes, triticale, whole wheat, wheat bran, wheat germ, refined white flour, flour tortillas, breads (French, Italian, multi-grain, oat, corn, corn/rye, rye, sprouted grain), bagels, croissants, English muffins, crackers (oat, rye, saltines), couscous, pasta, vegetable pasta, udon noodles, Chinese rice noodles, cream of rye, cream of wheat
VEGETABLES	Avocados, lima beans, raw cabbage, cauliflower, celery, cucumber, garlic, lettuce (butter, iceberg, red leaf, romaine), cooked onions (chives, green, brown, red, white, yellow, vidalia), parsley, parsnips, bell peppers (green, red, yellow), chili peppers, pimentos, potatoes (red, white rose, russet, yukon gold, purple), pumpkin, radishes, daikon radishes, rutabaga, sea vegetables (arame, dulse, kelp, nori, wakame), shallots, spinach, sprouts (alfalfa, clover, radish, sunflower), sauerkraut, squash (acorn, banana, butternut, yellow [summer], spaghetti, zucchini), cooked tomatoes (canned, hot-house, vine-ripened), turnips, watercress
VEGETABLE JUICES	Celery, carrot, carrot/celery, carrot/celery/parsley, parsley, spinach, tomato, V-8®
FRUITS	Apples (Golden or Red Delicious, Granny Smith, Jonathan, McIntosh, Pippin, Rome Beauty), apricots, bananas, blackberries, blueberries, boysenberries, cranberries, gooseberries, raspberries, guavas, kiwi, kumquats, lemons, limes, loquats, mangos, melons (casaba, crenshaw, honeydew, watermelon), papayas, peaches, pears, Fuju or Hychia persimmons, rhubarb, tangelos, tangerines, raisins
FRUIT JUICES	Apple, apple cider, apple/apricot, apricot, cherry, black cherry, cranapple, cranberry, grapefruit, guava, lemon, orange/mango, papaya, pear, pineapple, pineapple/coconut, tangerine, watermelon
VEGETABLE OILS	All-blend, almond, avocado, canola, coconut, corn, flaxseed, olive, safflower, sesame, soy, sunflower
SWEETENERS	Barley malt syrup, brown rice syrup, ReVita®, stevia
CONDIMENTS	Salsa, tahini, vinegar, salt, sea salt, Vege-Sal®
SALAD DRESSINGS	Vinegar and oil, lemon juice and oil
BEVERAGES	Herbal tea, Chinese oolong tea, green tea, Japanese tea; mineral water, sparkling water

Balanced

RARELY FOODS	No more than once a month
DENSE PROTEIN	Beef broth, beef liver, buffalo, venison, lamb, ham, bacon, sausage, pork; turkey, chicken, chicken broth, chicken livers, cornish game hen, duck; sea bass, trout; calamari (squid), lobster, scallops, shrimp
DAIRY	Whole milk, 2% milk, goat milk, buttermilk, kefir, regular or low fat yogurt (cinnamon apple, apricot, boysenberry, raspberry, strawberry, black cherry, lemon, pineapple/coconut, vanilla), nonfat yogurt (mandarin orange, banana/strawberry), frozen yogurt, most ice creams
NUTS and SEEDS	Almonds (raw), cashews (roasted, no salt), cashew butter, water chestnuts, filberts, macadamias (raw, roasted), macadamia butter, peanuts (raw, roasted), peanut butter, pecans, pine nuts (raw, roasted), walnuts (black, English), raw or roasted pumpkin or sesame seeds, sesame seed butter
LEGUMES	Beans (adzuki, black, butter [lima], garbanzo, great northern, red, soy), black-eyed peas, split peas
GRAINS	Amaranth, barley, buckwheat, millet, quinoa, long or short grain brown rice, polished rice, rye, breads (garlic, rice, 7-grain, sourdough, white, whole wheat), bagel, wheat crackers
VEGETABLES	Artichokes, arugula, asparagus, bamboo shoots, yellow wax beans, beets, bok choy, broccoflower, broccoli, brussels sprouts, cooked cabbage (green, napa, red), cauliflower, chard, cilantro, corn, eggplant, greens (beet, collard, mustard, turnip), kale, kohlrabi, leeks, lettuce (Boston, endive), mushrooms, okra, olives (green, ripe), raw onions, green peas, snow pea pods, raw tomatoes
VEGETABLE JUICES	Beet, carrot/celery/beet, green juices
FRUITS	Grapefruits (red, white), grapes (black, green, red), oranges, plums (black, purple, red), strawberries, prunes
FRUIT JUICES	Grape (purple, red, white), orange, prune
VEGETABLE OIL	Peanut
CONDIMENTS	Catsup, mustard, mayonnaise, barbecue sauce, horseradish, pesto sauce, soy sauce, margarine
SALAD DRESSINGS	Blue cheese, French, ranch, creamy Italian, creamy avocado, thousand island
SWEETENERS	Honey, molasses, sorghum, brown sugar, date sugar, raw sugar, refined cane sugar, maple syrup, corn syrup, fructose, saccharin, succonant, aspertame, Equal®, Sweet'n Low®, NutraSweet ®
DESSERTS	Chocolate, desserts containing chocolate, custards, tapioca, puddings, pies, cakes, raspberry sherbet, orange sherbet
CHIPS	Bean, corn (blue, white, yellow), potato
BEVERAGES	Coffee; black tea; wine (red, white), beer, barley malt liquor, margaritas, champagne, gin, Scotch, vodka, whiskey; regular Pepsi,® diet Pepsi®, diet Coke®, diet sodas, root beer, regular sodas

Balanced

MENUS

DIETARY EMPHASIS:

- Rotation essential, ideally allow 4 days before repeating a food.
- Balance choices from all food groups.
- Balance raw and cooked vegetables.
- Emphasize carbohydrates with moderate fat for breakfast, protein for lunch, and grain and vegetables for dinner.
- Avoid fruit for either lunch or dinner, check for personal sensitivity.

WEIGHT LOSS:

- Avoid caffeine, stimulants (including Ma Huang and alcohol) and sugar.
- Limit fats to 25-30% of total caloric intake. Caution: fat levels below 20% inhibit weight loss (see fats).
- Limit portion size.
- Eat fruit only for breakfast.
- Eat a light dinner, consuming most of calories at breakfast and lunch.
- Avoid snacking after dinner.
- Eliminate starches (especially breads and grains with wheat) at dinner.
- Reduce dairy.
- Emphasize protein and vegetables with 15% of total caloric intake from chicken, turkey, eggs, fish, or beef.
- Rotate foods.
- To keep weight off, lose it slowly.

WEIGHT GAIN:

- Increase protein when underweight; if at ideal weight or above, sugar, (including dried fruit and honey), and dairy (especially ice cream and milk) will add extra pounds.

VEGETARIAN DIET:

- Inadequate, since require 10-30% of total calories from dense protein (meats).

FATS:

- 20-30% of caloric intake.
- Best sources are butter, chicken, turkey, eggs, fish, and beef.

KEY

—all menus may be used by healthy persons
( ) around foods means that they're optional
L denotes weight loss menus
S denotes sensitive menus
G denotes weight gain menus

S		
		BREAKFAST: 7-8 a.m. Light-to-moderate, with grain and/or fruit, vegetables, dairy, nuts and/or seeds. Emphasize carbohydrates, with moderate fat.
S		Cream of rice
	G	Amaranth w/dates
	G	Oatmeal and oat bran w/whole milk or butter
S		Oatmeal (banana, applesauce, and/or butter)
S		Raw oatmeal w/Re-Vita® and butter
S		Special K w/apple juice
S	G	Corn grits w/dates or pineapple
S		Muffin and peaches
		Muffin, peach, and coffee w/Re-Vita®
		Bran muffin and butter
		Blueberry muffin
	G	Buckwheat pancakes w/raspberries
S		Corn bread w/butter
S		Rice and vegetable, such as green beans or squash
S	G	White basmati rice w/dates
S		Basmati rice (sunflower seed butter and/or fruit)
S		Eggs and rice or potato cake
	G	Omelette w/cheese, mushrooms, onions, and chili
		Brown rice (almond butter or sunflower seed butter, and/or fruit)
S		Rice cakes w/sunflower seed butter (cherry or blueberry jam)
S		Rice cakes w/cream cheese or kefir cheese

Balanced

L	S	G	Food
			Rice cakes and avocado
	S		Oat bread toast (butter)
	S		Fruit, toast (jelly), no butter
		G	Almond butter and banana on bagel
	S		Fruit – rotate – choice of apple, mango, nectarine, pineapple, cantaloupe, raspberries, cranberries, or blueberries
L			Fruit – rotate – choice of apple, mango, banana, pineapple, plums, pear, or peach
L			Cantaloupe or watermelon
			Granola bar
	S		Cottage cheese and pineapple or apple
		G	Fruit yogurt
	S		Sweet potato or yam (butter)
			Potatoes, carrots, and zucchini
			Baked potato (butter) or hash browns

MID-MORNING SNACK:
(Optional) Grain, vegetables, fruit.

L	S	G	Food
			Carrots, jicama, or bell pepper
	S		Apple juice w/protein powder
	S		Cantaloupe, blueberries, or pineapples
			Rice cakes

LUNCH:
12-2 p.m. Moderate, with protein, grain, vegetables and/or dairy. Emphasize protein.

L	S	G	Food
	S	G	Shark and rice (salad: carrots, tomatoes, and iceberg lettuce w/ranch dressing)
L			Shrimp and salad
	S		Tuna salad or salmon and salad
			Shrimp salad (potato and/or green salad)
L	S		Tuna, avocado, and green onion
L			Tuna on rye bread (cole slaw)
L	S		Tuna on oat bread (cole slaw)
	S	G	Red snapper and rice or potatoes
	S		Swordfish, white basmati rice, and spinach
			Trout w/cornmeal and spinach
	S	G	Beef, basmati rice, and carrots
L			Chicken and brown rice
L		G	Chicken, white basmati rice, and broccoli
L		G	White chicken and peanut sauce, basmati rice, and carrots
L		G	Teriyaki chicken, potato, and carrots
L		G	Turkey and pasta salad
L		G	Turkey sandwich on rye or oat bread, (w/romaine lettuce or cole slaw)
L			White turkey and lettuce salad w/vinaigrette dressing
L		G	Eggs, brown basmati rice, onion, and broccoli

MID-AFTERNOON SNACK:
(Optional) Protein, vegetables, grain, nuts.

L	S	G	Food
	S	G	Almonds
	S		Rice cake or rye cracker w/avocado (vegetable broth powder)

LUNCH or DINNER:
Chicken w/salsa or spices is good, but beef w/salsa, spices, or pepper is not, as this combination can actually cause muscle pain.

L	S	G	Food
L	S	G	Salmon, pasta, and zucchini
L		G	Shark and rice
L		G	Tuna and Italian salad dressing on bagel
L	S	G	Tuna, avocado, and romaine lettuce or rye crackers
L	S	G	Tuna, avocado, and sesame garlic dressing (raw carrots)
L		G	Swordfish, rice, asparagus, and carrots
L	S	G	Fillet of sole and brown basmati rice
L		G	Chicken salad on rye bread
L		G	Chicken fajita w/rice
		G	Chicken, salsa, and spices (rice and/or green beans)
		G	Tostada: corn tortilla, refried pinto beans, shredded Jack cheese, lettuce, and chicken
			Turkey and salad: romaine lettuce, carrots, sunflower sprouts, and sesame garlic dressing
	S	G	Pot roast, potatoes, onions, garlic, carrots, and celery

Balanced

	S	G	Meat loaf and mashed potatoes
	S		Eggs and potatoes
	S		Caesar salad or bean salad and seeds
	S		Sweet potatoes or yams and green beans
	S		Yellow squash, rice, carrots, and sunflower seeds
	S	G	Lasagna
	S		Pasta w/marinari sauce and cheese
	S		Pasta salad w/carrots, bell peppers, and Italian dressing (white cheese)
	S	G	Spaghetti w/ground beef, tomato sauce and paste, garlic, and Italian seasoning
L			Spaghetti w/tomato sauce
	S		Scalloped potatoes and lima beans
			Stir fry: broccoli, red bell pepper, onions, and celery on rice
	S	G	Kefir cheese on rye bread
	S		Lentil soup, seeds, and rye crackers

DINNER:
7-9 p.m. Moderate, with grain, vegetables, legumes, protein, and/or dairy. Emphasize grain and vegetables.

	S	G	Red snapper, basmati rice, and Chinese pea pods
L			Eggplant, (brown) basmati rice, bell peppers, onion, and garlic
L		G	Eggs and rice
		G	Omelette w/cheese and vegetables
L	S		Basmati rice and kidney beans
	S	G	Pasta, Monterey Jack cheese, and raw carrots
L			Pasta, eggplant, garlic, and olive oil
L	S		Pasta (butter and/or vegetables)
L	S		Pasta w/marinara sauce
	S		Corn bread (rice and beans)
L	S	G	Vegetable rotelle w/green beans, basil, olive oil, garlic, and parmesan/romano cheese
L			Stir-fry vegetables: carrots, green beans, onions, zucchini, celery w/tomato base and low-sodium ginger sauce (rice)
L			White basmati rice and peas or pea pods
L			Curry rice (squash)
L			Mexican rice (pinto beans)
L			Rice and steamed carrots, broccoli, and cauliflower
L			Vegetarian burrito (beans)
L	S		Cottage cheese and sunflower seeds
L			Baked potato w/butter and broccoli
L			Sweet potatoes (w/Bragg™ aminos and Spike®) (butter)
L			Sweet potato, green beans, and almonds
L	S		Rye crackers or rice cakes w/hummus and celery sticks
		G	Cheese sandwich w/lettuce, avocado, and tomato on sprouted sourdough, or French bread w/garlic and roasted, ground, salted sesame seeds
L			Bean or lentil soup
			Black cherry or raspberry yogurt
	S		Tofu, rice, carrots, green beans, green onions, and rye crackers (sunflower seeds)
L	S		Baked potato, green beans, and carrots
			Baked potato and steamed vegetables – any combination, such as broccoli and cauliflower, carrots, or peas (sesame garlic dressing)
L			Lettuce salad w/tofu cheese
		G	Vegetable salad w/chicken or fish (pasta or rice)
L			Salad: romaine lettuce, peppers, and tomato w/low fat dressing
			Lettuce salad: lettuce, red peppers, mushrooms, sunflower seeds, and avocado w/Caesar salad dressing and toast
			Lentil soup and rye crackers
			Black bean soup or potato leek soup
L			Vegetable soup

EVENING SNACKS:
(Optional) 10 p.m.-2 a.m. Three hours after dinner. Vegetables, fruit, seeds, grain, sweets.

	S		Rice cake w/avocado
	S		Popcorn
		G	Frozen yogurt w/almonds, macadamias, pecans, or sunflower seeds
		G	Ice cream

BLOOD

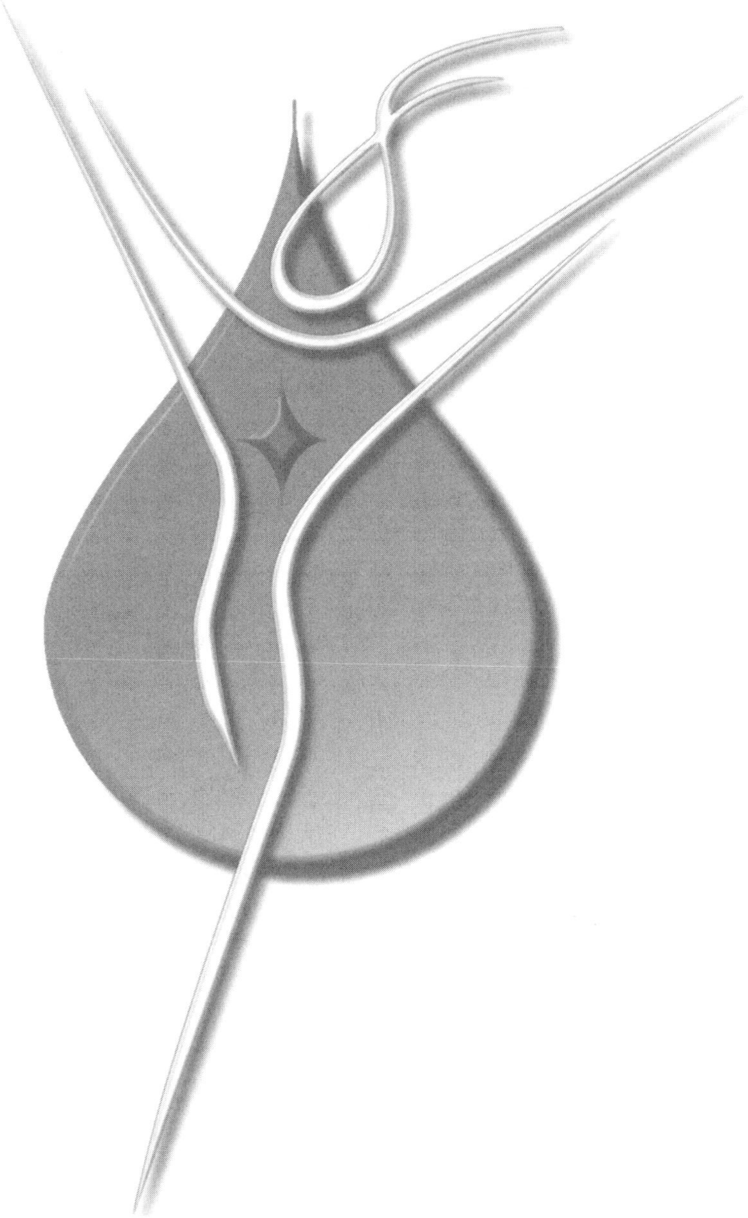

The "Blood Body Type"
is symbolized by a drop of blood.
Blood maintains harmony by carrying oxygen and nutrients and by removing wastes. Greatly affected by emotional and environmental stress, they go to great lengths to maintain harmony.

Blood

BODY TYPE PROFILE

LOCATION	Throughout entire body, circulating through heart, arteries, capillaries, and veins.
FUNCTION	Essentially serves as transport mechanism, consisting of plasma, red blood cells (which specifically carry oxygen and nutrients to cells throughout body), white blood cells (designed to fight infection), and platelets.
POTENTIAL HEALTH PROBLEMS	Basically, positive mental attitude toward health and relationships, mild-mannered, and even-tempered. Physically, prone to headaches. When energy is low, fatigue experienced first as difficulty concentrating. Sleeping difficulties. Skin rashes and outbreaks. Cardiovascular problems (e.g., arteriosclerosis, even triple by-pass surgery) may occur when chronic conflicts left unresolved.
RECOMMENDED EXERCISE	Exercise may be helpful or doesn't make much difference, making it optional. Its benefit is emotional. It gets energy moving in body and also provides a means of clearing the mind and releasing emotional stress. Moderate exercise is beneficial in losing or maintaining weight and vascular integrity. Heavy exercise is often contra-indicated. Ideal activities include walking, bicycling and dancing.

WOMEN'S CHARACTERISTICS

DISTINGUISHING FEATURES	Expressive, receptive eyes that immediately draw attention to face. Known for going to great lengths to maintain harmony. More than any other type, social and environmental harmony are essential to their health and well-being.
ADDITIONAL PHYSICAL CHARACTERISTICS	Buttocks relatively flat-to-rounded. Low back curvature average-to-swayed. Breasts average-to-large. Shoulders relatively even with hips. Torso solid with straight-to-defined waist, often short-waisted. Height generally average, but can range from petite-to-tall. Bone structure typically medium, but can vary. Average, elongated musculature with little definition. Average or broad, square hands. Average rectangular or oval face, often with low forehead.
WEIGHT GAIN AREAS	Lower body with initial gain in lower abdomen, upper hips, waist, and upper inner to outer 2/3rds of thighs. Secondary weight gain in entire upper 2/3rds of thighs, entire abdomen, buttocks, middle back, upper back under arms, upper arms, breasts, face, and under chin. Weight gain of more than 20 pounds is carried mainly in torso, including entire back, but not lower hips.

Blood

DIETARY GUIDELINES

"HEALTHY"	SCHEDULING MEALS: Breakfast: Light-to-moderate, with vegetables, protein, dairy, grain, and/or fruit. Lunch: Moderate-to-heavy, with protein, nuts, seeds, grain, and/or vegetables. Dinner: Moderate, with protein, nuts, seeds, dairy, grain, legumes, and/or vegetables. Emphasize carbohydrates.
"SENSITIVE"	Breakfast: Light-to-moderate, with vegetables, protein, dairy, grain, and/or fruit. Lunch: Moderate-to-heavy, with protein and/or grain. Dinner: Light-to-moderate, with protein and/or grain.
DIETARY EMPHASIS	• Following foods, when combined, support body; when eaten by themselves, they do not: eggs and Swiss cheese; beef and eggs; beef and rice; and ham and tomato (but no more than once a week per combination); turkey with celery, mustard, or bacon, however, may be consumed up to five times a week. • For weight loss, eliminate dairy (including butter); limit fats to 20% of calories, and avoid vegetable oils; substitute creamy Italian dressing for mayonnaise; and possibly use metabolic stimulant. • For weight gain, include dairy and increase total food quantity. • Vegetarian diets inadequate, since require 5-35% of calories from dense protein. • Fats, 20-30% of caloric intake, derived from avocados, chicken, fish, cheese, and pumpkin seeds.
KEY SUPPORTS FOR SYSTEM	Protein, such as white chicken breast (experience fatigue when don't get enough protein); carbohydrates, such as pasta, noodles, or rice; and vegetables, such as tomatoes, raw or steamed zucchini, steamed carrots, or cauliflower.
COMPLEMENTARY GLANDULAR SUPPORT	Lymph, through daily walking; nervous system, through consuming at least 2 oz. of dense protein three times per week.

Blood

FOODS CRAVED	*(When energy is low)* Sweets – e.g., ice cream (especially chocolate), cookies, chocolates. Carbohydrates – pasta, spaghetti, popcorn. Sometimes spicy foods, as they act as stimulants.
FOODS TO AVOID	Beef, ham, turkey, or eggs by themselves. However, certain combinations including these foods are acceptable – see "Dietary Emphasis."
RECOMMENDED CUISINE	Italian, Mexican, Chinese, Soup and Salad. Pasta dishes, including fish and pasta combinations.

PSYCHOLOGICAL PROFILE

ESSENCE

Just as the blood maintains harmony throughout the body by carrying oxygen and nutrients to all parts, Blood body types need to maintain harmony. They are greatly affected by what others think of them and will readily become physically ill when emotionally upset. They are noted for going to great lengths to maintain social and environmental harmony. Their strength lies in their ability to make people aware of the effect disharmony has on people and the earth.

CHARACTERISTIC TRAITS

Easy going and personable, Bloods are social beings whose basic nature is warm, receptive, and nurturing. Sensitive and considerate, they have a genuine concern for others, particularly those who aren't able to speak out on their own behalf. They are intensely drawn to the young, the old or disabled and to animals and nature.

Extremely sensitive to their physical and emotional environment, Bloods are at their best when they can maintain harmony, balance and tranquility. The slightest bit of disharmony, such as a minor misunderstanding, can have adverse effects on Blood types, physically as well as emotionally. Since emotional conflict affects them so profoundly, they are unable to let it slide. Conflict usually interferes with their sleep first, making them unable to sleep or rest well until the problem is resolved.

The Bloods' acute emotional sensitivity is evident in their ability to read others and their need to please them to keep peace. Being so conscious of others makes Blood types extremely aware of even the slightest bit of disharmony, even amidst much harmony. Wanting to make people feel comfortable, they often have a good sense of humor and are generally optimistic.

With their strong desire to experience life, Bloods are generally open-minded and willing to try new things, including the unorthodox. Internally driven to find a greater meaning in life, they will often study a subject in depth and

Blood

become totally immersed in it, getting so caught up with it that other things get ignored or forgotten. They may even concentrate so much on individual details that they temporarily lose sight of the whole. However, being practical and flexible, once Bloods have experienced it, they will let go of what isn't right for them and keep what works.

While Bloods are supported by social interaction and contact, they are highly task-oriented, self-motivated, and very responsible. When they commit to a project, they will make it their main focus, getting it done well with utmost efficiency. They can even be so meticulous as to border on the obsessive/ compulsive. In their efforts to understand something, they will do much analyzing and processing of events and the situations concerning them.

MOTIVATION

Harmony is of utmost importance to Bloods, so they will do almost anything to achieve and maintain it. All too often, they will compromise long term harmony with short term peace, choosing to suppress their feelings rather than confront conflict. When they do find the courage to speak up and things are not resolved, after having said their piece, they will go into denial of the problem to keep outside appearances calm. Unfortunately, unresolved conflict eventually undermines their inner tranquility and sense of well-being preventing them from experiencing true harmony. Suppressing unresolved conflict causes the stress and tension to be turned inward, and more so than with any of the other types, causes physical problems.

When unable to deal with a situation, or process the feelings, the tendency is to deny them or to stop expressing, denying parts of themselves. Unfortunately, these blocked emotions – especially those stemming from anger or confrontation – back up in the veins and arteries of the body, particularly around the heart and eventually result in coronary heart disease.

Respect is a motivating factor for Bloods – respect of themselves, respect for others, as well as respect from others. Self-respect can be a challenge for Bloods as they are often torn between being true to themselves and giving others what they want in order to maintain harmony. Often raised in a family where they were not allowed to express anger, many learned they needed to repress parts of themselves to get their needs met.

Placing their value in outside appearances, Bloods will try to please by over-committing physically, financially, or emotionally and overtax themselves. Needing social approval, the world's perception of them is extremely important, so making a favorable impression on others is essential. Consequently, their outward presentation is generally cordial and obliging - even when their true feelings are less congenial. Not only is harmony essential in their emotional world, but in their physical world as well. Having things in their life clear, ordered, and balanced provides them with a sense of security and well-being.

Blood

"AT WORST"

Highly emotional, Bloods will react without knowing why. They experience the feelings, but are unable to mentally grasp their basis. Unable to connect the words and to logically verbalize, they often express their feelings through tears. Crying is a way of dissipating or shutting off feelings. Frequently there is underlying anger, hurt, or sadness. Not knowing what they are feeling, Bloods will react in ways they have programmed themselves to react, which may be by becoming irritable, critical, short-tempered, or irrational.

Refusing to take personal responsibility for their feelings, they will react in a childlike fashion by easily letting their feelings be hurt and turning the hurt into inappropriate anger. They can become nit-picky, demanding, grouchy, and extremely impatient. They can get into an "I don't care," or "Whatever you do is not enough" attitude. When fear sets in they can become paranoid, anxious, compulsive, overly emotional and unreasonable.

Confrontation only aggravates the situation, so wanting to maintain harmony and not make waves, their tendency is to stuff the emotions into the body (later to be expressed through the body), and simply lose confidence in themselves. Unwilling to stand up in the world, they become co-dependent in relationships, living off someone else and stifling their own identity. A common defense is drinking, as alcohol numbs the emotions and creates isolation. Another more subtle form of isolation is through environmental sensitivities, as this leads to being controlled by outside sources.

Having a plan provides a sense of mental security. By knowing the plan, the rules and what to expect, they feel more secure. This can cause them to be obsessive about details, such as time schedules, with no flexibility. They want to know the rules and what to expect. While they start out being very accommodating and in complete agreement with the plan for the day or trip, if things don't go the way they had planned, particularly when things take longer than expected, they become irritable, nit-picky, demanding, paranoid, emotional and unreasonable.

"AT BEST"

Being personally responsible and recognizing that true harmony can only exist when there is complete harmony within one's self, Bloods will first examine themselves. Knowing they can't just let something go until they've gotten the message from it, Blood types will use their determination to do what they need to do to get to the bottom of the problem. By stepping back from a situation, they create the flexibility necessary to give the other person their space and provide themselves with a chance to honestly examine their true feelings.

By discovering what is true for them, they can know themselves, and honor and respect themselves by being true to themselves. This is what produces spiritual harmony and harmony within one's self. True integration occurs when they are able to move the energy from the emotional to the spiritual to the mental and express it physically. Being in harmony provides a sense of security that allows them to experience genuine happiness and freedom.

Blood

Positive and easygoing, Blood body types maintain harmony by carrying optimism and encouragement throughout their sphere of influence. With their ability to read others and their good sense of humor, it's easy for them to make others feel at ease. Having superior social skills, they're one of the most companionable of all the body types. More than socially adaptive, they contribute to the cohesiveness of the group, as well as tending to the needs of the individual members. Being sensitive to others' feelings, they are adept at "reading people". Genuinely interested in helping others, they are at their best when they express their well-developed humanitarian impulses.

Having learned to confront their anger by stopping and getting in touch with their feelings, they are able to communicate in a calm, loving fashion without getting caught up in the situation. Once they are able to release and let go, the Universe supports them. By "letting go and letting God", trusting their own inner knowing, and being true to themselves, they are able to truly be the Peace Makers and bring peace on earth.

Blood

FOOD LISTS

HEALTHY FOOD LIST

FREQUENTLY FOODS	3-7 meals per week – refers to each food, rather than category.
DENSE PROTEIN	Buffalo, lamb; turkey, chicken, chicken livers, chicken broth, cornish game hen; anchovy, bass, bonita, catfish, cod, flounder, haddock, halibut, herring, mackerel, mahi-mahi, perch, red snapper, roughy, salmon, sardines, shark, swordfish, trout; clams, eel, mussels, octopus
DAIRY	Goat milk, sweet cream, sour cream, kefir
CHEESE	Camembert, cream, goat, Parmesan, Romano
NUTS and SEEDS	Almonds (raw, roasted), coconut, macadamias (raw, roasted), peanuts (raw, dry roasted), pine nuts (raw, roasted), pistachios, pumpkin seeds (raw, roasted)
GRAINS	Rice (white or brown basmati), popcorn
VEGETABLES	Avocados, celery, eggplant, garlic, parsley, spinach
FRUITS	Melons (cantaloupe, watermelon), raisins
CONDIMENTS	Tahini
SWEETENERS	Re-Vita®, stevia
BEVERAGES	Coffee with Re-Vita®; black tea
MODERATELY FOODS	1-2 meals per week – refers to each food, rather than category.
DENSE PROTEIN	Beef liver, beef broth, bacon, pork, ham, sausage, veal, venison, organ meats (heart, brain); duck; sole, tuna; abalone, calamari (squid), crab, lobster, oysters, scallops, shrimp; eggs
DAIRY	Buttermilk, plain or flavored yogurt, frozen yogurt, ice cream (Breyers®, Ben & Jerry's®, Dreyer's), butter
CHEESE	American, blue, brie, Colby, cottage, Edam, feta, Gouda, Jack, kefir, Limburger, mozzarella, Muenster, ricotta, Swiss
NUTS and SEEDS	Almond butter, Brazils, cashews (raw, roasted), cashew butter, waterchestnuts, filberts, hazelnuts, macadamia butter, pecans, peanuts (roasted/salted), peanut butter, walnuts (black, English), raw or roasted seeds (caraway, sesame, sunflower), sesame seed butter, sunflower seed butter
LEGUMES	Beans (adzuki, black, lima [butter], garbanzo, kidney, navy, great northern, pinto, red, soy), lentils, black-eyed peas, split peas, tofu, soy milk, hummus, miso
GRAINS	Amaranth, barley, buckwheat, corn, corn bread, corn grits, corn tortillas, hominy grits, millet, oats, quinoa, rice (long or short grain brown, wild, Japanese), rice bran, rice cakes, triticale, rye, whole wheat, wheat bran, wheat germ, refined wheat flour, flour tortillas, breads (corn, corn/rye, French,

Blood

GRAINS (Continued)	garlic, Italian, multi-grain, oat, rice, rye, 7-grain, sourdough, sprouted grain, whole wheat, white), bagels, croissants, English muffins, crackers (saltines, wheat, oat, rye), couscous, pasta, Chinese rice noodles, udon noodles, cream of rice, cream of rye, cream of wheat
VEGETABLES	Artichokes, asparagus, bamboo shoots, green beans, yellow wax beans, lima beans, beets, bok choy, broccoflower, broccoli, brussels sprouts, cabbage (green, napa, red), carrots, cauliflower, chard, cilantro, corn, cucumbers, greens (beet, collard, mustard, turnip), hominy, jicama, kale, kohlrabi, leeks, lettuce (Boston, butter, endive, iceberg, red leaf, romaine), mushrooms, okra, olives (green, ripe), onions (chives, green, brown, red, white, vidalia), parsnips, peas, snow pea pods, bell peppers (green, red, yellow), chili peppers, pimentos, potatoes (red, russet, white rose, yukon gold, purple), pumpkin, radishes, daikon radishes, rutabaga, seaweed (arame, dulse, kelp, nori, wakame), sauerkraut, shallots, sprouts (alfalfa, clover, radish, mung bean, sunflower), squash (acorn, banana, butternut, spaghetti, yellow [summer], zucchini), sweet potatoes, tomatoes (vine-ripened, canned), turnips, watercress, yams
VEGETABLE JUICES	Carrot, carrot/celery, celery, tomato, V-8®
FRUITS	Apples (Golden or Red Delicious, Granny Smith, Jonathan, Pippin, McIntosh, Rome Beauty), apricots, bananas, blackberries, blueberries, boysenberries,cranberries, gooseberries, raspberries, cherries, grapes (black, green, red), grapefruits (red. white), guavas, kiwi, kumquats, lemons, limes, loquats, mangos, nectarines, oranges, papayas, peaches, pears, persimmons, pineapples, pomegranates, plums (black, purple, red), rhubarb, tangelos, tangerines, dates, figs (fresh, dried), prunes
FRUIT JUICES	Apple, apple cider, apple/apricot, apricot, black cherry, red cherry, cranapple, cranberry, grape (purple, red, white), grapefruit, guava, lemon, orange, papaya, pear, pineapple, pineapple/coconut, prune, tangerine, watermelon
VEGETABLE OILS	All-blend, almond, avocado, canola, coconut, corn, peanut, flaxseed, sesame, sunflower
SWEETENERS	Molasses, sorghum, brown sugar, raw sugar, brown rice syrup, barley malt syrup, corn syrup, fructose, succonant
CONDIMENTS	Catsup, mustard, horseradish, soy sauce, green chiles, barbecue sauce, pesto sauce, salsa, margarine, vinegar, ginger, lemon pepper, salt, sea salt, Vege-sal®, MSG
SALAD DRESSINGS	Blue cheese, French, ranch, creamy Italian, creamy avocado, thousand island, vinegar and oil, lemon juice and oil
DESSERTS	Custards, tapioca, puddings, pies, cakes, chocolate, desserts containing chocolate, raspberry sherbet, orange sherbet
CHIPS	Bean, blue corn, potato
BEVERAGES	De-caf coffee, Swiss mocha; herbal teas, mint tea, raspberry tea, green tea, Japanese tea, Chinese oolong tea; plain or flavored mineral water; white wine, chardonnay or zinfandel, champagne; tonic water w/lime.

Blood

RARELY FOODS	No more than once a month
DENSE PROTEIN	Beef
DAIRY	Milk (raw, whole, 2%, low fat, nonfat), half & half, most ice creams
CHEESE	Cheddar
NUTS and SEEDS	Trail mix
GRAINS	Polished rice
VEGETABLES	Arugula, hot-house tomatoes
VEGETABLE JUICES	Spinach, parsley
FRUITS	Strawberries, melons (casaba, crenshaw, honeydew)
VEGETABLE OILS	Olive, safflower, soy
SWEETENERS	Honey, date sugar, refined cane sugar, maple syrup, saccharin, aspertame, Equal®, Sweet'n Low,® NutraSweet®
CONDIMENTS	Mayonnaise
CHIPS	Corn (white, yellow)
BEVERAGES	Regular coffee; carbonated sparkling water; red wine, sherry, sake, liquers, beer, barley malt liquor, gin, Scotch, vodka, whiskey, margaritas; root beer, Coke®, sodas (diet, regular)
OTHER	Salty and fried foods

SENSITIVE FOOD LIST

FREQUENTLY FOODS	3-7 meals per week – refers to each food, rather than category.
DENSE PROTEIN	Chicken, chicken broth, chicken livers, cornish game hen; bonita, catfish, cod, flounder, haddock, herring, mackerel, red snapper
GRAINS	Rice (white or brown basmati), popcorn
VEGETABLES	Celery, eggplant
FRUITS	Cantaloupe, watermelon, raisins
MODERATELY FOODS	1-2 meals per week – refers to each food, rather than category.
DENSE PROTEIN	Beef broth, beef liver, buffalo, pork, ham, bacon, sausage, veal, organ meats (heart, brain); duck, turkey; bass, halibut, mahi-mahi, perch, orange roughy, salmon, sardines, shark, sole, swordfish, trout, tuna; abalone, calamari (squid), clams, crab, eel, lobster, octopus, oysters, scallops

Blood

DAIRY	Sweet cream, sour cream, kefir, frozen yogurt, butter
CHEESE	American, blue, brie, Camembert, cream, cottage, Edam, goat, Gouda, Jack, kefir, Limburger, Muenster, Parmesan, Romano, ricotta, Swiss
NUTS and SEEDS	Almonds (raw, roasted), Brazils, cashews (raw, roasted), coconut, macadamias (raw, roasted), peanuts (raw, roasted), pine nuts (raw, roasted), pistachios, walnuts (black, English), raw or roasted seeds (caraway, pumpkin, sesame, sunflower), sesame seed butter, sunflower seed butter
LEGUMES	Beans (adzuki, black, lima [butter], garbanzo, kidney, navy, great northern, pinto, red, soy), black-eyed peas, lentils, split peas, hummus, miso, soy milk, tofu
GRAINS	Amaranth, barley, buckwheat, millet, oats, quinoa, rice (long or short grainbrown, wild, Japanese), rice bran, rice cakes, rye, triticale, whole wheat, wheat bran, wheat germ, multi-grains, refined wheat flour, flour tortillas, breads (raisin, rice, honey wheat), couscous, pasta, Chinese rice noodles, udon noodles, cream of rice, cream of rye, cream of wheat
VEGETABLES	Artichokes, asparagus, avocados, bamboo shoots, green beans, yellow wax beans, lima beans, beets, bok choy, broccoli, brussels sprouts, cabbage (green, napa, red), carrots, cauliflower, cilantro, corn, cucumbers, garlic, greens (beet, collard, mustard, turnip), jicama, kale, kohlrabi, leeks, lettuce (Boston, butter, endive, red leaf, romaine), mushrooms, okra, olives (green, ripe), onions (chives, green, brown, red, white, vidalia), parsley, parsnips, peas, snow pea pods, bell peppers (green, red, yellow), chili peppers, pimentos, potatoes (red, white rose, russet, yukon gold, purple), pumpkin, daikon radishes, rutabaga, sauerkraut, seaweed (arame, dulse, kelp, nori, wakame), shallots, spinach, sprouts (alfalfa, clover, mung bean, radish, sunflower), squash (acorn, banana, butternut, spaghetti, yellow [summer], zucchini), sweet potatoes, tomatoes (canned, vine-ripened), turnips, watercress, yams
VEGETABLE JUICES	Celery, carrot, carrot/celery, tomato, V-8®
FRUITS	Apples (Golden or Red Delicious, Granny Smith, Jonathan, McIntosh, Pippin, Rome Beauty), apricots, blackberries, blueberries, boysenberries, cranberries, gooseberries, raspberries, cherries, grapes (black, green, red), grapefruits (white, red), guavas, kiwi, kumquats, lemons, loquats, mangos, papayas, pears, pineapples, plums (black, purple, red), pomegranates, rhubarb, tangelos, dates, figs (fresh, dried)
FRUIT JUICES	Apple cider, apple/apricot, apricot, black cherry, red cherry, cranapple, cranberry, grape (purple, red, white), guava, lemon, orange, papaya, pear, pineapple, pineapple/coconut, prune, watermelon
VEGETABLE OILS	All-blend, avocado, coconut
SWEETENERS	Brown rice syrup, barley malt syrup, Re-Vita®, stevia
CONDIMENTS	Vinegar, salt, sea salt, salsa, Vege-Sal®, spices

Blood

SALAD DRESSINGS	Vinegar and oil, lemon juice and oil
BEVERAGES	Coffee with Re-Vita®; herbal tea, green tea, mint tea, Japanese tea, Chinese oolong tea; plain or flavored mineral water
RARELY FOODS	No more than once a month
DENSE PROTEIN	Beef, lamb, venison; anchovy; mussels, shrimp; eggs
DAIRY	Milk (raw, whole, 2%, low fat, nonfat), goat milk, buttermilk, half & half, plain or flavored yogurt, most ice creams
CHEESE	Cheddar, Colby, feta, mozzarella
NUTS and SEEDS	Water chestnuts, filberts, hazelnuts, pecans, nut butters (almond, cashew, macadamia, peanut), trail mix
GRAINS	Corn, corn bread, corn grits, corn tortillas, hominy grits, polished rice, breads(French, Italian, 7-grain, multi-grain, corn, corn/rye, rye, sprouted grain, oat, garlic, sourdough, white, rice, whole wheat), bagels, croissants, English muffins, crackers (saltines, oat, rye, wheat)
VEGETABLES	Arugula, broccoflower, chard, hominy, iceberg lettuce, radishes, hot house tomatoes
VEGETABLE JUICES	Parsley, spinach
FRUITS	Bananas, strawberries, limes, melons (casaba, crenshaw, honeydew), nectarines, oranges, peaches, persimmons, tangerines, prunes
FRUIT JUICES	Apple, grapefruit, tangerine
VEGETABLE OILS	Almond, canola, corn, peanut, flaxseed, olive, safflower, soy, sesame, sunflower
SWEETENERS	Honey, date sugar, refined cane sugar, maple syrup, molasses, sorghum, brown sugar, raw sugar, corn syrup, fructose, succonant, saccharin, Equal®, aspertame, Sweet'n'Low®, Nutra-Sweet®
CONDIMENTS	Mayonnaise, soy sauce, tahini, catsup, mustard, horseradish, barbecue sauce, pesto sauce, margarine, MSG
SALAD DRESSINGS	Blue cheese, French, ranch, creamy Italian, creamy avocado, thousand island
DESSERTS	Custards, tapioca, puddings, pies, cakes, chocolate, desserts containing chocolate, raspberry sherbet, orange sherbet
CHIPS	Corn (blue, white, yellow), potato, bean
BEVERAGES	Coffee; hot chocolate; black tea; carbonated sparkling water; wine (red,white), sake, sherry, liqueurs, champagne, beer, barley malt liquor, gin, Scotch, vodka, whiskey; root beer, Coke, sodas (diet, regular)
OTHER	Salty and fried food

Blood

MENUS

DIETARY EMPHASIS:

- Protein, such as white chicken breast (generally experience fatigue when don't get enough protein).
- Consume at least 2 oz. of dense protein 3 times per week.
- Carbohydrates, such as pasta, noodles, or rice;and vegetables, such as tomatoes, raw or steamed zucchini, steamed carrots, or cauliflower.

KEY COMBINATIONS :

When combined, these foods support the body; when eaten by themselves, they do not.
Eat these foods no more than 1 x/wk per combination

- Eggs and Swiss cheese
- Beef and eggs
- Beef and rice
- Ham and tomato
- Turkey with celery, mustard, or bacon may be eaten up to 5x/wk.

WEIGHT LOSS :

- Eliminate all dairy including butter, cheese, yogurt, milk.
- Limit fats to 20% of calories.
- Avoid vegetable oils.
- Good substitute for mayonnaise is creamy Italian dressing.
- May use a metabolic stimulant.

WEIGHT GAIN:

- Include dairy.
- Increase quantity of food.

VEGETARIAN DIET:

- Inadequate, since require 5-35% of calories from dense protein.

SENSITIVE:

- Limit lunch and dinner to protein and/or grain.

FATS:

- 20-30% of caloric intake.
- Best sources are avocados, chicken, fish, cheese, and pumpkin seeds.

KEY

—all menus may be used by healthy persons
( ) around foods means that they're optional
L denotes weight loss menus
S denotes sensitive menus
G denotes weight gain menus

BREAKFAST:
7-9 a.m. Light-to-moderate, with vegetables, protein, dairy, grain, and/or fruit.

Fruit or juices (cold or warm) such as apple, grape, grapefruit, or orange, then protein or grain.

L	S	G	Menu
	S		Carrot/celery juice (beet)
			Apples and bananas
	S		Apricots and kiwi
		G	Grapefruit and blueberry muffin w/butter
L			Oranges or grapefruit – alone
L			Papaya, watermelon, or cantaloupe
L			Cantaloupe alone; grain 30 minutes later
L			Fruit, then oatmeal
			Oat bread or sourdough bread and almond butter
			Deli rye toast w/orange marmalade
			Toast or muffin and banana
L			Oat bran muffin (tea, such as spice, mint, orange or peppermint)
			Multi-grain pancakes w/blueberries or butter and peaches
L			Multi-grain pancakes w/Re-Vita® as syrup
		G	Pancakes w/blueberries and cream
L			Oat bran waffles w/Re-Vita®
L			Oatmeal w/Re-Vita®
	S		Oatmeal w/raisins
L			Cream of rice w/banana or peach
	S		Cream of rice and butter
L			Baked potato w/salsa (chives)

Blood

L	S	G	
	S		Baked potato w/broccoli and white cheddar cheese
		G	Kefir cheese and celery
		G	Yogurt w/frozen, thawed raspberries or blackberries
			BEEF & EGGS – Key combination
		G	Beef and eggs and V-8® juice
L		G	Beef and eggs with fruit or toast
	S	G	Roast beef, Yorkshire pudding, and apple sauce
			EGGS & SWISS CHEESE – Key combination
	S	G	Eggs, Swiss cheese, and spicy hot V-8® juice
		G	Eggs, Swiss cheese, and salsa or toast
		G	Omelette eggs, mushrooms, Swiss cheese, and onions (green chiles and salsa, shrimp, or crab)
	S	G	Halibut, scalloped potatoes, and asparagus
		G	Chicken, oriental vegetables, and rice
	S		Salad w/blue cheese dressing
L	S		Re-Vita® w/cranberry concentrate
			Mint tea or regular tea w/breakfast
			Swiss Mocha (Re-Vita®)

MIDMORNING SNACK:
(Optional) Fruit, vegetables, grain, nuts, seeds.

L	S	G	
	S		Fruit or fruit juice until 3 p.m.
			Red clover, cammomile, or raspberry patch tea
	S		Apricots, kiwi, or grapes

LUNCH:
12-2 p.m. Moderate-to-heavy, with protein, nuts, seeds, grain, and/or vegetables.

SENSITIVE: Moderate-to-heavy, with protein and/or grain.

L	S	G	
L		G	Chinese or Mexican food w/chicken
L		G	Chicken, mushrooms, and broccoli (rice)
L		G	Chicken and bell peppers
L	S	G	Chicken and rice
L		G	Chicken and rice w/salad romaine lettuce, tomato, carrots, and artichoke hearts w/creamy Italian dressing
L		G	Chinese chicken and stir-fry vegetables – no MSG
			BEEF & RICE – Key combination
L		G	Carne asada burrito and rice
			TURKEY & CELERY or MUSTARD or BACON – Key combination
		G	Turkey, celery (raw or in dressing), cranberries, mashed potatoes, and gravy
		G	Turkey, white cheese, and mustard on pasta and lettuce salad
L		G	Turkey, mustard, and lettuce on sourdough bread
L			Tuna on tomato or green salad
		G	Tuna w/pasta and avocado
		G	Tuna, eggs, and dill pickles w/creamy Italian dressing, celery and peanut butter, and fruit yogurt
L		G	Fish, rice pilaf, and vegetables
	S		HAM & TOMATO – Key combination
		G	Ham, tomato, and mustard on French roll w/salad romaine lettuce or spinach, carrots, cucumbers, and Italian dressing
			Tofu, rice, and stir-fry vegetables
		G	Cottage cheese and peaches
L			Pasta w/pesto sauce and spinach salad w/rice vinegar
			Beans and rice (tofu and/or avocado)
			Lentil soup w/corn bread (salad)

AFTERNOON or ANYTIME SNACK: (Optional) Dairy, nuts, seeds, grain, legumes, vegetables.

L	S	G	
L			Carrots and celery or bell pepper
		G	Celery (cream cheese)
	S	G	Apples and cheese
L	S		Rice cakes
L			Rice cakes and sesame tahini
	S		Re-Vita® w/cranberry concentrate
			Almonds
			Cammomile tea at 4-5 p.m.

Blood

LUNCH or DINNER:

- S G — Lamb chops and wild rice
- L G — Chicken, boiled red potatoes, peas, and carrots
- S G — Chicken, rice, and black beans
- G — Chicken taco (tomato, onion, black olives, cheese) w/sour cream
- L G — Chicken or turkey pot pie
- G — Chicken or bean and cheese burritos
- L — Chicken and corn tortilla
- L — Chicken rice soup and crackers
- G — Halibut and scalloped potatoes (asparagus)
- S — Halibut or tuna and pasta
- Halibut, rice, and green beans
- S — Salmon and brown rice
- L S — Re-Vita® w/cranberry concentrate
- L — Baked potato w/dill dressing
- L — Spanish rice

DINNER:

6-9 p.m. Moderate, with protein, nuts, seeds, dairy, grain, legumes, and/or vegetables. Emphasize carbohydrates.

SENSITIVE Light-to-moderate, with protein and/or grain.

- G — Steak and eggs w/hash browns
- L — Orange roughy w/mushrooms and rice or pasta
- L — Orange roughy and brussels sprouts, spinach, or zucchini
- L G — Salmon, asparagus, and rice pilaf
- L G — Tuna or salmon fillet, potatoes, and asparagus
- L — Tuna, rice, and peas or celery
- L — Tuna, rice, garlic, and onions
- L S — Fish and wild rice
- L G — Fish, potatoes, and asparagus
- G — Calamari, vegetable, and sourdough bread
- G — Mahi-mahi, rice, and salad w/creamy Italian dressing
- L — Mahi-mahi, steamed rice, carrots, and zucchini

TURKEY & CELERY – Key combination

- L G — Turkey, potatoes, peas, and celery (butter lettuce salad w/sesame seeds)
- L — Turkey, basmati and/or wild rice, and celery (spinach salad)
- L G — Turkey sausage, basmati rice, green beans, and celery
- L — Chef salad w/turkey, celery, and bell peppers
- L — Turkey or chicken in stir-fry vegetables
- S — Chicken and pasta
- L — Chicken, pasta, and eggplant or spinach salad
- L S G — Rosemary chicken and couscous
- S G — Chicken enchiladas
- G — Chili rellenos, rice, beans
- G — Bean burrito, (rice, beans, avocado, and/or salsa)
- L — Spinach salad w/walnuts (dill dressing)
- L — Lamb chops, wild rice, and broccoli
- G — Gyro (Greek salad and feta cheese)
- L S — Grape leaves w/ground lamb, onions, and rice
- L — Baked potato w/chili, turkey, tuna, or chicken
- G — Potato w/sour cream
- L — Rice and broccoli (spinach)
- L G — Lentil soup (rye bread)
- L — Couscous and steamed vegetables
- L G — Vegetable lasagna and spinach salad w/rice vinegar
- L — Angel hair pasta w/Thai spices (vegetables, such as broccoli, red peppers, onions and/or mushrooms)
- L — Vegetarian spaghetti
- L — Rice (soy sauce) and salad spinach, carrots, and green pepper (tomato and/or Italian salad dressing)
- S — Oatmeal w/Re-Vita®
- Alcohol with dinner or evening (optional) – white wine, chardonnay, or zinfandel, tonic water and lime, or champagne

Blood

EVENING SNACK:

(Optional) 10 p.m.-2 a.m. Dairy, nuts, seeds, grain, vegetables, fruit, sweets, desserts.

Swiss Mocha (Re-Vita®)

Peppermint tea

L Unbuttered air-popped popcorn

S Fruit smoothie

G Ice cream (chocolate syrup and cherries)

G Frozen yogurt w/almonds, coconut, or other nuts

Chocolate chip cookies w/nuts

Watermelon

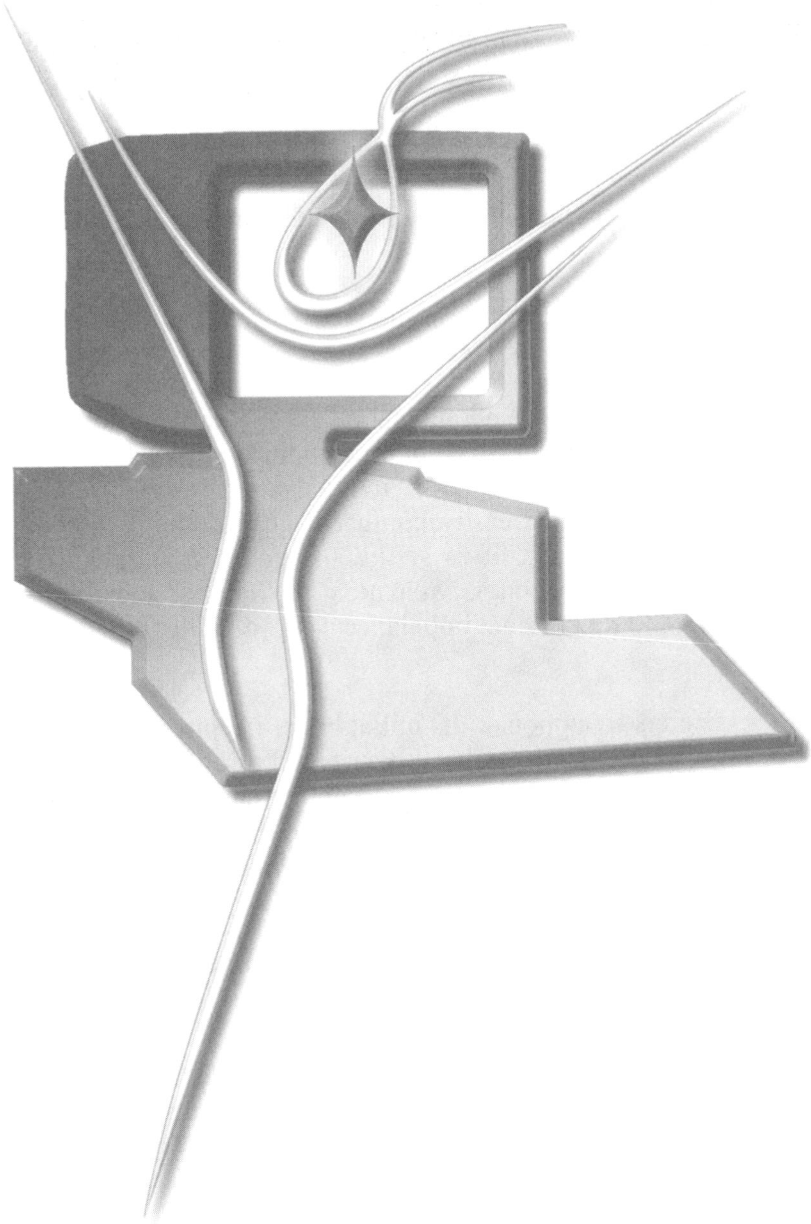

The "Brain Body Type"
is symbolized by a computer.
Meticulously collecting and storing
data for ready access, they like to have
all the information before making a
decision. With a strong desire to
do everything right, they are
extremely precise in their
speech and actions.

BRAIN

Brain

BODY TYPE PROFILE

LOCATION	Nervous tissue within cranium, including cerebrum, cerebellum, and pons.
FUNCTION	Controls and directs conscious activities of mind and body.
POTENTIAL HEALTH PROBLEMS	High energy – generally more energy early in the day. Often enjoy cold weather. When tired, brain is first area to reflect fatigue, so any thought process, particularly involving decisions, is too difficult. Brain fog – hard to make decisions, easily confused. Digestion is directly affected by stress. Nervous tension often settles in neck and shoulders. Sugar intolerance; migraine headaches; weakness in kidneys, low blood pressure; poor fat digestion; hormonal imbalances; sensitivity to chemicals and pollutants.
RECOMMENDED EXERCISE	Exercise is optional. Its initial benefit is physical, as it's essential to move to get energy from the head distributed throughout the body. Dance, aerobics, tennis, walking, biking, and moderate weight training are good basics. Important to connect the feelings to the intellect, so exercise needs to be fun or nurturing, such as getting up early and going for a meditative walk.

WOMEN'S CHARACTERISTICS

DISTINGUISHING FEATURES	Dominant forehead, often high. Frequently have dominant striking face, with piercing or commanding eyes. Known for intensely gathering information in detail. Precise in speech and actions with strong desire to do things right. Usually endowed with large breasts which are also area of initial weight gain.
ADDITIONAL PHYSICAL CHARACTERISTICS	Buttocks relatively flat-to-rounded. Low back curvature can range from straight-to-swayed. Breasts average-to-large. Shoulders relatively even with, to broader than, hips. Relatively slender torso. Either straight or well-defined waist. Average to short-waisted. Height petite-to-average. Bone structure small-to-medium. Average, elongated musculature. Slender legs. Hands average with short fingers. Average oval or rectangular face.
WEIGHT GAIN AREAS	Upper body with initial gain in breasts, upper hips, waist, lower abdomen, and possibly upper inner thighs. Secondary weight gain in entire back, buttocks, inner to entire upper 2/3rds of thighs, upper arms, face, under chin, then all over. May have difficulty gaining or maintaining weight, especially if food sensitivities are present. Low weight often associated with inadequate protein intake or poor assimilation.

Brain

DIETARY GUIDELINES

SCHEDULING MEALS:

"HEALTHY"

Breakfast: Moderate, with grain and fruit (not fruit alone). Protein after 11 a.m.

Lunch: Moderate, with protein, nuts, seeds, dairy, legumes, grain, and/or vegetables.

Dinner: Moderate, with protein, nuts, seeds, dairy, legumes, grain, vegetables, and/or fruit.

"SENSITIVE"

Breakfast: Moderate, with grain and fruit, vegetables, or yogurt and fruit.

Lunch: Moderate, with protein, nuts, seeds, dairy, legumes, grain, and/or vegetables.

Dinner: Moderate, with grain, legumes, vegetables, and/or fruit.

DIETARY EMPHASIS

- Protein such as eggs 2 times a week, and daily fruits and vegetables for vitamin C.
- For weight loss, reduce food quantity and limit fat consumption to 20% of total calories. Protein and carbohydrates should not be combined, such as bread with protein. Best times for meals are 10 a.m. for breakfast, 2 p.m. for lunch, and 6-7 p.m. for dinner.
- For weight gain, increase food quantity.
- Vegetarian diet recommended when healthy, although 15% may consist of dense protein.
- Fats, 20% for weight loss, 25% for maintenance. Best sources are pistachios, pecans, sunflower seeds, olive oil, dairy (including yogurt and cottage cheese), eggs, chicken and turkey.

KEY SUPPORTS FOR SYSTEM

Parsley assists kidneys. Use soy sauce in place of salt. Soy sauce may assist in bowel regulation.

Connect feelings with intellect by nurturing and pampering self.

Weight loss is mostly mental; need to get a mind set about being thin, discipline self to stop eating the moment you feel full, and never deny yourself anything, let go of rigid restrictive rules – because being told you can't have something only increases the desire. Make lunch biggest meal, be particularly careful about not having large meals for breakfast or dinner, and avoid the stuffed feeling. Smaller meals are best. May include snacks such as Spiru-tein® bar at mid-morning and smoothie or fruit at mid-afternoon. Salads are ideal.

Brain

KEY SUPPORTS FOR SYSTEM (Continued)	Need to satisfy "little kid" with something nourishing that also provides an emotional fix, as does the combination of caffeine, sugar, milk, and chocolate, as found in cafe' mocha. Drinking cafe' mocha in morning effectively satisfies little kid so you aren't compelled to do "acting-out eating" the rest of day. Something else that works for "cafe'-fix" is 1/2 cup of "fake coffee" consisting of 1/2 decaf and 1/2 regular coffee with cream. Sometimes Yoga or Chinese herb tea will also satisfy morning ritual. Use fun foods – those that are crunchy, or crackle, like air-popped popcorn or salads. Be careful to get enough protein.
COMPLEMENTARY GLANDULAR SUPPORT	Adrenals, through protein like eggs two times a week, and daily fruits and vegetables for vitamin C. Kidneys by building courage through doing something new at least two times a week, which could be as simple as taking a new route home from work.
FOODS CRAVED	*(When energy is low)* Sweets and carbohydrates, like chocolate, pie, cookies, breads, popcorn, potatoes; sweet fruits; creamy foods, such as cheese, sauces, ice cream, frozen yogurt, pudding; or almost all foods.
FOODS TO AVOID	Fried foods, hormone-fed beef, chicken or turkey, and caffeine.
RECOMMENDED CUISINE	Thai, Soup and Salad bars (Soup Plantation), Japanese, Italian, Greek, Mexican. Rarely – fast foods, French.

Brain

PSYCHOLOGICAL PROFILE

ESSENCE

Just as the brain is the information storage center of the body, Brain body types collect and store data. Brains are noted for intensely gathering information in detail, as they like to have all possible knowledge on a subject before making a decision. Memory, logical thought, and control of voluntary muscle responses are the brain's primary duties. It's the brain that is responsible for moving the body safely through the world. Since so many of our routine daily activities are done by automatic muscle memory, the brain knows the value of doing everything right. This desire to do everything right leads them to be very precise in their speech and actions.

CHARACTERISTIC TRAITS

Mentally oriented, Brain types are most comfortable when they have all the information available before they make a decision. Inclined to precision, they apply themselves conscientiously to whatever they undertake. Typically self-directed and independent, they can be quite diligent and persevering in carrying out projects. Brains tend to think in ways less conventional and more creative than most other types. Being quite analytical, they enjoy investigating a variety of topics, and will do so with adept resourcefulness and a lively curiosity. Sensitive and intuitive, as well, Brains are comfortable dealing with abstracts and conceptual realities.

Brains usually have a strong drive to find the meaning of life, and specifically, their personal direction. Their reason for being here may take the form of needing to feel they are needed, being involved in a worthwhile project, doing something where there is a mental challenge, or feeling their skills are well utilized in their job or career. Personal identity is often associated with their career, and academic recognition often provides the desired type of society status.

It is extremely important for Brains to do things right. They are not comfortable unless they can function at the highest possible level. Consequently, before embarking on any new theories or developments, they want to make sure it is scientifically proven with sufficient reasons, explanations and facts to support it.

Since the brain is the dominant organ or strongest system, it has the responsibility of carrying the greatest load and consequently fatigues first. Energy loss in the brain manifests as "brain fog", and makes even routine decisions difficult. Something as simple as deciding what to fix for dinner can be overwhelming. The tendency is to not eat dinner unless someone else fixes it, as it's "too hard to fix it myself", or to simply eat whatever happens to be in sight. Keeping weight on can be a problem because of not eating. Brains often get too busy and forget to eat, as it's not a high priority for them, or are extremely weight conscious and fearful of gaining weight, so they consciously restrict their food intake.

Brain

MOTIVATION

Brains are overly concerned with the possibility of making mistakes or appearing stupid. Consequently, they are thorough, meticulous, hard working, and inscrutably honest with a high desire for accuracy. They have a tendency to talk around things, without ever coming to a clear resolution. Brains may also belabor their points, assuming that otherwise people won't listen or understand them, or that they'll be perceived as naive, or even stupid. By being verbose, they can come across as cold and hard, without warmth. While their intention is not to be antagonistic, their mode of delivery often comes across as such. In reality, they are generally really nice people who have a genuine concern for others, and are usually very sweet and endearing.

Soft-spoken and not wanting to make waves, Brains would much prefer to avoid conflict, which tends to upset their rather delicate equilibrium, than to confront it. In wishing to get along with others, Brains are apt to acquiesce to the ideas of those around them. They may even withhold certain communications because of their desire to please others or win approval. Their apprehension about the possibility of doing something wrong can sometimes cause them to be passive or indecisive.

Basically sensitive and often somewhat shy or timid, Brains will use their strong intellect to provide a buffer from the unknown. While they prefer to handle life in a harmonious manner, they can be quite tenacious when it comes to getting what they want. Generally self-contained with active minds, they are perfectly content to stay at home or in their ivory tower research centers. Unfortunately, they get bored and need to get out into the world. To feel safe they gather as much information as they can. There is a tendency to spend too much time intellectualizing concepts and not enough time applying them, which causes Brains to thwart their basic need to produce tangible results.

"AT WORST"

Brains can become extremely rigid, locked into their own belief structures with a bias against anything new or different and a "Prove it to me" attitude. They intellectualize too much, needing to know every detail about something before making a decision, which others find extremely annoying. Their excessive mental activity can result in their getting lost in the details rather than seeing the whole picture. They can easily get side tracked by distractions, or withdraw into their own world or "Ivory Tower".

They can become mentally defiant to the extent that the mental realm becomes an arena for challenge or opposition. An example is insisting that everything have scientific, documentable "proof". They will confront anything that doesn't fit into their reality as a way of responding to a threat, rather than accept or allow other realities to co-exist. Their initial attitude toward anything that is not their idea is negative, pessimistic, and cynical. They will use the mental area to compensate for their basic underlying insecurities.

Easily stressed by mental or emotional upsets, once exhausted, they go brain dead and aren't able to make even the simplest decision. Their fear of being

Brain

"AT WORST"

wrong and appearing stupid or "doing something wrong" immobilizes them. Wary of taking risks, they will shy away from new adventures and experiences. Brains can easily stay too long in the ordinary, and wind up feeling dissatisfied. Unless they have outside support and encouragement, their fear of failure makes it difficult for them to make the needed changes.

Without strong physical contact, it's easy for Brains to get spaced out and lose touch with practical reality. Their lack of self-worth leads to perfectionism and compulsive aloofness. Depression is common, as is playing the role of the victim, and constantly asking why. With low self-esteem, it's easy for them to get caught in a feeling of hopelessness and become addicted to food, alcohol, drugs, or co-dependent relationships. Feelings of insecurity and self-doubt, will keep them distanced from the physical and social worlds causing them to miss out on opportunities that would give them their sense of direction.

"AT BEST"

Intuitive, sensitive, and empathic, Brains can be very effective in working with people. Since they typically use language with precision, they can be outstanding communicators and frequently excel in the teaching and counseling fields. In addition to being good at transmitting knowledge, Brains are also able to guide others in finding self-knowledge.

Gifted in the ability to tune into the needs of those around them, Brains are able to use this sensitivity and understanding to guide others in productive ways. They have good minds, and can be very focused, able to take the information they receive and carefully and precisely articulate it. Insightful and inventive, they're often able to explain things so they make sense to others, helping them see what had previously been cloudy or confusing.

Intuitive and practical, Brains can take the information they receive and distill it, putting it into a tangible form. They are likely to excel in academics, and pursuits that appeal to their inquiring nature, and are often found among distinguished researchers and scientists. Though especially good at abstract analysis, they can also be quite imaginative and artistic. Recognizing the power the mind has in controlling their lives, they maintain a positive attitude. Once Brains are clear about who they are and what they want, they have the direction they need to be quite successful, both professionally and socially. They are a lot of fun, supportive to others, and willing to be out in front. With their innate patience, perseverance, and tenacity, Brain types can effectively apply themselves and resolve the most intricate problems that they may encounter.

Brain

FOOD LISTS

HEALTHY FOOD LIST

FREQUENTLY FOODS	3-7 meals per week – refers to each food, rather than category.
DENSE PROTEIN	Beef broth, beef liver; chemical-free turkey, chicken broth; anchovy, sea bass, bonita, catfish, cod, flounder, haddock, halibut, herring, mackerel, mahi-mahi, perch, orange roughy, salmon, sardines, shark, red snapper, sole, swordfish, trout; calamari (squid), clams, eel, lobster, mussels, octopus, oysters, scallops
DAIRY	Half & half, butter
CHEESE	Kefir, Limburger
LEGUMES	Beans (adzuki, garbanzo, butter [lima], pinto, red, soy), lentils, hummus, tofu
GRAINS	Pasta, popcorn, brown or white basmati rice, English muffins
VEGETABLES	Brussels sprouts, carrots, celery, red leaf lettuce, parsley, zucchini
FRUITS	Cooked apples, bananas, raspberries, grapes (black, green, red), grapefruits (red, white), guavas, red plums
FRUIT JUICES	Apple/apricot, grape (purple, red, white)
SWEETENERS	Re-Vita®, stevia
CONDIMENTS	Soy sauce
BEVERAGES	Tea (mint, peppermint, Tension Tamer)
MODERATELY FOODS	1-2 meals per week – refers to each food, rather than category.
DENSE PROTEIN	Buffalo, pork, bacon, ham, sausage, lamb, veal, venison, organ meats (heart, brain); chemical-free chicken, chicken livers, cornish game hen, duck; tuna (fresh or canned); abalone, crab, shrimp; eggs
DAIRY	Milk (whole, 2%, nonfat, raw, goat) sweet cream, sour cream, kefir; regular, low fat, or nonfat yogurt (plain or flavored), frozen yogurt with nuts, ice cream (Dreyer's, or Ben & Jerry's®)
CHEESE	American, blue, brie, Camembert, Cheddar, Colby, cottage, cream, Edam, feta, goat, Gouda, Jack, mozzarella, Muenster, Parmesan, ricotta, Romano, Swiss
NUTS and SEEDS	Almonds (raw, roasted), almond butter, Brazils, cashews (raw, roasted), cashew butter, water chestnuts, coconuts, filberts, hazelnuts, macadamias (raw, roasted), macadamia butter, peanuts (raw, roasted), peanut butter, pecans, pine nuts (raw, roasted), pistachios, walnuts (black, English), raw or roasted seeds (caraway, pumpkin, sesame, sunflower), sesame seed butter, sunflower seed butter
LEGUMES	Beans (black, kidney, great northern), black-eyed peas, split peas, soy milk, miso

Brain

GRAINS	Amaranth, barley, buckwheat, corn, corn bread, corn grits, corn tortillas, hominy, millet, oats, quinoa, rice (long or short grain brown, wild, Japanese), rice bran, rice cakes, rye, triticale, refined wheat flour, flour tortillas, whole wheat, wheat bran, wheat germ, breads (French, garlic, Italian, sourdough, 7-grain, multigrain, oat, corn, corn/rye, rye, rice, sprouted grain, whole wheat, white), croissants, bagels, crackers (rye, saltines, wheat, oat), couscous, udon noodles, Chinese rice noodles, whole wheat noodles, cream of rice, cream of rye, cream of wheat
VEGETABLES	Artichoke, arugula, asparagus, avocados, bamboo shoots, green beans, lima beans, yellow wax beans, beets, bok choy, broccoli, broccoflower, cabbage (green, napa, red), cauliflower, chard, cilantro, corn, cucumbers, eggplant, garlic, greens (beet, collard, mustard, turnip), jicama, kale, kohlrabi, leeks, lettuce (Boston, butter, endive, iceberg, romaine), mushrooms, okra, olives (green, ripe), onions (chives, green, brown, red, white, yellow, vidalia), parsnips, peas, snow pea pods, bell peppers (green, red, yellow), chili peppers, pimentos, potatoes (all varieties), pumpkin, radish, daikon radish, rutabaga, sauerkraut, sea vegetables (arame, dulse, kelp, nori, wakame), shallots, spinach, sprouts (alfalfa, clover, mung bean, radish, sunflower, wheat), squash (acorn, banana, butternut, yellow [summer], spaghetti), sweet potatoes, tomatoes (canned, hot-house, vine-ripened), turnips, watercress, yams
VEGETABLE JUICES	Celery, carrot, carrot/celery, parsley, spinach, tomato, V-8®
FRUITS	Raw apples (all varieties), apricots, blackberries, blueberries, boysenberries, cranberries, gooseberries, strawberries, kiwi, kumquats, lemons, limes, loquats, mangos, melons (cantaloupe, casaba, crenshaw, honeydew, watermelon), nectarines, oranges, papayas, peaches, pears, persimmons, pineapples, plums (black, purple), pomegranates, rhubarb, tangelos, tangerines, dates, figs (fresh, dried), prunes, raisins
FRUIT JUICES	Apple, apple cider, apricot, black cherry, red cherry, cranapple, cranberry, grapefruit, guava, lemon, orange, papaya, pear, pineapple, pineapple/coconut, prune, tangerine, watermelon
VEGETABLE OILS	All-blend, almond, avocado, canola, coconut, corn, olive, peanut, flaxseed, safflower, sesame, soy, sunflower
SWEETENERS	Molasses, sorghum, brown sugar, date sugar, raw sugar, refined cane sugar, brown rice syrup, barley malt syrup, corn syrup, fructose, succonant, maple syrup
CONDIMENTS	Horseradish, pesto sauce, tahini, vinegar, Vege-Sal®, sea salt
SALAD DRESSINGS	Blue cheese, French, ranch, creamy Italian, creamy avocado, thousand island, vinegar and oil, lemon juice and oil
DESSERTS	Custards, tapioca, puddings, pies, cakes, raspberry or orange sherbet
CHIPS	Bean, corn (blue, white, yellow), potato
BEVERAGES	Coffee; herbal tea, black tea, green tea, Japanese tea, Chinese oolong tea; mineral water, sparkling water; wine (red, white), sake, beer, barley malt liquor, sherry, liqueurs, champagne, gin, Scotch, vodka, whiskey; root beer, regular sodas, diet sodas

Brain

RARELY FOODS	No more than once a month
DENSE PROTEIN	Chemical-fed chicken, turkey; beef
DAIRY	Buttermilk, most ice creams, frozen yogurt (alone)
GRAINS	Polished rice
FRUITS	Cherries
SWEETENERS	Honey, saccharin, aspertame, Equal®, NutraSweet®, Sweet'n Low®
CONDIMENTS	Barbecue sauce, catsup, mustard, salsa, mayonnaise, margarine, salt
DESSERTS	Chocolate, desserts containing chocolate

SENSITIVE FOOD LIST

FREQUENTLY FOODS	3-7 meals per week – refers to each food, rather than category.
DENSE PROTEIN	Chemical-free turkey
LEGUMES	Beans (adzuki, butter [lima], garbanzo, pinto, red, soy) lentils, hummus, tofu
GRAINS	Brown or white basmati rice, popcorn
VEGETABLES	Brussels sprouts, carrots, celery, parsley, zucchini
FRUITS	Bananas, raspberries, guavas, grapes (black, green, red), red plums
FRUIT JUICES	Grape (purple, red, white)
CONDIMENTS	Soy sauce
MODERATELY FOODS	1-2 meals per week – refers to each food, rather than category.
DENSE PROTEIN	Beef broth, beef liver, buffalo, veal, venison, organ meats (heart, brain); chemical-free chicken, chicken broth, chicken livers, cornish game hen, duck; anchovy, sea bass, bonita, catfish, cod, flounder, haddock, halibut, herring, mackerel, mahi-mahi, perch, orange roughy, salmon, sardines, shark, red snapper, sole, swordfish, trout, tuna (fresh or canned); abalone, calamari (squid), clams, crab, eel, lobster, mussels, octopus, oysters, scallops, shrimp; eggs
DAIRY	2% milk, nonfat milk, half & half, sweet cream, sour cream, butter, kefir; regular, low fat, or nonfat yogurt (plain or flavored), frozen yogurt with nuts
CHEESE	American, blue, brie, Camembert, Cheddar, cottage, cream, Edam, feta, goat, Gouda, kefir, Limburger, Muenster, Parmesan, ricotta, Romano, Swiss
NUTS and SEEDS	Almonds (raw, roasted), almond butter, Brazils, cashews (raw, roasted), cashew butter, water chestnuts, coconuts, filberts, hazelnuts, macadamias (raw, roasted), macadamia butter, peanuts (raw, roasted), peanut butter, pecans pine nuts (raw, roasted), pistachios, walnuts (black, English), raw or roasted seeds (caraway, pumpkin, sesame, sunflower), sesame seed butter, sunflower seed butter

Brain

LEGUMES	Beans (black, kidney, great northern), black-eyed peas, split peas, soy milk, miso
GRAINS	Amaranth, barley, buckwheat, corn, corn grits, corn bread, corn tortillas, hominy grits, millet, oats, quinoa, rice (long or short grain brown, wild, Japanese), rice bran, rice cakes, rye, triticale, refined wheat flour, flour tortillas, whole wheat, wheat bran, wheat germ, breads (French, garlic, Italian, sourdough, 7-grain, multigrain, oat, corn, corn/rye, rye, rice, sprouted grain, whole wheat, white), croissants, bagels, English muffins, crackers (rye, saltines, wheat, oat), pasta, couscous, udon noodles, Chinese rice noodles, whole wheat noodles, cream of rice, cream of rye, cream of wheat
VEGETABLES	Artichokes, arugula, avocados, bamboo shoots, green beans, lima beans, yellow wax beans, beets, bok choy, broccoli, broccoflower, cabbage (green, napa, red), cauliflower, chard, cilantro, corn, cucumbers, eggplant, garlic, greens (beet, collard, mustard, turnip), hominy, jicama, kale, kohlrabi, leeks, lettuce (Boston, butter, endive, iceberg, red leaf, romaine), mushrooms, okra, olives (green, ripe), onions (chives, green, brown, red, white, yellow, vidalia), parsnips, peas, snow pea pods, bell peppers (green, red, yellow), chili peppers, pimentos, potatoes (white rose, yukon gold, purple), pumpkin, radish, daikon radish, rutabaga, sauerkraut, sea vegetables (arame, dulse, kelp, nori, wakame), shallots, spinach, sprouts (alfalfa, clover, mung bean, radish, sunflower, wheat), squash (acorn, banana, butternut, yellow [summer], spaghetti), sweet potatoes, cooked tomatoes (canned, hot-house, vine-ripened), turnips, watercress, yams
VEGETABLE JUICES	Celery, carrot, carrot/celery, parsley, spinach, tomato, V-8®
FRUITS	Cooked apples (all varieties), apricots, blackberries, blueberries, boysenberries, cranberries, gooseberries, strawberries, grapefruits (white, red), kiwi, kumquats, lemons, limes, loquats, mangos, melons (cantaloupe, casaba, crenshaw, honeydew, watermelon), nectarines, oranges, papayas, peaches, pears, persimmons, plums (black, purple), pomegranates, rhubarb, tangelos, tangerines, dates, figs (fresh, dried), prunes, raisins
FRUIT JUICES	Apple, apple cider, apple/apricot, apricot, black cherry, red cherry, cranapple, grapefruit, guava, lemon, orange, papaya, pear, pineapple/coconut, pineapple, prune, tangerine, watermelon
VEGETABLE OILS	All-blend, avocado, coconut
SWEETENERS	Brown rice syrup, barley malt syrup, Re-Vita®, stevia
CONDIMENTS	Sesame tahini, vinegar, Vege-Sal®, sea salt
SALAD DRESSINGS	Vinegar and oil, lemon juice and oil
BEVERAGES	Herbal tea, mint tea, green tea, Japanese tea, Chinese oolong tea; mineral water, sparkling water

Brain

RARELY FOODS	No more than once a month
DENSE PROTEIN	Beef, lamb, pork, bacon, ham, sausage; chemical-fed chicken, turkey
DAIRY	Whole milk, raw milk, goat milk, buttermilk, ice cream, frozen yogurt (alone)
CHEESE	Colby, mozzarella, Jack
GRAINS	Polished rice
VEGETABLES	Raw tomatoes, asparagus, red or russet potatoes
FRUITS	Cherries, raw apples (all varieties), pineapples
FRUIT JUICES	Cranberry
SWEETENERS	Honey, molasses, sorghum, corn syrup, maple syrup, brown sugar, date sugar, raw sugar, refined cane sugar, fructose, saccharin, succonant, aspertame, Equal®, NutraSweet®, Sweet'n Low®
VEGETABLE OILS	Almond, canola, corn, olive, peanut, flaxseed, safflower, sesame, soy, sunflower
CONDIMENTS	Barbecue sauce, catsup, mustard, salsa, mayonnaise, horseradish, pesto sauce, margarine, salt
SALAD DRESSINGS	Blue cheese, French, ranch, creamy Italian, creamy avocado, thousand island
DESSERTS	Chocolate, desserts containing chocolate, custards, tapioca, puddings, pies, cakes, raspberry or orange sherbet
CHIPS	Bean, corn, blue corn, potato
BEVERAGES	Coffee; black tea; wine (red, white) sake, sherry, liqueurs, champagne, beer, barley malt liquor, gin, Scotch, vodka, whiskey; root beer, diet sodas, regular sodas
OTHER	Fried foods

Brain

MENUS

DIETARY EMPHASIS:

- Protein such as eggs 2 times a week, and daily fruits and vegetables for vitamin C.
- Parsley assists kidneys.
- Use soy sauce in place of salt.
- Make lunch largest meal, be particularly careful about not having large meals for breakfast or dinner to avoid the stuffed feeling.
- Smaller meals are best. May include snacks.
- Salads are ideal.

WEIGHT LOSS:

- Reduce food quantity.
- Limit fat consumption to 20% of total calories.
- Protein and carbohydrates should not be combined, such as bread with protein.
- Best times for meals are 10 a.m. for breakfast, 2 p.m. for lunch, and 6-7 p.m. for dinner.

WEIGHT GAIN:

- Increase food quantity.

VEGETARIAN DIET:

- Recommended when healthy, or may include up to 15% of calories from dense protein.

SENSITIVE:

- May include vegetables or yogurt for breakfast.
- Include dense protein, nuts, seeds, and/or dairy for lunch, but not dinner.

FATS:

- 20% for weight loss, 25% for maintenance.
- Best sources are pistachios, pecans, sunflower seeds, olive oil, dairy (including yogurt and cottage cheese), eggs, chicken and turkey.

KEY

—all menus may be used by healthy persons

( ) around foods means that they're optional

L denotes weight loss menus

S denotes sensitive menus

G denotes weight gain menus

BREAKFAST:
10 a.m. Moderate, with grain and fruit — not fruit alone. Protein after 11 a.m.

SENSITIVE: Moderate, with grain and fruit, vegetables, or yogurt and fruit.

L	S	G	Menu
L	S	G	Oatmeal and raspberries
L	S	G	Oatmeal and bananas
L		G	Oatmeal and raw apple
L	S	G	Oatmeal and applesauce or apple juice
		G	Oatmeal, apple, and pecans
	S	G	Oatmeal w/butter, and fruit
L	S	G	Oatmeal and Re-Vita®
L	S		Re-Vita® oatmeal treat: Re-Vita®, oats, butter, and oat flour
L	S	G	Cream of wheat and cooked apples
		G	Shredded wheat and rice milk (raisins and/or banana)
		G	Baked shredded wheat w/maple syrup and butter
			Cheerios® and juice – apple or tangerine
			Low fat granola w/nonfat yogurt
L			Basmati white or brown rice (butter) w/tangerine or tangerine juice
L			Basmati rice w/apple or pear, or apple or pear juice
	S		Basmati rice or potatoes (soy sauce)
L	S	G	Corn grits and bananas or raspberries
	S	G	Corn grits and ReVita® (butter)
		G	Corn bread and fruit juice – apricot or apple/apricot
	S	G	Pancakes w/maple syrup
L	S	G	Waffles w/strawberries
	S	G	Toasted English muffin w/strawberry jelly
L		G	Sprouted grain bread and fruit
		G	Bagel and jam or banana
	S	G	Plain yogurt w/Re-Vita® and strawberries, blueberries, orange, apple, or prunes

Brain

L	S	G	Food
	S		Baked white rose or yukon gold potato w/butter
	S		Spaghetti squash w/butter

SNACK:
(Optional): 12 p.m. Fruit, vegetables.

L	S	G	Food
	S		Carrots
	S		Celery
	S		Bell peppers
	S		Vegetable juice
L			Protein bar
L		G	Spiru-tein® Bar

LUNCH:
2 p.m. Moderate, with protein, nuts, seeds, dairy, legumes, grain, and/or vegetables.

L	S	G	Food
	S	G	Chemical-free turkey and avocado (pasta or corn tortilla)
	S	G	Chemical-free turkey, rice, and broccoli
	S	G	Chemical-free turkey, pasta, and zucchini or lettuce salad
	S	G	Chemical-free turkey, potato, and beets or spinach
		G	Chemical-free chicken, pinto beans, rice, and avocado
L			Tuna, cheese, and red leaf lettuce w/Hain™ Creamy Italian dressing
L			Tuna and avocado
L	S		Fish and steamed carrots, onions, and lima beans
L	S		Fish, and spinach salad: raw spinach, parsley, tofu, alfalfa, sunflower or wheat sprouts, raw carrots, broccoli, and kelp powder (ginger root)
		G	Cheese and spinach tortolini (cauliflower and broccoli)
		G	Cheddar cheese and corn or flour tortilla or rye Triscuits® (spinach salad: spinach, [radishes], and olive oil and vinegar dressing)
L	S	G	Brussels sprouts, tofu, and rice
L		G	Soybeans, broccoli, and cauliflower (plain yogurt)
L		G	Adzuki beans and corn or flour tortilla (avocado)
L	S	G	Chicken vegetable soup: chicken, chicken broth, chard, carrots, celery, zucchini, and corn
L	S		Chicken broth soup and raw vegetables: carrots, chard, radishes, broccoli, beets, and parsley
	S	G	Beans and rice w/avocado
L			Beans and rice
	S	G	Corn grits, eggs, and broccoli
L	S	G	Corn grits, tofu, and carrots
	S	G	Steamed brussels sprouts and celery w/almond butter
L	S		Steamed carrots, onions, and lima beans
L			Salad w/lowfat dressing
L	S	G	Soybeans and plain yogurt
L	S		Spinach salad: raw spinach, parsley, tofu, and sprouts – wheat, alfalfa or sunflower – raw carrots, broccoli, and kelp powder (ginger root)
L	S	G	Re-Vita® w/yogurt
L	S	G	Protein drink
L	S	G	Plain kefir w/almonds (Re-Vita®)

MID-AFTERNOON SNACK:
(Optional) Grain, nuts, seeds, dairy, fruit, vegetables.

L	S	G	Food
		G	Bagels w/cream cheese and fruit juice
		G	English muffin w/butter, goat cheese, and fruit juice or fruit jam
		G	Rice cakes and nut butter or cheddar cheese
		G	Tahini and cashew butter w/celery
L		G	Re-Vita® oatmeal treat: Re-Vita®, oatmeal, oat flour, and butter
	S	G	Re-Vita® and kefir or yogurt
L		G	Yogurt (butternut or berry Re-Vita®)
		G	Frozen yogurt w/nuts
		G	Kefir
L			Fruit: apples, grapes, raspberries, guavas, or red plums
		G	Apple and nut butter or cheese
			Tangerine juice

Brain

L	Smoothie
L	Vegetable juice

LUNCH or DINNER:

G	Chemical-free turkey, pasta, peas, and cranberry sauce
G	Chemical-free turkey, basmati white or brown rice, and peas
G	Chemical-free turkey, cornbread dressing, and cranberry sauce (pumpkin pie)
L G	Chemical-free turkey, broccoli, cauliflower, zucchini, and carrots
G	Turkey loaf, corn, mashed or baked potato, and vegetable juice
G	Chemical-free chicken, potato salad, and celery sticks
G	Chemical-free chicken and rice w/teriyaki sauce
G	Fish, rice, and corn on the cob
G	Tuna, rice, fajita mix, and salad: lettuce, carrots, bell pepper, Italian dressing
L	Lentils, rice, and yams (green beans, or zuccchini, or carrots, or brussels sprouts, or salad)
S	Millet and chicken broth
G	Cornish game hen, potato or rice, and green beans
G	Duck, yams, peas, zucchini, and broccoli
G	Chemical-free chicken, rice, and vegetable juice – carrot, or carrot/celery/spinach/beet/ginger/garlic
G	Chemical-free chicken, spanish rice, pinto beans, and vegetable juice
L G	Thai chicken and vegetables
L	Spaghetti w/tomato sauce, zucchini, mushrooms, onions and garlic, and vegetable juice
L S	Rice, and raw corn on the cob
S G	Rice, soaked raw garbanzo beans, tofu, and parsley
S G	Rice and eggs
L S	Tofu, lettuce, cucumber, and carrots
L S	Tofu and spinach
L S G	Tofu, manicotti or lasagna, and zucchini
L S G	Tofu loaf, raw carrots, and celery
G	Hot and sour soup, and stir-fry vegetables w/tofu, soy sauce, and rice
S G	Vegetarian chili and corn bread
L	Vegetarian chili
L S	Hummus and celery
L S	Steamed vegetables
S	Re-Vita® and kefir or yogurt

DINNER:
6-7 p.m. Moderate, with protein, nuts, seeds, dairy, legumes, grain, vegetables, and/or fruit.

SENSITIVE: Moderate with grain, legumes, vegetables, and/or fruit

L S G	Beans, rice, and avocado
L G	Beans and corn bread
L G	Lentils w/steamed broccoli, cauliflower, and carrots
G	Chemical-free chicken and pasta
G	Chemical-free chicken, potato, and peas
G	Chicken tamales and beans
G	Chemical-free chicken, basmati rice, and carrots
G	Cornish game hen, wild rice, and lettuce salad
G	Duck and white basmati rice
G	Venison, red potatoes, parsley, and butter
G	Tuna and spinach pasta
L	Tuna and salad
G	Burrito: flour tortilla, refried black beans, lettuce, Jack cheese, and sour cream
L	Brown basmati rice and adzuki beans
G	Corn grits and eggs
L	Rice, summer squash, and peas
G	Macaroni and cheese, and peas
L S G	Beans, rice, and brussels sprouts
L S G	Pinto beans, rice, and carrots

Brain

L S G Soybeans, rice, and cucumber or carrots

L S Baked butternut squash w/butternut Re-Vita®, and rice

L S Steamed carrots, onions, and lima beans

L S Brussels sprouts, tofu, and rice

L S G Adzuki beans and corn or flour tortilla

MID-AFTERNOON or EVENING SNACK:
(Optional) Dairy, nuts, seeds, grain, vegetables, fruit, sweets.

L G Plain kefir w/almonds and/or Re-Vita®

L G Yogurt w/butternut or berry Re-Vita®

G Cookies w/nuts

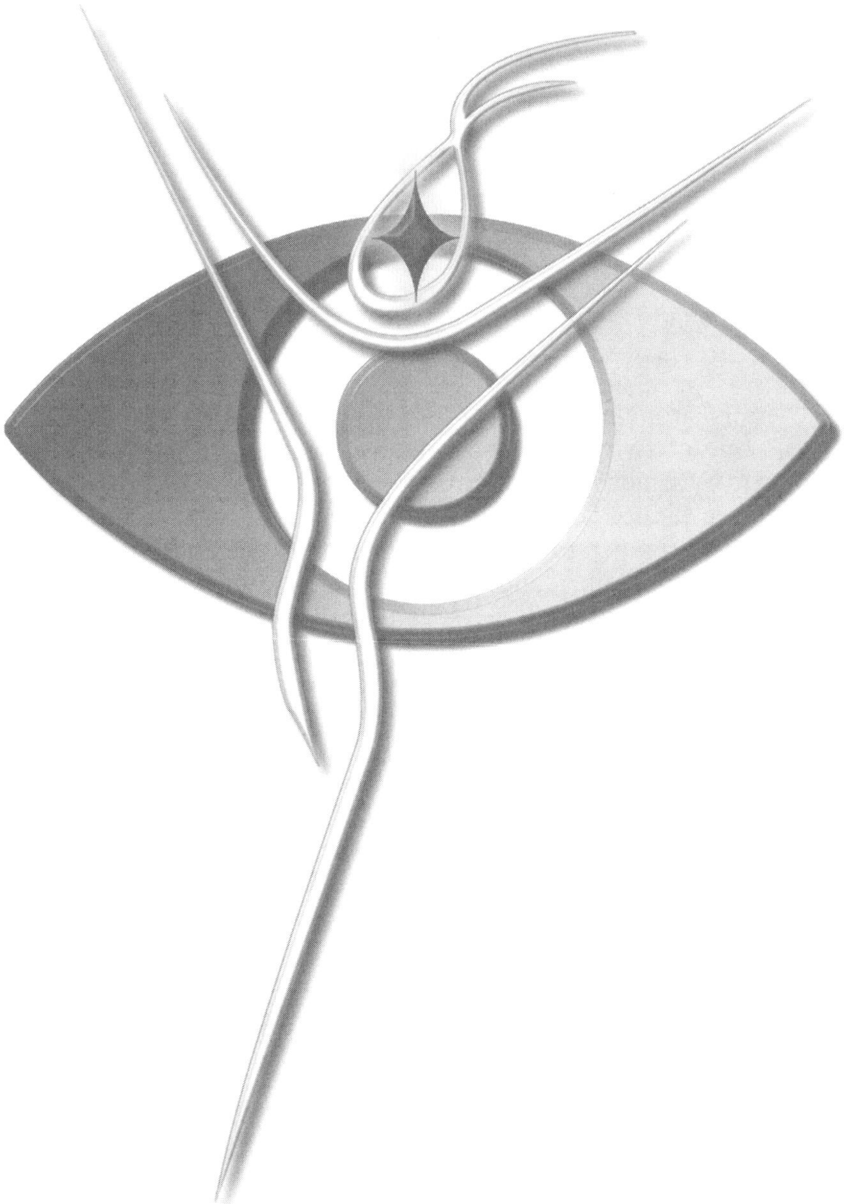

The "Eye Body Type" is symbolized by an eye. Just as our eyes link us to our outer world, Eye body types link the world by implementing their visions. Witty and creative, they have the ability to see the good in even the bleakest of situations.

EYE

Eye

BODY TYPE PROFILE

LOCATION

In bony orbits of the face.

FUNCTION

Organ of vision (sight).

POTENTIAL HEALTH PROBLEMS

Generally strong body with good stamina and endurance. Basic health tends to be one of two extremes–either very sound or with multiple problems. Prone to hyperactivity or excessive nervous energy when not eating adequate protein, respiratory weakness, asthma, chronic sinus congestion, arthritis, or gout. Body temperature often colder than average, often due to low thyroid. Problems with gums and teeth, like sensitivities and excessive cavities. Vascular weakness, such as severe headaches or blood pressure problems. Ear problems, like earaches or infections as children; ringing, pressure. Tend to internalize emotional stress, so predisposed to cancer.

RECOMMENDED EXERCISE

Exercise is essential, as it activates the immune system. A minimum of 1 hour every other day is required to provide continuous activation. Exercise benefits all levels, and in particular, helps activate the nervous system to organize information resulting in mental clarity. It aids digestion, and is an effective way of reducing stress. When stress is particularly high, may need physical activity 4-6 times a week and include activities such as 10 minutes of stomping and karate kicking to discharge anger held in lower body. Other good activities are free-style dancing, callanetics, yoga, treadmill, water sports, skiing, roller blading, walking, skipping, jumping rope, and biking.

WOMEN'S CHARACTERISTICS

DISTINGUISHING FEATURES

Eyes dominant or hooded. Vision is dominant sense and can be reflected in excellent eyesight and/or the ability to see what others don't notice. Awareness may also extend to other senses. Characteristic protrusion on upper 1/3rd of outer thighs.

ADDITIONAL PHYSICAL CHARACTERISTICS

Buttocks relatively flat-to-rounded. Low back curvature straight-to-average. Breasts small-to-average. Shoulders narrower than, to relatively even with, hips. Straight to well-defined waist. Average to long-waisted. Height ranges from very petite to tall. Bone structure small-to-medium. Average, elongated musculature, or layers of softness covering muscle. Small-to-average hands, often have broad, square palms with short fingers. Average-to-long oval face, often with high forehead. Body may be at least full size smaller above waist than below.

Eye

WEIGHT GAIN AREAS	Lower body with initial gain in upper 1/3rd of outer thighs, upper inner thighs, lower abdomen, and lower buttocks. Alternative weight gain pattern: minimal gain on upper 1/3rd of outer thighs with soft layer of fat covering entire body. Secondary weight gain in face, under chin, upper arms, breasts, waist, upper and/or lower hips, and eventually entire back. Some may have difficulty gaining or maintaining weight.

DIETARY GUIDELINES

SCHEDULING MEALS

Breakfast, lunch, and dinner: Light-to-heavy with protein, nuts, seeds, dairy, grain, legumes, vegetables, and/or fruit. Have extreme flexibility. Rotation and variety important. For weight loss or sensitive individuals, most foods should be limited to no more than twice a week. Breakfast for sensitive persons should be heavy.

DIETARY EMPHASIS

- Shellfish and foods high in vitamin A, including carrots, kelp, sweet potatoes, spinach, and yams. At least 10% of caloric intake from dense protein should be consumed daily. Fish or meat and vegetables, chicken or meat and rice.
- Variety and rotation essential. Frequently foods may be used in multiple combinations, limiting the same dish to 2 times a week.
- Vegetables best steamed or stir-fried in sesame oil, or alternately in all-blend, almond, avocado, flaxseed, soy, or sunflower oils.
- For weight loss, consume 25-35% of caloric intake from dense protein daily. Avoid caffeine, limit sugar including fruit, fruit juices, fructose, and refined carbohydrates, to 2 times a week. Avoid breads. Often helpful to use weight loss menus for five consecutive days, then regular menus for two days.
- For weight gain, consume minimum of 30% of calories from dense protein and increase food quantities. Resolve deep-seated emotional stress.
- Drink 3/4 gallon of water per day; if you wish, drink water before or after, but not with, meals.
- Vegetarian diet inadequate. 10-40% (3-10 oz. per day) of diet should be dense protein.
- Fats, 20-30% of calories should be derived from dense protein, butter, olive oil: for 30-35% fats, add nuts and seed.

KEY SUPPORTS FOR SYSTEM

Variety and rotation essential – eating same food no more than 2 times a week. Adequate exercise, particularly that undertaken individually, as Eyes need alone-time physical activity.

Eye

COMPLEMENTARY GLANDULAR SUPPORT	Thyroid, through consuming at least 2 oz. of dense protein (fish, eggs, chicken, or turkey) with a grain, such as rice or pasta, 5 times a week. Gallbladder, through consuming adequate fats.
FOODS CRAVED	*(When Energy is Low)* Sweets and carbohydrates, fats (e.g., ice cream and creamy sauces), or any food including spicy or salty foods, and such proteins as meats, shellfish, nuts, and cheese
FOODS TO AVOID	Black walnuts, broiled shrimp, roasted garlic, and charbroiled foods, charred toast. If sensitive, whole wheat, sugar – refined or fruit – no more than 2 times a week, caffeine (as it's a stimulant).
RECOMMENDED CUISINE	Seafood, Chinese, Japanese, Thai, standard American fare; Mexican, Italian, Greek, Indian (curry), home-style cooking, and highly seasoned, spicy foods. Fish or meat and vegetables, chicken or meat and rice.

PSYCHOLOGICAL PROFILE

ESSENCE

Just as our eyes link us to our outer world and environment, and provide a window to our soul, Eye body types link the world with themselves by connecting the inner and outer worlds through implementing visions. The world of the human body is connected and activated by the eyes, as they are responsible for integrating the body's intelligence throughout all the cells. It's our hands that reach out into the outside world and provide the main physical link to the environment. Use of the hands is connected with the eyes, as there is a direct link between the brain and the motor reflexes in the hands. Eye body types are typically known for implementing a vision. They visualize what they want to manifest and then set out to make it happen.

CHARACTERISTIC TRAITS

Since the main function of the eyes is to see, Eye body types are distinguished by their acute vision, both inner and outer. They'll access their inner vision through daydreaming or visualization, while externally, Eyes tend to see things that others don't notice. Besides discerning visual details, they pick up on subtle differences in voice, body language, and even intuitive information. Often visionaries, they have a unique ability to see the big picture and the myriad of options available on a project they are involved in, or anything else that catches their eye.

While the basic nature of Eyes tends to be quiet, gentle, and controlled; underneath there's a witty, rebellious side just waiting to surface. Eyes have their own particular sense of humor that is often described as being dry and a bit on the "far side", with the ability to see the good in even the bleakest of situations.

Eye

CHARACTERISTIC TRAITS

Eye types are intuitive, yet practical. Their ability to "see" is closely linked to heir being able to bring their visions into practical reality. They are exceptionally adept with their hands and will often find that their creativity comes through doing or implementing what they see needs to be done. Known for making things work, Eyes are also proficient in the realms of analysis and the abstract. The common thread of expertise between the practical and the theoretical is an eye for details, and the ability to see how they connect to create a whole system. Eyes are both conscientious about the components and able to perceive the big picture.

MOTIVATION

Eyes need personal experiences to integrate what they see into the physical world around them. Because they see the larger picture, and are constantly looking for ways to make life better, they need to see how much of their vision can be implemented. This leads them to wanting to do things differently, or their way, as this is what enables them to implement or express their vision. It's their rebellious side that stimulates growth and motivates them to move out of their previous restrictions. Refusing to follow directions is a form of quiet rebellion that leads them into discovering new ways of doing things. This initiates creative expression and raises the question, "Is there a better way?"

Being self-motivated and determined, Eyes often channel their creative energy through work. Applying themselves to a task for many hours at a time is quite normal for Eyes, and they can show great perseverance in completing endeavors that are elaborate or complex. True to type, Eyes will see that their projects are completed when they look right. While they derive satisfaction from visually seeing the fruits of their labor, in order to feel validated, they need occasional reassurance. Seeing all the little imperfections, the outside pat on the back helps them to focus on what is right and what has already been accomplished.

As a particularly sensitive type, Eyes often have problems dealing with elements of harshness in the world. In particular, issues of personal insecurity can cause difficulties in their relating to other people. Not knowing how to effectively deal with their negative emotions or feelings of vulnerability, Eyes will internalize their emotions. This internalization then in turn leads to physical problems, illness, or the emotional stress of feelings of emptiness and frustration due to the inability to deeply connect and establish true intimacy.

"AT WORST"

Stumped or overly stressed, generally from physical ailments, fatigue, or blocked emotions, Eyes go into overwhelm. This is when they'll sit on a stump in a daze, and wait to be rescued. Mentally exhausted, they are unable to see a way out of their dilemma. The problem looks too big, so working toward a solution is hopeless and they'll go into a depression. Then they'll wait to be taken by the hand and led through step-by-step, expecting constant approval and reassurance along the way.

Eye

"AT WORST"
(Continued)

Seeing multiple options, but unable to recognize the reality of what lies ahead, they get stuck in indecisiveness. Lacking confidence in their ability to pick the best course or to carry it out, Eyes are reluctant to make a commitment to any single alternative. They may even hold themselves back for the lack of courage of their convictions or become complacent, seeing what needs to be changed, but feeling the situation is hopeless. As a result, Eyes often postpone taking action or making a decision for as long as possible, waiting to be pushed into it by something or someone else.

When unable to express what they see, their visual energy can turn inward, causing them to be short-sighted or stuck in limited viewpoints, seeing only their side of things rather than the whole picture. Their tendency is to withdraw. Since this pattern is present during childhood, it can manifest physically in their requiring glasses early on when they've closed down their sight to minimize seeing what they don't want to see. Closing down can cause Eyes to retreat into the mental world, becoming too serious, rigid, and skeptical. If they get stuck in worry, they can manifest their fears. They may escape into work with an over-emphasis on production as a means of gaining personal recognition, making them even more emotionally unavailable in their relationships.

"AT BEST "

Not only are Eyes able to see the big picture and all the available options, they are able to effectively reach their goals. Being able to sort through a profusion of details and figure out a variety of problems, their ability to see more than one option for solving a problem enables them to make decisions quickly and act upon them. Eyes are resourceful, flexible, and adaptable. Meticulous, persevering, logical, and strong in common sense, Eyes are not afraid of hard work and are willing to do whatever it takes to accomplish what they set out to do.

Inner directed, Eyes work well independently and often prefer to do so. Being intuitive as well as practical and efficient, they are able to see what needs changing, make the changes, and bring the project into manifestation. With their heightened capacity for intuition and discernment, they tend to be quite efficient, and are able to get to the heart of the matter. Eyes are manually adept and are usually able to figure out how to repair, fix, or build almost anything.

Sensitive and compassionate, Eyes are fair-minded, giving, and responsive to others. They're gifted in their ability to speak, to empower, and to manifest. When they trust in their intuitive guidance, they can be comfortable out in the public eye, going where they need to go, and doing what they are guided to do. The emotional fire to manifest their desires comes through their passion about what they believe in. For Eyes, there is nothing more exhilarating than making a difference in the world, and particularly in the lives of everyone they encounter.

Eye

FOOD LISTS

HEALTHY FOOD LIST

FREQUENTLY FOODS	3-7 meals per week – refers to each food, rather than category.
DENSE PROTEIN	Beef, beef liver, beef broth, buffalo, lamb; chicken, chicken livers, chicken broth), cornish game hen, turkey; anchovy, cod, flounder, haddock, herring, mackerel, mahi-mahi, orange roughy, perch, smoked salmon, sardines, red snapper, sea bass, shark, swordfish, trout; calamari (squid), eel, clams, lobster, mussels, octopus, oysters, scallops; eggs
DAIRY	Butter
CHEESE	American, brie, Cheddar, Colby, cream, feta, Jack, mozzarella, Muenster, Parmesan, ricotta, Romano, Swiss
NUTS and SEEDS	Cashews (raw, roasted), cashew butter, filberts, macadamias (raw, roasted), macadamia butter, pine nuts (raw, roasted), pistachios, water chestnuts, sesame seeds (raw, roasted), sesame seed butter
GRAINS	Amaranth, buckwheat, rice (brown or white basmati, long or short grain brown, wild, Japanese), rice bran, rice cakes, refined wheat flour, white bread, yeastless wild rice spelt bread, Kavli® Crispbread, croissants, cream of rice, cream of rye
VEGETABLES	Artichoke, avocados, bamboo shoots, green beans, yellow wax beans, beets, bok choy, brussels sprouts, carrots, chard, corn, greens (beet, collard, mustard, turnip), eggplant, jicama, kale, kohlrabi, leeks, mushrooms, okra, olives (green, ripe), onions (chives, green, red, white, vidalia), parsley, peas, snow pea pods, pumpkin, rutabaga, scallions, seaweed (arame, dulse, kelp, nori, wakame), spinach, sprouts (alfalfa, clover, mung bean, radish, sunflower), acorn squash, sweet potatoes, watercress, yams
FRUITS	Apples (Red or Golden Delicious, Granny Smith, Jonathan), gooseberries, strawberries, grapes (black, green, red), guavas, kiwi, limes, mangos, nectarines, papayas, pears, pineapples, pomegranates, tangerines, tangelos, prunes
FRUIT JUICES	Black cherry, grapefruit, papaya
VEGETABLE OILS	Flaxseed, sesame
SWEETENERS	Honey, maple syrup, Re-Vita®, stevia
CONDIMENTS	Pickled ginger, sweet pickles, hot mustard, barbecue sauce, Bragg™ aminos
BEVERAGES	Coffee with Re-Vita®; Japanese tea; barley malt liquor; ginger ale, root beer

Eye

MODERATELY FOODS	1-2 meals per week – refers to each food, rather than category.
DENSE PROTEIN	Pork, ham, bacon, sausage, veal, venison, organ meats (heart, brain); duck; bonita, catfish, halibut, sole, tuna; abalone, crab, shrimp
DAIRY	Milk (whole, 2%, nonfat, raw, goat), buttermilk, sweet cream, sour cream, half & half, kefir; regular, low fat, or nonfat yogurt (plain or flavored), frozen yogurt, ice cream (Ben & Jerry's®, Dreyer's, Swensen's®)
CHEESE	Blue, Camembert, cottage, Edam, goat, Gouda, kefir, Limburger
NUTS and SEEDS	Almonds (raw, roasted), almond butter, Brazils, coconuts, hazelnuts, peanuts (raw, roasted), peanut butter, pecans, English walnuts, raw or roasted seeds (caraway, pumpkin, sunflower), sunflower seed butter
LEGUMES	Beans (adzuki, black, garbanzo, lima [butter], navy, kidney, great northern, pinto, red, soy), black-eyed peas, lentils, split peas, soy milk, tofu, hummus, miso
FRUITS	Fuju persimmons
GRAINS	Barley, corn, corn bread, corn grits, corn tortillas, hominy grits, millet, oats, popcorn, quinoa, rye, triticale, whole wheat, wheat bran, wheat germ, flour tortillas, breads (corn, rye, corn/rye, sprouted grain, 7-grain, multi-grain, French, garlic, Italian, oat, rice, sourdough, whole wheat), English muffins, bagels, crackers (wheat, saltines, oat, rye), pasta, couscous, udon noodles, Chinese rice noodles, cream of wheat
VEGETABLES	Arugula, asparagus, lima beans, broccoli, broccoflower, cabbage (green, napa, red), cauliflower, celery, cilantro, cucumber, garlic, lettuce (Boston, butter, endive, iceberg, red leaf, romaine), onions (brown, white, yellow), parsnips, bell peppers (green, red, yellow), chili peppers, pimentos, potatoes (red, russet, white rose, yukon gold, purple), radish, daikon radish, sauerkraut, shallots, squash (banana, butternut, spaghetti, yellow [summer], zucchini), tomatoes (canned, hot-house, vine-ripened), turnips
VEGETABLE JUICES	Carrot, carrot/celery, celery, parsley, spinach, tomato, V-8®
FRUITS	Apples (McIntosh, Pippin, Rome Beauty), apricots, bananas, blackberries, blueberries, boysenberries, cranberries, raspberries, cherries, grapefruits (red, white), kumquats, lemons, loquats, oranges, Fuju persimmons, melons (cantaloupe, casaba, crenshaw, honeydew, watermelon), peaches, plums (black, purple, red), rhubarb, dates, figs (fresh, dried), raisins
FRUIT JUICES	Apple, apple cider, apple/apricot, apricot, red cherry, cranapple, cranberry, grape (purple, red, white), guava, lemon, orange, pear, pineapple, pineapple/coconut, prune, tangerine
VEGETABLE OILS	All-blend, almond, avocado, canola, coconut, corn, olive, peanut, safflower, soy, sunflower
SWEETENERS	Brown sugar, date sugar, raw sugar, refined cane sugar, molasses, sorghum, barley malt syrup, corn syrup, brown rice syrup, fructose, succonant, saccharin

Eye

	barley malt syrup, corn syrup, brown rice syrup, fructose, succonant, saccharin
CONDIMENTS	Catsup, mayonnaise, mustard, horseradish, soy sauce, fish sauce, oyster sauce, pesto sauce, salsa, tahini, dill or sweet pickles, vinegar, salt, sea salt, Vege-Sal®
SALAD DRESSINGS	Blue cheese, creamy Italian, French, ranch, creamy avocado, thousand island, vinegar and oil, lemon juice and oil
DESSERTS	Custards, tapioca, puddings, pies, cakes, chocolate, desserts containing chocolate, raspberry sherbet, orange sherbet
CHIPS	Bean, corn (blue, white, yellow), potato
BEVERAGES	Coffee; herbal tea, mint tea, black tea, green tea, Chinese oolong tea; mineral water, sparkling water; wine (red, white), sake, liqueurs, champagne, gin, Scotch, vodka, whiskey, beer; regular sodas

RARELY FOODS	No more than once a month
DAIRY	Most ice creams
NUTS	Black walnuts
VEGETABLES	Roasted garlic
SWEETENERS	Aspertame, Equal®, Sweet'n Low®, NutraSweet®
CONDIMENTS	Margarine
BEVERAGES	Pepsi®, diet sodas
OTHER	Broiled and char-broiled foods/fish, e.g., broiled shrimp, charred toast

SENSITIVE FOOD LIST

FREQUENTLY FOODS	3-7 meals per week – refers to each food, rather than category.
DENSE PROTEIN	Mahi-mahi, shark, swordfish; clams, lobster, mussels, octopus, oysters, scallops, shrimp
CHEESE	Brie, feta, Parmesan, Romano
VEGETABLES	Beets, carrots, chard, jicama, kale, kelp, onions (chives, green, red), sweet potatoes, scallions, spinach, yams
VEGETABLE OIL	Sesame
BEVERAGES	Coffee with Re-Vita®; Japanese tea

Eye

MODERATELY FOODS	1-2 meals per week – refers to each food, rather than category.
DENSE PROTEIN	Beef, beef liver, beef broth, buffalo, lamb, pork, ham, bacon, sausage, veal, venison, organ meats (heart, brain); turkey, chicken, chicken broth, chicken livers, cornish game hen, duck; anchovy, bonita, sea bass, catfish, cod, flounder, haddock, halibut, herring, mackerel, perch, orange roughy, salmon, sardines, red snapper, sole, trout, tuna; abalone, calamari (squid), crab, eel; eggs
DAIRY	Milk (whole, 2%, nonfat, raw), half & half, sweet cream, sour cream, butter, kefir; regular, low fat, or nonfat yogurt (plain or flavored), frozen yogurt
CHEESE	American, blue, Camembert, Cheddar, Colby, cottage, cream, Edam, goat, Gouda, Jack, kefir, Limburger, mozzarella, Muenster, ricotta, Swiss
NUTS and SEEDS	Almonds (raw, roasted), almond butter, Brazils, cashews (raw, roasted), cashew butter, water chestnuts, coconuts, filberts, hazelnuts, macadamias (raw, roasted), macadamia butter, peanuts (raw, roasted), peanut butter, pecans, pine nuts (raw, roasted), pistachios, English walnuts, raw or roasted seeds (caraway, pumpkin, sesame, sunflower), sesame seed butter, sunflower seed butter
LEGUMES	Beans (adzuki, black, garbanzo, kidney, great northern, pinto, red, soy), black-eyed peas, split peas, soy milk, tofu, hummus, miso
GRAINS	Amaranth, barley, buckwheat, corn, corn bread, corn grits, corn tortillas, hominy grits, millet, quinoa, oats, popcorn, rice (brown or white basmati, long or short grain brown, wild, Japanese), rice bran, rice cakes, rye, triticale, whole wheat, wheat bran, wheat germ, refined wheat flour, flour tortillas, breads (French, garlic, Italian, rice, sourdough, 7-grain, multi-grain, oat, corn, corn/rye, rye, sprouted grain, white, whole wheat, yeastless wild rice spelt bread), croissants, Kavli® Crispbread, crackers (oat, wheat, rye, saltines), bagels, English muffins, couscous, pasta, udon noodles, Chinese rice noodles, cream of rice, cream of rye, cream of wheat
VEGETABLES	Artichoke, arugula, asparagus, avocados, bamboo shoots, green beans, lima beans, yellow wax beans, bok choy, broccoli, broccoflower, brussels sprouts, cabbage (green, napa, red), cauliflower, celery, cilantro, corn, cucumbers, greens (beet, collard, mustard, turnip), hominy, kohlrabi, leeks, lettuce (Boston, butter, endive, iceberg, red leaf, romaine), mushrooms, okra, olives (green, ripe), white onions, parsley, parsnips, peas, snow pea pods, bell peppers (green, red, yellow), chili peppers, pimentos, potatoes (red, white rose, russet, yukon gold, purple), pumpkin, radish, daikon radish, rutabaga, sauerkraut, seaweed (arame, dulse, nori, wakame), shallots, sprouts (alfalfa, clover, mung bean, sunflower, radish), turnips, squash (acorn, banana, butternut, spaghetti, yellow [summer], zucchini), watercress
VEGETABLE JUICES	Carrot, carrot/celery, celery, parsley, spinach, tomato, V-8®

Eye

FRUITS	Apples (Golden or Red Delicious, Granny Smith, Jonathan, McIntosh, Pippin, Rome Beauty), apricots, bananas, blackberries, blueberries, boysenberries, cranberries, gooseberries, raspberries, strawberries, cherries, grapes (black, green, red), guavas, kiwi, kumquats, grapefruits (red, white),lemons, limes, loquats, mangos, melons (cantaloupe, casaba, crenshaw, honeydew, watermelon), nectarines, oranges, papayas, peaches, pears, Hychia persimmons, pineapples, plums (black, purple, red), pomegranates, rhubarb, tangelos, tangerines, dates, figs (fresh, dried), prunes, raisins
FRUIT JUICES	Apple, apple cider, apple/apricot, apricot, cherry, cranapple, cranberry, grape (purple, red, white), grapefruit, guava, lemon, orange, papaya, pear, pineapple, pineapple/coconut, prune, tangerine
VEGETABLE OILS	All-blend, avocado, coconut
SWEETENERS	Brown rice syrup, barley malt syrup, Re-Vita®, stevia
CONDIMENTS	Salsa, tahini, dill or sweet pickles, vinegar, salt, sea salt, Vege-Sal®
SALAD DRESSINGS	Vinegar and oil, lemon juice and oil
BEVERAGES	Herbal tea, mint tea, green tea, Chinese oolong tea; mineral water, sparkling water
RARELY FOODS	No more than once a month
DAIRY	Buttermilk, goat milk, most ice creams
NUTS	Black walnuts
LEGUMES	Beans (lima [butter], navy), lentils
VEGETABLES	Eggplant, garlic (raw, roasted), onions (brown, vidalia, yellow), tomatoes (canned, hot house, vine-ripened)
VEGETABLE OILS	Almond, canola, corn, flaxseed, olive, peanut, safflower, soy, sunflower
FRUITS	Fuji persimmons
SWEETENERS	Honey, molasses, sorghum, brown sugar, date sugar, raw sugar, refined cane sugar, maple syrup, corn syrup, fructose, succonant, saccharin, aspertame, Equal®, Sweet'n Low®, NutraSweet®
CONDIMENTS	Margarine, mayonnaise, catsup, mustard, horseradish, soy sauce, barbecuesauce, fish sauce, oyster sauce, pesto sauce
SALAD DRESSINGS	Blue cheese, French, ranch, creamy Italian, creamy avocado, thousand island
DESSERTS	Custards, tapioca, puddings, pies, cakes, chocolate, desserts containing chocolate, raspberry sherbet, orange sherbet
CHIPS	Bean, corn (blue, white, yellow), potato
BEVERAGES	Coffee; black tea; wine (red, white), sake, champagne, beer, barley malt liquor, gin, Scotch, vodka, whiskey; Pepsi®, diet sodas, regular sodas, root beer
OTHER	Broiled and char-broiled foods (including fish and charred toast)

Eye

MENUS

DIETARY EMPHASIS:

- Shellfish and foods high in vitamin A including carrots, kelp, sweet potatoes, spinach and yams.
- At least 10% of caloric intake from dense protein daily.
- Fish or meat and vegetables; chicken or meat and rice.
- Variety and rotation essential. Frequently foods may be used in multiple combinations, limiting the same dish to 2 meals a week.
- Drink 3/4 gallon of water per day. If you wish, drink water before or after, but not with, meals.

WEIGHT LOSS and SENSITIVE:

- Consume 25-35% of caloric intake from dense protein daily.
- Avoid caffeine.
- Limit sugar (including fruit, fruit juices, fructose, and refined carbohydrates) to 2 meals per week.
- Avoid breads, especially whole wheat.
- Emphasize variety by eating most foods only one to two times per week.
- For weight loss, follow "Sensitive" meals and snacks.
- Often helpful to use weight loss menus for five consecutive days, then regular menus for two days.

WEIGHT GAIN:

- Consume minimum of 30% of calories from dense protein.
- Increase food quantities.
- Resolve deep-seated emotional stress.

VEGETARIAN DIET:

- Inadequate since require 10-40% (3-10 oz. per day) of calories from dense protein.

FATS:

- 20-30% of total calories.
- Best sources are dense protein, butter, olive oil; for 30-35% fats, add nuts and seeds.

KEY

—all menus may be used by healthy persons

( ) around foods means that they're optional

L denotes weight loss menus

S denotes sensitive menus

G denotes weight gain menus

BREAKFAST: 9-11 a.m. Light-to-heavy, with protein, nuts, seeds, dairy, grain, legumes, vegetables, and/or fruit.

SENSITIVE: 6-8 a.m. Heavy.

L	S	G	Menu
		G	Eggs, sausage, whole wheat toast, hash browns, orange juice, and coffee
		G	Cheese omelette and toast
		G	Eggs, bacon, pancakes, and hash browns
		G	Eggs, potatoes, broccoli, and toast
		G	Eggs, pinto, adzuki or black beans, and toast
L			Hamburger patty and 2 eggs (barbecue sauce)
		G	Turkey, rice w/turkey gravy, and toast
L			White or dark turkey and three bean salad
		G	Chicken and corn bread w/butter or chicken gravy
L			Chicken breast, egg, and cheese (teriyaki or barbecue sauce)
L			Canadian bacon w/melted cheese or eggs
L			Ham and white or black beans, or black-eyed peas
L			Shellfish w/another fish and stir-fry vegetables: celery, onions, squash with teriyaki sauce
		G	Biscuits and sausage gravy
	S		Multigrain cereal w/rice milk
	S		Puffed Kashi®, rice milk, and strawberries
			Corn flakes w/milk (orange juice)
L			Grape-nuts® w/milk (tomato juice)
L			Cream of wheat w/milk

Eye

			Oatmeal (juice and/or milk)
		G	Granola and apple/papaya/carrot juice
		G	Carrot muffin (butter) and grapes
		G	Pancakes and fruit: w/applesauce (cinnamon) papaya and/or pineapple, apple, coconut, banana, coconut and papaya, passion fruit, cantaloupe, or honeydew melon
	S		Sweet potato, carrots, or broccoli
	S		Baked potato, peas, eggplant, or cauliflower

LUNCH: 11:30 a.m.-2 p.m. Light-to-heavy, with protein, nuts, seeds, dairy, grain, legumes, vegetables and/or fruit.

		G	Grilled chicken, white potato, green beans, carrots, and white bread
		G	Barbecued chicken, potatoes, broccoli, and hot rolls
L			Chicken or shrimp stir-fry over rice
L			Chicken and noodles
L			Enchilada – chicken, beef or turkey
			Pasta w/chicken, olives, and tomato sauce (carrot sticks and/or sour cream dip)
		G	Hamburger steak w/barbecue sauce and potato salad
	S		Banana and peanut butter (trail mix)
	S	G	Peanut butter on toast (jam)
	S	G	Peanut butter on bran muffin
		G	Egg salad sandwich w/sweet pickle
L			Hard-boiled eggs (cauliflower and/or melted cheese)
			Tuna salad: pickle relish, mayonnaise, hard boiled egg, and onion on saltine, club or cheese crackers (grapes)
L			Tuna salad w/egg, iceberg lettuce, and sweet pickle
		G	Deviled ham sandwich w/lettuce and butter (raisins)
		G	Bacon, lettuce, and tomato sandwich
		G	Reuben sandwich: Swiss cheese, corned beef, and sauerkraut on rye w/potato salad
		G	Hamburger sandwich, pinto beans, and mozzarella cheese
		G	Gyro sandwich (grapes)
	S		Rice cake and cheese
	S		Shredded vegetables w/sunflower or sesame seeds, wrapped in flour tortilla
			Broccoli, rice, and cheese
			Lettuce salad w/tomatoes, carrots, and green onions
L		G	Spinach pasta w/spaghetti sauce (meat)
L			Pasta w/vegetables and tofu
L			Amaranth pasta w/melted Cheddar and Jack cheese
	S		Amaranth pasta w/Parmesan, Romano cheese, and olive oil
L			Wheat-free crackers w/avocado, tuna, or egg salad
	S	G	Carrot muffin w/apple
L			Pinto beans and flour tortilla (salsa and/or guacamole)
L		G	Beef and bean burrito
L	S		Bean w/bacon soup
	S		Split pea soup
			Vegetable soup (cornbread)
	S	G	Potato soup (brie cheese on sourdough bread)
L			Chili (w/beans, cheese, and/or onions)
L			Black bean soup w/cheese and onions
L			Onion soup (melted cheese)
L	S		Minestrone soup
	S		Chicken noodle soup (basmati rice)
		G	Chicken rice soup w/Colby cheese and ranch dressing sandwich, carrot sticks, apple, and/or celery
	S	G	Frozen yogurt w/almonds or trail mix
	S	G	Plain yogurt, raspberries, nuts, or trail mix

LUNCH or DINNER:

	S	G	Fish tacos
L			Sushi
L	S		Calamari, rice, and peas
L	S		Tuna and noodles, and green beans
	S		Tuna, avocado, and hard-boiled egg (spinach and/or grapes)

Eye

L S G	Salmon or mahi-mahi, potato, and carrot salad
G	Turkey, green beans or peas, and bread
L S	Turkey, rice, and broccoli or spinach
S G	Turkey, mozzarella cheese, and rice
L S	Baked chicken, rice, and peas
S G	Chicken, broccoli, and boiled white potatoes w/butter and parsley
L S G	Chicken and rice or pasta (green beans, cauliflower or corn)
L S	Chicken and rice (cooked or raw carrots)
S G	Chicken and potato salad: basil, yogurt, onion, celery, and potato w/white bread
S G	Chicken enchilada, chili relleno, and beans
S G	Chicken tamale
L S	Stir-fry: chicken, mushrooms, onions, tomato sauce, peas, and celery over steamed rice
G	Meat loaf, potato, and green beans
	Hamburger patty, baked potato, and coleslaw
S G	Bean burrito: flour tortilla w/pinto or black beans
G	Beef and bean burrito or taco (rice)
S	Beef ribs, potato, and peas (raw salad)
L S	Beef, rice, and green beans
G	Beef, red potatoes, and broccoli
S	Corned beef, sauerkraut, and potatoes
S	Liver and onions w/green peas
	Chili and bean chips
G	Navy bean soup and corn bread
S	Beef stew
G	Beef vegetable soup and corn bread
S	Clam chowder
S G	Ham, navy beans, and corn bread (butter)
S G	Pinto beans, rice, and corn bread
S	Beans – pinto, garbanzo, black, adzuki or split peas – and basmati, Japanese or wild rice
	Brown rice or pasta w/Parmesan and Romano cheese
L S	Brown rice, cooked in chicken broth, and vegetable salad: carrots, celery, green onions, broccoli, zucchini, and romaine lettuce w/blue cheese dressing
	Lasagna: noodles, tomato sauce, mozzarella cheese, and cottage cheese w/celery
G	Fettuccini alfredo w/scallops and garlic bread

MID-MORNING OR MID-AFTERNOON SNACK:
(Optional) Fruit, vegetables, grain, nuts, seeds, dairy, protein.

SENSITIVE & WEIGHT LOSS:
Mid-morning: None.
Mid-afternoon: Fruit, fruit juice.

L S G	Frozen cherries or mangos
L S G	Dried cherries, cranberries, or mangos
	Juice – grapefruit, black cherry, or papaya

DINNER:
7-8 p.m. Light-to-heavy, with protein, nuts, seeds, dairy, grain, legumes, vegetables, and/or fruit.

S G	Chicken or turkey, baked potato w/butter, and green peas
L S	Mahi-mahi, brown rice, and green beans
L S	Shark, baked potato, and mixed green salad
S	Salmon w/asparagus and blue cheese dressing
L S	Salmon, sardines, calamari, crab, or shrimp and rice
L S	Vegetarian chili and basmati rice w/cucumber salad
S	Meat loaf, rice, green beans w/onions and garlic, raw green bell peppers, and/or celery
S G	Pork chops, baked potato w/butter, broccoli, and white onions
S	Spaghetti (meat balls)
L	Stir-fry: onions, garlic, squash, carrots, and celery (rice)

Eye

L		Stir-fry: bamboo shoots, green peas, and snow pea pods (rice)
L		Green or yellow wax beans (garlic)
L	S	Lettuce salad w/carrots, green onions, broccoli, and celery (garlic)
L		Three bean salad w/kidney, green, and yellow wax beans and onions
L		Baked squash – no butter (onions)
		Baked pumpkin w/maple syrup (cinnamon and/or nutmeg)
L		Yam (peas)
L		Baked potato (pepper w/bean juice)
L		Green peas w/onions
L		Brussels sprouts
L		Spinach salad w/bacon and eggs

EVENING SNACK:
(Optional) 9 p.m.-2 a.m. Sweets, fruit, vegetables, grain, nuts, seeds, dairy.

SENSITIVE & WEIGHT LOSS: Sweets, fruit, dairy.

	S		Apple and cheese
	S	G	Blackberries or red or black raspberries and sour cream
	S	G	Banana, apple, applesauce, cantaloupe, or honeydew melon
			Juices – grapefruit, black cherry, or papaya
	S	G	Cookies
		G	Cherry pie, apple pie, or baked apple w/cheese
	S	G	Pumpkin pie or cheesecake
L		G	Hot chocolate w/2% milk
L	S		Carrots and/or celery (salsa)
L			Popcorn

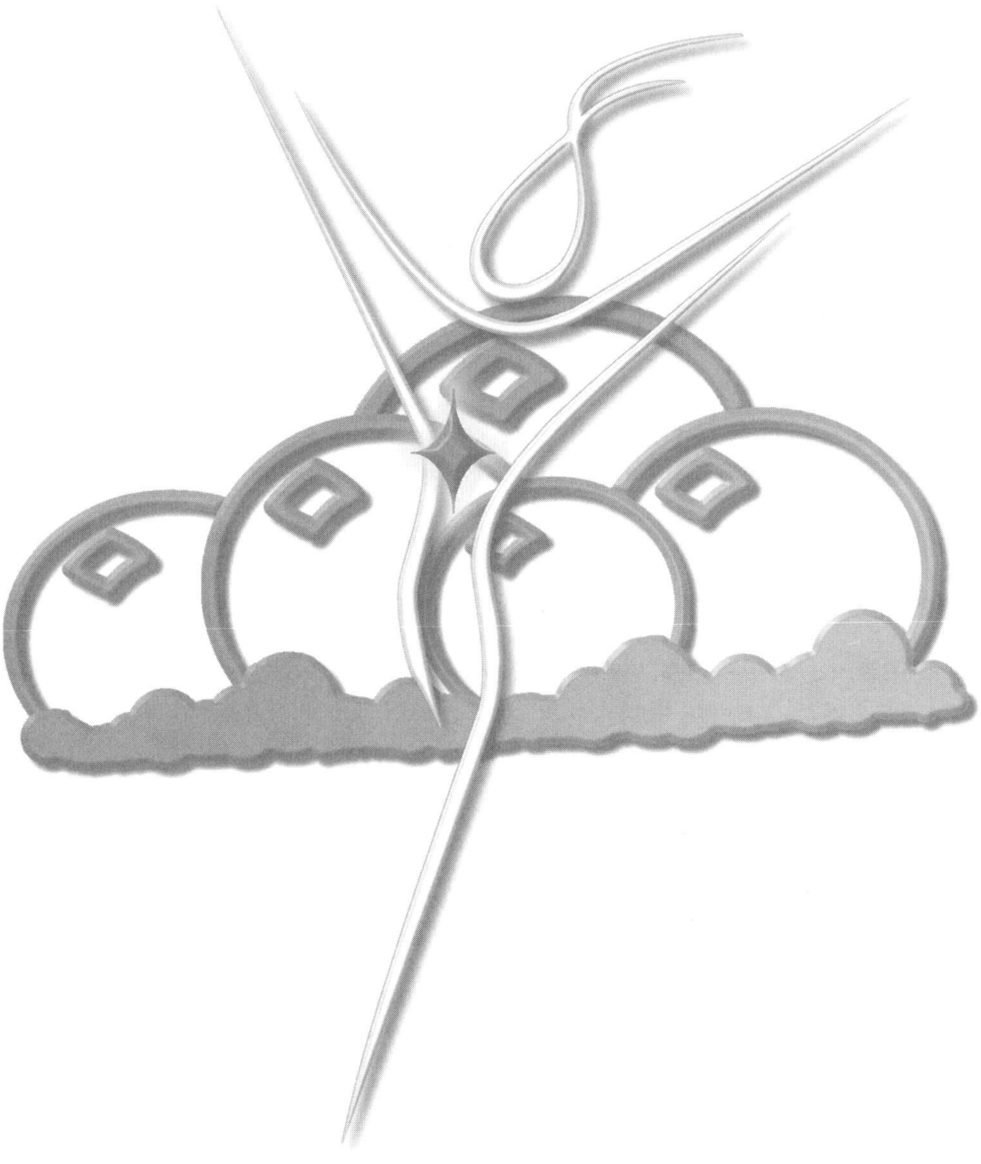

The "Gallbladder Body Type" is symbolized by soap suds. Like soap, bile is necessary to break down fats and the digestion of fats is essential to all other functions. Reliable, loyal and dependable, they are most fulfilled when they are being useful.

Gallbladder

BODY TYPE PROFILE

LOCATION	Right side of abdomen, under right side of liver.
FUNCTION	Reservoir for bile (produced by liver) which acts like soap in breakdown and absorption of fats. Bile is necessary for assimilation of fat-soluble vitamins and for preventing putrefaction of intestinal contents.
POTENTIAL HEALTH PROBLEMS	Generally healthy body with good stamina and strong immune system. Prone to respiratory conditions (i.e., colds, flu, throat virus, pneumonia), digestive difficulties (e.g., intestinal bloating, gas, constipation), gallbladder pain, and eye problems (e.g., fatigue, headache, aching behind eyes). Tension accumulates at base of skull when under stress. Tend to retain water.
RECOMMENDED EXERCISE	Exercise is optional. Its effect is primarily mental, as it clears the mind and provides a sense of doing something useful. Consequently, useful, productive activities such as gardening, yard work, cleaning windows or carpets are ideal. Walking, skiing – snow or water, treadmill, bicycling, rubberband exercises, callanetics, swimming or rebounding are good if they're enjoyable.

WOMEN'S CHARACTERISTICS

DISTINGUISHING FEATURES	Solid torso with most of weight gain in lower abdomen. Practical, helpful, down-to-earth personality. Consistent, reliable, and dependable. Often timid, preferring to work behind scenes.
ADDITIONAL PHYSICAL CHARACTERISTICS	Buttocks relatively flat-to-rounded. Low back curvature straight-to-average. Breasts small-to-large. Shoulders relatively even with hips. Average to short-waisted. Straight-to-defined waist. Height petite-to-average. Bone structure small-to-medium. Average, elongated musculature. Calves thin-to-muscular. Slender legs with little or no weight gain in thighs except upper inner. Hands average. Oval or rectangular head. May have small, deep-set eyes. Body may be at least a full size smaller above waist than below.
WEIGHT GAIN AREAS	Lower body with initial gain in lower abdomen, waist, and upper hips. Secondary weight gain in torso as general thickening, face, under chin, breasts, upper arms, entire abdomen, middle back, and possibly upper, inner thighs. Little or no weight gain in thighs, legs, lower hips, and buttocks. When weight gain is over 5 pounds, breasts may also increase, only to decrease when weight is lost.

Gallbladder

DIETARY GUIDELINES

SCHEDULING MEALS	Breakfast: Moderate, with fruit, grain, vegetables, protein, dairy, nuts, and/or seeds. Lunch: Moderate-to-heavy, with protein, legumes, dairy, grain, and/or vegetables. Dinner: Moderate, with protein, legumes, dairy, vegetables, grain, and/or fruit.
DIETARY EMPHASIS	• Consume more cooked than raw vegetables. • For weight loss, reduce breads, whole grains, crackers, dairy, and fruit; eliminate sugar and dried fruit; eat heaviest meal at lunch; include 15% of diet as dense protein; and limit fats to 25-30% of caloric intake (if below 20-25%, will actually gain weight). • For weight gain, 15% of caloric intake should be dense protein; include breads and dairy. • Vegetarian diet recommended when at ideal weight, although 10-30% of diet may consist of dense protein, preferably at breakfast and/or lunch. • Fats necessary to digest raw vegetables, particularly salads. 25-35% of caloric intake should be from butter, safflower, avocado or olive oil, sesame seeds, sunflower seeds, and avocados.
KEY SUPPORTS FOR SYSTEM	Couscous, white basmati rice, pinto beans, arugula, and chicken soup; watercress as liver stimulant. Kombucha tea (preferably made with Chinese oolong tea) after meals aids digestion, assimilation, and regulation of bowels. To support immune system, include at least 3 oz. dense protein.
COMPLEMENTARY GLANDULAR SUPPORT	Liver, through emotional support; and thymus, through consuming at least 3 oz. of dense protein daily.
FOODS CRAVED	*(When Energy is Low)* Carbohydrates, primarily bread with butter; beans; sweets, such as chocolate chip cookies or frozen yogurt; fats, like ice cream; mildly spicy foods, like Italian or Mexican.
FOODS TO AVOID	Whole wheat, cakes, cookies, pork. Breads should be used in moderation.
RECOMMENDED CUISINE	Homestyle cooking, Mexican, Italian, Thai, and Chinese.

Gallbladder

PSYCHOLOGICAL PROFILE

ESSENCE

Just as the gallbladder can be depended upon to store bile manufactured by the liver (which is essential for the breakdown of fats) and release it as needed, the Gallbladder body type is dependable. Known for being helpful, loyal and consistent, Gallbladder types create a steady, stable environment. They prefer to work behind the scenes, doing the jobs that are essential to keep a home or business running. Their quiet, steady strength is often expressed in what appears to be a timid or shy nature. They are exceptionally reliable and loyal, and feel most fulfilled when they are being useful.

CHARACTERISTIC TRAITS

Placing a high value on peace and tranquility, Gallbladder types are generally patient, calm, and easygoing. Typically soft-spoken, they impress others as being kind, gentle, and congenial. Social harmony is a high priority, so they generally get along well with others. While Gallbladders enjoy connecting with people, they are basically timid and shy, preferring to be around their families and close friends. There are a few Gallbladder types who have developed an outgoing nature, but the majority tend to be quiet and reserved around people, unless they know them well.

With a general lack of experience in knowing how to express emotions or connect on an emotional level, there's a reluctancy to venture into new social situations. However, they will go if someone takes them. Relating best to what can be physically seen and touched, and deriving a great deal of personal fulfillment from being useful, they feel very comfortable nurturing others by doing. Much of their satisfaction comes from making themselves useful to those around them.

Task-oriented, Gallbladders would rather undertake a task or project that is well-defined and already laid out for them, than generate one on their own. Careful, practical, and dependable, they show comparatively little interest in leadership positions. They're not really interested in standing out or making waves – or, for that matter, doing anything that might possibly wind up being disruptive.

MOTIVATION

Gallbladder types process information or make decisions by taking in information, letting it digest, and then seeing how it feels. They prefer life to be steady and consistent, structured and dependable. Feeling safe around what is known, changes are usually gradual. While open-minded, Gallbladders are generally skeptical about the myriad of claims, assertions, and changing perceptions that permeate the socio-cultural environment. Nevertheless, they are still open to new ideas that make good sense or can be validated.

Typically quite cautious, their views lean toward the traditional, conservative, or conventional side. Not especially intuitive or individualistic, Gallbladders frequently experience the need to rely on external standards to guide their

Gallbladder

MOTIVATION

thinking or action. There's a tendency to follow what they think they "should do", rather than trust their intuition or feelings. Acceptance of new ideas is relatively slow, so they typically prefer to stay with the "tried and true" or what they are used to.

In an attempt to feel safe when they feel frightened or intimidated, they will try to control their environment by closing down and withdrawing or acting out. There is a tendency to control others in a manipulative, dominating, restrictive manner, which is usually done subtly through persuasion, often as a defense against being controlled by someone else. Gallbladders can also be quite persevering, even stubborn, in their attempts to get others to do what they think is important, or to fully appreciate their beliefs and convictions.

"AT WORST"

When stressed, usually from physical imbalances, their mental processes become overloaded and mental acuity is impaired. Feeling overwhelmed and lethargic, it's hard for them to concentrate, routine tasks are not done as efficiently, and anything that requires focused thought is difficult. They have trouble understanding what others are communicating, so Gallbladders will ask them to explain the same thing several different ways before they can begin to grasp it.

Emotionally they will get into a state of depression, feeling low, melancholy, or generally frustrated. Since expressing anger doesn't fit their picture of how they "should" be, they will often suppress their anger, holding it in as resentment or bitterness. It's easy for them to fall into the victim role, feeling they are at the mercy of their circumstances. Feeling impatient, picky, or emotional, they don't want to be around people, unless it's someone who will support them. Being basically self-contained, they prefer to withdraw from their own feelings, disconnecting from people and situations.

Since Gallbladder types have difficulty dealing with emotions – theirs as well as others' – they're apt to "control" their emotions by suppressing them. This may take the form of denying their existence or responding to negative emotions with either stock, ready-made words of reassurance or by "prescribing" some ethical rule, or "should" that the other person had better follow. These "shoulds" come from what they have been taught rather than from their own experience, so they may come across as rigid or dogmatic.

"AT BEST"

When they find themselves in situations or faced with problems that they can do nothing about, they are able to turn them over to a higher power, get into a meditative state and allow their intuition to come forth. From here they are able to allow for new awarenesses, solutions and opportunities to manifest, enabling them to be expansive, creative and even adventurous, able to embrace new ideas and concepts.

Connecting with their quiet, inner strength, they are able to take personal responsibility for themselves and what they are creating, knowing that there

Gallbladder

"AT BEST"

are no victims and that everyone chooses their experiences. This is what it means to be personally empowered. By staying connected to their feelings and inner knowing, they are able to express their true nature, which is steady and dependable.

With an altruistic nature, Gallbladders are at their best when they are being of service to those in their world. They are conscientious, practical, dependable, and task-oriented. Their strengths include hard work, orderliness, common sense, and persistence. They are careful, steady, and reliable, with good stamina and follow-through. They can be depended upon to get things done in a timely manner, and are excellent support people. Gallbladders are also calm, congenial, and considerate. They like to fit in with those around them, and generally get along well with others. Being self-contained, they're not easily swayed by outside circumstances and are generally true to themselves.

Gallbladder

FOOD LISTS

HEALTHY FOOD LIST

FREQUENTLY FOODS	3-7 meals per week – refers to each food, rather than category.
DENSE PROTEIN	Buffalo, veal, beef broth; chicken broth, cornish game hen; bass, catfish, flounder, haddock, herring, red snapper, orange roughy, perch, sardines in oil, trout; crab, eel, octopus
DAIRY	Buttermilk, goat milk, regular plain or vanilla yogurt, kefir, butter,
CHEESE	Cream, mozzarella, Muenster, Parmesan, ricotta, Romano
NUTS and SEEDS	Coconuts (raw), filberts (raw or dry roasted), macadamias (raw), pine nuts(raw), water chestnuts, sesame seeds (raw or dry roasted), sesame seed butter
LEGUMES	Beans (adzuki, black, butter [lima], pinto), black-eyed peas, split peas
GRAINS	Millet, rice, (white basmati, Japanese, wild), rice cakes (unsalted), sesame rice cakes, couscous
VEGETABLES	Artichokes, arugula, bamboo shoots, cooked green beans, yellow wax beans, broccoli, brussels sprouts, carrots, chard, cauliflower, cucumbers, eggplant, garlic, kohlrabi, leeks, red leaf lettuce, mushrooms, okra, green and ripe olives, onions (chives, green, red, white, brown, yellow, vidalia), parsley, parsnips, peas, potatoes (all varieties), pumpkin, rutabaga, spinach, squash (acorn, banana, butternut, spaghetti), turnips, watercress, yams
FRUITS	Apples (all varieties), blackberries, cranberries, gooseberries, grapefruits (white, red), guavas, kiwi, mangos, papayas, plums (black, purple, red), pomegranates, tangelos, watermelons, dates, figs (Black Mission), stewed or dried prunes, raisins
FRUIT JUICES	Apple, grapefruit
SWEETENERS	Re-Vita®, stevia
VEGETABLE OILS	All-blend, avocado, corn, safflower, sesame, sunflower, soy
BEVERAGES	Herbal teas (peppermint, cammomile), Kombucha tea
MODERATELY FOODS	1-2 meals per week – refers to each food, rather than category.
DENSE PROTEIN	Beef, beef liver, liverwurst, lamb, venison, organ meats (brain, heart); chicken, chicken livers, turkey, beef or turkey bacon, duck; anchovy, bonita, cod, halibut, mackerel, mahi-mahi, salmon, sardines in tomato sauce, shark, sole, swordfish, tuna; abalone, calamari (squid), clams, lobster, mussels, oysters, scallops, shrimp; eggs
DAIRY	Milk (whole, 2%, low fat, raw), half & half, sweet cream, sour cream, low fat plain and flavored yogurt, regular flavored yogurt, frozen yogurt, ice cream (Dreyer's, Ben & Jerry's®, Swensen's®)

Gallbladder

CHEESE	American, blue, brie, Camembert, Cheddar, Colby, cottage, Edam, feta, goat, Gouda, Jack, kefir, Limburger, Swiss
NUTS and SEEDS	Raw or dry roasted, unsalted nuts almonds, almond butter, Brazils, cashews, cashew butter, hazelnuts, macadamia butter, pistachios, peanuts, peanut butter, pecans, walnuts (black, English), raw or dry roasted seeds (caraway, pumpkin, sunflower), sunflower seed butter
LEGUMES	Beans (garbanzo, great northern, navy, soy), lentils, hummus, miso, soy milk, tofu
GRAINS	Amaranth, barley, corn, corn bread, corn grits, blue corn, corn tortillas, hominy grits, oats, oat bran, popcorn, quinoa, short or long grain brown rice, brown basmati rice, rice bran, salted rice cakes, popcorn rice cakes, rye, triticale, wheat bran, raw or toasted wheat germ, refined wheat flour, flour tortillas, breads (French, Italian, sourdough, garlic, white, oat, corn, corn/rye, rice, rye, sprouted grain), croissants, bagels, English muffins, crackers (saltines, oat, rye), pasta, udon noodles, Chinese rice noodles, cream of rice, cream of rye, cream of wheat
SOUPS	Chicken vegetable, vegetable, clam chowder, bean with ham, beef vegetable, cream of broccoli, chili, asparagus, pumpkin, egg drop, corn chowder, miso
VEGETABLES	Asparagus, avocados, raw green beans, lima beans, beets, bok choy, cabbage (green, red, napa), celery, cilantro, corn, greens (beet, collard, mustard, turnip), hominy, jicama, kale, lettuce (Boston, butter, endive, iceberg, romaine), snow pea pods, bell peppers (green, yellow, red), chili peppers, pimentos, daikon radish, radish, sauerkraut, seaweed (dulse, nori, wakame), shallots, squash (yellow [summer], zucchini), sprouts (alfalfa, mung bean, clover, radish, sunflower), sweet potatoes, taro root, tomatoes (canned, hot-house, vine-ripened
VEGETABLE JUICES	Carrot, celery, parsley, carrot/celery, spinach/parsley/celery, spinach, tomato, V-8®
FRUITS	Apricots, bananas, blueberries, boysenberries, raspberries, strawberries, cherries, grapes (black, green, red), kumquats, lemons, limes, loquats, melons (cantaloupe, casaba, crenshaw, honeydew), nectarines, oranges, peaches, pears, persimmons, pineapples, rhubarb, tangerines
FRUIT JUICES	Apple cider, apple/apricot, apricot, cherry (black, red), cranapple, cranberry, grape (purple, red, white), guava, lemon, orange, papaya, pear, pineapple, pineapple/coconut, prune, tangerine, watermelon
VEGETABLE OILS	Almond, canola, coconut, flaxseed, olive, peanut
SWEETENERS	Honey, molasses, sorghum, brown sugar, date sugar, raw sugar, refined cane sugar, brown rice syrup, barley malt syrup, corn syrup, fructose, succonant, saccharin
CONDIMENTS	Salt, sea salt, Vege-Sal®, Bragg™ aminos, brewer's yeast, horseradish, mustard, soy sauce, barbecue sauce, pesto sauce, salsa, tahini, dill or sweet pickles
SALAD DRESSINGS	Blue cheese, French, ranch, creamy Italian, creamy avocado, thousand island, vinegar and oil, lemon juice and oil

Gallbladder

DESSERTS	Custards, tapioca, puddings, pies, chocolate, desserts containing chocolate, raspberry sherbet, orange sherbet
CHIPS	Bean, corn (blue, white, yellow), potato
BEVERAGES	Coffee, coffee with Re-Vita®; black tea, regular tea, Japanese tea, Chinese oolong tea; mineral water, sparkling water; wine (red, white), champagne, sake, liqueurs, beer, barley malt liquor, gin, Scotch, vodka, whiskey; root beer, regular sodas
RARELY FOODS	No more than once a month
DENSE PROTEIN	Pork, pork bacon, pork sausage, ham; sardines in mustard or chili
DAIRY	Nonfat milk, nonfat plain or flavored yogurt, most ice creams
NUTS and SEEDS	All roasted, salted
LEGUMES	Kidney or red beans
GRAINS	Buckwheat, polished rice, whole wheat, breads (7-grain, multi-grain, whole wheat), whole wheat crackers
VEGETABLES	Broccoflower, seaweed (arami, hyjikai, kelp)
SWEETENERS	Maple syrup, aspertame, Equal®, NutraSweet®, Sweet'n Low®
CONDIMENTS	Mayonnaise
DESSERTS	Cakes, cookies
BEVERAGES	Diet sodas

SENSITIVE FOOD LIST

FREQUENTLY FOODS	3-7 meals per week – refers to each food, rather than category.
DENSE PROTEIN	Buffalo, veal, beef broth; chicken broth, cornish game hen; flounder, haddock, herring, red snapper, orange roughy, sardines in oil; crab, eel, octopus
DAIRY	Goat milk, regular plain or vanilla yogurt
CHEESE	Muenster, Parmesan, ricotta
LEGUMES	Beans (adzuki, pinto), black-eyed peas
GRAINS	Japanese or wild rice, unsalted rice cakes, couscous
VEGETABLES	Artichokes, arugula, cooked green beans, yellow wax beans, broccoli (steamed), brussels sprouts, carrots, cauliflower, chard, eggplant, garlic, kohlrabi, leeks, red leaf lettuce, mushrooms, olives (green, ripe), onions (chives, green, brown, red, white, yellow, vidalia), parsley, parsnips, peas, potatoes (all varieties), pumpkin, rutabaga, squash (acorn, banana, butternut, spaghetti), turnips, watercress

Gallbladder

FRUITS	Apples (all varieties), cranberries, gooseberries, grapefruits (white, red), guavas, kiwi, mangos, papayas, plums (black, purple, red), pomegranates, tangelos, dates, figs (Black Mission), stewed prunes, raisins
FRUIT JUICES	Apple, grapefruit
VEGETABLE OILS	All-blend, avocado, corn, safflower, sesame, soy, sunflower
BEVERAGES	Herbal teas (peppermint, cammomile)
MODERATELY FOODS	1-2 meals per week – refers to each food, rather than category.
DENSE PROTEIN	Beef, beef liver, liverwurst, lamb, venison, organ meats (brain, heart); chicken, chicken livers, turkey, duck; anchovy, bass, bonita, catfish, cod, halibut, mackerel, mahi-mahi, perch, salmon, sardines in tomato sauce, shark, sole, swordfish, trout, tuna; abalone, calamari (squid), clams, lobster, mussels, oysters, shrimp, scallops; eggs
DAIRY	Buttermilk, kefir, milk (whole, 2%, low fat, raw), half & half, sweet cream, sour cream, butter, ice cream (Dreyer's, Swensen's®, Ben & Jerry's®)
CHEESE	American, blue, brie, Camembert, Cheddar, Colby, cottage, cream, Edam, feta, goat, Gouda, Jack, kefir, Limburger, mozzarella, Romano, Swiss
NUTS and SEEDS	Raw or dry roasted, unsalted nuts almonds, Brazils, cashews, cashew butter, water chestnuts, coconuts, filberts, hazelnuts, macadamias, macadamia butter, peanuts, pecans, pine nuts, pistachios, walnuts (black, English), raw or dry roasted, unsalted seeds (caraway, pumpkin, sesame)
LEGUMES	Beans (black, lima [butter], garbanzo, great northern, navy, soy), split peas, hummus, miso, soy milk
GRAINS	Millet, popcorn, quinoa, white or brown basmati rice, refined wheat flour, flour tortillas, wheat germ, breads (French, garlic, Italian, rice, sourdough, white), bagels, croissants, English muffins, Chinese rice noodles, cream of rice
SOUPS	Chicken vegetable, vegetable, bean with ham, chili, beef vegetable, clam chowder, cream of broccoli, asparagus
VEGETABLES	Asparagus, avocados, bamboo shoots, lima beans, beets, bok choy, cabbage, celery, cilantro, corn, cucumbers, greens (beet, mustard, turnip), hominy, jicama, lettuce (Boston, endive, butter, romaine), okra, snow pea pods, bell peppers (green, yellow, red), chili peppers, pimentos, radish, daikon radish, sauerkraut, shallots, spinach, yellow (summer) squash, sweet potatoes, tomatoes, yams
VEGETABLE JUICES	Celery, carrot, carrot/celery, parsley, spinach, tomato, V-8®, green juice
FRUITS	Bananas, blackberries, blueberries, boysenberries, raspberries, kumquats, lemons, limes, loquats, pears, persimmons, pineapples, melons (cantaloupe, crenshaw, honeydew, watermelon), rhubarb, tangerines

Gallbladder

FRUIT JUICES	Apple cider, apple/apricot, apricot, cherry, black cherry, cranapple, cranberry, grape (purple, red, white), guava, lemon, orange, papaya, pear, pineapple, pineapple/coconut, prune, tangerine, watermelon
VEGETABLE OILS	Coconut, olive
SWEETENERS	Barley malt syrup, corn syrup, Re-Vita®, stevia
CONDIMENTS	Salt, sea salt, Vege-Sal®, brewer's yeast, Bragg™ aminos, salsa, tahini, vinegar, dill pickles
SALAD DRESSINGS	Vinegar and oil, lemon juice and oil
BEVERAGES	Green tea, Japanese tea, Chinese oolong tea, Kombucha tea; mineral water, sparkling water
RARELY FOODS	No more than once a month
DENSE PROTEIN	Pork, ham, pork bacon or sausage; sardines in mustard or chili
DAIRY	Nonfat milk, nonfat plain or flavored yogurt, frozen yogurt, most ice creams
NUTS and SEEDS	Almond butter, peanut butter, sunflower seeds, sunflower seed butter, all roasted, salted nuts and seeds.
LEGUMES	Beans (kidney, red), lentils, tofu
GRAINS	Amaranth, barley, buckwheat, corn, corn bread, corn grits, corn tortillas, hominy grits, oats, long or short grain brown rice, polished rice, popcorn rice cakes, rye, triticale, whole wheat, wheat bran, breads (7-grain, multi-grain, whole wheat, oat, corn, rye, corn/rye), rye or whole wheat crackers, pasta, noodles, cream of rye, cream of wheat
VEGETABLES	Broccoflower, iceberg lettuce, sprouts (alfalfa, mung bean, clover, radish, sunflower), collard greens, kale, seaweed (all varieties), zucchini
FRUITS	Apricots, strawberries, peaches, nectarines, cherries, grapes (black, green, red), oranges, casaba melon
VEGETABLE OILS	Almond, canola, flaxseed, peanut
SWEETENERS	Honey, molasses, sorghum, brown sugar, raw sugar, refined cane sugar, date sugar, maple syrup, brown rice syrup, fructose, succonant, saccharin, aspertame, Equal®, NutraSweet®, Sweet'n Low®
CONDIMENTS	Mayonnaise, margarine, barbecue sauce, pesto sauce, soy sauce, sweet pickles, catsup, mustard, horseradish
SALAD DRESSINGS	Blue cheese, French, ranch, creamy Italian, creamy avocado, thousand island
DESSERTS	Cakes, cookies, custards, tapioca, puddings, pies, chocolate, desserts containing chocolate, raspberry sherbet, orange sherbet
CHIPS	Bean, corn (blue, white, yellow), potato
BEVERAGES	Black coffee; black tea; red wine, white wine, champagne, sake, beer, barley malt liquor, gin, Scotch, vodka, whiskey; diet sodas, root beer, regular sodas

Gallbladder

MENUS

DIETARY EMPHASIS :

- Fats necessary to digest raw vegetables, particularly salads. Good sources are avocados, olive oil, and sunflower seeds.
- More cooked than raw vegetables.
- Couscous, white basmati rice, pinto beans, arugula, and chicken soup.
- Watercress is a liver stimulant.
- Kombucha tea after meals aids digestion.
- To support immune system, include at least 3 oz. dense protein.

WEIGHT LOSS:

- Reduce breads, whole grains, crackers, dairy, and fruit.
- Eliminate sugar and dried fruit.
- Eat heaviest meal at lunch.
- Include 15% of caloric intake from dense protein.
- Limit fats to 25-30% of caloric intake (if below 20-25%, will actually gain weight).

WEIGHT GAIN :

- Include 15% of caloric intake from dense protein.
- Include breads and dairy.

VEGETARIAN DIET:

- Recommended when at ideal weight, although 10-30% of diet may consist of dense protein, preferably at breakfast and/or lunch.

FATS:

- Necessary to digest raw vegetables, particularly salads; include avocado, olive oil, and/or sunflower seeds.
- 25-35% of caloric intake.
- Best sources are butter, safflower, avocado or olive oil, sesame seeds, sunflower seeds, and avocados.

KEY

—all menus may be used by healthy persons

( ) around foods means that they're optional

L denotes weight loss menus

S denotes sensitive menus

S* denotes very sensitive menus

G denotes weight gain menus

BREAKFAST:
7-8 a.m. Moderate with fruit, grain, vegetables, protein, dairy, nuts, and/or seeds.

L	S*		Couscous and cooked parsley (butter)
L			Couscous or oatmeal and Re-Vita® (butter)
L	S		Grapefruit or grapefruit juice, then couscous or cream of rice and butter
	S	G	Apples and filberts w/cream
			Stewed prunes or raisins and walnuts
		G	Raspberries and/or blackberries w/sour cream
L	S*		Cream of rice w/butter and/or Re-Vita® – no milk
L	S		Basmati rice (butter and/or apple)
L			Sesame rice cakes w/apple butter or avocado (tea)
		G	Rice cake or rice bread w/macadamia butter or peanut butter
		G	English muffin w/peanut butter and banana
L			Cooked millet w/parsley and butter
L			Grapefruit or grapefruit juice, then oatmeal (butter)
		G	Oatmeal, half & half, and Re-Vita®
		G	Oatmeal, strawberries, and yogurt
		G	Shredded wheat w/half & half
		G	Bagels (garlic and onion), cream cheese, and pear
L		G	Corn bread w/butter or turkey or chicken gravy (egg)
		G	Egg and cheese omelette and corn tortilla
		G	Egg, waffles, butter, and/or Re-Vita®
	S	G	Eggs and rice
L			Eggs and onions (garlic)
L	S		Eggs, broccoli, and cauliflower
		G	Eggs, potatoes, and strawberries
		G	Orange roughy, halibut, sea bass, or sole w/rice
	S*		Buttermilk
	S		Liver or chicken

Gallbladder

L Liver and onions

S G Baked potato w/butter and/or sour cream

L Yam w/butter and peas

L Pineapple/coconut juice

MID-MORNING SNACK:
(Optional) 10-11 a.m.
Fruit, grain, protein, dairy.

G Fruit or fruit juice: grapefruit, banana, dates, raisins, black Mission figs, apple, prune, papaya, and/or pineapple

L S Rice cake w/butter, sesame butter, apple butter, or avocado

G White chicken or cheese (cracker)

LUNCH:
12-2 p.m. Moderate-to-heavy with protein, legumes, dairy, grain, and/or vegetables. Watercress or arugula (raw or steamed) may be added to menus.

L G Chicken, rice, and cooked or raw carrots

L G Chicken, basmati and wild rice, and green beans (onions)

L S Chicken or eggs, spinach, beet greens w/lemon or vinegar, and beets

L G Chicken, pasta, cooked tomatoes, and broccoli

L Chicken salad chicken, celery, onions, avocado or Hain™ Avocado salad dressing served w/raw celery, cucumber, olives, and carrots

L Cornish hen roasted w/onions and carrots

L G Turkey, rice, cranberry sauce, and peas or spinach

L Turkey, green beans, and onions

L G Yellowtail tuna, asparagus, and pasta

L G Yellowtail tuna, rice, steamed cauliflower, and broccoli

L G Salmon w/green onions, lemon juice, rice, and green peas

L Tuna stuffed tomato, and lettuce w/avocado or Hain™ Avocado dressing

L G Meat loaf, potatoes, and salad romaine lettuce, tomatoes, and cucumber

L G Lamb chops cooked w/thyme and asparagus

L S Liver and red onions w/green peas (butter)

L Liver and onions w/salad red leaf lettuce, carrots, peas, and red onions with Hain™ Avocado dressing

L G Beef, potatoes, and green beans

S G Black beans and yogurt – no sugar

S G Pinto beans and mozzarella cheese

L Split pea soup and corn bread (butter)

L Spaghetti, tomato sauce, (meat) and salad romaine lettuce, green onion, and avocado

L G Pasta, chicken or turkey, green beans, and onions (mushrooms and/or broccoli)

MID-AFTERNOON SNACK:
(Optional) 4-5 p.m. Protein, nuts, seeds, grain, dairy, vegetables.

SENSITIVE: Protein, nuts, seeds, grain.

L G Sunflower seeds

L G Plain or vanilla yogurt

L S G Chicken, turkey or chicken livers

S G Buttermilk or kefir

LUNCH or DINNER:

Lobster (butter), rice, broccoli, and carrots

S Salmon or chicken w/baked or mashed potatoes

L S Salmon and peas (spinach or beet greens)

L Tuna salad, avocado, and sesame rice cakes

G Tuna, celery, and onions on oat bread

L S Stir-fry chicken, mushrooms, onions, tamari sauce, peas, and celery over steamed rice

L S G Chicken and rice

L Chicken, green beans, carrots (onions)

L S Vegetable soup

L S Split pea soup, rice cake, and butter

S Boston clam chowder

L S Baked potato and cauliflower (w/Bragg™ aminos and/or butter)

S Baked potato and sour cream

Gallbladder

L	S	G	
L	S		Butternut, spaghetti, or acorn squash w/Re-Vita® (onions, green beans, or carrots)
		G	Macaroni and cheese w/peas (pearl onions)
L			Noodles – egg, udon, or Top Ramen® w/tuna and/or broccoli (butter)
L			Spinach or seminola pasta w/butter or white sauce
	S		Rice, butter, and cauliflower
	S		Rice and broccoli or green peas
L	S		Pinto beans and rice
		G	Pinto beans, rice, and yogurt
		G	Beans, cornbread, avocado, and/or cream cheese
	S		Plain or vanilla yogurt (Re-Vita®)

DINNER:
6-7 p.m. Moderate with protein, legumes, dairy, vegetables, grain, and/or fruit.

L	S	G	
L			Pinto beans and avocado
		G	Bean burrito and sour cream (rice)
L			Navy beans and onions w/corn bread and butter
L			Baked potato, Jack cheese, chard, and/or mustard greens
L	S		Baked potato w/butter and green peas
L	S		Yam w/butter (green peas)
L			Chicken burrito or tamale (celery)
L	S	G	Chicken, broccoli, parsley, rice, and butter
L			Chicken, corn, and cucumbers
L			Chicken, potatoes, and peas, or carrots and onions
L			Chicken, Japanese noodles, pea pods, and spinach salad
		G	Turkey sausage, navy beans, and lettuce salad
L		G	Orange roughy, rice, peas, and onions
L			Salmon, rice, broccoli, and carrots
L		G	Sole, rice, onions, garlic, and carrots
		G	Shrimp or chicken, fettucini alfredo, and spinach salad, or raw cucumbers
		G	Tuna and noodles, green beans, onions, and garlic
L		G	Fish, basmati rice, and spinach salad
	S		Rice, green beans, onions, garlic, raw green bell peppers, and/or celery
L			Rice, yellow squash, and carrots (Bragg™ aminos)
L			Basmati rice, broccoli, onions, mushrooms, cauliflower, and carrots
L			Rice and eggs (salsa)
L		G	Pasta (beef, chicken, or turkey), tomato sauce, and olives
L			Pasta, pesto sauce, basil, and spinach salad
L			Spinach or semolina pasta and salad red and green pepper, green onion, and carrots
L			Spinach pasta, tomato sauce, and carrots
L			Green pea soup w/carrots and celery
	S		Chili and basmati rice w/cucumber salad
L			Vegetable beef soup
L		G	Turkey stew ground turkey, tomatoes, zucchini, pinto beans, and pasta
L		G	Chicken noodle soup (basmati rice)
L		G	Chicken rice soup
L			Chinese sizzling rice soup
L			Steamed artichokes and romaine salad w/olives and cheese
	S	G	Apples or pears and cheese
	S	G	Blackberries or raspberries and sour cream or cream cheese

EVENING SNACK:
(Optional) At least 1/2 hour after dinner. Seeds, nuts, dairy, vegetables, fruit, grain, desserts.

L	S	G	
		G	Peaches and cottage cheese
L			Rhubarb cooked w/tapioca (Re-Vita®)
	S		Cooked carrots
	S	G	Brazil nuts, pecans, or walnuts
L	S	G	Vanilla, lemon or plain yogurt (berry Re-Vita®)
L		G	Pumpkin pie or cheese cake

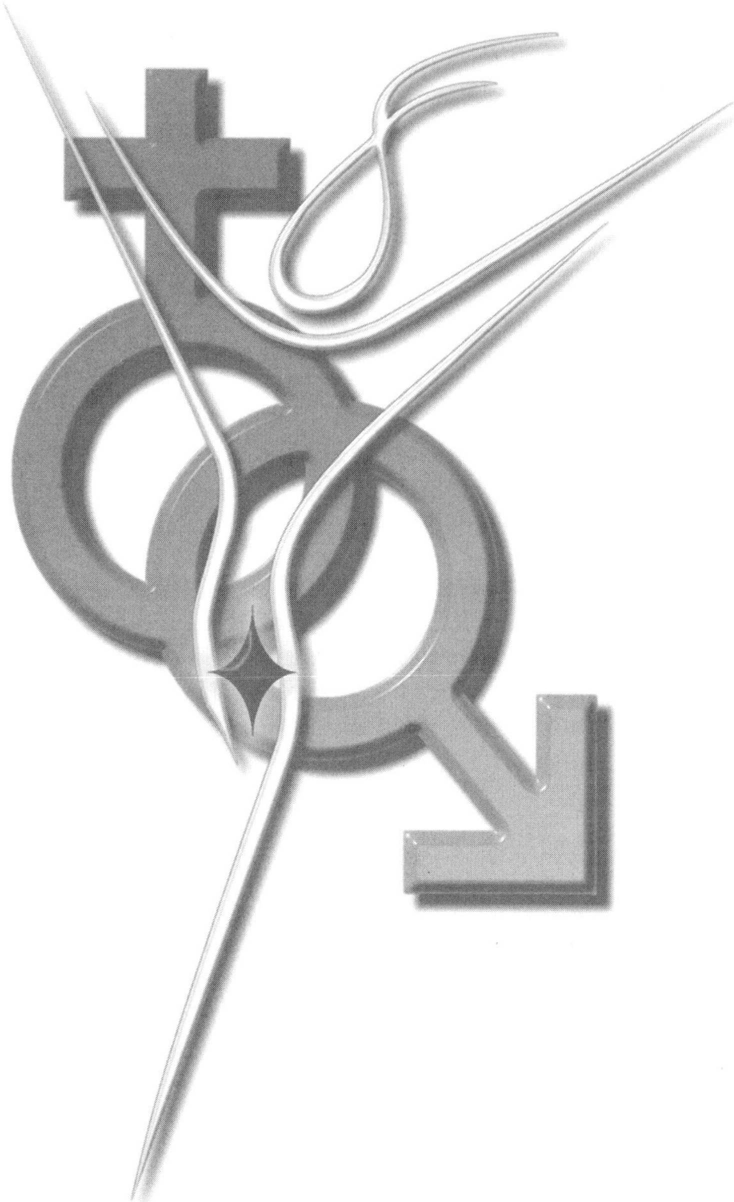

The "Gonadal Body Type" is symbolized by the male/female symbol. Sexuality is expressed through the gonads and is associated with pleasure and being playful. Highly emotional, they bring a light, playful, spontaneous quality to all aspects of their lives.

GONADAL

Gonadal

BODY TYPE PROFILE

LOCATION	Reproductive organs – ovaries.
FUNCTION	Reproduction, and secretion of hormones.
POTENTIAL HEALTH PROBLEMS	Early puberty. Typically healthy libido. Generally feels best when pregnant, both physically and psychologically. Digestive distress, such as difficulty digesting fats, low blood sugar, food allergies. Hormonal imbalances. Tendency toward edema (water retention), urinary tract infections.
RECOMMENDED EXERCISE	Exercise is helpful. Its benefit is initially emotional, then physical. It gives a sense of accomplishment and gets energy moving. Callanetics, exercises that work and develop upper body, aerobic dance or jog 2 times/week, massage for legs, walking very helpful, Nordic Track, sunlight important. Do well with vigorous exercise.

WOMEN'S CHARACTERISTICS

DISTINGUISHING FEATURES	Prominent muscular buttocks, often with sway back and relatively flat stomach. Characteristic muscular thighs that appear developed to the knees. Bright, attractive, oval, or rectangular face, often with delicate features. Loss of mental clarity is usually first sign of stress; to compensate, will search for and do "no brainer" jobs, like housework or shopping, until clarity returns. Generally light and playful.
ADDITIONAL PHYSICAL CHARACTERISTICS	Buttocks prominent-to-rounded. Low back curvature average-to-swayed. Breasts small-to-average. Shoulders narrower than, to relatively even with, hips. Hour-glass figure with defined to well-defined waist. Average to long-waisted. Height petite-to-average. Bone structure small-to-medium. Average, elongated musculature. Hands average, or long and slender. Oval or rectangular face. Body often at least a full size smaller above waist than below.
WEIGHT GAIN AREAS	Lower body with initial gain in buttocks, lower hips and entire thighs with main protrusion on upper outer 1/3rd and entire inner thighs continuing to inner knees, and possibly waist. Secondary weight gain in upper arms, middle back, lower-to-entire abdomen, waist, breasts, face, under chin, and upper hips. Cellulite formation is common. Weight often varies from 25 pounds over-weight to 15 pounds underweight.

Gonadal

DIETARY GUIDELINES

	SCHEDULING MEALS:
"HEALTHY"	Breakfast: Light, with fruit or moderate, with protein, nuts, seeds, grain, fruit, and/or dairy. Lunch: Light-to-heavy, with protein, legumes, grain, nuts, seeds, fruit, dairy, and/or vegetables. Dinner: Moderate-to-heavy, with protein, legumes, grain, vegetables, nuts, seeds, and/or dairy.
"SENSITIVE"	Avoid fruit, nuts, and seeds for lunch and dinner.
DIETARY EMPHASIS	• Include more cooked than raw vegetables in diet. • For weight loss, reduce fats to 15% of calories and select them from the recommended sources. Avoid bread for lunch; avoid spices; and minimize grain at dinner. • To gain weight, increase food intake. • Vegetarian diet is adequate, although up to 30% may consist of dense protein. • Fats, 25% of caloric intake for maintenance should be from nuts (almonds, Brazils, cashews, hazel nuts, pecans, macadamias, walnuts), seeds (pumpkin, sunflower), oils (avocado, olive, safflower, sesame), and butter.
KEY SUPPORTS FOR SYSTEM	Fruit (peaches, bananas, Gala apples, cranberries, dates, raisins, prunes), vegetables (avocados, yams, tomatoes), cottage cheese, fish, turkey, and brown rice.
COMPLEMENTARY GLANDULAR SUPPORT	Liver through emotional support. Pineal with sunlight.
FOODS CRAVED	*(When Energy is Low)* Spicy foods, like Mexican, Italian, Indian, or Thai. Sweets and sweet fruits like peaches and strawberries. Fats such as pastries, ice cream, chocolate, butter, and creamy salad dressings.
FOODS TO AVOID	Peanut butter, russet potatoes, casaba and honeydew melons, orange juice. Since fats and spices stimulate the gonads, best to use in moderation or avoid when wanting to lose weight.
RECOMMENDED CUISINE	Mexican, Italian, Seafood, Chinese, Japanese, Thai, Indian, Moroccan, Continental, French, English, or Irish 1-2 times/week.

Gonadal

PSYCHOLOGICAL PROFILE

ESSENCE

Just as the gonads are a pleasure center, the nature of the Gonadal body type is to create pleasure and be playful. They bring a light, playful spontaneous quality to their work, relationships, and to all aspects of their lives. to create pleasure and be playful. They bring a light, playful, spontaneous Integration, balance, and enjoyment create genuine playfulness. Highly emotional, Gonadals are prone to being controlled by their emotions. Difficulty focusing or concentrating is typical when tired or stressed. To compensate, Gonadals will look for and do "no-brainer" jobs like shopping, gardening, or routine tasks. Playtime or time to completely relax is essential, as it allows them to re-connect with their essence.

CHARACTERISTIC TRAITS

While Gonadals generally have fine symmetrical features, it's their strong sexual energy that makes them exceptionally physically attractive. Beauty is of vital importance, whether it's in their personal appearance, environment, or the beauty they see in everyone and everything.

Oriented primarily through their emotions, Gonadals are extremely sensitive to the emotional needs of others. Family is of utmost importance to them, since they often link their personal identity with their intimate relationships. Consequently, bonding with their family and friends, as well as maintaining their approval and acceptance, is essential. Gonadals are often the glue that holds the family together and binds relationships. Highly emotional and physically expressive, Gonadals quickly show their anger and hurt, as well as their affection, nurturing, and joy. Their nature is to be playful, as it's through play that they are able to access their inner joy.

Social interaction, whether it's parties, family gatherings, or connections with customers and co-workers, allows them to bring out the best in people. They have a special ability to recognize and appreciate the feelings of others; and being sensitive and caring, Gonadals offer emotional support to those who need it. They derive much of their gratification simply through harmonious interactions. Being more people than task-oriented, Gonadals thrive on substantial human contact.

Responding to situations primarily with their feelings rather than with their reasoning, makes Gonadals far more susceptible to stress reactions than other types. Consequently, they tend to easily feel overwhelmed when things don't go well. If Gonadals have too much on their mind or are experiencing conflict or frustration, or even when having a hormonal imbalance, their ability to think clearly can be significantly impaired. Their usual response is to take time out to recover or look for a "no-brainer" task that has a minimal requirement for concentration. Shifting gears for a while allows Gonadal types to renew their center of balance. Since they don't handle stress well, playtime is essential in maintaining a positive outlook.

Gonadal

MOTIVATION

Inspired by beauty, Gonadals see beauty as an undeniable aspect of God that exists in everything. Beauty and music provide an emotional lift. Becoming the music incorporates another dimension that allows for self-expansion and a sense of freedom. For Gonadals, beauty is what is seen as a person's essence. It's apparent in the way they look, the expression of their talents and through the kindness they show to others. Beauty is a quality free from judgement; and because it is the essence of everything, it can't be relative to anything else.

Gonadals nurture by helping others recognize and express their inner beauty. They want others to see what they see, so they enjoy enhancing someone's physical appearance or making their environment more beautiful. Emotionally sensitive, they feel another's pain and will do whatever they can to assist and nurture them.

Being result oriented, Gonadals want to see the physical results of their efforts. They tend to prefer the big picture to the details, meaning they like to quickly see that their efforts are making a difference. With the idea in their mind of what they want to create, Gonadals will often enthusiastically jump into a project without fully considering what they need to do to finish it. Their level of maturity will dictate how well or whether the project gets completed.

For Gonadal types, self-worth is often associated with how their accomplishments make them appear to others. This search for self-worth can lead them to be very conscientious, even to the point of perfectionism. While their basic nature is not especially industrious, they have the ability to apply themselves to a project with great determination when they feel it is relevant to their life. Establishing a sense of identity can lead them to be quite focused on business, while still maintaining their emotional focus in their personal lives.

Basing their identity on their family's and friends' responses and expectations of them, Gonadals can deny their own self-expression or easily fall into self-sacrifice. Their personal insecurity tends to lead them to be overly concerned about their physical appearance. Gonadals are usually the first to follow fashion trends and group activities, since they often rely on others for personal validation.

"AT WORST"

When frustrated, exhausted, or life gets difficult, Gonadal types often become stubborn and self-centered. Highly reactive to those around them, they may cry, yell, or explode in anger. Gonadals may be impatient, irritable, and difficult to deal with, and they will "lose it" or go "brain dead" when the stress becomes too much. It is easy for them to harbor bad feelings when a situation has been unpleasant and they haven't openly expressed their displeasure. If they have learned to "control" their emotions and hold back their impulses, their negative tendencies tend to manifest as secret hostility and resentment, or victim syndrome.

Gonadal

"AT WORST" (Continued)

For men, self-worth is often associated with how much in control of their families they appear to be to their friends. This can lead to "macho" behavior, which is an immature attempt to display masculine strength by dominating or controlling someone else. Depending on their degree of development, they may be more concerned about getting credit for work than on doing the job, and on getting it done as soon as possible rather than making sure it's done right. They will look for short cuts, and generally choose the easiest way to completion rather than the best way. Preferring to get started right away and learn what they need to know only when they need to know it, Gonadals often do not take enough time for preparation or deliberation of the details.

"AT BEST"

Gonadals are at their best once they have found their personal identity. By creating and maintaining their own safe environment, they are free to fully express themselves. They are able to see the beauty in everything, especially themselves, and bring it out so everyone else can see it. The real purpose of their nurturing is to bring forth and allow the other person to express their essence. Beauty is the essence of all that is, the part of everything that is real, the element of truth. Sharing the inspiration beauty brings makes beholding the beauty an emotional experience.

Activating the emotions ignites the creative spark. Being emotional requires being open and vulnerable. Creativity is a receptive state that requires a safe, protected environment. A nurturing environment allows them to be light, spontaneous, and playful. Creativity is an experience rather than a mental process which requires letting go of the mind to access the creative source.

Gonadals recognize their feelings as the activating energy that leads them back to their magical essence – God – their creative source. Creativity comes when they bring the magic back into their lives through adventure, fun and feeling unlimited. Accessing the magical child within allows the dream or make believe to become real. Gonadals nurture by creating an atmosphere or environment where everyone enjoys being themselves and can have fun, which releases the creative energy in everyone.

Gonadal

FOOD LISTS

HEALTHY FOOD LIST

FREQUENTLY FOODS	3-7 meals per week – refers to each food, rather than category.
DENSE PROTEIN	Beef liver, buffalo, beef broth (as a base); chicken livers, chicken broth, turkey, cornish game hen; catfish, cod, flounder, haddock, herring, mackerel, mahi mahi, perch, red snapper, yellow-tail tuna, mussels
DAIRY	Buttermilk, yogurt (plain, strawberry, raspberry, spiced apple), butter
CHEESE	Low fat or nonfat cottage, cream, feta, kefir, Muenster, Parmesan, ricotta, Romano, Swiss
NUTS and SEEDS	Brazils, water chestnuts, filberts, macadamias (raw, roasted), salted peanuts (raw, roasted), pecans, pine nuts (raw, roasted), walnuts (black, English), raw or roasted seeds (caraway, pumpkin, sesame, sunflower)
LEGUMES	Beans (black, lima [butter], garbanzo, great northern, kidney, navy, red, soy), black-eyed peas, split pea
GRAINS	Corn, rice (brown basmati, short grain brown), faccia (Italian bread), vegetarian flour tortillas, bran muffins, oat bran bagels, pasta (all varieties), pasta with oil (safflower, canola, or olive), couscous, udon noodles, Chinese rice noodles, cream of rice, cream of rye
VEGETABLES	Green beans, broccoli, carrots, cucumber, garlic, white rose potatoes, seaweed (arame, dulse, kelp, nori, wakame)
VEGETABLE JUICES	Carrot/celery/cucumber
FRUITS	Strawberries, bananas, nectarines, mixed fruit, cantaloupes, pineapples, dates, raisins
FRUIT JUICES	Cran/raspberry, mango, orange/pineapple
SWEETENERS	Re-Vita®, stevia
VEGETABLE OILS	Almond, avocado, all-blend, canola, corn, olive, safflower, sesame, soy, sunflower
CONDIMENTS	Sea salt
BEVERAGES	Herbal iced tea
MODERATELY FOODS	1-2 meals per week – refers to each food, rather than category.
DENSE PROTEIN	Lean beef, lamb, pork, ham, bacon, sausage, veal, venison, organ meats (heart, brain); chicken, duck; anchovy, bass, bonita, halibut, orange roughy, salmon, sardines, shark, sole, swordfish, trout, tuna; abalone, calamari (squid), clams, crab, eel, lobster, octopus, oysters, scallops, shrimp; eggs

Gonadal

DAIRY	Milk (whole, low fat, nonfat, raw), half & half, sweet cream, sour cream, kefir, flavored yogurt, ice cream (Ben & Jerry's®, Dreyer's, Swensen's®)
CHEESE	American, blue, brie, Camembert, Cheddar, Colby, Edam, goat, Gouda, low fat Jack, Limburger, part skim mozzarella
NUTS and SEEDS	Almonds (raw, roasted), almond butter, cashews (raw, roasted), cashew butter, coconuts, hazelnuts, macadamia butter, unsalted peanuts in shell (raw, roasted), pistachios, sesame seed butter, sunflower seed butter
LEGUMES	Beans (adzuki, pinto), lentils, hummus, miso, soy milk, tofu
GRAINS	Amaranth, barley, buckwheat, corn bread, corn grits, corn tortillas, hominy grits, millet, oats, popcorn, quinoa, rice (white basmati, long grain brown, wild, Japanese), rice bran, rice cakes, rye, triticale, whole wheat, wheat bran, wheat germ, refined wheat flour, breads (French, garlic, Italian, sourdough, oat, corn, corn/rye, rye, rice), croissants, bagels, English muffins, flour tortillas, sprouted wheat tortillas, whole wheat tortillas, crackers (saltines, wheat, oat, rye), cream of wheat
VEGETABLES	Artichokes, asparagus, avocados, bamboo shoots, yellow wax beans, lima beans, beets, bok choy, broccoflower, brussels sprouts, cabbage (green, napa, red), cauliflower, celery, chard, cilantro, corn, eggplant, greens (beet, collard, mustard, turnip), jicama, kale, kohlrabi, leeks, lettuce (Boston, butter, endive, iceberg, red leaf, romaine), mushrooms, okra, olives (black, green, ripe), onions (brown, red, white, yellow, vidalia), parsley, parsnips, peas, snow pea pods, bell peppers (green, red, yellow), chili peppers, pimentos, potatoes (red, yukon gold, purple), sweet potatoes, pumpkin, radish, daikon radish, rutabaga, sauerkraut, shallots, spinach, sprouts (alfalfa, clover, mung bean, radish, sunflower), squash (acorn, banana, butternut, spaghetti, yellow [summer], zucchini), tomatoes (canned, hot-house, vine-ripened), turnips, watercress, yams
VEGETABLE JUICES	Celery, carrot, carrot/celery, parsley, spinach, tomato, V-8®
FRUITS	Apples (Golden or Red Delicious, Gala, Granny Smith, Jonathan, McIntosh, Pippin, Rome Beauty), apricots, blackberries, blueberries, boysenberries, cranberries, gooseberries, raspberries, cherries, grapes (black, green, red), grapefruits (white, red), guavas, kiwi, kumquats, lemons, limes, loquats, mangos, melons (crenshaw, watermelon), oranges, papayas, peaches, pears, persimmons, plums (black, purple, red), pomegranates, rhubarb, tangerines, tangelos, figs (fresh, dried), prunes
FRUIT JUICES	Apple, apple cider, apple/apricot, apricot, black cherry, red cherry, cranapple, cranberry, grape (purple, red, white), grapefruit, guava, lemon, papaya, pear, pineapple, pineapple/coconut, prune, tangerine, watermelon
VEGETABLE OILS	Coconut, peanut, flaxseed
SWEETENERS	Honey, molasses, sorghum, brown sugar, date sugar, raw sugar, refined cane sugar, maple syrup, brown rice syrup, barley malt syrup, corn syrup, fructose, succonant, saccharin

Gonadal

CONDIMENTS	Dijon mustard, mustard, catsup, horseradish, soy sauce, barbecue sauce, pesto sauce, salsa, tahini, vinegar, salt, Vege-Sal®, pickles
SALAD DRESSINGS	Blue cheese, French, ranch, creamy Italian, creamy avocado, thousand island, vinegar and oil, lemon juice and oil
DESSERTS	Custards, tapioca, puddings, pies, cakes, chocolate, desserts containing chocolate, raspberry sherbet, orange sherbet
CHIPS	Bean, corn (blue, white, yellow), potato
BEVERAGES	Coffee, coffee with Re-Vita®; herbal tea, black tea, green tea, Japanese tea, Chinese oolong tea; mineral water, sparkling water; white wine, red wine, sake, liqueurs, champagne, beer, barley malt liquor, gin, Scotch, vodka, whiskey; regular sodas, root beer

RARELY FOODS	No more than once a month
DAIRY	Frozen yogurt, goat milk, most ice creams
NUTS and SEEDS	Peanut butter
GRAINS	Polished rice, breads (7-grain, multi-grain, sprouted grain, whole wheat)
VEGETABLES	Arugula, russet potatoes, green onions, chives
FRUITS	Melons (casaba, honeydew)
FRUIT JUICES	Orange
SWEETENERS	Aspertame, Equal®, NutraSweet®, Sweet'n Low®
CONDIMENTS	Mayonnaise, margarine
BEVERAGES	Diet sodas

SENSITIVE FOOD LIST

FREQUENTLY FOODS	3-7 meals per week – refers to each food, rather than category.
DENSE PROTEIN	Turkey
CHEESE	Low fat or nonfat cottage cheese
NUTS and SEEDS	Salted peanuts (raw, roasted), pecans, walnuts (black, English), raw or roasted seeds (pumpkin, sunflower)
GRAINS	Corn, vegetarian flour tortillas, pasta (all varieties), couscous, udon noodles
VEGETABLES	Green beans, carrots, cucumbers
FRUITS	Bananas, cantaloupes, nectarines, mixed fruit, pineapples, dates, raisins
VEGETABLE OILS	Olive, canola
CONDIMENTS	Sea salt
BEVERAGES	Herbal iced tea

Gonadal

MODERATELY FOODS	1-2 meals per week – refers to each food, rather than category.
DENSE PROTEIN	Beef broth, beef liver, buffalo, lamb, pork, ham, bacon, sausage, veal, venison, organ meats (heart, brain); chicken, chicken broth, chicken livers, cornish game hen, duck; anchovy, bass, bonita, catfish, cod, flounder, haddock, halibut, herring, mackerel, mahi-mahi, perch, orange roughy, salmon, sardines, shark, red snapper, sole, swordfish, trout, tuna; abalone, calamari (squid), clams, crab, eel, lobster, mussels, octopus, oysters, scallops, shrimp; eggs
DAIRY	Milk (whole, 2%, low fat, nonfat, raw), half & half, sweet cream, sour cream, kefir, plain and flavored yogurt, butter
CHEESE	American, blue, brie, Camembert, Cheddar, Colby, cream, Edam, feta, Gouda, low fat Jack, kefir, Limburger, part skim mozzarella, Muenster, Parmesan, ricotta, Romano, Swiss
NUTS and SEEDS	Almonds (raw, roasted), almond butter, Brazils, cashews (raw, roasted), cashew butter, water chestnuts, coconuts, filberts, hazelnuts, macadamias, (raw, roasted), macadamia butter, unsalted peanuts in shell (raw, roasted), pine nuts (raw, roasted), pistachios, raw or roasted seeds (caraway, sesame), sesame seed butter, sunflower seed butter
LEGUMES	Beans (adzuki, black, lima [butter], garbanzo, great northern, kidney, navy, pinto, red, soy), black-eyed peas, split peas, hummus, miso, soy milk, tofu
GRAINS	Amaranth, barley, corn bread, corn grits, corn tortillas, hominy grits, millet, oats, popcorn, quinoa, rice (brown and white basmati, long and short grain brown, wild, Japanese), rice bran, rice cakes, rye, triticale, whole wheat, wheat bran, wheat germ, refined wheat flour, flour tortillas, sprouted wheat tortillas, whole wheat tortillas, breads (French, garlic, Italian (faccia), oat, corn, corn/rye, rye, rice, white), croissants, bagels, oat bran bagels, bran muffins, English muffins, crackers (saltines, wheat, oat, rye), pasta with oil (safflower, canola or olive), Chinese rice noodles, cream of rice, cream of rye, cream of wheat
VEGETABLES	Artichokes, asparagus, avocados, bamboo shoots, lima beans, yellow wax beans, beets, bok choy, broccoli, broccoflower, brussels sprouts, cabbage (green, napa, red), cauliflower, celery, chard, cilantro, corn, eggplant, garlic, greens (beet, collard, mustard, turnip), jicama, kale, kohlrabi, leeks, lettuce (Boston, butter, endive, red leaf, romaine), mushrooms, okra, olives (green, ripe), parsley, parsnips, snow pea pods, bell peppers (green, red, yellow), chili peppers, pimentos, potatoes (red, white rose, yukon gold, purple), pumpkin, radish, daikon radish, rutabaga, sauerkraut, seaweed (arame, dulse, kelp, nori, wakame), shallots, spinach, sprouts (alfalfa, clover, mung bean, radish, sunflower), squash (acorn, banana, butternut, spaghetti, yellow [summer], zucchini), turnips, watercress
VEGETABLE JUICES	Celery, carrot, carrot/celery, parsley, spinach, tomato, V-8®
FRUITS	Apples (Golden or Red Delicious, Gala, Granny Smith, Jonathan, McIntosh, Pippin, Rome Beauty), apricots, blackberries, blueberries, boysenberries, cranberries, gooseberries, raspberries, strawberries, cherries, grapes (black,

Gonadal

	green, red), grapefruits (white, red), guavas, kiwi, kumquats, lemons, limes, loquats, mangos, melons (crenshaw, watermelon), oranges, papayas, peaches, pears, persimmons, pomegranates, rhubarb, tangelos, tangerines, figs (fresh, dried), prunes
FRUIT JUICES	Apple, apple cider, apple/apricot, apricot, black cherry, red cherry, cranapple, cranberry, grape (purple, red, white), grapefruit, guava, lemon, papaya, pear, pineapple, pineapple/coconut, prune, tangerine, watermelon
VEGETABLE OILS	All-blend, avocado, coconut, corn, safflower, sesame
SWEETENERS	Barley malt syrup, Re-Vita®, stevia
CONDIMENTS	Salsa, tahini, vinegar, salt, Vege-Sal,® pickles
SALAD DRESSINGS	Vinegar and oil, lemon juice and oil
BEVERAGES	Herbal tea, green tea, Japanese tea, Chinese oolong tea; mineral water, sparkling water
RARELY FOODS	No more than once a month
DENSE PROTEIN	Lean beef
DAIRY	Buttermilk, goat milk, goat cheese,most ice creams, frozen yogurt
NUTS and SEEDS	Peanut butter
LEGUMES	Lentils
GRAINS	Buckwheat, polished rice, breads (sourdough, whole wheat, 7-grain, multi-grain, sprouted grain)
VEGETABLES	Arugula, onions (chives, green, brown, red, vidalia, white, yellow), russet potatoes, sweet potatoes, peas, iceberg lettuce, tomatoes (canned, hot-house, vine-ripened), yams
FRUITS	Plums (black, purple, red), melons (casaba, honeydew)
FRUIT JUICES	Orange
VEGETABLE OILS	Almond, peanut, flaxseed, soy, sunflower
SWEETENERS	Honey, molasses, sorghum, brown sugar, refined cane sugar, raw sugar, date sugar, corn syrup, maple syrup, brown rice syrup, fructose, saccharin, succonant, aspertame, Equal®, NutraSweet®, Sweet'n Low®
CONDIMENTS	Catsup, mayonnaise, mustard, soy sauce, margarine, dijon mustard, horseradish, barbecue sauce, pesto sauce, margarine
SALAD DRESSINGS	Blue cheese, French, ranch, creamy Italian, creamy avocado, thousand island
DESSERTS	Custards, tapioca, puddings, pies, cakes, chocolate, desserts containing chocolate, raspberry sherbet, orange sherbet
CHIPS	Bean, corn (blue, white, yellow), potato
BEVERAGES	Coffee; black tea; white wine, red wine, champagne, beer, barley malt liquor, gin, Scotch, vodka, whiskey; root beer, diet sodas, regular sodas

Gonadal

MENUS

DIETARY EMPHASIS:

- Fruit (peaches, bananas, Gala apples, cranberries, dates, raisins, prunes), vegetables (avocados, yams, tomatoes).
- Vegetables – more cooked than raw.
- Cottage cheese, fish, turkey, and brown rice.

WEIGHT LOSS:

- Reduce fats to 15% of calories and select them from the recommended sources.
- Avoid bread for lunch.
- Avoid spices.
- Minimize grain at dinner.

WEIGHT GAIN:

- Increase food intake.

VEGETARIAN DIET:

- Recommended when healthy, although up to 30% of caloric intake may consist of dense protein.

FATS:

- 15% of caloric intake for weight loss, 25% for maintenance.
- Best sources are nuts (almonds, Brazils, cashews, hazel nuts, pecans, macadamias, walnuts), seeds (pumpkin, sunflower), oils (avocado, olive, safflower, sesame), and butter.

SENSITIVE:

- Avoid fruit, nuts and seeds at lunch and dinner.

KEY

—all menus may be used by healthy persons
( ) around foods means that they're optional
L denotes weight loss menus
S denotes sensitive menus
G denotes weight gain menus

BREAKFAST:

7-9 a.m. Light, with fruit or moderate, with protein, nuts, seeds, grain, fruit, and/or dairy.

L	S	G	Menu
L	S		Banana
	S		Banana w/yogurt
L			Apple, strawberries or pineapple
L			Watermelon or cantaloupe
L			Cherries or nectarine
			Pear or mango
			Fruit dish apple, banana, nectarine, and cantaloupe
		G	Avocado
L			V-8® juice
			Cantaloupe or pineapple (cottage cheese)
L		G	Strawberry yogurt w/pine nuts and sunflower seeds
L			Yogurt w/strawberries
L	S		Plain yogurt w/raspberries
		G	Apple and cheese
L			Nonfat cottage cheese and nectarine
			Fruit smoothie banana, strawberries, and apple juice (nectarine)
			Cranberry concentrate, berry Re-Vita®, and water
		G	Eggs, date/nut toast w/butter, and milk (w/Re-Vita®)
L		G	Scrambled egg, nonfat cheddar cheese, and couscous
		G	Boiled egg and banana or apple
L		G	Eggs and turkey (apple)
			Egg, puffed millet, cran/raspberry juice, and ginseng tea
		G	French toast
L		G	Turkey, white rose potatoes, and pear
L			Chicken, brown basmati rice, peas, tomatoes, and capers
	S	G	Granola and strawberry or raspberry kefir
	S	G	All Bran® or muesli and kefir
			Puffed cereal and kefir
		G	Oatmeal and raisins or banana or apple
L			Oatmeal (fruit yogurt)
	S		Cream of rice or cream of rye
			Cooked wheat cereal
			Danish apple bread (apple)
		G	Date nut raisin bread (banana)

Gonadal

L Bran muffin w/nonfat cream cheese and cantaloupe
L Toasted oat bran bagel w/nonfat cream cheese and pineapple
L Rice cakes and hummus
G Italian bread, cashew butter, and banana
G Italian bread w/almond butter (raisins)
S Waffles or pancakes and Re-Vita®
L Coffee or tea

MID-MORNING SNACK:
(Optional) Fruit, dairy.
Fruit or fruit juice
Yogurt

LUNCH:
1-3 p.m. Light-to-heavy, with protein, legumes, grain, nuts, seeds, fruit, dairy and/or vegetables.

SENSITIVE: Avoid nuts, seeds, and fruit.

L G Beef, baked potato, and carrots and peas, or raw carrots and celery
S G Turkey on Italian bread w/red leaf lettuce, and tomato
L Turkey or chicken and salad w/vinaigrette dressing
G Turkey and Cheddar cheese on flour tortilla
L Turkey and lowfat cheese on tortilla
S Ground turkey lasagna, and salad: romaine lettuce, tomato, carrot, celery, and Italian dressing
Tuna salad in tomato
S G Tuna salad on oat bread
S Tuna, Chinese noodles, mushroom soup, celery, and onion
L S Tuna, cottage cheese, and red leaf lettuce
S G Tuna, alfalfa sprouts, and rye bread
L Fish vericruse – fish, tomato sauce, and vegetables w/rice
Shrimp cocktail and crab salad w/butter lettuce, onions, avocado, and yogurt dressing
S Taco salad w/butter lettuce, kidney beans, tomato, swiss and cheddar cheeses, and turkey
G Bean, or bean and cheese burrito (rice)
G Carne asada burrito, (rice) (beans)
S G Pinto beans, flour tortilla, romaine lettuce, tomato, and Jack and Cheddar cheeses
S Spinach quiche
Pasta, broccoli, and cheese sauce
Spaghetti w/tomato or cream sauce
S G Spaghetti and Italian bread
S Pasta, green and red peppers, onion, tomato, artichoke, olives, lemon, and pesto sauce
G Grilled Cheddar cheese on rye w/tomato or dill pickle
G Italian bread, Cheddar cheese, and Hain Creamy Italian or Avocado dressing
G Submarine sandwich lunch meat, cheese, lettuce, tomato, and oil and vinegar sauce
L Salad carrots, tomatoes, butter lettuce, cucumber, any cheese, and creamy garlic dressing
L S Salad: carrots, tomatoes, garbanzos, cucumber, and creamy garlic dressinr
Salad: carrots, romaine lettuce, red cabbage, cucumbers, broccoli, red or yellow bell peppers, sunflower seeds, and olive oil or vinegar and oil
S Salad: romaine lettuce, tomato, carrots, celery, and Italian dressing w/Italian bread
L Salad: cucumber, bell pepper, beets, romaine lettuce, oil and vinegar dressing, and low fat cottage cheese
L Salad: romaine lettuce, cucumber, bell pepper, shoestring beets, turkey or chicken, and vinaigrette dressing
Steamed vegetables: broccoli, cauliflower, and carrots
Minestrone soup
S G Zucchini bread

MID-AFTERNOON SNACK:
(Optional) Grain, dairy, nuts, seeds, vegetables.
Carrot/celery/cucumber juice
Colby, mozzarella, or Cheddar cheese and Ritz® crackers
Rice cakes (cashew butter)

Gonadal

Corn chips (salsa)
Popcorn (butter)

LUNCH or DINNER:

G Sea bass, carrots, and rice
Shrimp, peas, and white basmati rice
L Tuna salad, avocado, lettuce, and tomato
Crab, pasta, and salad
G Chicken or fish tacos w/lettuce, guacamole, salsa, and onions, and beans and rice
Chicken, basmati rice, butter, yellow squash, and peas or brussels sprouts
Turkey, broccoli, and pasta
Eggs, Cheddar cheese, red potatoes, and onions
G Italian bread, salami, and cheese
Cheese enchiladas, and chili rellenos (medium salsa) (rice) (beans)
Quesedilla: flour tortilla w/Cheddar cheese, onions, guacamole, and sour cream (carne asada burrito)
Flour tortilla, beans, cheese, and salsa
L Flour tortilla, pinto beans, and onions
G Corn tortilla, pinto beans, and cheese (lettuce and/or salsa) (rice)
Tostadas
L Rice, black beans, and onions
Sweet potatoes, peas, and salad (fish)
Spaghetti w/tomato sauce (meat balls)
G Lasagna or manicotti (garlic bread)
L Tuna and broccoli

DINNER:
8-12 p.m. Moderate-to-heavy, with protein, legumes, grain, vegetables, nuts, seeds and/or dairy.

SENSITIVE: Avoid fruit, nuts and seeds.

G Fillet of sole, green beans, and rice or pasta
G Swordfish, rice pilaf, and salad
L Tuna and broccoli
G Turkey, broccoli, and rice
G Turkey, provolone cheese, and horseradish on rye
L Turkey, potatoes, green beans, and mushrooms
S Turkey and corn on the cob
S Tacos w/lettuce, tomato, onion, ground turkey, and cheese
S Chicken enchiladas
Chicken, pasta, yellow squash, brussels sprouts, carrots, and onions
G Chicken breast, rice, and brussels sprouts
L Chicken, potatoes, carrots, and onions or peas
L Beef, yukon gold potatoes, and peas
L Beefsteak or roast beef, zucchini, tomatoes, and spinach salad raw spinach, celery, carrots, and Italian dressing
S Porcupine balls: hamburger, rice, and egg in tomato sauce w/salad
L S Yukon gold potato w/yogurt, green beans, and salad
S Baked yukon gold potato, yogurt, corn, and green beans
L Vegetable soup in turkey broth w/celery, carrots, onions, small amount of corn (barley)
Vegetarian pizza
S G Pasta, spinach, corn, and Italian bread
S Angel hair pasta w/sun-dried tomatoes, Parmesan cheese, tomato sauce, and salad
S G Angel hair pasta w/butter and Parmesan cheese
S Mock ravioli: lasagna, spinach, egg, garlic, onion, Parmesan cheese, and meat sauce

EVENING SNACK:
(Optional) Fruit, grain, dairy, vegetables, protein, sweets.
Healthy may include nuts and seeds.

S Apple, blueberries, strawberries, raspberries, red grapes, or orange
Fruit juice
L Nonfat cream cheese roll
L Oatmeal raisin cookies
L Chocolate chip cookies w/out nuts
Peach cobbler
Ice cream

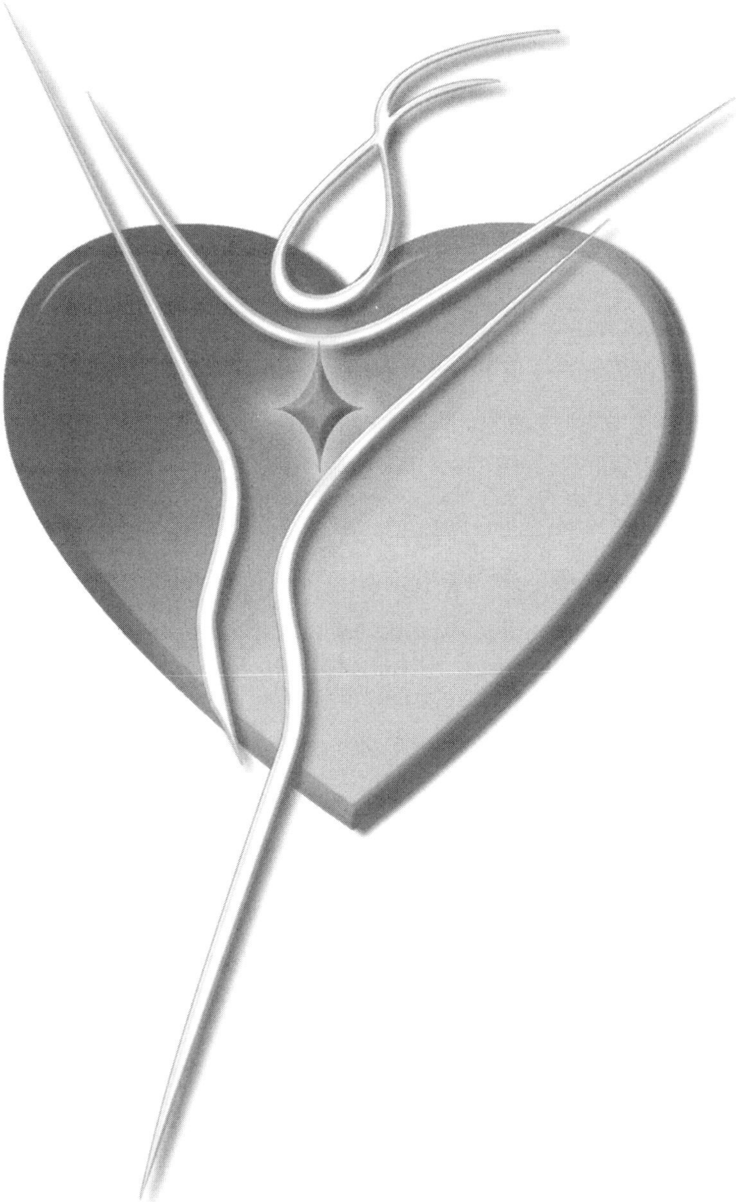

The "Heart Body Type"
is symbolized by a heart. Huggable and approachable, they set the beat by getting in step with their environment and then shifting it to their desires. Like the heart, they bring their own rhythm or music to their environment.

Heart

BODY TYPE PROFILE

LOCATION	Left side of upper chest, between lungs.
FUNCTION	Circulates blood through body.
POTENTIAL HEALTH PROBLEMS	Earaches, weak kidneys, gets chilled easily. Certain foods such as corn and kidney beans may cause digestive stress. Prunes or pineapple are helpful for constipation.
RECOMMENDED EXERCISE	Exercise is optional. Its effect is initially emotional. It acts as a mood elevator and provides a means of connecting with people. For weight loss, exercise a minimum of 30 minutes (up to an hour) daily. Running, biking, brisk walking, isometric exercises, karate, and tennis may be done daily; yoga, stretching or weight lifting, 1 to 2 times a week.

WOMEN'S CHARACTERISTICS

DISTINGUISHING FEATURES	Soft, round, heart-shaped appearance. Generally sweet, gentle, warm, and approachable, with energy radiating predominantly from heart. Like the heart, they bring their own rhythm or music to their environment, readily influencing others' moods. Maintains a round, shapely appearance, even when large amounts of weight are gained.
ADDITIONAL PHYSICAL CHARACTERISTICS	Firm, shapely, rounded-to-prominent buttocks. Low back curvature straight-to-swayed. Breasts average-to-large. Shoulders narrower than, to relatively even with, hips. Waist defined to well-defined. Average to short-waisted. Height petite-to-average. Bone structure small-to-medium. Layer of softness covering muscle resulting in little definition. Small-to-average hands and feet. Heart-shaped or oval, full face. Body is often at least full size smaller above waist than below.
WEIGHT GAIN AREAS	Lower body with initial gain in lower abdomen, upper 2/3rds of thighs including upper inner thighs, inner knees, waist, middle back, and upper hips. Alternative weight gain pattern: lower abdomen, lower hips, and thighs. Secondary weight gain in face, under chin, upper arms, breasts, buttocks, and entire back.

Heart

DIETARY GUIDELINES

	SCHEDULING MEALS:
"HEALTHY"	Breakfast: Moderate, with grain, fruit, dairy, and/or limited protein. Lunch; Heavy, with protein, dairy, grain, and/or vegetables. Fruit for dessert. Dinner: Moderate, with grain, vegetables, protein, dairy, nuts, seeds, and/or legumes.
"SENSITIVE"	Breakfast: Moderate, with grain, and/or fruit. Lunch: Moderate, with grain, vegetables, legumes (beans, tofu), and/or limited protein (fish, eggs). Dinner: Early. Moderate-to-heavy, with grain, vegetables, protein (fowl, beef, lamb), nuts, seeds, and/or legumes.
DIETARY EMPHASIS	• For weight loss, eliminate all dairy except butter. • For weight gain, emphasize dairy. • Vegetarian diets inadequate, since require 10-25% of calories from dense protein. • Fats, 25-35% of total caloric intake from butter, dense protein (chicken, fish, eggs, beef, pork, lamb), and seeds (pumpkin, sesame, sunflower).
KEY SUPPORTS FOR SYSTEM	Eating fruit after lunch is very supportive. It acts as digestive aid and often eliminates the craving for sweets. Calli® tea after lunch and/or dinner helps digestion.
COMPLEMENTARY GLANDULAR SUPPORT	Thyroid, through consuming 2 oz. of dense protein with rice or pasta 5 times a week. Blood, through maintaining harmony.
FOODS CRAVED	*(When Energy is Low)* Sweets and carbohydrates, such as cookies and fruit. Creamy foods, such as ice cream and yogurt. Salty foods.
FOODS TO AVOID	Refined sugar, as it causes fatigue of muscles and brain. Also avoid honey and whole wheat bread.
RECOMMENDED CUISINE	Greek, German, Seafood, English, Oriental, Chinese

Heart

PSYCHOLOGICAL PROFILE

ESSENCE

Just as the heart beat regulates the flow of the blood throughout the body, Heart body types regulate the beat of their environment. Heart types can walk into a room and create either harmony or discord within a group, even causing conflict when they so desire. Their approach can be quite subtle, especially when they are in a new environment; first getting in step with what is going on, and then deciding whether to shift it. Being able to set the beat, they have the natural ability to influence the moods of those around them. Physically softer than most other types, they impress others as being sweet and lovable. Women are often round and heart-shaped, while men and boys are huggable like teddy bears. Like the heart, they bring their own rhythm or music to their environment.

CHARACTERISTIC TRAITS

The body type that especially inspires hugs is the Heart. Distinguished by an approachability that is hard to define but easy to recognize, Hearts are typically soft, gentle, and giving. They project a sensitivity and caring that makes others feel at ease. Gentle and supporting, Heart types are usually easy to be around. Home and family are particularly important to them, and they tend to provide the glue that creates cohesiveness in their families.

The Heart personality has a unique ability to influence the moods of others. While some are extroverted, most tend to be shy and cautious with strangers and in new situations. Very approachable, they are usually warm and receptive to others, yet passive when it comes to initiating relationships. People are drawn to them, and because of their sensitivity to others' needs, it's easy for Hearts to direct the conversation or activity.

Seeking the approval and acceptance of others, they can be very accommodating, going out of their way to avoid hurting anyone's feelings, striving to maintain peace and harmony or gently guide the situation to get their needs and desires met. Their influence is often subtle and largely non-verbal, merely a radiation of an emotional tone that others unconsciously follow. Just as the heart is central to the body's circulatory system, the Heart type becomes central to the emotional dynamics of a group or gathering.

Highly emotional and strongly connected to their feelings, Hearts are sensitive, intuitive, and expressive. With a passive, accommodating, blending-in nature, Hearts are prone to stress and can easily get uptight. Creative endeavors like music and art allow their intuitive side to express mentally. Music is particularly effective in releasing excess emotional energy, whether it be playing, listening, or dancing. Since music accurately expresses their essence, it is most effective when they let go and allow the music to move them. Other creative endeavors like painting, flower arranging or computer graphics and cartoon creation, promote a feeling of peace.

Heart

MOTIVATION

Hearts are worriers, especially men, and they worry about everything. Worry is a means of protection, and the belief is that thinking about what could happen somehow makes it less threatening. Unfortunately, putting large amounts of emotional energy into a negative pattern can sometimes attract it, or at least create stress.

Hearts react to situations, exaggerating their worst fears, traits, and mistakes. They blow things out of proportion because their feelings are so amplified, and this puts them on an emotional roller-coaster. Once they get caught in their emotions, it's hard to be objective and view anything from the outside.

In an attempt to create safety and stability, they will mentally cover as many bases as possible. When they become fatigued, or the next step becomes evasive, they will mentally go over and over the same material. This creates a mental loop that blocks intuition or creativity. Breaking the cycle can easily be accomplished by doing something physical, such as simply walking around the house or getting up to get a drink of water.

Unsure of the value or effectiveness of what they have done, Hearts will often seek outside approval and validation. The belief is that if they do everything perfectly, they'll be safe. Consequently, it's easy for them to get bogged down in details, spending too much time on a project. The desire to be thought well of will often motivate them to be reliable, competent, and responsible.

"AT WORST"

When stressed, Hearts can easily become anxious, fearful, over-emotional, and worry over everything. They can suffer from low self-esteem, reflected as "I'm not good enough." Getting caught in a feeling of failure, they will amplify anything negative and make it worse. By personifying the negative, reflecting and magnifying it, they accelerate a negative spiral. They then believe that what they see on the outside is the way it is.

Setbacks and criticism can cause Hearts to retreat within themselves where they dwell excessively on negative experiences until they feel like failures, lose their motivation, and eventually give up on life. They may become couch potatoes, eating primarily junk food and expecting others to take care of them. When it comes to food, or life in general, Hearts will often satisfy their senses, taking the easiest way, and doing what is most convenient. Food or drugs are easy ways of sedating their emotions.

Emotionally oriented, the approval of others is often the basis of their self-approval. Not wanting to do anything that would make them stand out or appear to be in error, they are likely to "go with the flow" to gain acceptance, denying their feelings and intuition in the process. Since self-worth is often connected with how other people respond to them, there is a tendency to tell people what they want to hear, or withhold information that could upset someone, and then fail to follow through on agreements.

When Hearts are not at peace with themselves, their natural ability to influence others' moods can produce discord and conflict. Two Hearts in the

Heart

"AT WORST"

same house, particularly boys, usually experience a need to establish their own identity and demonstrate some form of control. This is when they are apt to express opposite poles, such as positive or negative and introverted or extroverted. The result can be either balanced or destructive, harmony or chaos, or positive or negative emotions and exchanges.

In an attempt to do what is best, protect from harm and control their environment, Hearts can become too persistent. This control element comes into play when Hearts feel that their solution is what's best for the other person. To get someone else to do what they want, they will verbally wear them down to where they give in just to shut the Heart up, also known as nagging.

"AT BEST"

Hearts at their best bring a gentle, harmonious, peaceful atmosphere into their environment. Their calm, positive, good natured, supportive attitude is encouraging to others and helps them find the best in themselves.

Having found their own sense of self-worth within, rather than looking for it outside in the way others react to them, allows these basic positive qualities to naturally surface. Once they have learned to open their hearts to themselves, to give and nurture themselves, self-approval is easy and peace is the result.

Intuitive and emotionally sensitive, Hearts are extremely aware and considerate of the feelings of others. Loyal in relationships, and family-oriented, nurturing and supportive, they are easy to talk to and readily listen to others, providing strength and comfort. By their very nature, they tend to draw out the best in those who associate with them.

Their real gift lies is in manifesting the spiritual principles of peace, harmony, love and emotion into the practical, physical world. Good-natured, conscientious and self-sufficient, they excel in what they set out to do and do it well, being particularly aware of the details. Sensitive and caring, they can be models of success in both business and personal relationships.

With their exceptional ability to manifest whatever they focus on, and the emotional energy to propel it, Hearts need to be particularly vigilant about what they allow their minds to dwell upon. Not only do they affect their own lives, but they readily influence the moods of others. When love is the dominant feeling, peace and harmony prevail.

Heart

FOOD LISTS

HEALTHY FOOD LIST

FREQUENTLY FOODS	3-7 meals a week – refers to each food, rather than category.
DENSE PROTEIN	Beef, beef liver, beef broth, buffalo, lamb, pork, ham, bacon, sausage, organ meats (heart, brain) veal, venison; turkey, chicken, chicken broth, chicken livers, cornish game hens, duck; anchovy, bass, bonita, catfish, cod, flounder, haddock, halibut, herring, mackerel, mahi-mahi, perch, roughy, salmon, sardines, shark, red snapper, sole, swordfish, trout, tuna; abalone, calamari (squid), clams, crab, eel, lobster, mussels, octopus, oysters, scallops, shrimp; eggs
DAIRY	Butter
CHEESE	Nonfat cottage cheese, cream cheese
NUTS and SEEDS	Almonds without skin, cashews (raw, roasted), cashew butter, pistachios, pumpkin seeds, sesame seeds, sesame seed butter, raw sunflower seeds
LEGUMES	Beans (adzuki, black, lima [butter], navy, great northern, red, soy), black-eyed peas
GRAINS	Amaranth, barley, buckwheat, oats, popcorn, quinoa, rice (all varieties), rice cakes, rice bran, rye, wheat germ, breads (oat, rice, rye), cream of rice, cream of rye, cream of wheat
VEGETABLES	Green beans, yellow wax beans, lima beans, beets, broccoli, carrots, celery, onions (chives, green, brown, red, white, yellow, vidalia), peas, snow pea pods, potatoes (all varieties), seaweed (arame, dulse, kelp, nori, wakame)
VEGETABLE JUICES	Carrot,carrot/beet, carrot/celery, celery, spinach
FRUITS	Apples (Red or Golden Delicious, Granny Smith, Jonathan, McIntosh, Pippin, Rome Beauty), apricots, blackberries, blueberries, boysenberries, cranberries, gooseberries, raspberries, strawberries, grapes (black, green, red),grapefruits (red, white), guavas, kiwi, kumquats, lemons, limes, loquats, mangos, nectarines, oranges, papayas, peaches, pears, pineapples, plums (black, red, purple), tangerines, dates, figs, prunes, raisins
FRUIT JUICES	Apple, apple cider, apple/apricot, apricot, cranberry, grape (white, purple, red), grapefruit, guava, lemon, papaya, pear, pineapple, pineapple/coconut, prune, tangerine
SWEETENERS	Molasses, sorghum, barley malt syrup, barley malt powder, Re-Vita®, stevia
MODERATELY FOODS	1-2 meals a week – refers to each food, rather than category.
DAIRY	Whole milk, raw milk, half & half, sweet cream, sour cream, buttermilk, goat milk, kefir, yogurt (plain, flavored), ice cream (Dreyer's, Ben & Jerry's®, Swensen's®, Alta Dena®)

Heart

CHEESE	American, blue, brie, Camembert, Cheddar, Colby, low fat and regular cottage, Edam, Feta, goat, Gouda, Jack, kefir, Limburger, mozzarella, Muenster, Parmesan, ricotta, Romano, Swiss
NUTS and SEEDS	Almonds (raw, roasted), almond butter, Brazils, water chestnuts, coconuts, filberts, hazelnuts, macadamias (raw, roasted), macadamia butter, peanuts (raw, roasted with or without salt), peanut butter, pecans, pine nuts (raw, roasted), walnuts (black, English), roasted sunflower seeds, nut milk, sunflower seed butter
LEGUMES	Pinto beans, lentils, split green peas, soy milk, tofu, miso
GRAINS	Corn, corn bread, corn grits, corn tortillas, hominy grits, millet, triticale, refined wheat flour, flour tortillas, wheat bran, breads (French, Italian, corn, corn/rye, garlic, sourdough, 7-grain, multi-grain, white bread), croissants, bagels, English muffins, crackers (oat, rye, wheat, saltines), couscous, pasta, udon noodles, Chinese rice noodles
VEGETABLES	Artichokes, avocado, bamboo shoots, bok choy, broccoflower, brussels sprouts, cabbage (green, napa, red), cauliflower, chard, cilantro, cucumbers, eggplant, garlic, greens (beet, collard, mustard, turnip), hominy, jicama, kale, kohlrabi, leeks, lettuce (Boston, butter, red leaf, romaine), mushrooms, okra, olives (green, ripe), parsnips, bell peppers (green, red, yellow), chili peppers, pimentos, sweet potato, pumpkin, radish, daikon radish, rutabaga, sauerkraut, shallots, spinach, sprouts (alfalfa, clover, mung bean, radish, sunflower), squash (acorn, banana, butternut, spaghetti, yellow [summer], zucchini), tomatoes, turnips, watercress, yams
VEGETABLE JUICE	V-8®
FRUITS	Bananas, cherries, melons (cantaloupe, casaba, crenshaw, honeydew, watermelon), persimmons, pomegranates, rhubarb, tangelos
FRUIT JUICES	Black cherry, red cherry, cranapple, orange
VEGETABLE OILS	All-blend, almond, avocado, canola, coconut, corn, flaxseed, olive, peanut, safflower, sesame, soy, sunflower
SWEETENERS	Brown sugar, date sugar, raw sugar, corn syrup, maple syrup, brown rice syrup, fructose, succonant
CONDIMENTS	Salt, sea salt, Vege-Sal®, tahini, salsa, soy sauce, barbecue sauce, pesto sauce, mayonnaise, horseradish, mustard, vinegar
SALAD DRESSINGS	Blue cheese, French, ranch, creamy Italian, creamy avocado, thousand island, vinegar and oil, lemon juice and oil
DESSERTS	Custards, tapioca, puddings, pies, cakes, chocolate, desserts containing chocolate, raspberry sherbet, orange sherbet
CHIPS	Bean, corn (blue, white, yellow), potato
BEVERAGES	Coffee with Re-Vita®; herbal tea, black tea, green tea, Japanese tea, Chinese oolong tea; mineral water, sparkling water; barley malt liquor, champagne, gin, Scotch, vodka, whiskey; root beer, regular sodas

Heart

RARELY FOODS	No more than once a month
DAIRY	Nonfat or low fat milk, frozen yogurt, most ice creams
LEGUMES	Garbanzo and kidney beans, hummus
GRAINS	Whole wheat, sprouted grain bread, whole wheat bread
VEGETABLES	Arugula, asparagus, corn, lettuce (iceberg, bib, endive), parsley
VEGETABLE JUICES	Parsley, tomato
SWEETENERS	Honey, refined cane sugar, saccharin, aspertame Equal,® Sweet'n Low®, NutraSweet®
CONDIMENTS	Catsup, margarine
BEVERAGES	Coffee; wine (red, white), sake, liqueurs, beer; diet sodas

SENSITIVE FOOD LIST

FREQUENTLY FOODS	3-7 meals a week – refers to each food, rather than category.
DENSE PROTEIN	Pork, ham, bacon, sausage, organ meats (heart, brain); eggs
DAIRY	Butter
CHEESE	Nonfat cottage cheese, cream cheese
NUTS and SEEDS	Cashews, cashew butter, pistachios, pumpkin seeds, sesame seeds, sesame seed butter
GRAINS	Oats, rye, rice (all varieties), rice cakes, breads (oat, rice, rye, pumpernickle)
VEGETABLES	Beets, broccoli, carrots, celery, peas, snow pea pods, potatoes (all varieties)
VEGETABLE JUICES	Carrot, celery, carrot/celery
FRUITS	Blueberries, grapes (purple, green, red), papayas, pineapples, dates, prunes
FRUIT JUICES	Grape (purple, red, white), papaya, pineapple, pineapple/coconut, prune
SWEETENERS	Molasses, sorghum, barley malt syrup, barley malt powder
MODERATELY FOODS	1-2 meals a week – refers to each food, rather than category.
DENSE PROTEIN	Beef, beef broth, beef liver, buffalo, lamb, veal, venison; turkey, chicken, chicken broth, chicken livers, cornish game hens, duck; anchovy, bass, bonita, catfish, cod, flounder, haddock, herring, mackerel, mahi-mahi, perch, roughy, salmon, sardines, shark, red snapper, sole, swordfish, trout, tuna; abalone, calamari (squid), clams, crab, eel, lobster, mussels, octopus, oysters, scallops, shrimp
DAIRY	Whole milk, raw milk, half & half, goat milk, sweet cream, sour cream, buttermilk, plain kefir
CHEESE	American, blue, brie, Camembert, Cheddar, Colby, Edam, feta, goat, Gouda, Jack, kefir, Limburger, mozzarella, Muenster, Parmesan, ricotta, Romano, Swiss

Heart

NUTS and SEEDS	Almonds (raw or roasted without skin), almond butter, Brazils, water chestnuts, coconuts, filberts, hazelnuts, macadamias (raw, roasted), macadamia butter, peanuts (raw or roasted with or without salt), peanut butter, pecans, pine nuts (raw, roasted), walnuts (black, English), caraway seeds (raw, roasted), sunflower seeds (raw, roasted), sunflower seed butter, nut milk
LEGUMES	Beans (adzuki, black, lima [butter], navy, great northern, red, soy), lentils, black-eyed peas, split green peas, soy milk, tofu, miso
GRAINS	Amaranth, barley, corn, corn bread, corn grits, corn tortillas, hominy grits, millet, popcorn, quinoa, rice bran, triticale, wheat germ, wheat bran, refined wheat flour, flour tortillas, breads (white, French, Italian, sourdough, garlic, corn, corn/rye), croissants, bagels, English muffins, crackers (oat, rye, saltines) pasta, couscous, udon noodles, Chinese rice noodles, cream of rice, cream of wheat, cream of rye
VEGETABLES	Artichokes, avocados, bamboo shoots, green beans, lima beans, yellow wax beans, bok choy, broccoflower, brussels sprouts, cabbage (green, napa, red), cauliflower, chard, cilantro, cucumbers, eggplant, garlic, greens (beet, collard, mustard, turnip), hominy, jicama, kale, kohlrabi, leeks, mushrooms, okra, olives (green, ripe), onions (chives, green, brown, red, white, yelllow, vidalia), parsnips, bell peppers (green, red, yellow), chili peppers, pimentos, sweet potatoes, pumpkin, radish, daikon radish, rutabaga, sauerkraut, seaweed (arame, dulse, kelp, nori, wakame), shallots, spinach, sprouts (alfalfa, mung bean, clover, radish, sunflower), squash (acorn, banana, butternut, spaghetti, yellow [summer], zucchini), tomatoes, turnips, watercress, yams
VEGETABLE JUICES	Spinach, V-8®
FRUITS	Apples (Red or Golden Delicious, Granny Smith, Jonathan, McIntosh, Pippin, Rome Beauty), apricots, bananas, blackberries, boysenberries, cranberries, gooseberries, raspberries, strawberries, cherries, grapefruits (white, red), guava, kiwi, kumquats, lemons, limes, loquats, mangos, melons (cantaloupe, casaba, crenshaw, honeydew), nectarines, oranges, peaches, pears, persimmons, plums (red, black, purple), pomegranates, rhubarb, tangelos, tangerines, figs, raisins
FRUIT JUICES	Apple, apple cider, apple/apricot, apricot, black cherry, red cherry, cranapple, cranberry, grapefruit, guava, lemon, orange, pear, tangerine
VEGETABLE OILS	All-blend, avocado, coconut
SWEETENERS	Re-Vita®, stevia
CONDIMENTS	Salt, sea salt, Vege-Sal®, vinegar
SALAD DRESSINGS	Vinegar and oil, lemon juice and oil
BEVERAGES	Herbal tea, green tea, Japanese tea, Chinese oolong tea; mineral water, sparkling water

Heart

RARELY FOODS	No more than once a month
DENSE PROTEIN	Halibut
DAIRY	Nonfat or low fat milk, plain or flavored yogurt, flavored kefir, frozen yogurt, most ice creams
LEGUMES	Beans (garbanzo, kidney, pinto), hummus
GRAINS	Buckwheat, whole wheat, breads (sprouted grain, whole wheat, 7-grain, multi-grain), whole wheat crackers
VEGETABLES	Arugula, asparagus, corn, eggplant, parsley, lettuce (all varieties)
VEGETABLE JUICES	Parsley, tomato
FRUITS	Watermelon
VEGETABLE OILS	Almond, canola, corn, flaxseed, olive, peanut, safflower, sesame, soy, sunflower
SWEETENERS	Brown sugar, raw sugar, refined cane sugar, date sugar, honey, corn syrup, maple syrup, brown rice syrup, fructose, saccharin, succonant, aspertame, Equal®, Sweet'n Low®, NutraSweet®
CONDIMENTS	Catsup, barbecue sauce, salsa, soy sauce, tahini, mustard, mayonnaise, margarine, horseradish, pesto sauce
SALAD DRESSINGS	Blue cheese, creamy Italian, creamy avocado, French, ranch, thousand island
DESSERTS	Custards, tapioca, puddings, pies, cakes, chocolate, desserts containing chocolate, raspberry sherbet, orange sherbet
CHIPS	Bean, corn (blue, white, yellow), potato
BEVERAGES	Coffee; black tea; wine (red, white), sake, liqueurs, beer, barley malt liquor, champagne, gin, Scotch, vodka, whiskey; diet sodas, root beer, regular sodas

Heart

MENUS

DIETARY EMPHASIS:

- Include fruit as dessert for lunch. It acts as a digestive aid and often eliminates sweet cravings.
- Avoid refined sugar, as it causes fatigue of muscles and brain.
- Avoid honey and whole wheat bread.
- Calli® tea after lunch and/or dinner helps digestion.

WEIGHT LOSS:

- Eliminate all dairy except butter.

WEIGHT GAIN:

- Emphasize dairy.

VEGETARIAN DIET:

- Inadequate, since require 10-25% of calories from dense protein.

FATS:

- 25-35% of total caloric intake.
- Best sources are butter, dense protein (chicken, fish, eggs, beef, pork, lamb), and seeds (pumpkin, sesame, sunflower).
- May use Hain™ creamy Italian or Avocado dressing instead of mayonnaise.

SENSITIVE:

- Grain and/or fruit at breakfast, light protein at lunch, and early dinner with heavy protein.

KEY

—all menus may be used by healthy persons

( ) around foods means that they're optional

L denotes weight loss menus

S denotes sensitive menus

G denotes weight gain menus

BREAKFAST:
7-8 a.m. Moderate, with cereal or grain and/or fruit, dairy, limited protein.

SENSITIVE: Moderate, with grain and/or fruit.

L	S		Grapefruit juice, then oatmeal, bagel, or English muffin
L	S		Orange, pear, or banana, then oatmeal
		G	Fruit or fruit juice, then oatmeal w/half & half or kefir
		G	Apple, then bagel (cream cheese)
L	S		Oatmeal with bananas, blueberries, or Re-Vita®
		G	Oat, raisin, and almond cereal w/plain kefir
L	S		Oatmeal w/butter
		G	Oatmeal w/whole milk, half & half, or kefir
		G	Oat bran, blueberries, and whole milk
L	S		Oat groats w/Re-Vita®
	S		Oat groats w/butter
		G	Granola, whole milk, and blueberries
			Granola and apple juice or pineapple/coconut juice11
		G	Puffed rice w/goat milk or kefir and apple, banana, or blueberries
	S		Puffed rice w/rice milk
	S		Cream of rice w/butter
	S		Brown rice (butter and Re-Vita® Lite w/pineapple juice)
	S		Rice and applesauce
		G	Cream of rye or rye flakes w/whole milk and banana
L			Wheat Farina and banana
L			Cream of wheat and orange or grapefruit
L			Cream of wheat and fresh pineapple
			Nectarine or peach and cream of wheat
	S		Apple, nectarine, strawberries, or pineapple w/or before brown rice
		G	Egg on English muffin, w/butter (bacon), and grapefruit juice
		G	Ham and eggs, oat or rye toast, and orange juice
	S		Blueberry, or apple pancakes
	S		Fruit and rye or oat toast (butter)
	S		Grapefruit and oat toast w/butter and raspberry jam

Heart

- S — Raisin bread w/butter
- Irish soda bread (butter) w/grapefruit juice, banana, or apple
- S — Apples, bananas, oranges, and/or strawberries
- L — Fresh mango, grapefruit, or cantaloupe

MID-MORNING SNACK:
(Optional) 10 a.m. Fruit.

- S — Orange juice or fruit salad
- S — Blueberries or banana

LUNCH:
12-2 p.m. Heavy, with protein, dairy, grain, and/or vegetables. Fruit for dessert.

SENSITIVE: Moderate, with grain, vegetables, legumes (beans, tofu) and/or limited protein (fish, eggs).

- L — Chicken and rice
- L — Chicken, raw celery, and apple
- Chicken and potato salad (grapes, kiwi fruit, or peach)
- L — Chicken, red leaf lettuce, and tomato (apple)
- Chicken on dark or light rye, avocado, and/or apple, kiwi, or orange
- G — Turkey, romaine lettuce, and Swiss cheese on rye
- Turkey, butter lettuce, and tomato on rye (mustard and/or orange, apple, grapes, or peach)
- Turkey sandwich on oat bread w/creamy avocado dressing or avocado (tomato) and apple, and/or orange, grapes, or banana
- L S — Salmon, spinach, and cucumber salad
- L S — Salmon, pasta, and peas
- L S — Shark steak and baked russet potato
- L S — Tuna and avocado dressing
- L S — Baked bass, boiled potato, and green beans
- Tuna salad on rye bread (apple, peach, grapes)
- L — Tuna, red leaf lettuce, and tomato
- G — Tuna, Swiss cheese, and romaine lettuce on rye
- Tuna, celery, carrots, pickles, rye bread, and/or apples, oranges, grapes, or kiwi
- S — Fish w/peas, carrots, and broccoli
- L — Pork chop, potato, and broccoli
- L — Lamb, pasta, and peas
- L — Lamb, rice, and applesauce
- Roast beef and butter lettuce on oat bread and carrots (apple, grapes, or peach)
- Reuben sandwich (strawberries and/or raspberries)
- Bacon, butter lettuce, and tomato on oat bread
- G — Ham, cheese, and romaine lettuce on oat bread w/mustard (apple, grapes, or peach)
- S G — Eggs and bagel w/cream cheese
- L S — Eggs, rice, and green beans, or crook-neck squash
- Quesadilla and raw carrots or salad: romaine lettuce, cabbage, and carrots (Italian dressing)
- Pizza and carrots or salad (orange or apple)
- G — Cottage cheese, romaine lettuce, and pineapple
- G — Grilled cheese sandwich on rye bread (apple, peach, grapes)
- G — Grilled cheese w/tomato or salsa
- L S — Tofu, vegetables, and rice
- L S — Red beans, rice, green beans, carrots, and onions
- L S — Green beans and pasta (vegetable juice)
- S — Pork and beans and cucumber (peas)
- L S — Red or russet potato and green beans

MID-AFTERNOON SNACK:
(Optional) 3 p.m. Fruit, vegetables, grain, protein, dairy, nuts, or seeds.

SENSITIVE: Fruit, vegetables, grain.

- Pineapple or strawberry kefir w/Re-Vita® – any flavor

Heart

L	S	G	
		G	Yogurt (fruit)
	S		Fruit

LUNCH or DINNER:

L	S	G	
			Pasta (pesto sauce and/or beef, turkey, chicken, or fish, and/or vegetables or salad)
		G	Spaghetti w/tomato sauce and cheese (meat)
		G	Lasagna (salad and/or rose wine)
			Hamburger w/butter lettuce (mustard, relish, pickles)
			Turkey sandwich on black rye bread (kiwi)
L			Turkey, potato, gravy, and green beans (mango)
L			Broiled or grilled fish, pasta, and peas
	S		Quesadilla and salad (raw tomato and/or raw carrots)
		G	Pizza topped w/cheese, pepperoni, sausage, or Canadian bacon w/carrots
			Red or russet potato (yogurt) and green beans
L	S		Vegetable soup
L	S		Split pea soup

DINNER:
7-9 p.m. Moderate, with grain, vegetables, protein, dairy, nuts, seeds, and/or legumes.

SENSITIVE: 6-7p.m. Early. Moderate-to-heavy, with grain, vegetables, protein (fowl, beef, lamb), nuts, seeds, and/or legumes.

L	S	G	
L	S	G	Sirloin, potatoes, and squash
	S		Mongolian beef
	S		Steak and turnips or cauliflower
	S	G	Steak, boiled potato, and salad
	S	G	Pork chops, baked potato, carrots, and broccoli
L	S	G	Lamb, pasta, and peas
	S		Lamb, potato or rice, and peas
L	S		Turkey w/onions and brown rice
L			Grilled chicken (raw carrots, lettuce, cucumber, and/or potato w/vegetable)
L		G	Chicken, potato, and mixed vegetables
L	S	G	Chicken, red or russet potato, and beets or broccoli
L		G	Chicken, beef, lamb, or duck, sunflower or sesame seeds, beans, and mushrooms
L			Chicken and rice
	S		Cashew chicken
L	S	G	Chicken, baked potato, and salad
	S		Chicken frank w/sauerkraut
			Chicken salad on rye bread
		G	Chicken and cheese on corn tortilla
L			Fish, rice, and vegetables
L			Fish, pasta, and vegetables (pasta primevera)
		G	Bacon and eggs, hash browns, and English muffin
	S		Bacon and eggs
	S		Rice (beef, turkey, chicken, or fish, and/or vegetables or salad)
	S		Pasta w/meat balls or meat sauce
		G	Corn tortilla w/cheese
	S		Turnips, potato, and pecans (broccoli)
L	S		Baked potato w/butter (chives and/or pepper) and green peas
		G	Pizza topped w/vegetables, cheese, any sausage, and pepperoni w/jicama
		G	Cheese pizza w/carrots
			Split pea soup and oat or rye bread
L	S		Vegetable beef soup
L	S		Rice, peas, and carrots w/pumpkin seeds

EVENING SNACK:
(Optional) Fruit , sweets or dairy 1 hour after dinner.

L	S	G	
L	S		Strawberries, fresh or frozen
		G	Dreyer's ice cream
			Fig cookies

NIGHT or MIDNIGHT SNACK:
(Optional) 10 p.m.-1 a.m. Protein, vegetables, grain, dairy, nuts, seeds, sweets.

L	S	G	
			Oatmeal cookies
L			Sushi

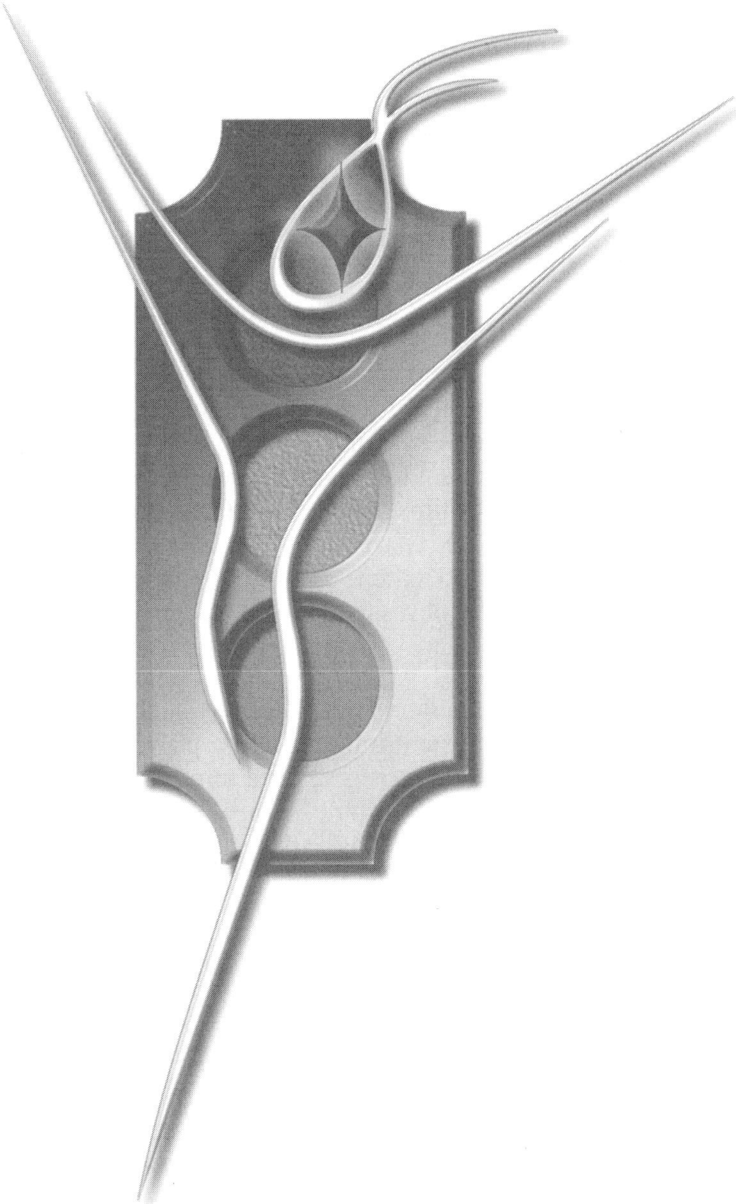

The "Hypothalamus Body Type" is symbolized by a traffic signal. In charge of keeping the body running, they have an intense sense of responsibility, and are therefore cautious about their decisions. They will extensively gather data and focus exclusively on what is at hand.

Hypothalamus

BODY TYPE PROFILE

LOCATION	At center of brain base, anterior to thalamus and including posterior pituitary.
FUNCTION	Controls visceral activities, such as water balance, temperature, and sleep.
POTENTIAL HEALTH PROBLEMS	Typically, either very healthy or extremely sensitive. Prone to allergies, respiratory, and immune system ailments, high blood pressure, and hearing problems. May be subject to bloating in waist and lower abdomen with fluid retention in upper hips, thighs, and face (especially around eyes). Also vulnerable to digestive distress and sluggish bowels, directly linked to appropriateness of food eaten. Prone to depression and self-destructive thoughts (which can be obsessive).
RECOMMENDED EXERCISE	Exercise is helpful. Its effect is initially physical and can be beneficial in all areas. It facilitates physical integration by providing a way to connect with and feel the physical body. It gives the mind a rest and allows centering to occur. Ideally, exercise 20 minutes every other day, e.g., walking, dancing, singing, callanetics, tennis, basketball, biking, and low impact aerobics. Exercise works best when done recreationally; otherwise, it's low priority.

WOMEN'S CHARACTERISTICS

DISTINGUISHING FEATURES	Height average-to-very tall. Head small-to-average, with long narrow, rectangular, or oval face. Often have wistful, distant look in eyes. Characterized by extremes: will completely immerse themselves in project or endeavor, then transfer all their energy onto something else, going through phases. Generally prefer hot and dry to moderately humid, temperate climate or very cold weather. If prefer hot climate, cold weather drains their energy.
ADDITIONAL PHYSICAL CHARACTERISTICS	Buttocks relatively flat-to-rounded. Low back curvature straight-to-average. Breasts small-to-average. Shoulders narrower than, to relatively even with, hips. Long, slender torso or broad chest and torso. Waist straight-to-defined. Average to long-waisted. Bone structure medium. Average, elongated musculature. Often have long arms and legs. Feet may be narrow.
WEIGHT GAIN AREAS	Lower body with initial gain in lower abdomen, entire upper 2/3rds of thighs including upper inner thighs, buttocks, upper hips, and waist. Alternative weight gain pattern: entire abdomen, waist, upper hips, and buttocks. Secondary weight gain in entire abdomen, middle-to entire back, breasts, upper arms, face, and under chin, with little gain in lower hips and legs. May have difficulty gaining or maintaining weight.

Hypothalamus

DIETARY GUIDELINES

	SCHEDULING MEALS
"HEALTHY"	Breakfast: Light, with protein, dairy, and/or fruit. Lunch: Moderate, with grain, raw vegetables, legumes, dairy, nuts, and/or seeds. Dinner: Moderate, with protein, dairy, legumes, cooked or steamed vegetables, and/or grain. Raw vegetables, as in salads, may be eaten with meat and pasta.
"SENSITIVE"	Breakfast: Light-to-moderate, with fruit, protein, dairy, and/or grain. Lunch; Moderate, with protein, dairy, and/or vegetables. Dinner: Moderate, with grain, dairy, legumes, and/or vegetables.
DIETARY EMPHASIS	• Raw vegetables best assimilated at lunch; cooked vegetables best for dinner. Broccoli, zucchini or yellow squash should always be eaten raw. Best when more raw than cooked vegetables are consumed. Emphasize cheese, nuts, seeds, and vegetables at lunch. Drink 1/2 gallon of water per day (with or without lemon). In general, good to rotate foods. • To detoxify system, upon arising drink Celestial or herbal tea, or hot water with lemon. Wait 2-3 hours before eating breakfast. • For weight loss, consume 15-30% of calories from dense protein other than beef or pork, limit fats to 25% of caloric intake with at least 15% from sources listed below under "Fats", limit dairy, frozen yogurt, fried foods, alcohol, caffeine, diet sodas, and breads with yeast, limit snacks to evening, and adhere to food and time schedule. May skip lunch and have light snack at mid-afternoon, or when hungry. • For weight gain, consume protein and fruit for breakfast, increase quantity of food and include snacks, and derive 35% of calories from fats in form of dairy, avocados, nuts, and seeds. Exercise essential to build muscle weight. • Vegetarian diet recommended when healthy, although diet may consist of up to 30% dense protein. • Fats: 15-25% for weight loss, 25-30% for maintenance, and 35% for weight gain from avocados, coconuts, seeds (pumpkin, sunflower, and sesame), tahini, and nuts (almonds, pecans, Brazils, macadamias, pistachios, and dry roasted cashews).

Hypothalamus

KEY SUPPORTS FOR SYSTEM	Brown rice, salads, fruits, and vegetables. Eat fruit in morning and, if desired, add midmorning snack. Kombucha tea and cashews before or after lunch regulate bowels; nuts activate movement. 8oz. plain water will often clear headaches or stomachaches. Connect feelings with intellect by nurturing self, through activities such as structured dance or playing musical instrument.
COMPLEMENTARY GLANDULAR SUPPORT	Thalamus, through getting sunlight and spending time "communing" with nature; and pituitary, through attempting to understand self, others, or life experiences generally.
FOODS CRAVED	(*When Energy is Low*) Sweets and fats, such as chocolate, caramel, frozen yogurt, ice cream, chewy cookies, doughnuts, cakes, and pies. (When feeling heavy or bloated, drawn toward carbonated beverages in attempt to relieve discomfort.)
FOODS TO AVOID	Ice cream, frozen yogurt, bagels, fried foods, and soft drinks.
RECOMMENDED CUISINE	Mexican, Thai, Chinese, Greek, Italian, French. (Prefer simple menus, including grains, noodles, salads, soups, and legumes; unless sensitive, like spicy foods.)

Hypothalamus

PSYCHOLOGICAL PROFILE

ESSENCE

Just as the hypothalamus gland is responsible for and in charge of the involuntary functions necessary for life, including regulating the heartbeat, body temperature, blood pressure, metabolism and blood-sugar levels, as well as directing the pituitary gland, Hypothalamus body types have an intense sense of responsibility for their behavior. They seem to be intuitively aware of the significance of their actions, and have a sense of responsibility for accuracy in all they do. Consequently, they approach life with a certain caution. They will generally gather all the necessary tools, study the directions, and formulate a plan before starting a project.

CHARACTERISTIC TRAITS

Being single minded, Hypothalamuses prefer to continue with a task until it is finished or until they reach a saturation point which causes their focus to change. Shifting gears, particularly from mental to emotional, can be difficult, so they prefer not to be interrupted or given multiple tasks.

Characterized by phases, Hypothalamuses will totally immerse themselves in an activity or endeavor, often to the point of becoming a crusader. However, once they complete what they need, they will switch to the next subject that catches their interest. These phases encompass all facets of reality including relationships, new developments, topics, inner probings, travel to unfamiliar places, and career changes.

It's not unusual for men to focus on business, retire, devote themselves to family and home, then abandon retirement to repeat the cycle. They seem most at home in the financial world, often as stock brokers or financial consultants. Money issues are common and they often experience the extremes of abundance and subsistence. Women, however, tend to have a better sense of money management.

With a deep innate curiosity about the nature and function of things, Hypothalamuses are comfortable in the world of concepts and ideas. Their basic strengths include logic, decisiveness, commitment, and determination (essential traits necessary to succeed professionally), especially in the business world. Generally quick-thinking and able to see the "big picture" of a project, they tend to work through steps 1-3, then leap ahead to 9-10, delegating to others the intermediate steps.

MOTIVATION

Hypothalamuses travel through different phases as a means of finding themselves. By immersing themselves in their point of interest, they are able to travel to their inner depths and connect integral parts of their being, thereby learning to rely on their own internal guidance rather than conventional standards and opinions. This self-integration is the key to their fulfillment. Although they may not stay focused on an experience or activity for long, while absorbed in something, they experience it fully.

Hypothalamus

MOTIVATION

The inherent nature of Hypothalamuses is self-contained and independent. Carried to the extreme, it may manifest as difficulties with self-disclosure. This behavior pattern usually forms in childhood with a suppressive family background. Many grew up in homes where their parents were either very critical or overly protective. Sensitive and fearful of failing, making mistakes, or otherwise losing their parents' support or approval, they often felt obliged to inhibit their self-expression. Their natural urges toward exploration of inner and outer worlds thus subdued, they may have developed (at least in the company of others) a certain habit of self-restraint. This is why, if they are to realize their full potential, they must be around people with whom they can feel safe. For the more they're able to experience external support, the more open they'll be about their thoughts and feelings, and the more they'll be able to embrace the changes that can enable them to realize their multifaceted nature.

"AT WORST"

At times Hypothalamuses have difficulty trusting their intuition. They may struggle with a problem for too long, trying to solve it logically, without loosening the reins of the intellect to create a space for the solution to manifest. In addition, they may also become stuck in a mental "loop" and fail to move outside themselves. Being mentally focused, they sometimes need other people to serve as sounding boards, particularly if they're to get in touch with what's going on with their own emotions. Focused inward mentally, they are unable to see what others are mirroring back, and remain within the limitations of their own thinking.

Frequently, Hypothalamuses almost seem to expect that outside forces will intervene and take charge of their lives in ways beyond anything they might have imagined. The assumption is that things will magically fall into place without their having to do anything about them. This is frequently the case when it comes to managing money. Hypothalamuses often become so focused on the situation in front of them, such as how to help their children with their immediate desires, that they fail to consider the long term effects of not setting financial boundaries. While they may be very good at managing other people's money, men often fail to do their own financial planning, feeling everything will be okay, so they're free to spend whatever they want. Unfortunately, this is where they can get sidetracked, especially by others. When they listen to outside voices rather than their own inner knowing, they can easily lose their way and fail to experience their abundant zest for life.

Intimate relationships are often a major challenge, women often find they have difficulty maintaining their identity and self-expression, and men have difficulty dealing with problems and sharing their emotions. Unresolved emotional stress usually manifests initially as depression. Alcohol and drugs are commonly used to avoid facing what often seems like problems that have no solution. Work can also be a means of escape, as can finding ways of neglecting an unfulfilling relationship.

Hypothalamus

"AT BEST"

Mentally adept, Hypothalamuses are good at analyzing things objectively. Decision-making comes naturally, since they are inclined to understand or relate to things through judging them. Hypothalamuses are effective at handling projects because they can easily grasp what needs to be done, devise an appropriate plan for accomplishing it, and responsibly see the job through. Typically, when embarking on a new project, they'll conscientiously study the written instructions (while other types will bypass them), and learn as much as they can before scrupulously following the plan they have developed.

Having thoroughly investigated a subject before taking action, Hypothalamuses will handle whatever obstacles arise and, if necessary, are comfortable having to redo things later on to achieve their desired results. They are generally receptive and flexible enough to change their approach to something as situations change or if they become aware of a better way of reaching their goals. Hypothalamuses are happiest when they can become creatively absorbed in their current challenge, whether professional or personal.

With active, inquiring minds, they're proficient not only in acquiring but also applying new knowledge. Receptive, sensitive, and intuitive, they are comfortable in the world of concepts and ideas. At times, they will throw themselves into life with intensity, willing to follow their enthusiasm wherever it may lead. While it's their curiosity that drives them to experience the world with immediacy and passion, it's their caution about being physically safe that holds them back. How well they're able to balance these aspects is reflected in the degree of their aliveness. It's when they dance with life that they excel.

At their best, Hypothalamuses are intuitive and receptive. They are able not only to explore and access information, but to manifest it in ways that often take the knowledge to a new level. Once they learn to trust their intuition, they'll rely more on their own internal guidance for answers than on conventional standards or opinions. One of their special gifts is the capacity to get the insights or solutions they require simply by raising a question to themselves and then waiting for the answer to come to them or pop into their head. When they're able to join this innate receptivity or intuitiveness to their inborn tenacity, their success in any endeavor is virtually assured.

Hypothalamus

FOOD LISTS

HEALTHY FOOD LIST

FREQUENTLY FOODS	3-7 meals per week – refers to each food, rather than category.
DENSE PROTEIN	Turkey; tuna; calamari (squid), clams, crab, lobster, mussels, oysters; eggs
CHEESE	Colby, Cheddar, Jack, mozzarella, Romano, raw cheese
NUTS and SEEDS	Cashews (roasted, unsalted), macadamias, macadamia butter, seeds (caraway, pumpkin, sunflower), sunflower seed butter
LEGUMES	Adzuki or pinto beans
GRAINS	Popcorn, rice (white or brown basmati, long or short grain brown or white), wheat bran, wheat germ, semolina pasta, breads (French, 7-grain, multi-grain)
VEGETABLES	Asparagus, fresh green beans, broccoli, carrots, cabbage (green, napa, red), cauliflower, chard, corn, garlic, leeks, mushrooms, peas, snow pea pods, bell peppers (green, red, yellow), pimentos, potatoes (white rose, russet), pumpkin, sauerkraut
VEGETABLE JUICE	Carrot
FRUITS	Bananas, strawberries, grapes (black, green, red), grapefruits (white, red), oranges, papayas, pineapples, dates, figs (fresh, dried), prunes, raisins, dried fruits
FRUIT JUICES	(Morning) Unfiltered raw apple, pear, grape (purple, red, white), orange
SWEETENERS	Re-Vita®, stevia
VEGETABLE OILS	Canola, olive, safflower
BEVERAGES	Decaf coffee
MODERATELY FOODS	1-2 meals per week – refers to each food, rather than category.
DENSE PROTEIN	Beef, beef broth, beef liver, buffalo, lamb, ham, pork, bacon, sausage, organ meats (heart, brain), venison, veal; chicken, chicken broth, chicken livers, cornish game hen, duck; anchovy, bass, bonita, catfish, cod, flounder, haddock, halibut, herring, mackerel, mahi-mahi, perch, roughy, salmon, sardines, shark, red snapper, sole, swordfish, trout; abalone, eel, octopus, scallops, shrimp
DAIRY	Kefir, plain or flavored yogurt, raw goat milk, milk (whole, 2%, lowfat, nonfat, raw), half & half, sweet cream, sour cream, butter, ice cream (Alta Dena®, Breyer's®, Ben & Jerry's®, Dreyer's, Haagen-Dazs®, Swensen's®, Baskin-Robbins™)
CHEESE	American, blue, brie, Camembert, cottage, cream, Edam, feta, raw goat, Gouda, kefir, Limburger, Muenster, Parmesan, ricotta, Swiss, pasteurized cheese

Hypothalamus

NUTS and SEEDS	Almonds, almond butter, Brazils, cashew butter, water chestnuts, coconuts, filberts, hazelnuts, peanuts, peanut butter, pecans, pine nuts, pistachios, walnuts (black, English), sesame seeds, sesame seed butter
LEGUMES	Beans (black, garbanzo, kidney, navy, great northern, lima [butter], red, soy), lentils, black-eyed peas, split peas, soy milk, tofu, hummus, miso
GRAINS	Amaranth, barley, buckwheat, corn, corn bread, corn tortillas, hominy grits, millet, oats, quinoa, rice (Japanese, wild, polished), rice bran, rice cakes, triticale, wheat, refined wheat flour, flour tortillas, breads (Italian, garlic, sourdough, white, corn, oat, whole wheat, sprouted grain), croissants, English muffins, crackers (oat, saltines, whole wheat), pasta (whole wheat, corn), couscous, udon noodles, Chinese rice noodles, cream of rice, cream of wheat
VEGETABLES	Artichokes, arugula, avocados, bamboo shoots, yellow wax beans, lima beans, beets, bok choy, broccoflower, brussels sprouts, celery, cilantro, cole slaw, cucumber, eggplant, greens (beet, collard, mustard, turnip), hominy, jicama, kale, kohlrabi, lettuce (Boston, endive, iceberg, red leaf, romaine), okra, olives (green, ripe), onions (chives, green, brown, red, white, yellow, vidalia), parsley, parsnips, chili peppers, potatoes (red, yukon gold), radish, daikon radish, rutabaga, sauerkraut, seaweed (arame, dulse, kelp, nori, wakame), shallots, spinach, sprouts (alfalfa, mung bean, clover, radish, sunflower), squash (acorn, banana, butternut, spaghetti, yellow [summer], zucchini), sweet potatoes, tomatoes, turnips, watercress, yams
VEGETABLE JUICES	Celery, carrot/celery, parsley, spinach, tomato, V-8®
FRUITS	Apples (Golden or Red Delicious, Granny Smith, Jonathan, McIntosh, Pippin, Rome Beauty), apricots, blackberries, blueberries, boysenberries, cranberries, gooseberries, raspberries, cherries, guavas, kiwi, kumquats, lemons, limes, loquats, mangos, melons (casaba, crenshaw, watermelon, honeydew), nectarines, peaches, pears, persimmons, plums (black, purple, red), pomegranates, rhubarb, tangelos, tangerines
FRUIT JUICES	(Morning) Apple cider, apricot, apple/apricot, black cherry, red cherry, cranapple, cranberry, grapefruit, guava, lemon, papaya, pineapple, pineapple/coconut, prune, tangerine
VEGETABLE OILS	All-blend, almond, avocado, coconut, corn, flaxseed, peanut, sesame, soy, sunflower
SWEETENERS	Honey, molasses, sorghum, brown sugar, date sugar, raw sugar, refined cane sugar, maple syrup, brown rice syrup, barley malt syrup, corn syrup, fructose, succonant
CONDIMENTS	Catsup, mustard, horseradish, soy sauce, barbecue sauce, pesto sauce, salsa, tahini, salt, sea salt, Vege-Sal®, vinegar
SALAD DRESSINGS	Blue cheese, French, ranch, creamy Italian, creamy avocado, thousand island, vinegar and oil, lemon juice and oil
DESSERTS	Custards, tapioca, puddings, pies, cakes, milk chocolate, desserts containing milk chocolate, raspberry sherbet, orange sherbet

Hypothalamus

CHIPS	Bean, corn (blue, white, yellow), potato
BEVERAGES	Coffee; herbal tea, black tea, green tea, Japanese tea, Chinese oolong tea; mineral water, sparkling water; wine (red, white), sake, liqueurs, champagne, beer, barley malt liquor, gin, Scotch, vodka, whiskey; root beer, diet sodas, regular sodas
RARELY FOODS	No more than once a month
DAIRY	Buttermilk, pasteurized goat milk, most ice creams, frozen yogurt
CHEESE	Pasteurized goat cheese
NUTS	Raw cashews
GRAINS	Rye, rye bread, rye crackers, cream of rye, bagels
VEGETABLES	Butter lettuce
FRUITS	Cantaloupes
FRUIT JUICES	Filtered, pasteurized apple juice
SWEETENERS	Saccharin, aspertame, Equal®, NutraSweet®, Sweet'n Low®
CONDIMENTS	Mayonnaise, margarine
DESSERTS	Dark chocolate

SENSITIVE FOOD LIST

FREQUENTLY FOODS	3-7 meals per week – refers to each food, rather than category.
NUTS and SEEDS	Macadamia nuts, pumpkin seeds
GRAINS	Popcorn
VEGETABLES	Fresh green beans, carrots
FRUITS	Cooked apples, red grapes, oranges, pineapples, papayas, dried bananas
FRUIT JUICE	Unfiltered raw apple
MODERATELY FOODS	1-2 meals per week – refers to each food, rather than category.
DENSE PROTEIN	Beef broth, beef liver, buffalo, veal, venison, lamb, organ meats (heart, brain); turkey, chicken, chicken broth, chicken livers, cornish game hen, duck; anchovy, bass, bonita, catfish, cod, flounder, haddock, halibut, herring, mackerel, mahi-mahi, perch, roughy, salmon, sardines, shark, red snapper, sole, swordfish, trout, tuna; abalone, calamari (squid), clams, crab, eel, lobster, mussels, octopus, oysters, scallops, shrimp; eggs
DAIRY	Raw goat milk, half & half, sour cream, sweet cream, kefir, plain or fruit flavored yogurt, butter

Hypothalamus

CHEESE	American, blue, brie, Camembert, Cheddar, Colby, cottage, cream, Edam, feta, raw goat, Gouda, Jack, kefir, Limburger, mozzarella, Muenster, Parmesan, raw cheese, ricotta, Romano, Swiss
NUTS and SEEDS	Almond butter, Brazils, cashews (roasted, unsalted), cashew butter, water chestnuts, coconuts, filberts, hazelnuts, macadamia butter, peanuts, peanut butter, pecans, pistachios, pine nuts, walnuts (black, English), seeds (caraway, sesame, sunflower), sesame seed butter, sunflower seed butter
LEGUMES	Beans (adzuki, black, garbanzo, navy, great northern, kidney, lima [butter], pinto, red), black-eyed peas, split peas, hummus, miso
GRAINS	Amaranth, barley, buckwheat, corn, corn bread, corn grits, corn tortillas, hominy grits, millet, oats, quinoa, rice (white or brown basmati, long or short grain brown or white, Japanese, wild), rice bran, rice cakes, refined wheat flour, flour tortillas, breads (French, Italian, garlic, sourdough, 7-grain, multi-grain, oat, corn, rice, sprouted grain), croissants, English muffins, crackers (oat, saltines), couscous, pasta, udon noodles, Chinese rice noodles, cream of rice
VEGETABLES	Artichokes, asparagus, avocados, bamboo shoots, yellow wax beans, lima beans, beets, bok choy, broccoli, broccoflower, brussels sprouts, cooked cabbage, cauliflower, celery, chard, cilantro, corn, cucumbers, eggplant, garlic, (beet, collard, mustard, turnip), jicama, kale, kohlrabi, leeks, lettuce (Boston, endive, iceberg, red leaf, romaine), mushrooms, okra, olives (green, ripe), onions (chives, green, brown, red, white, yellow, vidalia), parsley, parsnips,peas, snow pea pods, bell peppers (green, red, yellow), chili peppers, pimentos, potatoes (red, russet, white rose), pumpkin, radishes, daikon radishes, rutabaga, seaweed (arame, dulse, kelp, nori, wakame), shallots, spinach, sprouts (alfalfa, clover, mung bean, radish, sunflower), squash (acorn, banana, butternut, spaghetti, yellow [summer], zucchini), sweet potatoes, tomatoes, turnips, yams
VEGETABLE JUICES	Celery, carrot, carrot/celery, parsley, spinach, tomato, V-8®
FRUITS	(Golden or Red Delicious, Granny Smith, Jonathan, McIntosh, Pippin, Rome Beauty), apricots, blackberries, blueberries, boysenberries, cranberries, gooseberries, raspberries, strawberries, cherries, green or purple grapes, kiwi, kumquats, limes, loquats, mangos, melons (casaba, crenshaw, honeydew, watermelon), nectarines, pears, persimmons, pomegranates, rhubarb, tangelos, dates, figs, prunes, raisins
FRUIT JUICES	(Morning) Apple cider, apricot, apple/apricot, red cherry, black cherry, cranapple, cranberry, grape (purple, red, white), guava, orange, papaya, pear, pineapple, pineapple/coconut, prune, tangerine
VEGETABLE OILS	All-blend, avocado, coconut
SWEETENERS	Brown rice syrup, barley malt syrup, Re-Vita®, stevia
CONDIMENTS	Salsa, tahini, salt, sea salt, Vege-Sal®, vinegar
SALAD DRESSINGS	Vinegar and oil, lemon juice and oil

Hypothalamus

BEVERAGES	Decaf coffee with Re-Vita®; herbal tea, green tea, Japanese tea, Chinese oolong tea; mineral water, sparkling water
RARELY FOODS	No more than once a month
DENSE PROTEIN	Beef, ham, pork, bacon, sausage
DAIRY	Milk (whole, 2%, low fat, nonfat), buttermilk, pasteurized goat milk, most ice creams, frozen yogurt
CHEESE	Pasteurized goat cheese
NUTS	Almonds, raw cashews
LEGUMES	Soy beans, lentils, soy milk, tofu
GRAINS	Polished rice, rye, triticale, whole wheat, wheat bran, wheat germ, breads (rye, white, whole wheat), bagels, crackers (rye, whole wheat), cream of rye, cream of wheat
VEGETABLES	Arugula, raw cabbage, butter lettuce, yukon gold potatoes, sauerkraut, watercress
FRUITS	Bananas, cantaloupes, grapefruit, lemons, peaches, plums (black, purple, red)
FRUIT JUICES	Filtered pasteurized apple, grapefruit, lemon
VEGETABLE OILS	Almond, canola, corn, flaxseed, olive, peanut, safflower, sesame, soy, sunflower
SALAD DRESSINGS	Blue cheese, French, ranch, creamy Italian, creamy avocado, thousand island
SWEETENERS	Honey, molasses, sorghum, raw sugar, refined cane sugar, brown sugar, date sugar, corn syrup, maple syrup, fructose, succonant, saccharin, aspertame, Equal®, Nutra Sweet®, Sweet'n Low®
CONDIMENTS	Catsup, margarine, mayonnaise, soy sauce, sour pickles, mustard, horseradish, barbecue sauce, pesto sauce
DESSERTS	Custards, tapioca, puddings, pies, cakes, milk chocolate, desserts containing milk chocolate, dark chocolate, raspberry sherbet, orange sherbet
CHIPS	Bean, corn (blue, white, yellow), potato
BEVERAGES	Regular coffee; black tea; wine (red, white), sake, liqueurs, beer, barley malt liquor, champagne, gin, Scotch, vodka, whiskey; Pepsi®, root beer, diet sodas, regular sodas

Hypothalamus

MENUS

DIETARY EMPHASIS

- Vegetables and fruit, with fruit in the morning.
- Raw vegetables best assimilated at lunch.
- Cooked vegetables best for dinner.
- Broccoli, zucchini and yellow squash should always be eaten raw.
- More raw vegetables than cooked.
- Emphasize nuts, seeds, cheese and vegetables at lunch.
- Rotate foods.
- Drink 1/2 gallon of water (with or without lemon).
- To detoxify system, upon arising drink Celestial Seasonings® or herbal tea, or hot water with lemon. Wait 2-3 hours before eating breakfast.

WEIGHT LOSS:

- Consume 15-30% of calories from dense protein other than beef or pork.
- Limit fats to 25% of caloric intake with at least 15% from sources listed below under "Fats".
- Limit dairy, frozen yogurt, fried foods, alcohol, caffeine, diet sodas and breads with yeast.
- Limit snacks to evening.
- May skip lunch and have light snack at mid-afternoon or when hungry.
- Adhere to food and time schedule.

WEIGHT GAIN:

- Consume protein and fruit for breakfast.
- Increase quantity of food and include snacks.
- Derive 35% of calories from fats in the form of dairy, avocados, nuts, and seeds.
- Exercise essential to build muscle weight.

VEGETARIAN DIET:

- Recommended when healthy, although diet may consist of up to 20% dense protein.

FATS:

- 15-25% of caloric intake for weight loss, 25-30% for maintenance, 35% for weight gain.
- Best sources are avocados, coconuts, seeds (pumpkin, sunflower, and sesame), tahini, and nuts (almonds, pecans, Brazils, macadamias, pistachios, and dry roasted cashews).

KEY

—all menus may be used by healthy persons
( ) around foods means that they're optional
L denotes weight loss menus
S denotes sensitive menus
G denotes weight gain menus

BREAKFAST:
9-10 a.m. Light, with protein, dairy, and/or fruit.

SENSITIVE: Light-to-moderate, with fruit, protein, dairy, and/or grain.

	S	G	Eggs and grape juice
	S	G	Eggs and fruit (toast)
	S	G	Scrambled eggs w/cheese, or cheese omelette
L			Basted eggs and grapefruit
L			Hard-boiled egg and fruit juice
			Bacon or ham, and pineapple or pineapple juice
L		G	Chicken or cornish hen, w/grapes or white grape juice
L		G	Chicken w/pineapple chunks or pineapple juice
L		G	Turkey w/apples, applesauce, or unfiltered apple juice
L		G	Duck and cherries
L			Tuna w/lemon juice
L		G	Lobster and grapes, apples, cherries, or blackberries
L		G	Mussels and apples
L		G	Oysters and grapes
	S	G	Cottage cheese and pineapple, or green apples
		G	Plain yogurt and apple or banana
	S	G	Nonfat raspberry yogurt
	S	G	Yogurt or kefir and berry Re-Vita®
	S		Oatmeal w/raisins and butter
	S		Granola or muesli w/kefir
	S		Rice w/butter

Hypothalamus

	S		Basmati rice and mango, or papaya (plain yogurt)
	S		Couscous w/blackberries, blueberries, raspberries, or Re-Vita®
	S		Raisin bread toast and butter
	S		5-grain pancakes w/apple sauce
	S		Pancakes w/blueberries or strawberries and Re-Vita®
	S		Waffles and strawberries or blueberries (Re-Vita®)
	S		Baked apple w/cinnamon
	S		Grape juice

MID-MORNING SNACK:
(Optional). Grain, vegetables, fruit, dairy, nuts, seeds, protein, and/or legumes.

L			Carrot and beet juice
		G	Celery w/almond butter
	S		Popcorn, unsalted (parmesan cheese)
		G	Coconut
	S	G	Peanuts, walnuts, pistachios, or sunflower seeds
		G	Raw or roasted sunflower or pumpkin seeds, unsalted
	S		Pumpkin seeds and raisins
	S		Oat crackers and cheese
			Granola bar
			Pineapple/coconut juice

LUNCH:
1-2 p.m. Moderate, with grain, raw vegetables, legumes, dairy, nuts, and/or seeds.

SENSITIVE: Moderate, with protein, dairy, and/or vegetables.

		G	Corn tortilla, refried beans, and kefir or feta cheese
		G	Corn tortilla and mozzarella cheese
		G	Flour tortilla, cheese, and avocado
L			Pasta or couscous w/butter
L			Pasta and raw broccoli (Italian dressing)
L			Pasta w/pesto and raw carrots
		G	Chicken taquito w/guacamole and cheese
			Spinach lasagna and salad: romaine lettuce, tomato, cucumber, red bell pepper w/creamy Italian dressing
	S		Chicken, potatoes, and raw broccoli or spinach
L	S		Chicken, raw broccoli, and corn
	S		Orange roughy and raw broccoli or green beans
	S	G	Sole fillet, scalloped potatoes, and raw spinach
	S		Tuna and salad w/oil and vinegar or salad dressing
	S		Tuna and sunflower seed sprouts
L	S		Salmon, cauliflower, and raw broccoli or salad
L	S		Salmon and salad: cucumber, spinach, and green peas
	S	G	Salmon, red leaf lettuce, cucumber, carrots, and tomatoes w/creamy Italian dressing
	S		Lamb chops, peas, and mushrooms
	S		Steak, mushrooms, onions, and raw carrots
		G	English muffin w/avocado or peanut butter and honey
		G	Peanut butter and Re-Vita® sandwich
		G	Oatmeal muffin w/butter and swiss cheese
		G	Sourdough bread, Jack cheese, and jicama w/Hain™ Creamy Italian dressing
			Celery w/peanut butter and carrots
		G	Baked potato topped w/mozzarella cheese and sprouts
		G	Vegetable pasta and cream sauce
L			Bean burrito w/avocado or salad and low fat dressing
L			Bean burrito and salad: red leaf or romaine lettuce, tomato, onion, and mushrooms
L			Falafel, rice, and salad: green leaf lettuce, feta cheese, onions,and Greek salad dressing
		G	Pizza, cheese, (black olives), and raw carrots
		G	Vegetarian pizza w/cheese (salad)

Hypothalamus

L — Spinach salad
G — Spinach salad w/sunflower or pumpkin seeds
L S — Spinach leaves, cucumber, sesame oil, and sprouts
L — 3-bean salad and red leaf lettuce salad
S — Salad: jicama, carrots, red bell peppers, green onions, and spinach w/blue cheese dressing
S — Chef salad: 3 cheeses, turkey, romaine lettuce, alfalfa sprouts, and cherry tomatoes
L — Salad: romaine lettuce, alfalfa sprouts, cherry tomatoes, seeds, and ranch dressing
S — Carrot and beet juice

MID-AFTERNOON SNACK:
(Optional) 4 p.m. Dairy, nuts, seeds, grain, and/or vegetables.

S — String cheese
S — Rice cakes or rice crackers w/mozarella cheese
G — Muffin
G — Bread with tahini butter
G — Nuts and/or seeds
G — Protein bar
G — Cookies

DINNER:
6:30-9 p.m. Moderate, with protein, dairy, legumes, cooked or steamed vegetables, and/or grain. Raw vegetables, as in salads, may be consumed with meat and pasta.

SENSITIVE: 7-9 p.m. Moderate, with grain, dairy, legumes, and/or vegetables.

L — Turkey, white rose potatoes, and green beans
Curry chicken w/rice and noodles
Chicken, pasta, and garlic sauce
L — Chicken, spinach, and red potatoes
L G — Cashew chicken, water chestnuts, snow pea pods, and rice
L — Chicken, rice, and green beans or asparagus
L G — Barbecued chicken and Chinese vegetables
L — Chicken, pinto beans, and rice (butternut squash)
Chow mein, fried rice, hot and sour soup, and steamed vegetables
G — Sausage, pasta (cooked celery, green onions, and/or red and green peppers)
G — Steak and pasta (salad)
L — Steak and salad
G — Barbecued steak, mushrooms, onions, and carrots
G — Corned beef and sauerkraut
L G — Lamb chops, peas, and mushrooms
G — Swordfish, scalloped potatoes, and leeks
L — Cod, rice pilaf, and asparagus
L G — Rainbow trout, pasta, and raw broccoli
L — Halibut and asparagus
G — Halibut, pasta, and salad
L — Salmon, basmati rice, and asparagus
L G — Red snapper, pasta, and asparagus
Shrimp, tomato garlic pasta, and green beans
L — Scrambled eggs w/broccoli
S G — Pasta w/pesto
G — Pasta w/clam sauce
L — Pasta w/tomato marinara, mushrooms, and onions
Spaghetti and meat balls
S — Rice and beans
S — Refried beans and corn tortilla
L G — Cheese enchilada, rice, and beans (avocado, salsa)
Adzuki beans and rice (curry)
L — Lentils, onions, peppers (rice, beans, or cauliflower)
L — Pizza and hot spiced carrots
L G — Hawaiian pizza w/ham and pineapple
L S — Stir-fry: mushrooms, onions, carrots, celery, red peppers, and pasta
L S — Stir-fry: Chinese vegetables and rice
S — Baked pumpkin w/butter and cinnamon

Hypothalamus

S Spaghetti squash and green peas

S Carrots and cooked cabbage

S G Yams, peas, and butter

G Chili and cornbread

S Soup: cabbage, endive, and leek (onion)

L S Soup: red potatoes, cauliflower, and beets

L S Split pea soup

L S Bean soup

L Chicken noodle soup

Chicken vegetable soup

EVENING SNACK:
(Optional) 10 p.m.-1 a.m. Protein, dairy, vegetables, grain, nuts, seeds, sweets.

SENSITIVE: 9-11 p.m. Fruit, grain, sweets.

G Peanuts, walnuts, pistachios, roasted cashews, or sunflower seeds

L Popcorn w/olive oil

S G Milk chocolate

G Cake

S G Pumpkin pie

G Apple pie 1 hour after dinner

S Fruits: nectarine, pear, grapes, apple, or figs

G Dates or figs

S Sorbet w/strawberries, blueberries, or raspberries

S Toasted sourdough bread w/butter (before bed)

INTESTINAL

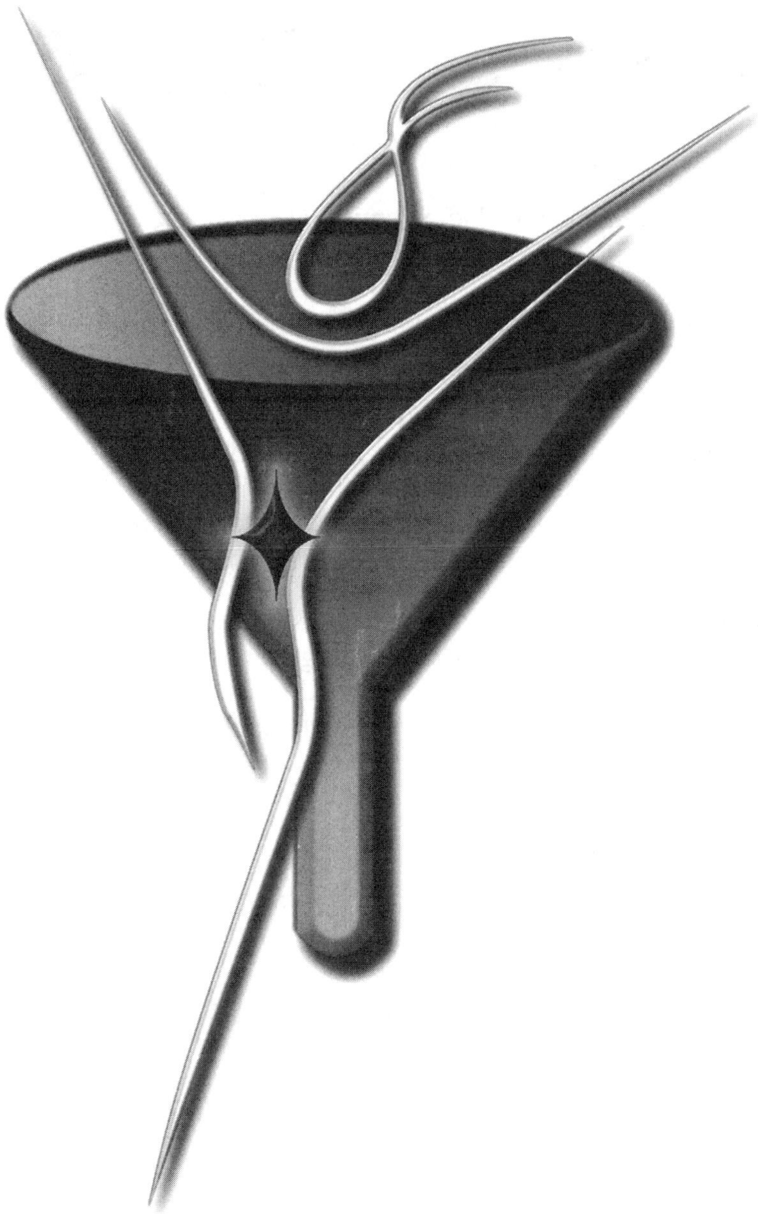

The "Intestinal Body Type" is symbolized by the funnel. They accept everything that comes in, and then discern what to keep and what to release. Constant new experiences are vital to their continued growth and expansion.

Intestinal

BODY TYPE PROFILE

LOCATION	Lower abdomen, including entire intestinal tract.
FUNCTION	Digestion and absorption of food, other nutrients, and water
POTENTIAL HEALTH PROBLEMS	Usually have strong, sturdy bodies with good stamina. Prone to digestive problems, intestinal distress, improper fat metabolism, hypoglycemia, and slow metabolism. Birth control pills can elevate blood pressure over time. Hormonal imbalances, depression, emotional stress.
RECOMMENDED EXERCISE	Exercise is optional. Its effect is initially emotional. Exercise relieves emotional stress and moves energy. It affects emotions, then affects the physical body by aiding digestion. For some, exercise can help in understanding how the physical world works. With Intestinals, time of day enhances effectiveness of exercise: optimal time is between 11 a.m. and 4 p.m., 20 minutes to 1 hour. Ideally, need to do some form of exercise at least 5 days a week. Maximum weekly frequency for each activity as follows: walking – 5 x/wk, swimming – daily, callanetics – 2 x/wk, biking – 2 x/wk, stretching – 2 x/wk, low impact aerobics – 2 x/wk. Most exercise is moderate. No heavy weight lifting, although light weights (5-10 lbs.) may be beneficial.

WOMEN'S CHARACTERISTICS

DISTINGUISHING FEATURES	Solid body, with layer of softness covering muscle, reducing muscle definition. Often have muscle weakness under chin which gives rise to double chin. Emotionally sensitive with an open approach to life. Need new experiences to grow mentally, emotionally, or spiritually; or will expand physically.
ADDITIONAL PHYSICAL CHARACTERISTICS	Buttocks relatively flat-to-rounded. Low back curvature straight-to-average. Breasts average-to-large. Shoulders narrower than, to relatively even with, hips. Waist straight-to-defined. Average-to-short waisted. Height average, although can range from petite to very tall. Bone structure small-to-medium. Often have relatively straight calves. Hands long, slender, or delicate. Generally have average-to-long oval or rectangular face, often with high forehead.

Intestinal

WEIGHT GAIN AREAS

Upper, lower, or entire body with initial gain in lower to entire abdomen, waist, upper hips, inner knees, entire inner and possibly entire upper 2/3rds of thighs. May gain initially in breasts. While weight may be gained in thighs, it is disproportionately less than on abdomen. Secondary gain in face, under chin, upper arms, entire back, buttocks, and extending throughout entire thighs; thengenerally all over. Capable of carrying large amounts of weight. Tend to carry more weight in front of body than back.

DIETARY GUIDELINES

SCHEDULING MEALS

"HEALTHY"

Breakfast: Light-to-moderate, with fruit, fruit juice, vegetables, and/or dairy. No dense protein or grain except with fruit, sweetener, or vegetable.

Lunch: Moderate, with grain, protein, dairy, legumes, cooked vegetables, and/or seeds. Raw vegetables may be eaten with protein, e.g., Caesar salad with chicken.

Dinner: Moderate, with grain, dairy, legumes, protein, raw vegetables, and/or seeds.

"SENSITIVE"

Breakfast: Moderate-to-heavy, with vegetables, protein, seeds, and/or grain.

Lunch: Moderate-to-heavy, with protein, cooked vegetables, and/or grain.

Dinner: Light-to-moderate, with vegetables, legumes, dairy, protein, and/or grain.

DIETARY EMPHASIS

- Legumes and squash. Intestinals do best with foods in combinations; it's also important for them to rotate foods.
- For weight loss, caloric intake of 15-20% dense protein and 10-15% fat daily recommended. Eliminate bread, yeast, mayonnaise, and caffeine. Also avoid the following: nuts (almonds, Brazils, cashews, coconut, filberts, peanuts, macadamias, pecans, walnuts); seeds (pumpkin, sesame, sunflower); beans (black, butter lima, garbanzo, great northern, kidney, red, soy); lentils, dried peas, corn; bananas; dried fruit (dates, raisins, pineapple); sweets (ice cream, cheese cake). Limit fruit juice.
- Vegetarian diet adequate, although 15% may consist of dense protein, 25% fat. When sensitive or rebuilding body, may increase dense protein to 40%.
- Fats, 20-25% of caloric intake should be from sesame seeds, tahini, butter, fish – halibut, orange roughy, salmon, shark, swordfish, lobster, shrimp; olive oil, and sesame oil.

Intestinal

KEY SUPPORTS FOR SYSTEM	Often need snacks to maintain blood sugar level. Grow mentally, spiritually, or emotionally or will expand physically.
COMPLEMENTARY GLANDULAR SUPPORT	Thyroid, through consuming 2 oz. of dense protein (chicken, turkey, eggs, or fish) with a grain, such as rice or pasta, 5 times a week. Kidney, through building courage by doing something new 2 times a week (such an activity can be as simple as taking a new route home).
FOODS CRAVED	*(When Energy is Low)* Sweets, primarily chocolate; secondarily, pastry and cookies. Carbohydrates, such as muffins. Secondarily, fats and creamy foods, such as ice cream. Salty foods, such as chips. Spicy foods.
FOODS TO AVOID	Breads containing yeast.
RECOMMENDED CUISINE	Mexican, Italian, Home-style cooking.

Intestinal

PSYCHOLOGICAL PROFILE

ESSENCE

Just as the intestines openly accept everything that comes in and then discern between nutrients and waste material or what to keep and what to release the Intestinal body type is discerning. They approach life with an openness, taking everything in, and then letting go of what isn't appropriate. This often leads to a thorough analysis of everything new and a prejudice ("pre-judge") against anything similar to something already analyzed in the past. While their initial response to life is emotional, they generally don't trust their emotions, so they gather as much information as possible to make a logical decision. New experiences are vital since expansion is essential, and if it doesn't occur mentally, emotionally, or spiritually, Intestinals will expand physically.

CHARACTERISTIC TRAITS

Sensitive and extremely emotional, Intestinals are typically gentle, loving and compassionate. Relationships are of utmost importance to them, particularly family and close friends. With their extreme sensitivity, they are exceedingly concerned about feelings. When they're not sure about how to deal with an uncomfortable situation, their tendency is to internalize it. Being acutely aware of the stress unresolved issues have on them personally, as well as on their relationships, they have a strong need to clear the air. Intestinals are usually the ones who will gingerly bring up the issue sometime later on, once they've had time to think about it.

They have high standards and self-expectations. With their strong desire to do things right, Intestinal types need to understand everything they encounter. Consequently, Intestinals are very good at responding to problems objectively and analytically. Responsible, orderly, methodical, and attentive to detail, Intestinal types are extremely capable and usually achieve whatever they set out to accomplish.

Intestinals are imaginative, and their active imaginations often escape into the creative world of daydreams. They are apt to daydream about what they'd like to have happen or about various "what-ifs" and may at times feel restricted by present-day realities. By nature free spirits, they are typically a bit conventional in their thinking and rarely bound by tradition. They're likely to be artistically inclined, both in their own expression through an artistic medium and also in their appreciation of the arts.

CHARACTERISTIC TRAITS

Creative and expansive, Intestinals enjoy working with others. They are inspired by group association and interaction with other people. Therefore, they generally function best when they can connect with others, as it provides a forum for inspiration and new ideas. Their inspiration often comes from the emotional boost they receive from being around people who are positive and enjoy what they are doing. For them, inspiration is a process that occurs within, not that others set out to inspire them, or the kind of inspiration that comes from a sales meeting or rally. With their strong emotional energy,

Intestinal

MOTIVATION (Continued)

Intestinals are good at motivating others and providing support where-ever needed. They are often an inspiration in themselves, as they can enliven a room by their presence alone.

While they enjoy working with others, they are highly capable and can just as easily work alone, often preferring to figure things out by themselves. Not being limited by tradition, being open to new or unconventional ideas, and stimulated by personal growth, Intestinals are able to let their creativity soar and develop new ways of dealing with problems.

Intestinals need variety and change to gain life experiences. They are intellectually curious, and mental stimulation satisfies their need to expand. Since expansion is essential in their lives, feelings of being restricted or held back are strong motivations for change. Change, however, is not easy because their sensitivity and feelings of insecurity in the world often cause an internal conflict. This is because order and consistency provide them with a sense of security. To feel safe, Intestinal types will often gather everything they can on a new subject, and analyze it in detail until they fully understand it.

Profusely gathering information and thoroughly analyzing whatever comes their way is another way of balancing their strong emotional responses. But having to explore all options before making a decision can be restrictive and conflict with their need to expand. The analysis process alone, can delay the implementation of beneficial changes in their lives. With limited real life experience, Intestinals need to rely more heavily on their free spirit, openness and willingness to explore non-conventional areas, or they can get caught in their fear of the unknown and miss out on really enjoying life.

"AT WORST"

Intestinal types will often block experiences and relationships by pre-judging future situations based on the past, when things didn't go the way they had planned. This causes them to become stuck or restricted. Once they have head or intellectual knowledge, Intestinals will often block new information or insights from coming in by saying, "I already know it." Not only does this block new experiences, but restricts their relationships when they discourage others from openly discussing or reflecting any limiting behavior Intestinals may inadvertently be expressing.

With their emotions so close to the surface, Intestinal types can be overly sentimental easily crying or laughing or swing to the opposite extreme of being abrasive. By letting people easily push their buttons, their soft-spoken demeanor quickly changes into suspicion and contentiousness. Prone to worry, when Intestinals are physically stressed, they get caught up in their negative emotions. Fatigue alone is often enough to trigger depression or pessimism. Not knowing how to deal with their emotions, they often retreat into fantasy or denial. There is a natural tendency to become suspicious and challenge all new information, especially if it can't be touched or proven. Lack of courage to face the fear of the unknown is common and can cause Intestinals to be skeptical and pessimistic, especially when they get stuck in worry and all the negative that accompany it.

Intestinal

They will hold themselves back in relationships because they don't like change. Because of a fear of loss or rejection, Intestinal types tend to get too attached to their families. With low self-esteem, they often find themselves in physically or emotionally abusive relationships. Lacking courage, they will go into or stay in a deficient situation too long, stuffing their emotions, and not having the nerve to speak out or make a change. Since confrontation is difficult, they will often avoid it at all costs.

Change is difficult for them to initiate or sustain without external support because of their tendency to procrastinate, their pessimism, and their being so hard on themselves. Needing outside validation to establish their self-worth, Intestinals will make negative assumptions about other's opinions of them and then get upset, wallowing in their own self-pity, become self-absorbed, or go into the victim role, wanting to be rescued. Their pessimism often translates into a distrust of people in authority and even of the world in general.

"AT BEST"

Intestinals have a good sense of humor and can be a lot of fun to be around. They can fill a room with their joy and vivaciousness. Dependable and reliable, they are able to get things done and will work until the job is finished. Idealistic and altruistic, Intestinals particularly enjoy helping others.

Good with people and in organizations, Intestinal types genuinely like everybody. They are excellent support people or coordinators, as they inspire others to do their best, and provide the cohesiveness needed to see things through. Having learned to trust and listen to their strong intuitive nature, Intestinals are able to quickly and accurately assess situations and projects, easily making the best decisions.

It's their strong intuitive side that causes them to be attracted to opportunities for new settings, situations and people, as well as what draws them to non-traditional experiences. They have fun with their physical expression, and are active, enjoying whatever experience shows up. Self-sufficient and introspective, they take care of themselves, setting limits and establishing boundaries as to what other people can expect from them. This way, they can protect their energies from becoming depleted. Self-nurturing often comes through personal growth.

Once Intestinals are able to effectively express their creative energies, by keeping the channel to their intuitive side open, and learning to observe their emotions by letting them pass, they seem to be intuitively connected and are able to be in the flow of life, listening telepathically. Intestinals have strong Universal support and intuitive guidance. Life works when they learn to trust, listen and follow their own intuitive sense. The secret is staying out of the mind and not getting too caught up in the mental by asking why or needing to understand.

Intestinal

FOOD LISTS

HEALTHY FOOD LIST

FREQUENTLY FOODS	3-7 meals per week – refers to each food, rather than category.
DENSE PROTEIN	Chicken, turkey
DAIRY	Raw whole milk, plain or flavored yogurt, plain kefir, butter
CHEESE	White low fat Cheddar cheese
NUTS and SEEDS	Cashews (unsalted, dry roasted), cashew butter, peanuts (unsalted, dry roasted), peanut butter, pecans, walnuts (black, English), roasted and unsalted seeds (pumpkin, sesame, sunflower), sesame seed butter, sunflower seed butter
LEGUMES	Beans (black, lima [butter], pinto), lentils
GRAINS	Amaranth, corn, corn bread, corn grits, hominy grits, millet, rye, rice (brown or white basmati, long or short grain brown, polished, Japanese, wild), rice bran, rice cakes, popcorn cakes, whole wheat, whole wheat tortillas, breads (whole wheat, corn), cream of rice, cream of rye, cream of wheat
VEGETABLES	Artichokes, beets, broccoli, brussels sprouts, cabbage (green, napa, red), corn, cucumbers, garlic, jicama, red leaf lettuce, mushrooms, onions (all varieties), peas, snow pea pods, potatoes (all varieties), sweet potatoes, pumpkin, seaweed (arame, dulse, kelp, nori, wakame), spinach, squash (acorn, butternut), yams
FRUITS	Apples (Golden or Red Delicious), bananas, blueberries, strawberries, grapes (black, red), cantaloupes (alone), black plums, dates, dried pineapples, raisins, apple, apple cider
FRUIT JUICES	Apple, apple cider, cranapple, cranberry, cranberry concentrate w/Re-Vita®
SWEETENERS	Brown rice syrup, sorghum, molasses, date sugar, Re-Vita®, stevia
CONDIMENTS	Spike®, pickles (dill, sweet)
BEVERAGES	Seltzer water
MODERATELY FOODS	1-2 meals per week – refers to each food, rather than category.
DENSE PROTEIN	Beef, beef broth, beef liver, buffalo, lamb, pork, ham, bacon, sausage, veal, venison, organ meats (heart, brain); chicken broth, chicken livers, cornish game hen, duck; anchovy, bass, bonita, catfish, cod, flounder, haddock, halibut, herring, mackerel, mahi-mahi, perch, orange roughy, salmon, sardines, shark, red snapper, sole, swordfish, trout, yellowtail tuna; abalone, calamari (squid), clams, crab, eel, lobster, mussels, octopus, oysters, scallops, shrimp; eggs
DAIRY	Milk (whole, low fat, nonfat, goat), half & half, sour cream, sweet cream, buttermilk, flavored kefir, frozen yogurt, ice cream (Dreyer's, Ben & Jerry's®, Swensen's®), Ice Bean®, Rice Dream®

Intestinal

CHEESE	American, blue, brie, Camembert, Cheddar, Colby, cottage, cream, Edam, feta, goat, Gouda, Jack, kefir, Limburger, mozzarella, Muenster, Parmesan, ricotta, Romano, Swiss
NUTS and SEEDS	Almonds (raw, roasted), almond butter, Brazils, raw cashews, water chestnuts, coconuts, filberts, hazelnuts, macadamias (raw, roasted), macadamia butter, raw peanuts, pine nuts (raw, roasted), pistachios, raw seeds (sesame, sunflower), raw or roasted caraway seeds
LEGUMES	Beans (adzuki, garbanzo, great northern, kidney, navy, red, soy), black-eyed peas, split peas, hummus, miso, soy milk, tofu
GRAINS	Barley, buckwheat, blue corn, corn tortillas, oats, oat flour pancakes, popcorn, quinoa, triticale, wheat bran, wheat germ, refined wheat flour, flour tortillas, breads (French, Italian, garlic, 7-grain, multi-grain, oat, corn/rye, rye, rice, sprouted grain, sourdough, white), croissants, bagels, English muffins, crackers (oat, oriental rice, rye, saltines, sesame seed, Carr's® Table Water®, whole wheat), pasta (plain, spinach, beet), couscous, udon noodles, Chinese rice noodles
VEGETABLES	Asparagus, avocados, bamboo shoots, green beans, yellow wax beans, lima beans, bok choy, broccoflower, carrots, cauliflower, celery, chard, cilantro, eggplant, greens (beet, collard, mustard, turnip), kale, kohlrabi, leeks, lettuce (Boston, butter, endive, curly leaf, romaine), okra, olives (black, green, ripe), parsley, parsnips, bell peppers (green, red, yellow), chili peppers, pimentos, radish, daikon radish, rutabaga, sauerkraut, shallots, sprouts (alfalfa, mung bean, clover, radish, sunflower), squash (banana, spaghetti, yellow [summer], zucchini), tomatoes (canned, hot-house, vine-ripened), turnips, watercress
VEGETABLE JUICES	Celery, carrot, carrot/celery, parsley, spinach, tomato, V-8®
FRUITS	Apples (Jonathan, Rome Beauty, McIntosh, Pippin, Granny Smith), blackberries, boysenberries, cranberries, gooseberries, raspberries, cherries, green grapes, grapefruits (red, white), guavas, kiwi, kumquats, lemons, limes, loquats, mangos, melons (casaba, crenshaw, honeydew, watermelon), nectarines, oranges, papayas, peaches, pears, persimmons, pineapples, plums (purple, red), pomegranates, rhubarb, tangelos, tangerines, figs (fresh, dried), prunes
FRUIT JUICES	Apple/apricot, apricot, black cherry, red cherry, grape (purple, red, white), grapefruit, guava, lemon, papaya, pear, pineapple, pineapple/coconut, prune, tangerine, watermelon
VEGETABLE OILS	All-blend, almond, avocado, canola, coconut, corn, flaxseed, olive, peanut, safflower, sesame, soy, sunflower
SWEETENERS	Honey, brown sugar, raw sugar, refined cane sugar, barley malt syrup, corn syrup, succonant
CONDIMENTS	Salt, sea salt, Vege-Sal®, catsup, mustard, horseradish, barbecue sauce, pesto sauce, soy sauce, tahini, salsa, vinegar
SALAD DRESSINGS	Blue cheese, French, ranch, creamy Italian, creamy avocado, thousand island, vinegar and oil, lemon juice and oil

Intestinal

DESSERTS	Chocolate, desserts containing chocolate, custards, tapioca, puddings, pies, cakes
CHIPS	Bean, corn (blue, white, yellow), potato
BEVERAGES	Coffee, coffee with Re-Vita®; tea blends (Bigelow®, Constant Comment®), peppermint tea, raspberry tea, herbal tea, black tea, green tea, Japanese tea, Chinese oolong tea; mineral water, sparkling water; wine (red, white), sake, liqueurs, champagne, beer, barley malt liquor, gin, Scotch, vodka, whiskey; root beer, regular sodas
RARELY FOODS	No more than once a month
DENSE PROTEIN	Tuna
SEEDS	Pumpkin (raw)
GRAINS	Tomato pasta
VEGETABLES	Arugula, iceberg (head) lettuce
FRUITS	Apricots
FRUIT JUICES	Orange
SWEETENERS	Maple syrup, fructose, saccharin, aspertame, Equal®, Sweet'n Low®, NutraSweet®
CONDIMENTS	Margarine, mayonnaise
DESSERTS	Raspberry sherbet, orange sherbet
BEVERAGES	Diet sodas

SENSITIVE FOOD LIST

FREQUENTLY FOODS	3-7 meals per week – refers to each food, rather than category.
NUTS	Walnuts (black, English)
LEGUMES	Pinto beans
GRAINS	Amaranth, brown or white basmati rice, rice cakes
VEGETABLES	Peas, snow pea pods, sweet potatoes, cooked spinach
FRUITS	Dried pineapples
FRUIT JUICES	Cranapple, cranberry concentrate with Re-Vita®
SWEETENERS	Brown rice syrup, sorghum, date sugar
CONDIMENTS	Pickles (dill, sweet), Spike®
MODERATELY FOODS	1-2 meals per week – refers to each food, rather than category.
DENSE PROTEIN	Beef broth, beef liver, buffalo, veal, venison, organ meats (heart, brain); chicken, chicken broth, chicken livers, turkey, duck; anchovy, bass, bonita,

Intestinal

DENSE PROTEIN (Continued)	catfish, cod, flounder, haddock, halibut, herring, mackerel, mahi-mahi, perch, orange roughy, salmon, sardines, shark, red snapper, sole, swordfish, trout; abalone, calamari (squid), clams, crab, eel, mussels, octopus, oysters, scallops, shrimp
DAIRY	Buttermilk, half & half, sour cream, sweet cream, plain or flavored kefir, plain or flavored yogurt, butter
CHEESE	American, blue, brie, Camembert, white low fat Cheddar, Colby, cottage, cream, Edam, feta, goat, Gouda, Jack, kefir, Limburger, mozzarella, Muenster, Parmesan, ricotta, Romano, Swiss
NUTS and SEEDS	Cashews (raw, dry roasted), cashew butter, water chestnuts, filberts, hazelnuts, macadamias (raw, roasted), macadamia butter, pine nuts (raw, roasted)
LEGUMES	Beans (adzuki, black, lima [butter], garbanzo, kidney, great northern, navy, red), lentils, black-eyed peas, split peas, hummus, miso
GRAINS	Blue corn, millet, oats, oat flour pancakes, popcorn, popcorn cakes, quinoa, rice (Japanese, polished), rye, triticale, whole wheat, wheat bran, wheat germ, refined wheat flour, yeast-free rye bread, onion bagels, plain bagels, English muffins, crackers (oat, oriental rice, rye, saltine, sesame seed, Carr's® Table Water®, wheat), pasta, couscous, udon noodles, Chinese rice noodles, cream of rice, cream of rye, cream of wheat
VEGETABLES	Artichokes, asparagus, bamboo shoots, green beans, yellow wax beans, lima beans, bok choy, broccoli, broccoflower, cabbage (green, napa, red), carrots, cauliflower, celery, chard, cilantro, eggplant, garlic, greens (beet, collard, mustard, turnip), jicama, kale, kohlrabi, leeks, lettuce (Boston, butter, endive, curly leaf, red leaf, romaine), mushrooms, okra, olives (green, ripe), brown onions, parsley, parsnips, potatoes (all varieties), pumpkin, radishes, daikon radishes, rutabaga, sauerkraut, seaweed (arame, dulse, kelp, nori, wakame), shallots, sprouts (alfalfa, mung bean, clover, radish, sunflower), squash (acorn, banana, butternut, spaghetti, yellow [summer], zucchini), cooked tomatoes, turnips, watercress, yams
VEGETABLE JUICES	Carrot, carrot/celery, celery, parsley, spinach, tomato, V-8®
FRUITS	Apples (all varieties), bananas, blackberries, boysenberries, cranberries, gooseberries, raspberries, strawberries, cherries, grapes (black, green, red), grapefruits (white, red), guavas, kiwi, kumquats, lemons, limes, loquats, mangos, melons (casaba, cantaloupe, crenshaw), nectarines, papayas, peaches, pears, persimmons, pineapples, plums (black, purple, red), pomegranates, rhubarb, tangelos, tangerines, dates, figs (fresh, dried), prunes, raisins
FRUIT JUICES	Apple, apple cider, black cherry, red cherry, cranberry, grape (purple, red, white), grapefruit, guava, lemon, papaya, pear, pineapple, pineapple/coconut, prune, tangerine, watermelon
VEGETABLE OILS	All-blend, avocado, canola, coconut, corn, flaxseed, olive, peanut, safflower, sesame, sunflower

Intestinal

SWEETENERS	Barley malt syrup Re-Vita® , stevia
CONDIMENTS	Salt, sea salt, Vege-Sal®, tahini, vinegar
SALAD DRESSINGS	Blue cheese, French, ranch, creamy Italian, creamy avocado, thousand island, vinegar and oil, lemon juice and oil
BEVERAGES	Tea blends (Bigelow®), peppermint tea, raspberry tea, herbal tea, green tea, Japanese tea, Chinese oolong tea
RARELY FOODS	No more than once a month
DENSE PROTEIN	Beef, lamb, pork, ham, bacon, sausage; cornish game hen; wild game; tuna; lobster; eggs
DAIRY	Milk (whole, 2%, low fat, nonfat, raw), goat milk, frozen yogurt, most ice creams
NUTS and SEEDS	Almonds (raw, roasted), almond butter, Brazils, coconuts, peanuts (raw, roasted), peanut butter, pecans, pistachios, raw or roasted unsalted seeds (caraway, pumpkin, sesame, sunflower), sesame seed butter, sunflower seed butter
LEGUMES	Soy beans, soy milk, tofu
GRAINS	Barley, buckwheat, corn, corn bread, corn grits, corn tortillas, hominy grits, rice (long or short grain brown, wild), rice bran, oat bran, flour tortillas, breads (French, Italian, 7-grain, multi-grain, oat, corn, corn/rye, sprouted grain, sourdough, rye, white, whole wheat), croissants, bagels (except plain or onion), spinach pasta, tomato pasta, beet pasta
VEGETABLES	Arugula, avocados, beets, brussels sprouts, corn, cucumbers, iceberg (head) lettuce, onions (chives, green, red, white, yellow, vidalia), bell peppers (green, red, yellow), chili peppers, pimentos, raw spinach, raw tomatoes
FRUITS	Apricots, blueberries, melons (honeydew, watermelon), oranges
FRUIT JUICES	Apricot, apple/apricot, orange
VEGETABLE OILS	Soy, almond
SWEETENERS	Honey, molasses, corn syrup, maple syrup, brown sugar, raw sugar, refined cane sugar, fructose, saccharin, succonant, aspertame, Nutra Sweet®, Equal®, Sweet'n Low®
CONDIMENTS	Mayonnaise, salsa, barbecue sauce, pesto sauce, soy sauce, catsup, mustard, horseradish, margarine
SALAD DRESSINGS	Blue cheese, French, ranch, creamy Italian, creamy avocado, thousand island
DESSERTS	Chocolate, desserts containing chocolate, orange sherbet, raspberry sherbet, custards, tapioca, puddings, pies, cakes
CHIPS	Bean, corn (blue, white, yellow), potato
BEVERAGES	Coffee; Constant Comment® tea, black tea; mineral water, sparkling water, Seltzer water; wine (red, white), sake, liqueurs, barley malt liquor, champagne, beer, gin, Scotch, vodka, whiskey; root beer, diet sodas, regular sodas

Intestinal

MENUS

DIETARY EMPHASIS:

- Legumes and squash.
- Balance cooked and raw vegetables.
- Cooked vegetables best at lunch.
- Raw vegetables best at dinner.
- Foods in combinations; rotate frequently.
- Consuming 2 oz. of dense protein (chicken, turkey, eggs, or fish) with a grain such as rice or pasta, 5 times a week supports the thyroid.

WEIGHT LOSS:

- Limit dietary fat to no more than 15% of total calories and include15-20% dense protein daily.
- Eliminate bread, yeast, mayonnaise, and caffeine.
- Avoid: nuts (almonds, Brazils, cashews, coconut, filberts, peanuts, macadamias, pecans, walnuts; seeds (pumpkin, sesame, sunflower); beans (black, butter [lima], garbanzo, great northern, kidney, red, soy); lentils; dried peas; corn; bananas; dried fruit (dates, raisins, pineapple); sweets (ice cream, cheese cake).
- Limit fruit juice.

WEIGHT GAIN:

- Increase fats and food quantity.

VEGETARIAN DIET:

- Recommended, although diet may consist of up to 15% dense protein.
- Maintain fat at 25% of total calories.

FATS:

- 10-15% of caloric intake for weight loss, 20-25% for maintenance.
- Best sources are sesame seeds, tahini, butter, fish (halibut, orange roughy, salmon, shark, swordfish, lobster, shrimp), olive oil, and sesame oil.

SENSITIVE:

- May increase dense protein to 40% of calories.

KEY

—all menus may be used by healthy persons
( ) around foods means that they're optional
L denotes weight loss menus
S denotes sensitive menus
G denotes weight gain menus

BREAKFAST:
8-9 a.m. Light-to-moderate, with fruit juice, fruit, vegetables and/or dairy. No protein or grain except with fruit, sweetener, or vegetable.

SENSITIVE: Moderate-to-heavy, with vegetables, protein, seeds, and/or grain.

L			Apple juice
L			Cranberry juice (Re-Vita®)
			Cranapple juice or grape juice
L			Apple or nectarine
			Grapefruit
	S		Acorn or butternut squash and green beans (w/butter)
L			Blueberries
			Cantaloupe
L			Baked yam, sweet potato, or squash w/butter (peas or green beans)
L			Baked yam, sweet potato, or butternut squash w/butter, soy sauce, or Italian seasonings
	S		Steamed peas
L			Oatmeal w/apples
			Oatmeal w/applesauce (butter)
L			Oatmeal w/Re-Vita® or sorghum
		G	Oatmeal w/Re-Vita® and/or banana
		G	Oatmeal w/raisins
		G	Cream of rye w/dates
L			Cream of rye w/strawberries
L			Cream of rice w/pears, strawberries, or molasses
L			Short grain brown rice sauteed in butter w/broccoli and onions
L			Millet w/broccoli

Intestinal

G Whole wheat raisin muffin and apple juice or sweet potato

G Sourdough English muffin w/fruit jam or fruit

L Blueberry pancake or waffle w/rice syrup

Nutri-Grain® Total and strawberries w/low fat or 2% milk

Nutri-Grain® Total and bananas w/low fat or 2% milk

L Shredded wheat w/blueberries

L Two eggs and broccoli or asparagus

Eggs and fruit or fruit salad

S Eggs chicken or steak and hash browns

S Steak and cauliflower

S Turkey, mushrooms and onions

S Chicken, steamed broccoli, and butternut squash

S Chicken and pasta or asparagus

S Chicken tamale (salsa) (avocado)

S Steak, potato, and mixed fruit

Cottage cheese and banana

L Cottage cheese and kiwi

L Flavored yogurt

S Plain or raspberry kefir

Protein drink w/milk and fruit

MID-MORNING SNACK:
(Optional) 10-11 a.m. Fruit, dairy, vegetables, nuts, seeds.

L S Fruit

S Yogurt and fruit or flavored yogurt

S Cheese

S Kefir

S Celery w/peanut butter

S Cashews

S Carrots or jicama

LUNCH:
12-2 p.m. Moderate, with grain, protein, dairy, legumes, cooked vegetables, and/or seeds. Raw vegetables may be eaten with protein, e.g., Caesar salad with chicken.

SENSITIVE: Moderate-to-heavy, with protein, cooked vegetables and/or grain.

S Chicken, potato, and peas or broccoli

S Chicken, rice and broccoli

L Chicken, yams, green beans, and raw carrot sticks

Chicken cacciatore w/pasta

Chicken, pinto beans, and corn bread

Chicken w/peanut sauce, bell pepper, tomato, and sorghum

Caesar salad w/chicken

L S Chicken soup: chicken, carrots, potatoes, garlic, peas, and brown onions

L Salad: turkey, butter lettuce, cucumber, jicama, cilantro, red onion, and red radish w/Italian dressing or vinegar and oil

L Turkey, (rice), red leaf lettuce, brown onion, and tomato

L Turkey, (rice), romaine lettuce, and tomato

L Turkey, red potatoes, and peas or pea pods

L Turkey, rice, and green beans

Turkey loaf, potatoes, and peas (salad)

S Turkey, brown basmati rice, and peas

S Turkey, basmati rice, pinto beans, and black pepper

L S Turkey, angel hair pasta, garlic, butter, and broccoli

G Chili w/turkey, beans, and corn bread

L Salmon and white basmati or Japanese rice (cilantro and/or lemon juice)

L Fish or bean burrito

L S Sushi

L Fish taco and taquito

Fish taco, refried beans, and taquito

L Swordfish and baked potato (salad)

L Grilled swordfish and broccoli (baked potato)

L Catfish, rice, and asparagus

Intestinal

Catfish, rice, and peas

L S Catfish broiled w/lemon juice, garlic, and pepper, and brown basmati rice, and peas, (pickles)

L Salmon, pasta, and green beans

L Thresher shark w/flour tortilla, lemon juice, and coleslaw

G Beef burrito and guacamole (rice) (beans)

Beef stew

Steak, peas, and cucumber

S Steak, potato, and corn

S Pot roast, potatoes, and carrots (onions)

L Meat loaf, zucchini, and red leaf or romaine lettuce

S Lamb chops, potatoes, and peas (onions)

L Eggs and potatoes (Indian seasoning)

L S Semolina pasta and peas, broccoli, zucchini, or asparagus

G Macaroni and Colby cheese w/peas

L S Spinach pasta w/tomato sauce (tofu)

Pasta w/mushrooms and artichokes

S Seasoned pinto beans w/onions, garlic, cilantro, and rice

Fried squash (Korean) and long grain brown rice

S Brown basmati rice and seaweed, sauteed in sesame oil

Hijihki, basmati and short grain brown rice, peas, carrots, lima beans, and white sesame seeds

L Rice, squash, onions, and garlic

Rice cakes w/cashew butter, and steamed broccoli

Butternut squash w/butter and pecans

L Squash, pea pods, carrots, and onions sauteed in butter, w/rice

S Butternut or acorn squash w/sesame tahini

L Baked potato

S Baked potato w/peas and/or pinto beans

S G Lentil soup

LUNCH or DINNER:

Pinto beans, cilantro, and corn bread

L S Whole millet cooked in chicken broth

G Cream of rye w/sunflower seeds

S G Chicken, beef or cheese burrito or enchilada, rice and beans (avocado), (salsa)

S Spaghetti, tomato sauce, and meat balls (vegetable soup)

Lasagna and green beans

S Turkey, noodles, and peas

S Fish – shark, sole, swordfish, or red snapper, rice, and mixed vegetables or green beans

MID-AFTERNOON SNACK:
(Optional) 3-4 p.m. Fruit or grain.

L Blueberries or cantaloupe

G Banana

Grapes – red or black

L Raspberry tea

SNACK:
(Optional) 4-5 p.m. Protein, nuts, seeds, dairy, vegetables

G Roasted sunflower seeds (raisins)

G Rice cakes w/cashew butter

Kefir cheese

DINNER:
7-9 p.m. Moderate, with grain, dairy, legumes, protein, raw vegetables, and/or seeds.

SENSITIVE: Light-to-moderate, with vegetables, legumes, dairy, protein, and/or grain.

L S Pinto beans and cheese

L Pinto beans, cheese, and corn tortilla

Eggs, fried rice, and raw vegetables

S Omelette with eggs, cheese, bell peppers, and onion

Soup – split pea, bean, vegetable, or chicken noodle

Intestinal

	S		Baked potato (butter) and broccoli (steamed)
	S		Eggplant parmesan (manicotti)
	S		Yam and/or squash and green beans
L			Salad: romaine lettuce, mushrooms, eggs, and low fat ranch dressing
			Cream lasagna: pasta, tomato sauce, cheese, and cream (tossed salad: romaine lettuce, tomato, green onion, and cucumber)
	S		Angel hair pasta and white Cheddar cheese (tossed salad)
		G	Tabouli, hummus, and whole wheat pita bread
	S		Plain bagel w/cream cheese
	S	G	Rice cakes w/cashew butter and raw carrots
L			Rye crackers, carrots, and celery
	S		Rye cracker w/white Cheddar cheese
			Rye crackers w/white Cheddar cheese, carrots, and celery
L			Plain yogurt w/Re-Vita®
			Wine w/dinner
			EVENING SNACK: (Optional) 10 p.m.-2 a.m. Nuts, seeds, vegetables, grain, protein, fruit, sweets.
	S	G	Cashews
		G	Peanuts, pecans, raw almonds, or sunflower seeds
			Yogurt or frozen yogurt w/nuts
		G	Bagel and cream cheese
L			Carrot juice
		G	Celery w/sour cream dip
L			Popcorn
		G	Ice cream
L	S		Raspberry tea

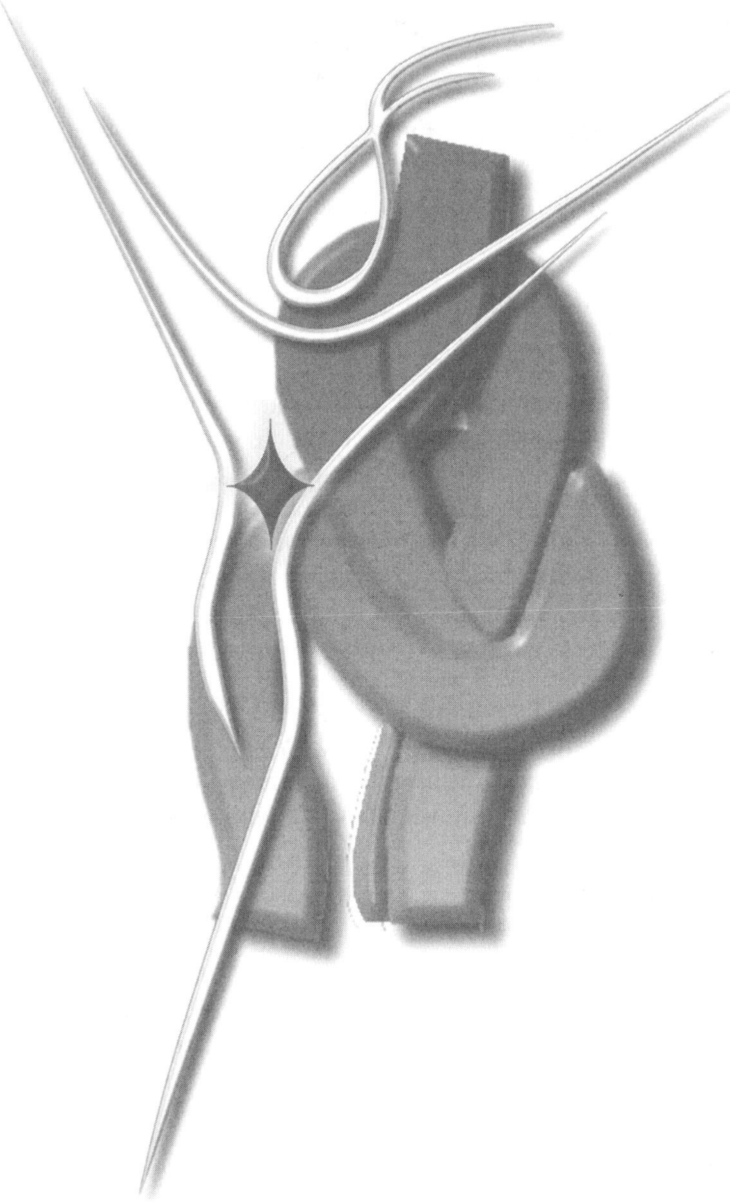

The "Kidney Body Type"
is symbolized by a bolan knot.
This unique knot takes hold when
under pressure and relaxes when the
pressure subsides. Procrastinating
until sufficient pressure builds
enables them to move further
than they ever imagined.

KIDNEY

Kidney

BODY TYPE PROFILE

LOCATION	Lower back, near lower ribs, about four inches on each side of spine.
FUNCTION	Filters blood and secretes urine.
POTENTIAL HEALTH PROBLEMS	Strong, solid body with good muscle tone. Unlike many other types, generally feel good when pregnant and have easy pregnancies. Prone to mood swings, emotional volatility, and excess nervous energy. As children, prone to attention deficits and hyperactivity (which often subside at puberty). Muscle tension and sensitivity. Digestive distress – diarrhea, gas. Chronic tooth plaquing. When unable to digest protein completely, dairy foods cause mucous. Prone to skin rashes and fungal infections.
RECOMMENDED EXERCISE	Exercise is helpful. Its benefit is initially physical. Allows movement in life and gets energy moving through body. Yoga, stretching, callanetics, tennis, running, and walking. Although may have difficulty getting motivated, exercise 4 times a week important for alleviation of stress.

WOMEN'S CHARACTERISTICS

DISTINGUISHING FEATURES	Long, oval face with V-shaped chin and high forehead. Strong, sturdy body. Large, muscular thighs. Tend to procrastinate, forcing themselves to excel when under pressure of deadlines, time, or performance.
ADDITIONAL PHYSICAL CHARACTERISTICS	Buttocks rounded-to-prominent. Low back curvature average-to-swayed. Breasts small-to-average. Shoulders relatively even with hips. Waist defined to well-defined. Average to long-waisted. Height generally petite-to-average. Bone structure medium. Average, elongated to dense, solid musculature. Hands often broad and square with short-to-average fingers. May have wide feet with short-to-average toes.
WEIGHT GAIN AREAS	Lower body with initial gain in entire upper 2/3rds of, including upper inner thighs, which can extend to knees, inner knees, lower hips, buttocks, and minimally, if at all, in abdomen. Secondary weight gain in legs (including calves and ankles) lower-to-entire abdomen, waist, upper hips, upper arms, face, and middle back. Prone to developing cellulite.

Kidney

DIETARY GUIDELINES

	SCHEDULING MEALS:
HEALTHY	Breakfast: Light-to-moderate, with light protein (dairy, eggs, nuts, seeds) and vegetables, legumes, grain, and/or fruit. Lunch: Heavy, with dense protein, dairy, nuts, seeds, legumes, vegetables, and/or grain. Dinner: Light, with light protein (eggs, dairy, cheese, nuts, seeds) vegetables, legumes, grain, and/or fruit.
SENSITIVE	Breakfast: Heavy, with dense protein and/or vegetables. Lunch: Heavy, with dense protein, legumes, vegetables, and/or grain. Dinner: Light, with vegetables, legumes, and/or vegetable juices.
DIETARY EMPHASIS	• For weight loss, observe the following intervals between meals: 6 hours between breakfast and lunch, 6 hours between lunch and dinner, 3 hours after breakfast for mid-morning snack, and 4 hours after lunch for mid-afternoon snack, consume 10-30% of calories from dense protein, and 20-25% from fats – fat calories below 15% actually inhibit weight loss. Decrease carbohydrates and increase protein. • For weight gain, increase food intake, emphasizing protein and carbohydrates; consume 25-30% of calories from dense protein, and 30-35% from fats. When at ideal weight or above (though not when underweight), creamy foods, such as ice cream, cream pie, and cheese cake, as well as all foods containing sugar and fat, will quickly increase weight. • Vegetarian diet recommended when healthy, although may have 10-15% dense protein (up to 30% when sensitive). • Fats, 20-35% of caloric intake, from olive oil, almonds, peanuts, butter, and dairy (cheese and yogurt).
KEY SUPPORTS FOR SYSTEM	Eating bananas, vegetables (tomatoes, broccoli, green beans, spinach, corn), olive oil (builds immune system) at least once a day; salsa and other spicy foods (which stimulate lymphatics); rotating foods. Minimizing refined grains. Eating meals only at scheduled times.
FOODS CRAVED	*(When Energy is Low)* Sweets, especially chocolate, ice cream, peppermint, mint chocolates. Carbohydrates, like pastry, pizza, doughnuts, cereals, corn, rice, wheat. Protein, such as peanut butter, yogurt, cheese, steak. Fruit, like bananas, oranges, apples, raisins, fruit juices. Coffee. Mexican foods.

Kidney

FOODS TO AVOID	Whole wheat bread, sugar, and certain fats such as ice cream, pie, and cheesecake since they'll cause weight gain. Also, try to stay away from each of the following foods unless eaten in these combinations: bologna and cucumber; eggs and tomato or catsup; turkey and cranberry sauce; tuna and lettuce.
KEY COMBINATIONS	When certain foods are combined, their digestibility and utilization increases. These key combinations consistently provide an enhancement that other foods are unable to match and can even increase the frequency that a food can be beneficially eaten. These combinations include: eggs with tomato, salsa or catsup; bologna with cucumber; turkey with cranberry sauce; and tuna with lettuce.
COMPLEMENTARY GLANDULAR SUPPORT	Skin, through stretching and sweating; lymphatic system, through exercise that moves lymph, such as walking or rebounding.
RECOMMENDED CUISINE	Mexican, frequently (3-7 times/wk); Thai, Chinese, Italian, Seafood, or Indian, moderately (1-2 times/wk).

Kidney

PSYCHOLOGICAL PROFILE

ESSENCE

Just as the kidneys regulate body fluid levels and are responsive to arterial pressure, Kidney body types rise to the occasion when under pressure. They respond and function best when they are needed, particularly if coupled with time or performance pressure. If sufficient outside pressure doesn't exist, they will create it, procrastinating until they get behind in their projects to the point of discomfort, which forces them to excel and move beyond their previous limits. Fearful by nature, successfully meeting challenges builds confidence and prepares them for their next experience, allowing them to move further than they had ever dreamed.

CHARACTERISTIC TRAITS

Kidneys are known for their procrastination. Their way of dealing with anything they don't feel they have all the answers for or can't do perfectly is to put it off. The pressure of a deadline forces them to do a task, even though they don't feel they are competent enough to do it. Pressure produces the stimulation needed to get busy and start a job. Ideally, successful completion then propels them to the next level. Realistically, too much procrastination causes them to fall behind, so their points of acceleration only bring them up to status quo.

Relationships are of paramount importance to Kidney types, whether it be with family, children or friends. In touch with their emotions, sensitive, and expressive, Kidneys are exceptionally good at helping others become more aware of their feelings and effectively communicate them. Being good listeners, they typically respond to the words of others accurately and objectively, rather than emotionally. Looking at things objectively, allows them to solve problems systematically, laying things out in steps. They will look a problem, size it up, and break it down, laying out the best approach.

Willing and supportive, many find that their friends frequently call them, and ask for assistance in dealing with their problems. Being generally optimistic and positive, they are usually nonjudgmental and look for the good qualities in people. Kidneys excel when working with others, particularly in a service or "teaching" capacity and find it extremely rewarding.

Kidneys need new experiences, options, and challenges. Highly creative, they are stimulated by variety, and need a wide range of choices to choose from, especially when confronted with life's challenges. Easily bored with conventional, routine, or repetitive activities, they are often drawn toward new, unproven ideas and technology. Generally practical and cautious, they need time to consider all their options.

MOTIVATION

Needing the stimulation of new concepts and projects, Kidneys experience the "routine, day-to-day stuff" boring. Not really wanting to do something, they procrastinate, feeling too tired, and have a hard time getting motivated. Craving variety, they welcome new ventures with extreme enthusiasm. Once

Kidney

MOTIVATION (Continued)

they get started, they tend to work in spurts, alternately giving their all until they either complete the task or collapse, too tired to work any longer. When motivated, they are persistent and tenacious. They will jump right in and go for it, even getting things done ahead of schedule. They actually like to complete things so they can be put in a "box" where they can be easily handled.

Kidneys control by controlling their environment. Putting things in a "box" is a way of being able to handle them and keep them under control. Needing to have a wide range of life experiences to sift through to find their purposes and ideals, Kidneys, in their sorting process, put things in "boxes" as a way of controlling and handling them. Completing jobs and doing the things that need to be done so they aren't hanging over their heads are ways of controlling their environment. In their attempt to control outcomes, they need to have everything appear perfect and all together. Unknown's are unnerving as they bring up the fear of not being able to handle a situation perfectly.

Unsure of themselves, Kidneys are fearful of making wrong decisions. In reality, since their life is about experience, the only wrong decision is no decision, because it causes them to miss opportunities or stay in situations too long. Kidneys often find themselves torn between wanting enough time to make the best decision and wanting to be in control where they are forced to make quick decisions. Being in leadership roles minimizes unknowns and adds to their sense of power and of feeling important. Deadlines force them to make a decision or accept someone else's decision. When situations become too uncomfortable or they feel trapped, Kidneys will venture into unknown areas, forcing them to excel and move beyond their previous limits.

Another reason Kidneys have such a hard time making decisions or getting started on projects is because they have such a hard time letting go. Being quite tenacious, they won't back down; so wanting to complete an experience, they tend to dwell on a situation for days on end. This often comes from their needing to get the essence, fullness, or lesson of the experience before they can release it. Ironically, the answer usually doesn't come until they are able to let it go and often appears as their ego needing to be right.

"AT WORST"

Kidneys are lazy, irresponsible or lackadaisical. They procrastinate too long or too much and get stuck. Fearful of making a mistake or being inadequate, they avoid taking any action. Lacking self-esteem they get stuck in abusive or co-dependent relationships. Being too hard on themselves or impatient, often results in their being impulsive or irrational. Their self-defeating and self-destructive behavior can affect all aspects of their lives. Lacking adequate self-confidence or knowledge of what they really want, they easily succumb to peer pressure, drugs or alcohol.

When their fear surfaces, the underlying pessimist appears, and they get caught in thinking the worst, "You know my luck" or "what if?" Being exceptionally good at visualization and creating what they focus their

Kidney

"AT WORST" (Continued)

attention upon, they manifest negative situations. Basically fearful, Kidneys will limit themselves by their own self-imposed limitations. Unresolved emotional stress tends to affect them physically, resulting in excess weight or restrictive health problems.

Kidneys are bored by routine, but without structure, they procrastinate. Seeking approval, they over commit or overextend themselves, making promises they can't keep or exhausting themselves trying to do it all. By spreading themselves too thin, their health eventually suffers or they lose significant opportunities by not prioritizing and following through on important projects. They spend an excessive amount of time getting ready to do something, and waste time in too much preparation. By not handling things as they come up, Kidneys allow the pressure to build until they are forced to act. They will then react to situations emotionally, either through activity without thought or direction, or fear, becoming lackadaisical.

"AT BEST"

Sensitive and expressive, Kidneys are in touch with their emotions. They love people and have a special gift for helping others connect with and communicate their own feelings. With their ability to listen and hear what a person is truly saying, as well as see viable, practical solutions, Kidneys make excellent mediators, counselors and teachers. Especially gratifying is serving others in ways that make significant differences in their lives.

Having developed their self-confidence to the point where they are no longer compelled to hold themselves back, Kidneys can be quite capable of making quick decisions and acting on their feelings. They are able to take advantage of new experiences, focusing on those that have a purpose or an ideal. Kidneys are extremely adaptable and are happiest when they are free to choose between several options. Flexibility comes when there are options, which only comes through multiple experiences. Of particular importance is truth, people and experiences with them.

Creative and intuitive, Kidneys are good at seeing and implementing practical solutions. Extremely visual, they are very good at visualizing expected results and outcomes before they happen. Self-confidence comes from pushing through their fears. By making conscious choices and pushing through the fear that holds them back, the world opens up and supports them in experiencing the fullness of life. Having learned to balance their feelings with their mind, and their receptive, feminine side with their active masculine side, Kidneys are able to visualize what they want and have it manifest. They are able to move beyond any limitation and assist others in doing the same. Being firmly connected with God or their spiritual Source gives them the courage to know and speak their truth.

Kidney

FOOD LISTS

HEALTHY FOOD LIST

FREQUENTLY FOODS	3-7 meals per week – refers to each food, rather than category.
DENSE PROTEIN	Beef; salmon, trout, tuna; crab, lobster, scallops
CHEESE	Cheese (blue, feta), sour cream, butter
NUTS	Almonds (raw, roasted), peanuts (raw, roasted), peanut butter, pine nuts (raw, roasted), walnuts (black, English)
LEGUMES	Beans (black, garbanzo, butter [lima], kidney, navy, pinto), hummus
GRAINS	Rice (white or brown basmati, Chinese or Japanese white), couscous, pasta, refined wheat breads (white, sourdough, Italian, French, dill/rye), croissants
VEGETABLES	Avocados, green beans, cabbage (green, napa, red), carrots, cucumbers, eggplant, garlic, iceberg lettuce, cooked onions, peas, snow pea pods, yellow bell peppers, potatoes (yukon gold, purple), sweet potatoes, radishes, daikon radishes, cherry tomatoes, tomatoes (canned, hot-house, vine-ripened), yams
FRUITS	Apples (all varieties), bananas, raspberries, grapefruits (white, red), kiwi, lemons, limes, loquats, cantaloupes, oranges, peaches
SWEETENERS	Re-Vita®, stevia
BEVERAGES	Tea (Good Earth®, peppermint, spearmint)
MODERATELY FOODS	1-2 meals per week – refers to each food, rather than category.
DENSE PROTEIN	Beef broth, beef liver, buffalo, lamb, ham, bacon, sausage, pork, organ meats (heart, brain), veal, venison, pastrami, pepperoni; chicken (dark, white, broth, livers), cornish hen, turkey, duck; ahi, anchovy, sea bass, bonita, catfish, cod, flounder, haddock, halibut, herring, mackerel, mahi-mahi, perch, orange roughy, sardines, shark, red snapper, sole, swordfish; abalone, calamari (squid), clams, eel, mussels, octopus, oysters, shrimp; eggs
DAIRY	Milk (nonfat, raw, half & half), goat milk, buttermilk, sweet cream, kefir, low fat or nonfat flavored yogurt, frozen yogurt, ice cream (Dreyer's, Ben & Jerry's®, Swensen's®)
CHEESE	American, brie, Camembert, Cheddar, Colby, cottage, cream, Edam, goat, Gouda, Jack, kefir, Limburger, mozzarella, Muenster, Parmesan, ricotta, Romano, Swiss
NUTS and SEEDS	Almond butter, Brazils, cashews (raw, roasted), cashew butter, water chestnuts, coconuts, filberts, hazelnuts, macadamias (raw, roasted), macadamia butter, pecans, pistachios, raw or roasted seeds (caraway, pumpkin, sesame, sunflower), sesame seed butter, sunflower seed butter
LEGUMES	Beans (adzuki, great northern, red, soy), split peas, soy milk, tofu, tempeh, miso

Kidney

GRAINS	Amaranth, barley, buckwheat, corn, corn bread, corn grits, corn tortillas, flour tortillas, millet, oats, oat bran, popcorn, quinoa, rice (long or short grain brown, wild), rice cakes, rice bran, rye, triticale, breads (7-grain, multi-grain, corn, English toasting, corn/rye, rye, sprouted grain), whole wheat, wheat bran, wheat germ, white flour, multi-grains, bagels, English muffins, crackers (saltines, wheat, oat, rye), vegetable pasta, udon noodles, cream of rice, cream of rye, cream of wheat
VEGETABLES	Artichokes, arugula, asparagus, bamboo shoots, yellow wax beans, beets, bok choy, broccoflower, broccoli, brussels sprouts, cauliflower, celery, chard, cilantro, corn, greens (beet, collard, mustard, turnip), jicama, kale, kohlrabi, leeks, lettuce (butter, endive, red leaf, romaine), mushrooms, okra, olives (black, green, ripe), raw onions (chives, brown, green, red, white, yellow, vidalia), parsley, parsnips, bell peppers (red, green), chili peppers, pimentos, potatoes (red, russet, white rose), pumpkin, rutabaga, sauerkraut, sea vegetables (arame, dulse, kelp, nori, wakame), shallots, spinach, sprouts (alfalfa, clover, mung bean, radish, sunflower), squash (acorn, banana, butternut, spaghetti, yellow [summer] zucchini), taro leaves, turnips, watercress
VEGETABLE JUICES	Carrot, carrot/celery, celery, parsley, spinach, tomato, V-8®
FRUITS	Apricots, blackberries, blueberries, boysenberries, cranberries, gooseberries, strawberries, mixed berries, mixed fruit, cherries, grapes (black, green, red, white), guavas, kumquats, mangos, melons (casaba, crenshaw, honeydew, watermelon), nectarines, papayas, pears, persimmons, pineapples, plums (black, purple, red), pomegranates, rhubarb, tangelos, tangerines, unsulphured dried apricots, dates, figs (fresh, dried), prunes, raisins
FRUIT JUICES	Rotate: Apple, apple cider, apple/apricot, apricot, black cherry, cherry, cranapple, cranberry, grape (purple, red, white), grapefruit, guava, lemon, orange, papaya, pear, pineapple, pineapple/coconut, prune, tangerine
VEGETABLE OILS	All-blend, almond, avocado, canola, coconut, corn, flaxseed, olive, peanut, safflower, sesame, soy, sunflower
SWEETENERS	Honey, molasses, sorghum, barley malt syrup, corn syrup, raw sugar,refined white sugar, brown sugar, fructose
CONDIMENTS	Pesto sauce, salsa, catsup, mustard, Miracle Whip®, soy sauce, barbecue sauce, tahini, sweet or dill pickles, vinegar, salt
SALAD DRESSINGS	Blue cheese, French, Italian, ranch, roquefort, creamy avocado, creamy Italian, thousand island, vinegar and oil, lemon juice and oil
DESSERTS	Custard, tapioca, raspberry sherbet, orange sherbet
CHIPS	Bean, corn (white, yellow)
BEVERAGES	Herbal tea, black tea, regular tea, Japanese tea; mineral water, sparkling water; wine (red, white), sake, beer, barley malt liquor, champagne, gin, Scotch, vodka, whiskey; root beer, regular sodas

Kidney

RARELY FOODS	No more than once a month
DAIRY	Plain yogurt, milk (whole, low fat), most ice creams
LEGUMES	Black-eyed peas, lentils
GRAINS	Polished white rice, breads (whole wheat, raisin, buckwheat, oat)
SWEETENERS	Brown rice syrup, maple syrup, date sugar, succonant, aspartame, Equal®, saccharin, Sweet'n Low®, NutraSweet®
CONDIMENTS	Horseradish, mayonnaise, margarine
DESSERTS	Chocolate, desserts containing chocolate
CHIPS	Blue corn, potato
BEVERAGES	Coffee; diet sodas
OTHER	Blue/green algae, acidophilus

SENSITIVE FOOD LIST

FREQUENTLY FOODS	3-7 meals per week – refers to each food, rather than category.
DENSE PROTEIN	Fresh tuna (raw, as in sushi, or cooked)
VEGETABLES	Avocados, string beans, peas
MODERATELY FOODS	1-2 meals per week – refers to each food, rather than category.
DENSE PROTEIN	Beef (broth, liver), steak, veal, venison, organ meats (heart, brain); chicken (broth, livers), cornish hen, turkey; ahi, sea bass, bonita, catfish, cod, flounder, haddock, halibut, herring, mackerel, mahi-mahi, perch, orange roughy, salmon, sardines, shark, red snapper, sole, swordfish, trout, tuna (water-packed albacore); abalone, calamari (squid), clams, eel, mussels, octopus, oysters; eggs in foods
DAIRY	Milk (nonfat, raw, half & half), sweet cream, sour cream, kefir, low fat or nonfat yogurt (plain, peach, vanilla), butter
CHEESE	American, brie, Camembert, Cheddar, Colby, cottage, Edam, feta, goat,Gouda, Jack, kefir, Limburger, mozzarella, Muenster, Parmesan, ricotta, Romano, Swiss
NUTS and SEEDS	Almond butter, cashews (raw, roasted), cashew butter, water chestnuts, filberts, hazelnuts, pecans, peanuts (raw, roasted), peanut butter, pine nuts (raw, roasted), pistachios, raw or roasted seeds (caraway, pumpkin, sesame, sunflower), sesame seed butter, sunflower seed butter
LEGUMES	Beans (adzuki, black, garbanzo, kidney, lima [butter], navy, great northern, pinto, red, soy), tofu, tempeh, soy milk, hummus, miso

Kidney

GRAINS	Amaranth, barley, flour tortillas, millet, popcorn, quinoa, rice (white or brown basmati, long or short grain brown, Japanese white, wild), rice bran, rice cakes, popcorn rice cakes, rye, triticale, white flour, wheat bran, wheat germ, breads (English toasting, French, Italian, sourdough, rye, sprouted grain, white), bagels, croissants, English muffins, couscous, udon noodles, pasta, vegetable pasta, hard wheat pasta without tomatoes, crackers (saltines, wheat, oat, rye), cream of rice, cream of rye, cream of wheat
VEGETABLES	Artichokes, bamboo shoots, green beans, yellow wax beans, bok choy, broccoflower, cabbage (green, napa, red), celery, chard, cilantro, cucumbers, greens (beet, collard, mustard, turnip), jicama, kale, kohlrabi, leeks, lettuce (butter, endive, green and red leaf, romaine), okra, olives (black, green, ripe), cooked (green, white) or raw onions (chives, brown, red, yellow, vidalia), parsnips, snow pea pods, yellow bell peppers, chili peppers, pimentos, potatoes (white rose, yukon gold, purple), sweet potatoes, pumpkin, radishes, daikon radishes, rutabaga, sauerkraut, seaweed (arame, dulse, kelp, nori, wakame), shallots, spinach, sprouts (alfalfa, clover, radish, sunflower), squash (acorn, banana, butternut, spaghetti, yellow (summer), turnips
VEGETABLE JUICES	Carrot, carrot/celery, celery, parsley, spinach, tomato, V-8®
FRUITS	Apples (Golden Delicious, Granny Smith, Jonathan, McIntosh, Pippin, Rome Beauty), bananas, blackberries, boysenberries, gooseberries, raspberries, cherries, grapes (black, green, red, white), grapefruits (red, white), guavas, kumquats, lemons, limes, loquats, melons (cantaloupe, casaba, crenshaw), nectarines, peaches, pears, persimmons, pineapples, plums (red, black, purple), pomegranates, rhubarb, tangelos, tangerines, unsulpured dried apricots, dates, figs (fresh, dried), raisins
FRUIT JUICES	(rotate): Apple, apple cider, apple/apricot, apricot, black cherry, cherry, cranapple, cranberry, grape (purple, red, white), grapefruit, guava, lemon, papaya, pear, pineapple, pineapple/coconut, tangerine, prune
VEGETABLE OILS	All-blend, almond, avocado, coconut, flaxseed, peanut, olive, safflower, sesame, soy, sunflower
SWEETENERS	Re-Vita®, stevia
CONDIMENTS	Salsa, tahini, vinegar, salt
SALAD DRESSINGS	Vinegar and oil, lemon juice and oil, creamy avocado
BEVERAGES	Good Earth® herbal tea, peppermint and spearmint tea, regular tea, Japanese tea;mineral water, sparkling water
RARELY FOODS	No more than once a month
DENSE PROTEIN	Buffalo, lamb, bacon, ham, sausage, pork, pastrami, pepperoni; duck; anchovies, tuna (oil packed); crab, lobster, scallops, shrimp; eggs
DAIRY	Cheese (blue, cream), milk (whole, low fat), buttermilk, goat milk, regular (whole milk) yogurt, strawberry yogurt, frozen yogurt, ice cream

Kidney

NUTS and SEEDS	Almonds (raw, roasted), Brazils, coconuts, macadamias (raw, roasted), macadamia butter, walnuts (black, English)
LEGUMES	Split peas, black-eyed peas, lentils
GRAINS	Buckwheat, corn, corn bread, corn grits, corn tortillas, oats, polished white rice, whole wheat, multigrains, breads (buckwheat, corn, corn/rye, dill/rye, multigrain, 7-grain, oat, raisin, whole wheat)
VEGETABLES	Arugula, asparagus, beets, broccoli, brussels sprouts, carrots, cauliflower, corn, eggplant, garlic, lettuce (iceberg), mushrooms, raw onions (green, white), parsley, bell peppers (red, green), potatoes (red, russet), mung bean sprouts, tomatoes, cherry tomatoes, watercress, yams, zucchini
FRUITS	Apple sauce, Red Delicious apples, apricots, blueberries, cranberries, mixed berries, strawberries, kiwi, mangos, melons (honeydew, watermelon), oranges, papayas, soaked prunes
FRUIT JUICES	Orange
VEGETABLE OILS	Canola, corn
SWEETENERS	Honey, molasses, sorghum, brown sugar, date, sugar, raw sugar, refined cane sugar, maple syrup, barley malt syrup, corn syrup, brown rice syrup, succonant, fructose, saccharin, aspartame, Equal®, Sweet'n Low®, NutraSweet®
CONDIMENTS	Catsup, mustard, soy sauce, barbecue sauce, pesto sauce, horseradish, mayonnaise, margarine, Miracle Whip®
SALAD DRESSINGS	Blue cheese, French, ranch, roquefort, creamy Italian, thousand island
DESSERTS	Custard, tapioca, raspberry sherbert, orange sherbert, chocolate, desserts containing chocolate
CHIPS	Bean, corn (blue, white, yellow), potato
BEVERAGES	Coffee; black tea; wine (red, white) sake, beer, barley malt liquor, champagne, gin, Scotch, vodka, whiskey; root beer, diet sodas, regular sodas
OTHER	Blue/green algae, acidophilus

Kidney

MENUS

DIETARY EMPHASIS:

- Bananas, vegetables (tomatoes, broccoli, green beans, spinach, corn).
- Olive oil at least once a day, as it builds immune system.
- Salsa and other spicy foods as they stimulate lymphatics.
- Minimize refined grains.
- Rotate foods.
- Key combinations make the first food much easier to digest.

WEIGHT LOSS:

- Breakfast, light with fruit and/or grain.
- Mid-morning snack, fruit.
- Lunch, heavy with protein, dairy, nuts, seeds, legumes, vegetables, and/or grain.
- Mid-afternoon snack, grain with butter.
- Dinner, light with vegetables and/or legumes.
- Observe the following intervals between meals: 6 hours between breakfast and lunch, 6 hours between lunch and dinner, 3 hours after breakfast for mid-morning snack, and 4 hours after lunch for mid-afternoon snack.
- Decrease carbohydrates and increase protein.
- 10-30% of caloric intake from dense protein.
- 20-25% from fats, below 15% inhibits weight loss.

WEIGHT GAIN:

- Increase quantity of food, emphasizing protein and carbohydrates.
- 25-30% of caloric intake from dense protein.
- 30-35% of caloric intake from fats.
- When at ideal weight or above (though not when underweight), creamy foods, such as ice cream, cream pie, and cheese cake, as well as all foods containing sugar and fat, will quickly increase weight.

VEGETARIAN DIET:

- Recommended when healthy, although may have up to 30% dense protein.

FATS:

- 20-35% of caloric intake.
- Best sources are olive oil, almonds, peanuts, butter, and dairy (cheese and yogurt).

KEY

—all menus may be used by healthy persons

( ) around foods means that they're optional

L denotes weight loss menus

S denotes sensitive menus

G denotes weight gain menus

BREAKFAST:
8-9 a.m. Light-to-moderate, with light protein (eggs, dairy, nuts, seeds) and vegetables, legumes, grain, and/or fruit.

SENSITIVE: Heavy, with dense protein and/or vegetables.

L	S	G	Menu
		G	Peanut butter on rice cakes or sourdough toast (carrots)
	S		Peanut butter and apples
			Peanut butter (on white or sourdough bread) and banana
			Nuts – peanuts, almonds, or walnuts (raisins)
		G	Cole slaw and unsalted peanuts
		G	French toast and bacon (syrup)
			EGGS, and TOMATO or CATSUP – Key combination
		G	Eggs, catsup, and sourdough bread
		G	Eggs and mashed potatoes w/tomato or catsup
		G	Egg and cheese omelette, tomato, or catsup (pancakes)
L			Oatmeal w/strawberries
	S		Cheerios or granola (nonfat milk or yogurt)
		G	Cheerios® or granola, banana or kiwi, and skim milk
L			Couscous (raisins)
		G	Couscous w/almonds or walnuts

Kidney

L	S	G	
L			Cream of rice w/banana
L			Corn grits or cornmeal mush
		G	Polenta – cornmeal w/cheese
			Banana smoothie w/protein powder, milk, and banana
			Smoothie: banana, strawberries, and apple juice
L			Smoothie: banana, raspberries, and grape juice
			Protein drink w/protein powder, apple, celery, and carrot juice
			Apples and cheese, Cheddar, mozzarella, Monterey Jack, Swiss, or brie
			Low fat or nonfat cottage cheese
			Low fat or nonfat yogurt and apple or banana
			Avocado and cauliflower or corn
			Apples and cheese
L			Bananas, kiwi, green apples, red apples, or orange
L			Cantaloupe
L			White basmati rice cooked in beef or chicken broth
L			Plain waffle
			Oat bran muffin or banana nut muffin
L			Oat bran toast w/butter, banana, and orange juice
L			English muffin (toasted) w/butter, peach and tea
			Cherry almond or raspberry scone
	S		Baked yukon gold potato and green beans
	S		Steamed vegetables (butter)
	S		Fish and carrots or broccoli
	S		Chicken and potato (gravy, and/or peas, or salad)
	S		Chicken and spinach salad
	S		Steak and white rose potato

MID-MORNING SNACK:
(Optional) 10 a.m. Fruit.

L	S	G	
L	S		Raisins
L			Apple, peach, banana, grapes, raspberries, blueberries, cantaloupe, or watermelon
L	S		Banana smoothie

LUNCH:
12-2 p.m. Heavy, with dense protein, dairy, nuts, seeds, legumes, vegetables, and/or grain.

SENSITIVE: Heavy, with dense protein, vegetables, legumes, and/or grain.

TUNA and LETTUCE – Key combination

L	S	G	
L	S	G	Tuna, avocado, lettuce, tomato, and sunflower seeds
L			Tuna and lettuce (carrots and/or cherry tomatoes).
		G	Tuna and lettuce on croissant or bread – white, French or Italian
	S		Tuna and hard-boiled egg (salad: romaine lettuce, avocado, and celery w/Italian dressing
L		G	Shrimp, Indian rice, and vegetables
L		G	Trout and rice (brussels sprouts)
L			Crab or shrimp sushi
L	S	G	Any fish and carrots or broccoli (rice)
			California roll
			BOLOGNA and CUCUMBER – Key combination
		G	Bologna on white bread, w/lettuce, tomato, and cucumber
		G	Bologna, cucumber, and raw onion on French or Indian bread
		G	Chili and corn bread
		G	Beef stroganoff (salad or cucumbers)
		G	Steak, eggs and catsup or tomato (potatoes)
L	S	G	Broiled steak and salad: romaine lettuce, radish, and onion
L		G	Beef or lamb, and broccoli or peas
L	S	G	Beef liver, potatoes, and carrots
L	S	G	Steak or chicken, potatoes, carrots, and onions
L		G	Liver and onions, broccoli or peas
		G	Chicken w/macaroni and cheese
L		G	Chicken, potatoes, and broccoli
	S	G	Chicken, potatoes, and green beans
	S	G	Chicken and baked yukon gold potato w/butter and chives
		G	Chicken, rice, and green beans

Kidney

L G	Chicken burrito w/beans and cheese
L S G	Chicken pot pie
L S G	Chicken chow mein
L S G	Chicken and salad
L G	Chicken, vegetables, and rice
	TURKEY and CRANBERRY SAUCE – Key combination
G	Turkey and cranberry sauce on white bread
	Turkey, cranberry sauce, and salad
L G	Pizza topped w/ham, cheese, and peppers
G	Pizza topped w/Canadian bacon and pineapple (cheese)
L S	Clam chowder
G	Ham and beans w/corn bread
L	Grilled or sauteed mushrooms, red bell peppers, zucchini, eggplant, and red onion over rice or pasta, w/salad
L	Caesar salad
L G	Beans and corn bread
L	Pasta w/olive oil, garlic, yellow bell pepper, and broccoli
L G	Pasta w/romano or parmesan cheese

LUNCH or DINNER:

L	Salad: lettuce, beans, corn, and peas
L	Cauliflower and avocado w/soy sauce, garlic powder, and pepper
	Avocado and sprouts on white bread
G	Bean burrito (salsa and/or avocado)
	Beans w/corn tortilla (corn)
	Quinoa w/any variety of squash (soy sauce)
	Basmati rice and green beans
S	Vegetarian chili

MID-AFTERNOON SNACK: (Optional) 4-5 p.m. Grain and butter.

L	Rice cake, crackers, or tortillas w/butter

DINNER: 6-8 p.m. Light, with light protein (eggs, dairy, cheese, nuts, seeds), vegetables, legumes, grain, and/or fruit.

SENSITIVE: Light with vegetables, legumes, and/or vegetable juices.

	Stir fry: yellow bell pepper, garlic, and parsley on white rice, and cantaloupe and honeydew melon slices
	Stir-fry: tofu, bean sprouts, mushrooms, almonds, garlic, onions fried in canola oil and served over rice
	Red bell peppers, zucchini, eggplant, and red onion over rice or pasta, and salad
	Eggplant parmesan, salad, and garlic bread
	Steamed carrots, pea pods, green beans, and white flour tortilla w/cheese
L S	Steamed carrots, pea pods, and string beans
L S	White rose potato and navy beans
L	Salad: lettuce, beans, corn, and peas
L S	Salad: lettuce, cucumber, beans, corn, tomatoes, and peas
L S	Salad: red leaf lettuce, sprouts, onion, garbanzo beans, spinach, sunflower seeds, and Italian dressing
L S	Salad: butter lettuce, yellow bell peppers, chives, and radish w/olive oil and lemon juice
L S	Spinach salad
S	Mixed green salad and baked potato w/butter, sour cream, and chives
L S	Raw vegetables
S	Vegetable juices
G	Pasta w/cheese (garlic bread)
G	Pasta and cheese w/peas and green beans
	Pasta w/olive oil, garlic, red bell pepper and/or green pepper, and broccoli
	Couscous and broccoli
	Couscous, raisins, cinnamon, and Rice Dream®
G	Cheese quesadilla on flour tortilla (salad and/or chips and salsa)
G	Corn tortilla w/Gouda cheese

Kidney

	G	Grilled cheese sandwich w/celery or lettuce salad
	G	Sourdough bread, brie cheese, and green apple
	G	Bagel, cream cheese, and raisins
		Millet w/onions and mushrooms (asparagus)
		White basmati rice in broth – beef, chicken or fish
		Wild rice, tofu, and chard (plum)
		Pinto or black beans and rice
		Beans and corn bread
	G	Pinto beans and rice (tortilla and/or cheese
	G	Bean burrito w/cheese
L	S	Lentils and green beans
L	S	Lentil soup
	G	Chicken noodle soup and egg salad sandwich
L	S	Baked potato and vegetables
L	S	Baked potato (cream cheese) and beans
	G	Yukon gold potatoes, mushrooms, plain yogurt, and sesame seeds
		Broccoli and cheese quiche
	G	Eggs and potatoes w/hot sauce (chard)
	G	Omelette w/cheese and tomato
		Eggs and salsa, cauliflower, and corn on the cob
	G	Vegetarian pizza
	G	Falafel vegeburger w/cheese and avocado, and banana/apple smoothie
		Tofu w/rice, vegetable, and salad
		Tofu, rice, soy sauce, and sprouts (tomatoes)
	G	Apples and cheese
	G	Apples or bananas and peanut butter
	G	Banana smoothie

DESSERTS: After lunch or dinner.

L		Apples, berries, cantaloupe, honeydew, or watermelon
	G	Fig Newtons®

EVENING SNACK:
(Optional) 10 p.m.-2 a.m. Protein, nuts, seeds, dairy, vegetables, grain, fruit, sweets.

			Cherry almond or raspberry scone
	S		Peanuts and raisins
			Peanuts, almonds, or walnuts
	S		Apples and peanut butter or cheese
	S		Grapes, raspberries, peaches, or pears
L			Pineapple upside down cake
		G	Macadamia chocolate chip cookies and milk
			Cherry pie
			New York style cheese cake
			Ice cream

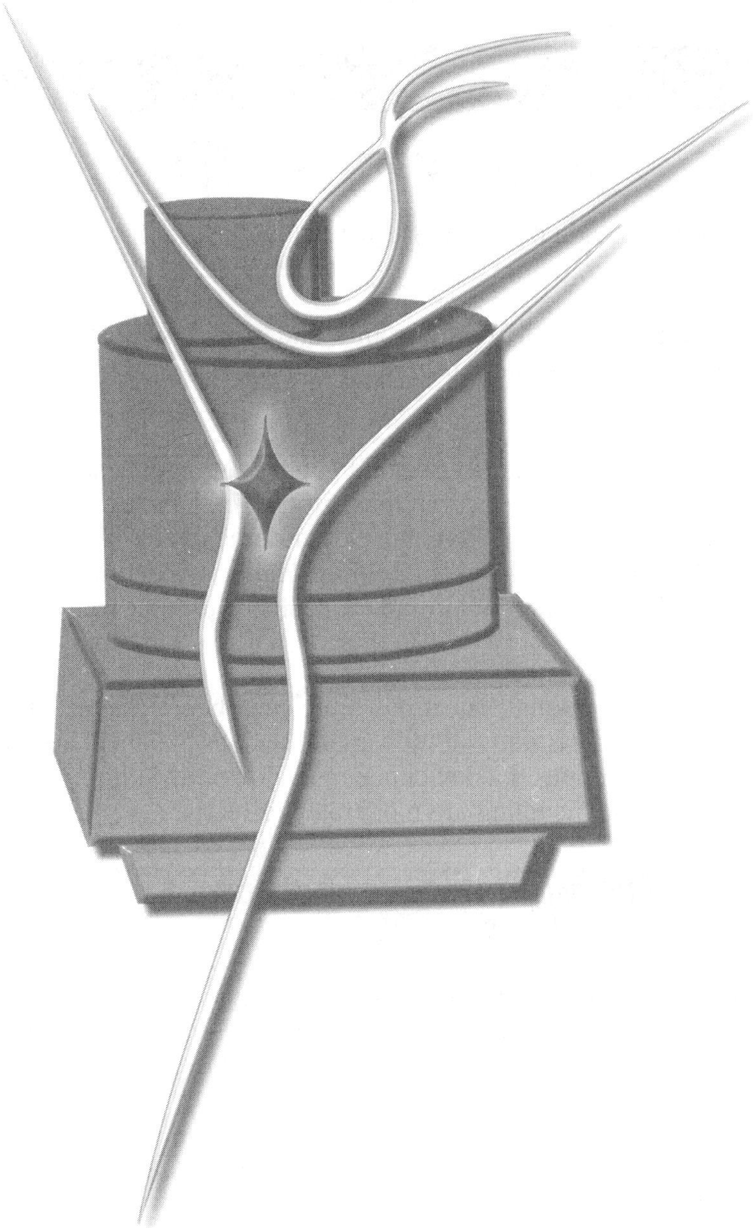

The "Liver Body Type" is symbolized by a food processor. Converting and processing sugars and protein is like putting the pieces together and fitting them into the flow of the day or project. Loyal and stable, they excel at helping with whatever needs to be done.

Liver

BODY TYPE PROFILE

LOCATION	Upper right side of abdomen, just below the diaphragm.
FUNCTION	Essential to life, it produces bile and converts most sugars into glycogen, which it stores for later use.
POTENTIAL HEALTH PROBLEMS	Basically strong, sturdy, healthy body with good stamina and endurance. Problems generally involve musculo-skeletal system with injuries involving joints and sore or sensitive muscles. Edema (water retention). Sensitive skin, resulting in rashes, hives, or itching. Hair may become coarse when suffering from adrenal stress. Migraine headaches; vascular weakness.
RECOMMENDED EXERCISE	Exercise is optional, but it has a physical benefit, as it burns calories. Best when there is a fluidity of movement, such as in dance, jazzercise, callanetics, Tai Chi, walking, backpacking, and downhill skiing. Exercise machines, weights, and bicycling are moderately effective.

WOMEN'S CHARACTERISTICS

DISTINGUISHING FEATURES	Broad, thick torso with little weight gain in thighs. Buttocks relatively flat-to-rounded. Often have well-defined muscular calves. Exceptionally loyal and family-oriented. Good teachers. Tend to put things together so they flow.
ADDITIONAL PHYSICAL CHARACTERISTICS	Generally low back curvature straight-to-average. Breasts average-to-large. Shoulders relatively even with, to broader than, hips. Straight-to-defined waist. Average to short-waisted. Height generally average, although can range from petite to very tall. Bone structure small-to-large. Strong, solid body with sturdy appearance. Dense, solid musculature, often with well-defined muscular calves. Typically, smaller lower body with narrow hips. May wear two sizes of clothes, with top larger than bottom. Average-to-thick or wide hands and feet. Round, oval, or rectangular face. Short, thick neck, with tendency toward double chin.
WEIGHT GAIN AREAS	Upper body with initial gain in lower to entire abdomen, waist, upper, middle, and entire back, upper hips, and upper inner thighs, with slight gain in entire upper 2/3rds of thighs. Alternative weight gain pattern: upper abdomen, waist, entire back, upper hips, upper inner thighs, upper arms, and face. Secondary weight gain as solid thickening in upper abdomen, upper and entire back, upper arms, entire inner and outer thighs, under chin, and breasts.

Liver

WEIGHT GAIN AREAS (Continued)	Weight gain results in a general thickening, noticeable on profile, rather than a widening. May have cellulite on upper arms and inner thighs. Little, if any, weight gain in thighs.

DIETARY GUIDELINES

SCHEDULING MEALS:

"HEALTHY"

Breakfast: Light, with grain, dairy, protein, vegetables, legumes, and/or fruit or fruit juice.

Lunch: Heavy, with protein, dairy, nuts, seeds, legumes, grain, vegetables, and/or limited fruit.

Dinner: Moderate-to-heavy, with legumes, grain, protein, dairy, and/or vegetables.

"SENSITIVE"

Breakfast: Moderate-to-heavy, with grain, dairy, protein, vegetables, legumes, and/or fruit or fruit juice.

Lunch: Light-to-moderate, with protein, dairy, nuts, seeds, legumes, grain, vegetables, and/or limited fruit.

Dinner: Moderate, with legumes, grain, protein, dairy, and/or vegetables

DIETARY EMPHASIS

- Alcohol: May affect sinuses and decrease energy. When sensitive, may experience depression or sleepiness after consumption, particularly with grain alcohols. Tequila, with lime or orange juice and without salt, can, if consumed in moderation, be more easily tolerated. Can usually tolerate, with no side effects, up to 1/2 glass (i.e., up to 4 oz) of wine with dinner, 2 meals per week.
- For weight loss, eliminate salt, reduce fats to 15%, exercise daily, get emotional support (weight loss groups are often appropriate), and avoid chocolate, sodas, and alcohol (although may use appetite suppressants).
- For weight gain, consume 25% of calories from dense protein, increase fats to 25%, and follow a balanced diet.
- Vegetarian diet nutritionally inadequate; need 10-25% of caloric intake from dense protein.
- Fats, 15-25% of total caloric intake, from butter, cheese, cottage cheese, fish, and chicken.

Liver

KEY SUPPORTS FOR SYSTEM	Rotation and variety – vegetables, fruits, protein (eggs, poultry, fish); moderate dairy. Since raw foods are generally supportive to system, more raw than steamed vegetables are recommended. Garlic supports immune system. Food is best assimilated when eaten in combinations. Need 8 glasses of water daily. Frequently require outside emotional support, for which support groups can be beneficial.
COMPLEMENTARY GLANDULAR SUPPORT	Adrenals, through consuming dense protein (best sources include eggs, poultry, and fish), fruits, and vegetables; lungs, through nurturing both self and others.
FOODS TO AVOID	Salt, pork, diet sodas, regular sodas, chocolate, and artificial sweeteners as they can all cause liver damage.
FOODS CRAVED	(*When energy is low*) Salty foods such as chips, nuts, bacon (as in BLT sandwich). Protein foods with sauces or gravy (chicken or beef), cheeses – including melted cheese such as on cheeseburgers. Creamy foods like ice cream, chocolate with creamy or caramel centers. Sweets, especially donuts, pastries, pies and sugary desserts.
RECOMMENDED CUISINE	Seafood; Chinese, Japanese, Thai, Indian; English, German, Irish, homestyle (meat and potatoes), foods prepared with gravies and sauces; Italian and Mexican. Spicy foods, including jalepeno and chili peppers, as well as curry, as they stimulate lymphatic system.

PSYCHOLOGICAL PROFILE

ESSENCE	Just as the liver is in charge of converting substances into usable forms and filtering out what can't be used, the Liver body type unifies life. Livers are noted for putting pieces together and fitting them into the flow of the day or project. Placing a high priority on family, loyalty, and stability, they excel at helping with whatever needs to be done. By seeing something in the flow, they create the desire, that when coupled with their tremendous physical strength, results in accomplishment or manifestation. Teaching, often through leader-ship, is their way of insuring the unity of life, as the knowledge gained by one generation can flow to the next.

Liver

CHARACTERISTIC TRAITS

Liver body types are family-oriented, and extremely loyal. Consistent and reliable, they can always be counted on to carry out their duties and obligations. Their strong family ties make them exceptionally devoted to their children. Faithful and dependable, Livers are known for being there through thick and thin. Supportive and caring, they can always be relied upon to help out with whatever needs to be done.

The basic nature of Livers is kind, patient, and considerate. People-oriented, they function well in most social situations. Needing to be needed, Liver types enjoy giving of themselves and being there for others. Teaching gives them an ultimate sense of fulfillment, as it enables them to give to others and experience themselves as being important and valuable.

Liver types are tough and resilient. They have a great deal of physical endurance and are able to see a job through to its completion. They enjoy seeing the physical results of their efforts. Livers have a strong sense of commitment, perseverance, and orderliness. They derive a great deal of enjoyment through the actual doing of their tasks or creative projects.

Known for their good organizational skills, Livers are attentive to detail, and have the ability to view problems systematically, as well as from a broad perspective. Pragmatic as well, they'll generally make the best decision available at the time without unduly anguishing over it or looking back afterwards and second-guessing themselves. Moreover, if they see a problem as irreparable, they have little difficulty putting it out of their mind rather than worrying about it.

MOTIVATION

With an intense desire to experience all that life has to offer, Livers have a strong need to know how and why things work. They enjoy physical activity that involves doing something constructive or accomplishing an objective, as this allows them to put ideas into a physical form that can be seen, felt, or experienced.

Liver types make good teachers because once they learn something, they really know it. It becomes integrated into their being. Learning is usually done through a step-by-step manner, mastering each step along the way. Teaching a subject allows them to learn it well, and to interact with and assist others. There's an intense desire to help others by giving them the guidance they themselves didn't receive. Their goal is to help their students avoid some of the predictable pitfalls of life.

Physically strong and emotionally based, Livers have a compelling need to experience life. Especially when young, they tend to follow their heart's desire and often go along with the group activities, without considering the consequences. This "do it first, think about it later" attitude leads to a certain impulsivity or rashness of behavior. Having made sufficient errors in judgement, many Livers will later resort to taking a safe observer role rather than striking out on their own to explore uncharted territories.Livers with self-esteem issues run the risk of becoming co-dependent in their relationships.

Liver

MOTIVATION

Being much better at physically and emotionally nurturing others than in identifying and adequately taking care of their own needs, there is often an unconscious belief that, "If I take care of someone else, they'll take care of me." The basis of this belief comes in part from the fact that outside support is often a vital motivator in their making major personal changes. Often coming from backgrounds where they were deprived of nurturing support or emotional intimacy, they may have developed a protective barrier that creates emotional distance from others, thus preventing them from getting the support they desire. Support is the motivating force for personal change. Fortunately, the lack of support is just as effective as receiving it.

Livers are prone to compulsive or addictive behavior and are at high risk for alcoholism or eating disorders, especially when they have grown up in an alcoholic or otherwise seriously dysfunctional family. With their low self-esteem, lack of functional role models, loyalty and strong family ties, Livers often find themselves trapped in codependent relationships. They can also sabotage themselves with shoulds and self-punishments, but refuse to take personal responsibility for themselves.

"AT WORST"

Better at nurturing others than taking care of their own needs, Livers remain stuck by shying away from relationships that could offer them the emotional support that they were deprived of in early life. To deal with the situation, Livers will often emotionally transfer their need to care for their family to work and become workaholics. Substance abuse is another means of escaping emotional pain. Alcohol is often used to take the edge off their emotions. It makes them less aware of their problems, allows them to relax with their friends, and releases their self-control. Unfortunately, alcohol can also release the suppressed anger stored in the liver, leading to emotional outbursts or violent behavior.

When in control, Livers tend to be rather soft-spoken and self-restrained, they may have difficulty locating and/or expressing negative feelings, especially anger. When they keep their emotions pent up, they often become depressed or addicted in an attempt to drown their feelings with excess food or alcohol consumption. Liver types are capable of blocking their emotions and continuing to function in the world without emotional involvement. Men in particular, often learn to hide behind an "I don't need anybody" attitude. Ultimately, this emotional suppression eventually erupts, causing them to display a fit of anger that can be just as surprising to themselves as to others.

"AT BEST"

Once they have been able to connect with their personal higher power, Livers have a sense of self-sufficiency. They project a real "can do" attitude, and are capable of handling things efficiently and effectively. They are able to magnify their natural creative abilities and knack for putting things together. When free of their emotional turmoil, they are able to access their excellent organizational skills, and provide stability to their work and family. This is

Liver

"AT BEST"
Continued

also when they are able to express their emotions in a positive manner, turning anger into laughter and hurt into creativity.

Having learned the hard way, Liver types are excellent teachers. Patient and genuinely concerned about others, they will often impart their knowledge to others in the concrete form of showing them how to do something, or the more abstract form of introducing them to new concepts and ideas. Teaching is ultimately their most rewarding endeavor.

Carrying this need to be efficient into their work environment, job satisfaction is far more important than monetary reward. If Livers don't have the authority to do what they feel is necessary to be effective, they will seek work where their ideals and efforts are more appreciated. They have the courage to move on when they feel like they're in a rut.

By being in tune with life, Liver types are able to be in the flow of life. Being in the flow means they seem to know what needs to be done and how to organize so the day flows with all the necessary items being completed. It's this being in the flow that enables Livers to sense things about people, places and things, like knowing when someone will call or a person's basic nature. It provides them with the ability to pick up on what's going on, gives them insight into the basic nature of those around them, and often allows them to predict others' behavior.

Liver

FOOD LISTS

HEALTHY FOOD LIST

FREQUENTLY FOODS	3-7 meals per week – refers to each food, rather than category.
DENSE PROTEIN	Beef liver, beef broth, buffalo; chicken (white), chicken livers, chicken broth; anchovy, bass, catfish, flounder, haddock, halibut, herring, mahi-mahi, roughy, sardines, red snapper, sole, trout; clams, eel, mussels, octopus, oysters, scallops
DAIRY	Plain or flavored low fat yogurt, butter
CHEESE	Brie, Camembert, Cheddar, Colby, low fat cottage cheese, feta, low fat Jack
NUTS and SEEDS	Brazils, filberts, coconuts, pine nuts, seeds (pumpkin, sesame)
LEGUMES	Beans (adzuki, lima [butter], great northern, navy, kidney, red, soy) black-eyed peas
GRAINS	Amaranth, buckwheat, millet, quinoa, white or brown basmati rice, cream of rice, couscous
VEGETABLES	Asparagus, beets, cabbage (green, napa, red), celery, chard, cucumber, eggplant, garlic, greens (beet, collard, mustard, turnip), jicama, kale, kohlrabi, okra, ripe olives, peas, potatoes (red, russet, white rose, yukon gold), pumpkin, rutabaga, sprouts (alfalfa, clover, mung bean, radish, sunflower), squash (butternut, spaghetti), turnips, watercress
FRUITS	Cranberries, cherries, guavas, kiwi, limes, mangos, melons (cantaloupe, casaba, crenshaw, honeydew, watermelon), pomegranates, rhubarb
FRUIT JUICES	Red cherry, pineapple/coconut, fruit juice with carbonated water
SWEETENERS	Re-Vita®, stevia
VEGETABLE OILS	Almond, avocado, all-blend, canola, corn, olive, safflower, sesame, soy
BEVERAGES	Berry Calistoga® water
MODERATELY FOODS	1-2 meals per week – refers to each food, rather than category.
DENSE PROTEIN	Beef, lamb, veal, venison, organ meats (heart, brain), bacon; turkey, chicken (dark), cornish game hen, duck; bonita, cod, mackerel, perch, salmon, shark, swordfish, tongle tuna; calamari (squid), crab, lobster, shrimp; eggs
DAIRY	Milk (low fat, nonfat, raw), goat milk, buttermilk, sweet cream, sour cream, kefir, frozen yogurt, ice cream (Dreyer's, Ben & Jerry's®, Swensen's®)
CHEESE	American, blue, cream, Edam, goat, Gouda, kefir, Limburger, mozzarella, Muenster, Parmesan, ricotta, Romano, Swiss
NUTS and SEEDS	Almonds, almond butter, cashews, cashew butter, water chestnuts, hazelnuts, macadamias, macadamia butter, peanuts, peanut butter, pecans, pistachios, walnuts (black, English), seeds (caraway, sunflower), sesame seed butter, sunflower seed butter

Liver

LEGUMES	Beans (black, garbanzo, pinto), lentils, split peas, hummus, miso, soy milk, tofu
GRAINS	Barley, corn, corn tortillas, corn bread, corn grits, hominy grits, millet, oats, air-popped popcorn, rice (long or short grain brown, Japanese, wild), rice bran, rice cakes, rye, cream of rye, triticale, wheat bran, wheat germ, refined wheat flour, flour tortillas, breads (Italian, French, garlic, corn, corn/rye, rye, rice, oat, 7-grain, multi-grain, sprouted grain, sourdough, white), croissants, bagels, English muffins, pasta (durum, semolina, vegetable, herbed – garlic, basil), udon noodles, rice noodles, Nutri-Grain®, granola, cream of wheat
VEGETABLES	Artichokes, avocados, bamboo shoots, green beans, yellow wax beans, lima beans, bok choy, broccoli, broccoflower, brussels sprouts, carrots, cauliflower, cilantro, corn, hominy, leeks, lettuce (Boston, butter, endive, iceberg, red leaf, romaine), mushrooms, green olives, onions (chives, green, brown, red, white, yellow, vidalia), parsley, parsnips, snow pea pods, bell peppers (green, red, yellow), chili peppers, pimentos, sweet potatoes, radishes, daikon radishes, sauerkraut, seaweed (arame, dulse, kelp, nori, wakame), shallots, spinach, squash (acorn, banana, yellow [summer], zucchini), tomatoes, yams
VEGETABLE JUICES	Celery, carrot, carrot/celery, parsley, spinach, tomato, V-8®
FRUITS	Apples (Red or Golden Delicious, Gala, Granny Smith, Jonathan, McIntosh, Pippin, Rome Beauty), apricots, bananas, blackberries, blueberries, boysenberries, gooseberries, raspberries, strawberries, grapes (black, green, red), grapefruits (red, white), kumquats, lemons, loquats, nectarines, oranges, papayas, peaches, pears, Fuju persimmons, plums (black, red, purple), pineapples, tangelos, tangerines, black Mission figs, dates, prunes, raisins
FRUIT JUICES	Apple, apple cider, apple/apricot, apricot, black cherry, cranapple, cranberry, grape (purple, red, white), grapefruit, guava, lemon, orange, papaya, pear, pineapple, prune, tangerine, watermelon
VEGETABLE OILS	Coconut, peanut, flaxseed, sunflower
SWEETENERS	Honey, molasses, sorghum, date sugar, brown sugar, raw sugar, refined cane sugar, brown rice syrup, barley malt syrup, corn syrup, maple syrup, fructose, succonant
CONDIMENTS	Catsup, mustard, soy sauce, barbecue sauce, pesto sauce, salsa, tahini, pickles, horseradish, sweet basil, rosemary, cinnamon, cloves, curry, dill weed, nutmeg, sage, thyme, pepper (black, cayenne, white), sea salt, Vege-Sal®
SALAD DRESSINGS	Blue cheese, French, ranch, creamy Italian, creamy avocado, thousand island, vinegar and oil, lemon juice and oil
DESSERTS	Custards, tapioca, puddings, pies, cakes, raspberry sherbet, orange sherbet
CHIPS	Bean, corn (blue, white, yellow)
BEVERAGES	Coffee, coffee with Re-Vita®; herbal tea, black tea, green tea, Japanese tea, Chinese oolong tea; mineral water, sparkling water; wine (red, white), sake, beer, barley malt liquor, champagne, gin, Scotch, vodka, whiskey; root beer

Liver

RARELY FOODS	No more than once a month
DENSE PROTEIN	Pork, ham, sausage; abalone
DAIRY	Whole or 2% milk, half & half, high fat yogurt, most ice creams
GRAINS	Whole wheat, whole wheat bread, grape-nuts®
VEGETABLES	Arugula
SWEETENERS	Saccharin, aspertame Equal®, NutraSweet®, Sweet'n Low®
CONDIMENTS	Salt, mayonnaise, margarine, Bragg™ aminos, MSG
DESSERTS	Chocolate, desserts containing chocolate
CHIPS	Salted potato chips
BEVERAGES	Regular and diet sodas

SENSITIVE FOOD LIST

FREQUENTLY FOODS	3-7 meals per week – refers to each food, rather than category.
DENSE PROTEIN	Chicken (white); bass, catfish, trout
NUTS	Coconuts
GRAINS	White or brown basmati rice
VEGETABLES	Asparagus, celery, chard, eggplant, garlic, greens (beet, collard, mustard, turnip), jicama, kale, kohlrabi, okra, ripe olives, potatoes (red, white rose, yukon gold)
FRUITS	Cherries, cranberries
VEGETABLE OILS	All-blend, almond, avocado, canola, safflower, sesame, soy
BEVERAGES	Calistoga® water
MODERATELY FOODS	1-2 meals per week – refers to each food, rather than category.
DENSE PROTEIN	Beef, beef liver, beef broth, buffalo, lamb, veal, venison, organ meats (brain, heart); duck, chicken livers, chicken broth, chicken (dark), chicken Italian sausage, cornish game hen; anchovy, bonita, cod, flounder, haddock, halibut, herring, mackerel, mahi-mahi, perch, roughy, salmon, sardines, shark, red snapper, sole, swordfish, tongle tuna; calamari (squid), clams, crab, eel, lobster, mussels, octopus, oysters, scallops, scampi, shrimp; eggs
DAIRY	Kefir, butter
CHEESE	American, blue, brie, Camembert, Cheddar, Colby, low fat cottage, cream, Edam, feta, goat, Gouda, low fat Jack, kefir, Limburger, mozzarella, Muenster, Parmesan, ricotta, Romano, Swiss

Liver

NUTS and SEEDS	Almonds, almond butter, Brazils, cashews, cashew butter, waterchestnuts, filberts, hazelnuts, macadamias, macadamia butter, peanuts, peanut butter, pecans, pine nuts, pistachios, walnuts (black, English), seeds (caraway, pumpkin, sesame, sunflower), sesame seed butter, sunflower seed butter
LEGUMES	Beans (adzuki, black, garbanzo, kidney, lima [butter], great northern, navy, pinto, red, soy), lentils, black-eyed peas, split peas, hummus, miso, soy milk, tofu
GRAINS	Amaranth, barley, buckwheat, corn, corn tortillas, corn bread, corn grits, hominy grits, millet, oats, air-popped popcorn, quinoa, rice (long or short grain brown or white, Japanese, wild), rice cakes, rice bran, rye, triticale, wheat bran, wheat germ, refined wheat flour, breads (French, Italian, sourdough, 7-grain, multi-grain, corn, corn/rye, rye, rice, garlic, oats, sprouted grain, white), croissants, bagels, English muffins, crackers (saltines, oat, rye), pasta, couscous, udon noodles, rice noodles, cream of rice, cream of rye, cream of wheat
VEGETABLES	Artichokes, avocados, bamboo shoots, green beans, yellow wax beans, lima beans, beets, bok choy, broccoli, broccoflower, cabbage (green, napa, red), carrots, cauliflower, chives, cilantro, corn, cucumbers, leeks, mushrooms, green olives, onions (all varieties), parsley, parsnips, peas, snow pea pods, bell peppers (red, yellow, green), chili peppers, pimentos, russet potatoes, sweet potatoes, pumpkin, radishes, daikon radishes, rutabaga, seaweed (arame, dulse, kelp, nori, wakame), sauerkraut, shallots, sprouts (alfalfa, clover, mung bean, radish, sunflower), squash (acorn, banana, butternut, spaghetti), turnips, watercress, yams
VEGETABLE JUICES	Carrot, celery, carrot/celery, parsley, spinach, tomato, V-8®
FRUITS	Apples (Red or Golden Delicious, Gala, Granny Smith, Jonathan, Pippin, McIntosh, Rome Beauty), apricots, bananas, blackberries, blueberries, boysenberries, gooseberries, raspberries, strawberries, grapes (black, green, red), grapefruits (red, white), guavas, kiwi, kumquats, lemons, limes, loquats, mangos, melons (cantaloupe, casaba, crenshaw, honeydew, watermelon), nectarines, peaches, Bosc pears, Fuju persimmons, plums (black, red, purple), rhubarb, pomegranates, tangelos, tangerines, dates, black Mission figs, prunes, raisins
FRUIT JUICES	Apple, apple cider, apricot, black cherry, red cherry, cranberry, cranapple, apple/apricot, grape (white, red, purple), grapefruit, guava, lemon, pear, pineapple/coconut, prune, tangerine, watermelon
VEGETABLE OILS	Corn, flaxseed, olive, coconut, peanut, sunflower
SWEETENERS	Re-Vita®, stevia
CONDIMENTS	Salsa, tahini, vinegar, pickles, sweet basil, rosemary, cinnamon, cloves, curry, dill weed, nutmeg, sage, thyme, pepper (black, cayenne, white), sea salt, Vege-Sal®
SALAD DRESSINGS	Creamy avocado, vinegar and oil, lemon juice and oil
BEVERAGES	Herbal tea, Japanese tea, Chinese oolong tea; mineral water, sparkling water

Liver

RARELY FOODS	No more than once a month
DENSE PROTEIN	Pork, bacon, ham, sausage; turkey; abalon
DAIRY	Milk (whole, 2%, raw, low fat or nonfat milk), goat milk, buttermilk, half & half, sweet cream, sour cream, plain or flavored yogurt, high fat yogurt, frozen yogurt, most ice creams
GRAINS	Whole wheat, flour tortillas, whole wheat bread, whole wheat crackers, grape-nuts®
VEGETABLES	Arugula, brussels sprouts, lettuce (Boston, butter, endive, iceberg, red leaf, romaine), spinach, yellow (summer) squash, tomatoes, zucchini
FRUITS	Oranges, papayas, pineapples
FRUIT JUICES	Orange, papaya, pineapple
SWEETENERS	Honey, molasses, sorghum, brown sugar, date sugar, raw sugar, refined cane sugar, brown rice syrup, barley malt syrup, corn syrup, maple syrup, fructose, succonant, saccharin, aspertame, Equal®, NutraSweet®, Sweet'n Low®
CONDIMENTS	Catsup, mustard, horseradish, barbecue sauce, pesto sauce, soy sauce, salt, Bragg™ aminos, MSG, margarine, mayonnaise
SALAD DRESSINGS	Blue cheese, French, ranch, creamy Italian, thousand island
DESSERTS	Custards, tapioca, puddings, pies, cakes, raspberry sherbert, orange sherbert, chocolate, desserts containing chocolate
CHIPS	Bean, corn (blue, white, yellow), potato
BEVERAGES	Coffee; black tea, green tea; wine (red, white) sake, beer, barley malt liquor, margaritas, champagne, gin, Scotch, vodka, whiskey; root beer, diet sodas, regular sodas

Liver

MENUS

DIETARY EMPHASIS:
- Rotation and variety – vegetables, fruits, protein (eggs, poultry, fish); moderate dairy.
- Raw foods are generally supportive to system.
- Include more raw than cooked vegetables.
- Food is best assimilated when eaten in combinations.
- Garlic supports immune system.
- Need 8 glasses of water daily.

WEIGHT LOSS:
- Eliminate salt.
- Reduce fats to 15%.
- Exercise daily.
- Emotional support (weight loss groups are often appropriate).
- Avoid chocolate, sodas, and alcohol, (although may use appetite suppressants).

WEIGHT GAIN:
- Consume 25% of calories from dense protein.
- Increase fats to 25%.
- Follow a balanced diet.

VEGETARIAN DIET:
- Inadequate, as require 10-25% of caloric intake from dense protein.

FATS:
- 15-25% of total caloric intake.
- Best sources are butter, cheese, cottage cheese, fish, and chicken.

SENSITIVE:

Moderate-to-heavy breakfast, light-to-moderate lunch, and moderate dinner.

ALCOHOL:
- May affect sinuses and decrease energy.
- When sensitive, may experience depression or sleepiness after consumption, particularly with grain alcohols.
- Tequila, with lime or orange juice and without salt, can, if consumed in moderation, be more easily tolerated.
- Can usually tolerate, with no side effects, up to 4 oz. of wine with dinner, 2 meals per week.

KEY

—all menus may be used by healthy persons

( ) around foods means that they're optional

L denotes weight loss menus

S denotes sensitive menus

G denotes weight gain menus

BREAKFAST:
6-9 a.m. Light, with grain, dairy, protein, vegetables, legumes and/or fruit or fruit juice.

SENSITIVE: Moderate-to-heavy.

L	S	G	
L			Cantaloupe or watermelon
L			Oatmeal (Re-Vita® – berry, butternut, or vanilla – and/or fruit banana, peaches, white raisins or blueberries)
	S		Couscous and Re-Vita®, then apple juice
	S		Amaranth and carrots (onions)
L			Amaranth w/fruit banana, peaches, or blueberries
			Raisin Bran® w/low fat milk
	S	G	Nutri-Grain® cereal w/kefir
L			Nutri-Grain® cereal w/low fat yogurt
	S	G	Muesli w/kefir
L			Cream of rye w/mocha milk
	S		Cream of rye or cream of rice (golden raisins, or Re-Vita®)
L			Cream of rice w/banana, peaches, or blueberries
			Cream of rice (low fat milk)
L			White basmati rice
	S		Rice (Re-Vita®, broccoli, peas, or carrots)
		G	Cinnamon raisin bagel w/cream cheese
		G	Peanut butter or almond butter on rice cakes, oat, rye, or sourdough bread
L	S		Carrot juice
L	S		Cranberry concentrate w/Re-Vita® and water
L			Apple

Liver

S G Eggs and rice

L S G Eggs, brown basmati rice, and purple onion

G Eggs, rice, onion, and salsa w/ corn tortilla

L Low fat or nonfat strawberry yogurt

L Fruit juice and Sunrider® Simply Herbs

L Apple, papaya or pineapple/papaya juice

L Watermelon

L Grapefruit

S Chicken breast and rice or asparagus

S Trout and rice

S Baked potato w/Cheddar cheese

MID-MORNING SNACK:
(Optional) 10 a.m. Vegetables, grain.

S Unsalted air-popped popcorn (butter)

L S Celery, cucumbers, bell peppers and/or radishes

LUNCH:
12-2 p.m. Heavy, with protein, dairy, nuts, seeds, legumes, grain, vegetables and/or limited fruit.

SENSITIVE: Light-to-moderate.

L G Chicken breast, cauliflower, and broccoli

L G Grilled chicken, corn or flour tortilla, and salad lettuce, avocado, and tomato

L G Chicken burrito w/cheese

L S Chicken and white basmati rice

L Breast of chicken and salad spinach, carrots, cucumbers, mushrooms, broccoli, and red peppers w/rice vinegar

L Chicken and beets

L Chicken livers and onions

G Turkey on onion roll w/mustard, lettuce, and tomato

S G Tuna, avocado, celery, and/or carrots, and onions

L G Tuna, pasta, and asparagus

G Tuna on rye bread

L Salmon or trout, rice or baked potato w/ 1/4 tsp/butter, and stir-fry carrots, broccoli, cauliflower, and cabbage

G Hamburger on white bun w/tomatoes and lettuce

G Liverwurst on rye bread

S Eggs, broccoli, cauliflower, and English muffin

S Pine nuts – up to 8 oz, and apple or cherries

S Quinoa or amaranth pasta w/Jack cheese and peas

S Pasta w/mushrooms, tomatoes, and olive oil

L Spaghetti and meatballs

L S Salad romaine lettuce, cucumber, carrots, tomato, onions, oil and vinegar w/blue cheese

L Salad w/vinaigrette dressing and baked potato w/1/4 tsp butter

S Beef vegetable soup (cornbread)

Lentil soup and salad or raw vegetable

S Lentils, couscous, and curry

L Nonfat cottage cheese and cantaloupe

L Nonfat yogurt and fruit

S Rice cakes w/butter

S Popcorn rice cakes

S Calistoga fruit juice

L Vegetable juices: carrot, carrot/celery, carrot/celery/beet, or parsley/spinach/celery

MID-AFTERNOON SNACK:
(Optional) 3 30-4 p.m. Vegetables, grain, fruit, dairy, protein, nuts, seeds.

L S Honeydew, cantaloupe, or cherries

L Apple, plum, or grapes

S Dates

Dried cranberries (nuts)

L Low fat or nonfat strawberry yogurt

L Granola bar

LUNCH or DINNER:

L G Swordfish or sole and rice (broccoli, cauliflower, and/or carrots)

S Fillet of sole w/cauliflower, broccoli, and low fat Jack cheese

Liver

S	Halibut and cooked carrots (long grain brown rice and parsley)
L G	Trout or sea bass fillets w/butter, garlic, and slivered almonds or pine nuts, asparagus pasta, and salad romaine lettuce, cucumbers, and red bell peppers
L G	Tuna, rice, and carrots, or green beans (celery)
L G	Red snapper w/lemon and rice, broccoli, peas, carrots, or asparagus
L S	California roll w/avocado, rice, and imitation crab
S G	Lamb, rice, and mint jelly
L S G	Ground sirloin and asparagus
S G	Steak and potato w/butter, chives, and/or broth gravy
L S G	Steak, broccoli, and baby carrots
L G	Turkey breast and cranberries (green beans)
L S G	Chicken breast w/brown basmati rice, onion, and mushrooms
L S G	Chicken and stuffing basmati rice, onion, celery, carrots, garlic, red bell pepper, and asparagus
L S G	Chicken, baked potato, raw carrots, and celery
L S G	Chicken, steamed cauliflower, and/or broccoli, mushrooms, and onions
L S G	Chicken, almonds, and water chestnuts w/white rice
L S G	Curried duck and rice
L S	Eggs, brown basmati rice, and purple onion
L S	Hard-boiled egg, raw carrots, and baked potato
L S G	Vegetable pasta w/pine nuts, low fat Cheddar cheese, celery, onions, broccoli, and parsley
L S G	Low fat cheese, broccoli, and mushrooms over brown basmati rice
L	Baked potato (cheese and/or bacon)
L S	Potato w/parsley and broccoli (butter)
L	Miso soup, green beans, and rice
L	Tofu, rice, and carrots

DINNER:
6-9 p.m. Moderate-to-heavy, with legumes, grain, protein, dairy, and/or vegetables.

SENSITIVE: Moderate.

L S G	Cheese enchilada w/corn tortilla, rice, and beans
L	Bean burrito and spinach (carrots, cucumbers, and/or red peppers)
L S	Butternut or spaghetti squash and broccoli
L S	Eggplant and green beans
L S G	Cauliflower w/melted low fat white Cheddar cheese (brown rice and/or pine nuts)
L S	Baked potato (green beans)
L	Baked potato or quinoa pasta w/broccoli and low fat cheese
S	Potato cheese soup w/corn bread
G	Barley soup stew meat, barley, crushed tomato, onions, carrots, and celery w/French roll
S G	Guacamole, black beans, and cilantro on corn tortilla
L S	Pinto or black beans and rice
L S	Green beans, cucumber, and cabbage salad
L S	Pasta and asparagus (olive oil, garlic, and herbs)
L	Plain or vegetable pasta, tomato sauce, mushrooms, onions, broccoli, and carrots
L S G	Chicken breast, baked potato or white basmati rice, carrots, broccoli, cauliflower, and onion
L G	Chicken and rice (green beans, cauliflower, broccoli, or peas)
L S G	Chicken, water chestnuts, and white rice
L S G	Turkey, green beans, and/or broccoli (baked potato) (cranberry sauce)
S G	Curried duck w/orange and rice
L S G	Beef liver, onions, and potatoes
L S G	Beef liver, broccoli, carrots, and cauliflower
S G	Beef, pinto beans, and rice

Liver

L G Ground sirloin and broccoli (plain or pickled beets)

Shrimp in salad w/romaine lettuce, cucumber, cabbage, and onion

L S Scallops and rice

L S Steamed crab and green beans, cauliflower, and carrots

L S Tuna or scallops and stir-fry in water green pepper, onion, and mushrooms

L S G Cod fish, carrots, green beans, brussels sprouts, and rice

L S G Sole or white fish and rice

S Bagel and artichoke or peas

L Salad sprouts, avocado, tomatoes, and cabbage w/avocado dressing

L Spinach salad spinach, carrots, bean sprouts, onion, mushrooms, and hard-boiled egg

EVENING or BEDTIME SNACK: (Optional) 9 p.m.-2 a.m. Fruit, vegetables, grain, dairy, limited protein. Sweets – 1 hour or more after dinner.

Spaghetti and meatballs

Ravioli

G Cheese custard w/whipped cream

L Nonfat yogurt and fruit

G Granola bar

L S G Frozen cherries

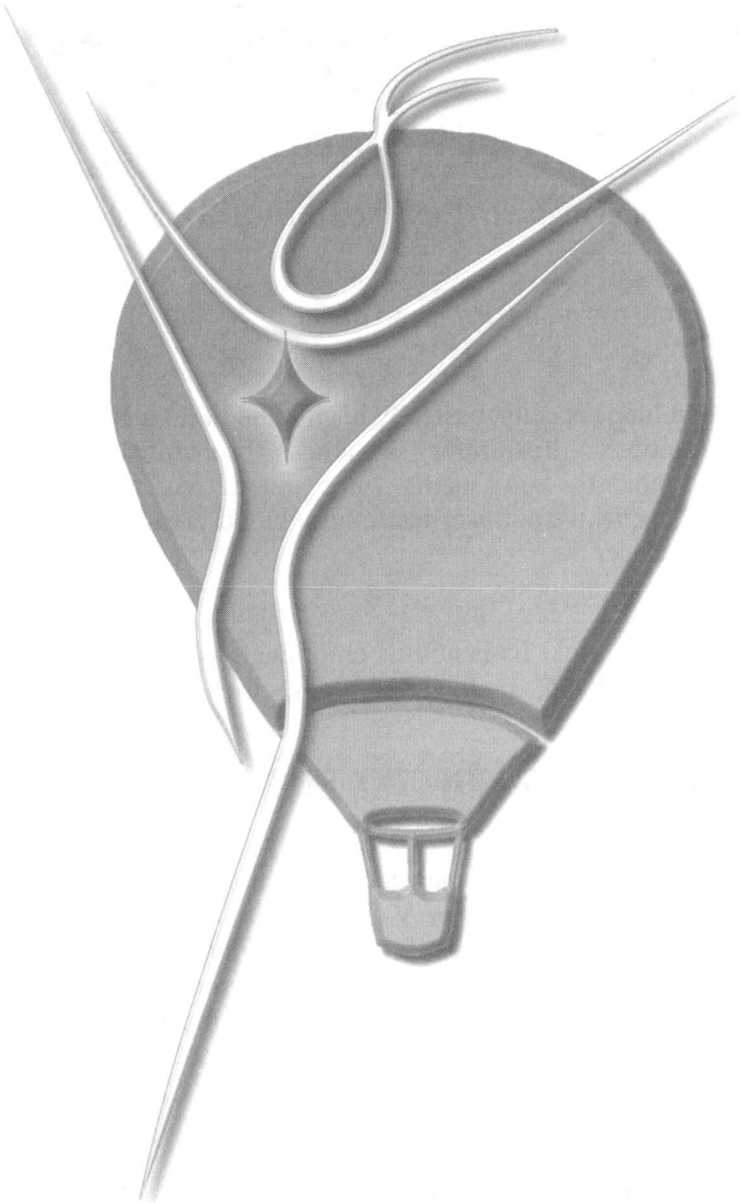

The "Lung Body Type"
is symbolized by the hot air
balloon. Air or oxygen creates
buoyancy and is necessary for life.
Nurturing and creative, Lungs give life
to their world by expressing positive,
supportive emotions, enabling
them to make the most
of the moment.

Lung

BODY TYPE PROFILE

LOCATION	Lateral cavities of chest. They are separated from each other by the heart.
FUNCTION	Respiration, providing oxygen to blood.
POTENTIAL HEALTH PROBLEMS	Excellent lung capacity, basically healthy bodies, and generally in touch with their emotions. Respiratory weakness, bronchitis, asthma, emphysema. Weak ligaments, body pains when not active, muscle pain. Delicate digestion, sensitive gums or teeth, high blood pressure, migraine headaches, and skin cancer.
RECOMMENDED EXERCISE	Exercise is helpful. Its benefit is emotional, as it calms the mind. Walking, swimming, dancing, any lower body exercise.

WOMEN'S CHARACTERISTICS

DISTINGUISHING FEATURES	Weight gain in lower abdomen and upper hips with little gain in thighs. High cheek bones with square or V-shaped jaw, often with prominent chin or average oval or rectangular face. Naturally creative and artistic with a practical flair. Mild-mannered, even-tempered, sensitive, and caring with strong nurturing qualities. Emotionally expressive, they are known for making the most of the moment. Generally excel in music, dance, or some creative physical expression.
ADDITIONAL PHYSICAL CHARACTERISTICS	Buttocks relatively flat-to-rounded. Low back curvature straight-to-average. Breasts small-to-average. Shoulders relatively even with hips. Average torso with defined waist. Height petite-to-average. Bone structure small-to-medium. Average, elongated musculature. Hands average-to-slender, long, or delicate. Feet may be narrow. Hair texture medium-to-thick. Body may be a full size smaller above the waist than below.
WEIGHT GAIN AREAS	Lower body with initial gain in lower abdomen, waist, and upper hips, with slight to no gain in thighs. Secondary weight gain primarily in entire abdomen, middle-to-entire back, upper arms, possibly breasts, buttocks, face, under chin, and minimally in entire upper 2/3rds of thighs.

Lung

DIETARY GUIDELINES

SCHEDULING MEALS	Breakfast: Heavy, with protein, grain, nuts, seeds, dairy, fruit, legumes, and/or vegetables. Lunch: Moderate, with grain, vegetables, legumes, dairy, nuts, seeds, protein and/or fruit. Dinner: Light, with small portions of protein, legumes, vegetables, and/or grain.
DIETARY EMPHASIS	• For weight loss, eliminate sugar, limit fats to 10-15% of caloric intake, include 15% dense protein, drink 64 oz. water daily, and exercise. • For weight gain, consume 30% of calories from dense protein, increase fats to 20-30%, include sugar (fruits), and drink 64 oz. daily to flush kidneys. • Vegetarian diet recommended when healthy, although up to 30% of calories may consist of dense protein. • Fats, 10-30% derived from nuts (almonds, pine nuts, pecans, coconuts, cashews), seeds, protein (beef, chicken, turkey, lamb, fish, eggs), olive oil, and butter.
KEY SUPPORTS FOR SYSTEM	Fruits (bananas, apples, grapes), pine nuts, sprouted rye bread, rice with steamed kale, and collards. Substantial breakfast with protein. Kombucha tea, made with green tea, aids digestion and assimilation.
COMPLEMENTARY GLANDULAR SUPPORT	Thyroid, through consuming a minimum of 2 oz. dense protein (eggs, chicken, turkey, or fish) with a grain, such as rice or pasta at least 2 times/week. Heart, through music, by playing or moving with it.
FOODS CRAVED	*(When Energy is Low)* Sweets, like chocolate candy bars, cakes, cookies, puddings. Fruit. Carbohydrates, such as breads, pasta. Dairy, like frozen yogurt, yogurt. Nuts, particularly walnuts or pine nuts, sandwiches, or chips. Coffee.
FOODS TO AVOID	Artificial sweeteners, diet or regular sodas, and milk because they aggravate the lungs. Carbonated beverages of all kinds as they affect oxygen uptake. Fried foods
RECOMMENDED CUISINE	Chinese, Thai, Sushi, vegetable style Mexican, or Italian. Soup and salad.

Lung

PSYCHOLOGICAL PROFILE

ESSENCE

Just as the lungs supply the oxygen needed for life, the Lung body type takes in life. Nurturing and creative, Lungs give life to their world by expressing positive, supportive emotions. Their strength lies in being able to shift emotional energy, like changing hurt into creativity. This allows them to express the energy of negative emotions in a safe, constructive or positive manner. By using emotions as an indicator rather than a response, respecting emotions, and getting the essence from them, emotions can be used to move into a greater richness and fullness of life, which is what enables Lungs to excel at making the most of the moment.

CHARACTERISTIC TRAITS

Lungs are generally sensitive, caring, idealistic, even tempered, and mild-mannered. Emotional by nature, Lung types tend to breathe in others' emotions, which can cause their own to snowball, or they'll go to the opposite extreme of suppressing their own and discounting others' emotions. In an attempt to avoid being driven entirely by emotions, there is a tendency to become too analytical and suppress them all together.

Systematic in their thought processes, Lungs like to think things through before taking any action. They like to understand what's taking place and feel sure about their choices before making any changes, which often inhibits their spontaneity. By being well-organized, and laying things out in advance, they are able to prevent their feelings from interfering with their ability to sort things through.

Lungs are naturally creative, as well as very practical. Being quite imaginative and gifted at working with their hands, Lungs can take abstract ideas and translate them into physical forms. With a well-developed sense of style, they can express these talents through drawing, sculpturing, design, or construction. With a good sense of rhythm and timing, they also tend to express their nurturing and creativity through music or dance.

MOTIVATION

Lungs have a strong need to nurture and be nurtured. This often leads them into service-oriented vocations where they can be expressive and establish emotional connections. Lungs tend to value the nurturing of relationships more than personal achievements. It's easy for them to become a caretaker or rescuer of those in need, often losing touch with their own needs in the process. Between their sense of responsibility and fear of change, Lungs are prone to stay in relationships much longer than is beneficial for them, and may at times find it difficult to let go and get on with their own lives.

Idealistic, Lungs basically have a high regard for peace. Not only will they work for peace in the outside world, but will do everything they can to establish it in their personal relationships. Even when a relationship has ended in divorce, they will often do everything they can to restore it to at least "friendship" status.

Lung

MOTIVATION

Lungs are persistent and loyal, particularly in their attempts to right wrongs or effect necessary reforms. It's not unusual for them to devote a great deal of energy helping the underdog. In social situations, they are the ones who will dance with the "wallflowers" and make sure no one is left out.

Creative expression is essential to balance their own energies, for self-expression and personal fulfillment. Self-expression provides the motivation to grow, develop, and make changes in their lives. Being creative as well as practical, their emotional sensitivity and drive to nurture others serves as a catalyst for the expression of their creativity. Work that is methodical and requires care is more appealing than that which requires making quick decisions and includes high responsibility, since Lung types are not comfortable taking risks that involve other people.

"AT WORST"

Lungs often experience difficulty finding balance in their lives. Their attention is often too focused on a single aspect of life, such as work, at the expense of others, particularly relationships. They may even ignore their personal needs for rest, relaxation, or play. Being overly concerned with the expectations of others, Lungs tend to take on more than they can realistically expect to accomplish. Even though they may be overwhelmed, they are still reluctant to back out of their commitments. Not wanting to openly decline, they then tend to withdraw, or "get too busy".

Strong-willed to the point of stubbornness and rigidity, Lungs tend to operate from gut feelings rather than outside information. There's a tendency to become narrow-minded and get stuck in the rut of a routine. They often have difficulty organizing their time, efficiently planning, prioritizing, and making decisions. It's easy for them to fritter their time away socializing or puttering around on a project.

Fearful of disapproval and rejection, with a strong need to please others, Lungs are often unsuccessful at pleasing themselves. Being extremely uncomfortable with conflict, they will often accommodate others to avoid it, and then end up resentful or disappointed, sad or depressed. By making themselves less important than others, they can actually deepen their own self-doubts. It's usually the lack of confidence and other internal barriers that interfere with their self-acceptance and self-respect.

Lungs will expend a great deal of time and energy on their interests, and serving humanity is their highest concern. Their emotional sensitivity, along with their burning drive to nurture others serves as a catalyst for the expression of their creativity. They are particularly sensitive to the needs of those around them, and will go to great lengths to fulfill those needs.

Lung

"AT BEST"

Practical, efficient, and aware of things that need to be done, Lungs are not only able to accurately analyze the potential effect that doing these things has on others, but they're also good at taking action and getting them done. Moreover, they're able to take charge of a situation when they need to. Tactful and indirect, rarely is their behavior perceived as pushy or offensive. They are honest, loyal, and can be trusted to honor their commitments while acting in the best interests of those they are serving.

Lung types are nurturing to others, as well as to themselves. They are basically self-sufficient and tend to regenerate best through sleep. Lungs are generally comfortable being alone, particularly since they need time to integrate and process to make their own decisions. They have their own sense of direction and are not led by what everyone else is doing.

Lungs are known for being creative, imaginative, and often vocally expressive. They can be quite persuasive and leave a lasting impression on people, making them quite effective as social reformers, speakers, or performers. They have the ability to connect with and activate others' emotional energy. By trusting their intuition and inner guidance, Lungs can be successful and influential in helping humanity.

Lung

FOOD LISTS

HEALTHY FOOD LIST

FREQUENTLY FOODS	3-7 meals per week – refers to each food, rather than category.
DENSE PROTEIN	Chicken, turkey, cornish game hen; salmon, shark, swordfish, tuna
DAIRY	Butter
CHEESE	Cheddar, cottage, Jack
NUTS	Almonds, cashews, coconut, pecans, pine nuts
LEGUMES	Great northern beans, split peas
GRAINS	Amaranth, barley, blue corn, millet, oats, quinoa, rice (white or brown basmati, long or short grain brown, Japanese, polished, wild), rye, rice cakes, rice bran, breads (sprouted rye, 7-grain sprouted, rice), rice noodles, cream of rice, cream of rye
VEGETABLES	Bamboo shoots, green beans, beets, bok choy, broccoli, brussels sprouts, cabbage (green, red, napa), carrots, cauliflower, celery, chard, corn, eggplant, greens (beet, collard, mustard, turnip), kale, kohlrabi, leeks, lettuce (Boston, butter, endive, iceberg, red leaf, romaine), mushrooms, okra, olives (green, ripe), parsnips, peas, bell pepper (green, red, yellow), yukon gold potatoes, pumpkin, radishes, daikon radishes, rutabagas, sauerkraut, seaweed (arame, dulse, kelp, nori, wakame), spinach, sprouts (alfalfa, clover, mung bean, radish, sunflower), squash (acorn, banana, butternut, yellow [summer], spaghetti), cherry tomatoes, turnips, watercress, yams
VEGETABLE JUICES	Carrot, carrot/celery, celery, spinach, tomato, V-8® (no salt)
FRUITS	Apples (Red or Golden Delicious, Granny Smith, Jonathan, McIntosh, Pippin, Rome Beauty), apricots, bananas, blackberries, blueberries, boysenberries, cranberries, gooseberries, raspberries, strawberries, cherries, grapes (black, green), guavas, kiwi, lemons, limes, loquats, nectarines, persimmons, pineapples, plums (red, purple, black), pomegranates, rhubarb, tangelos, tangerines, figs, raisins
FRUIT JUICES	Apple, black cherry, cranberry, cranapple, grape (purple, white), papaya, pineapple/coconut, pineapple, prune, tangerine
VEGETABLE OILS	Flaxseed, olive
SWEETENERS	Honey, maple syrup, Re-Vita®, stevia
MODERATELY FOODS	1-2 meals per week – refers to each food, rather than category.
DENSE PROTEIN	Beef, beef broth, beef liver, buffalo, lamb, pork, bacon, ham, sausage, veal, venison, organ meats (heart, brain); chicken livers, chicken broth, duck;anchovy, bass, bonita, catfish, cod, flounder, haddock, halibut, herring, mackerel, mahi-mahi, perch, roughy, sardines, red snapper, sole, trout; abalone, calamari (squid), clams, crab, eel, lobster, mussels, octopus, oysters, scallops, shrimp; eggs

Lung

DAIRY	Goat milk, buttermilk, half & half, sweet cream, sour cream, kefir, plain yogurt, frozen yogurt, ice cream (Dreyer's, Ben & Jerry's®, Swensen's®)
CHEESE	American, blue, brie, Camembert, Colby, cream, Edam, feta, goat, Gouda, kefir, Limburger, mozzarella, Muenster, Parmesan, ricotta, Romano, Swiss
NUTS and SEEDS	Almond butter, almond milk, Brazils, cashew butter, water chestnuts, filberts, hazelnuts, macadamias, macadamia butter, peanuts, peanut butter, pistachios, walnuts (black, English), seeds (caraway, pumpkin, sesame, sunflower), sesame seed butter, sunflower seed butter
LEGUMES	Beans (adzuki, black, lima [butter], garbanzo, kidney, navy, pinto, red, soy), lentils, black-eyed peas, hummus, miso, soy milk, tofu
GRAINS	Corn, corn bread, corn grits, corn tortillas, hominy grits, popcorn, triticale, refined wheat flour, flour tortillas, breads (French, Italian, garlic, sourdough, white, oat, rye, 7-grain, multi-grain, corn, corn/rye, sprouted grain), bagels, croissants, crackers (saltines, oat, rye), couscous, pasta, udon noodles, cream of wheat
VEGETABLES	Artichokes, asparagus, avocados, basil, yellow wax beans, lima beans, broccoflower, cilantro, cucumbers, garlic, jicama, onions (all varieties), parsley, snow pea pods, chili peppers, pimentos, potatoes (red, russet, white rose, purple), shallots, sweet potatoes, tomatoes, zucchini squash
VEGETABLE JUICE	Parsley
FRUITS	Red grapes, grapefruits (red, white), kumquats, mangos, melons (cantaloupe, casaba, crenshaw, watermelon), oranges, papayas, peaches, pears, rhubarb, dates, prunes
FRUIT JUICES	Apple cider, apple/apricot, apricot, red cherry, red grape, grapefruit, guava, lemon, orange, pear, prune, watermelon
VEGETABLE OILS	All-blend, almond, avocado, canola, coconut, corn, peanut, safflower, sesame, soy, sunflower
SWEETENERS	Molasses, sorghum, brown sugar, date sugar, raw sugar, refined cane sugar, barley malt syrup, corn syrup, rice bran syrup, fructose, succonant
CONDIMENTS	Salsa, catsup, mustard, dijon mustard, horseradish, barbecue sauce, pesto sauce, soy sauce, tahini, pickles, vinegar, salt, sea salt, Vege-Sal®
SALAD DRESSINGS	Blue cheese, French, ranch, creamy Italian, creamy avocado, thousand island, vinegar and oil, lemon juice and oil
DESSERTS	Custards, puddings, tapioca, pies, cakes, chocolate, desserts containing chocolate, orange sherbet, raspberry sherbet
CHIPS	Bean, corn (blue, white, yellow)
BEVERAGES	Coffee, coffee with Re-Vita®; peppermint tea, herbal tea, black tea, green tea, Japanese tea, Chinese oolong tea; mineral water, sparkling water; wine (red, white) sake, beer, barley malt liquor, champagne, gin, Scotch, vodka, whiskey, tequila; root beer

Lung

RARELY FOODS	No more than once a month
DAIRY	Milk, flavored yogurt, most ice creams
GRAINS	Buckwheat, whole wheat, English muffins, whole wheat bread, whole wheat crackers, wheat bran, wheat germ
VEGETABLES	Arugula
FRUITS	Honeydew melons
SWEETENERS	Aspertame, Equal®, NutraSweet®, Sweet'n Low®
CONDIMENTS	Mayonnaise, margarine
BEVERAGES	Regular or diet sodas
OTHER	French fries, fried foods

SENSITIVE FOOD LIST

FREQUENTLY FOODS	3-7 meals per week – refers to each food, rather than category.
GRAINS	7-grain sprouted bread
VEGETABLE	Carrots, bell pepper (green, red, yellow)
VEGETABLE JUICE	V-8® (no salt)
VEGETABLE OILS	Flaxseed, olive
MODERATELY FOODS	1-2 meals per week – refers to each food, rather than category.
DENSE PROTEIN	Beef broth, beef liver, buffalo, lamb, veal, venison, organ meats (heart, brain); chicken, chicken broth, chicken livers, turkey, cornish game hen, duck; bass, bonita, catfish, cod, flounder, haddock, halibut, herring, mackerel, mahi-mahi, perch, roughy, salmon, sardines, shark, red snapper, sole, swordfish, trout, tuna; abalone, calamari (squid), clams, crab, eel, lobster, mussels, octopus, scallops, shrimp; eggs
CHEESE	American, blue, brie, Camembert, Cheddar, Colby, cottage, Jack, kefir, Limburger, Muenster, Parmesan, ricotta, Romano
DAIRY	Kefir, butter
NUTS and SEEDS	Almonds, almond butter, almond milk, Brazils, cashew butter, water chestnuts, coconuts, filberts, hazelnuts, macadamias, macadamia butter, pecans, pine nuts, pistachios, seeds (caraway, pumpkin, sesame, sunflower), sesame seed butter, sunflower seed butter

Lung

LEGUMES	Beans (adzuki, black, garbanzo, lima [butter], great northern, navy, pinto, red), lentils, black-eyed peas, split peas, hummus, miso
GRAINS	Amaranth, barley, corn, corn bread, corn grits, hominy grits, millet, oats, popcorn, quinoa, rice (brown or white basmati, long or short grain brown or white, Japanese, polished, wild), rice bran, rice cakes, rye, triticale, refined wheat flour, breads (French, Italian, corn, corn/rye, garlic, oat, multi-grain, rice, rye, sourdough, white), bagels, croissants, crackers (saltines, oat, rye), couscous, pasta, udon noodles, rice noodles, cream of rice, cream of rye
VEGETABLES	Artichokes, asparagus, avocados, bamboo shoots, green beans, yellow wax beans, lima beans, beets, bok choy, broccoli, brussels sprouts, cabbage (green, napa, red), cauliflower, celery, chard, cilantro, corn, cucumbers, eggplant, garlic, greens (beet, collard, mustard, turnip), jicama, kale, kohlrabi, leeks, lettuce (Boston, butter, endive, iceberg, red leaf, romaine), mushrooms, okra, olives (green, ripe), onions (all varieties), parsley, parsnips, peas, snow pea pods, chili peppers, pimentos, potatoes (russet, white rose, purple, yukon gold), sweet potatoes, pumpkin, radishes, daikon radishes, rutabaga, sauerkraut, seaweed (arame, dulse, kelp, nori, wakame), shallots, spinach, sprouts (alfalfa, clover, mung beans, radish, sunflower), squash (acorn, banana, butternut, yellow [summer], spaghetti, zucchini), cherry tomatoes, turnips, watercress, yams
VEGETABLE JUICES	Celery, carrot/celery, parsley, spinach, tomato
FRUITS	Apples (Granny Smith, Jonathan, McIntosh, Rome Beauty), boysenberries, cranberries, gooseberries, raspberries, strawberries, cherries, grapefruits (white, red), guavas, kiwi, kumquats, lemons, limes, loquats, mangos, melons (casaba, crenshaw, watermelon), pineapples, plums (black, purple, red), pomegranates, rhubarb, tangelos, tangerines, dates, figs, prunes, raisins
FRUIT JUICES	Apple, apple cider, apple/apricot, apricot, black cherry, cranberry, cranapple, grape (purple, red, white), grapefruit, guava, lemon, pear, pineapple/coconut, papaya, pineapple, prune, tangerine, watermelon
VEGETABLE OILS	All-blend, almond, avocado, coconut, corn, rice bran, safflower, sesame
SWEETENERS	Honey, molasses, sorghum, date sugar, rice bran syrup, maple syrup, barley malt syrup, corn syrup, Re-Vita®, stevia
CONDIMENTS	Salsa, dijon mustard, horseradish, pesto sauce, tahini
SALAD DRESSINGS	Blue cheese, creamy Italian, creamy avocado, vinegar and oil, lemon juice and oil
DESSERTS	Pies, orange or raspberry sherbet
BEVERAGES	Peppermint tea, herbal tea, black tea, green tea, Japanese tea, Chinese oolong tea; mineral water, sparkling water

Lung

RARELY FOODS	No more than once a month
DENSE PROTEIN	Beef, pork, bacon, ham, sausage; anchovy; oysters
DAIRY	Milk, goat milk, buttermilk, half & half, sweet cream, sour cream, plain or flavored yogurt, frozen yogurt, ice cream
CHEESE	Cream, Edam, feta, goat, Gouda, mozzarella, Swiss
NUTS	Cashews, peanuts, peanut butter, walnuts (black, English)
LEGUMES	Beans (kidney, soy), soy milk, tofu
GRAINS	Buckwheat, corn tortillas, flour tortillas, whole wheat, wheat bran, wheat germ, whole wheat bread, English, muffins, whole wheat crackers, cream of wheat
VEGETABLES	Arugula, red potatoes, tomatoes, broccoflower
VEGETABLE JUICE	Carrot
FRUITS	Apples (Pippin, Red, or Golden Delicious), apricots, bananas, blackberries, blueberries, grapes (black, green, red), papayas, melons (cantaloupe, honeydew), nectarines, oranges, peaches, pears, persimmons
FRUIT JUICES	Red cherry, orange
VEGETABLE OILS	Canola, peanut, sunflower, soy
SWEETENERS	Refined cane sugar, brown sugar, raw sugar, fructose, succonant, saccharin, aspertame, Equal®, NutraSweet®, Sweet'n Low®
CONDIMENTS	Barbecue sauce, pickles, catsup, mustard, mayonnaise, margarine, soy sauce, salt, sea salt, vinegar
SALAD DRESSINGS	French, ranch, thousand island
DESSERTS	Custards, tapioca, puddings, cakes, chocolate, desserts containing chocolate, cheese cake
CHIPS	Bean, corn (blue, white, yellow), potato
BEVERAGES	Coffee; sake, wine (red, white), beer, barley malt liquor, champagne, gin, Scotch, vodka, whiskey, tequila; root beer, regular sodas, diet sodas
OTHER	French fries, fried foods

Lung

MENUS

DIETARY EMPHASIS:

- Fruits (bananas, apples, grapes), pine nuts, sprouted rye bread, rice with steamed kale and collards.
- Substantial breakfast with protein.
- Kombucha tea, made with green tea, aids digestion and assimilation.
- Consume a minimum of 2 oz. dense protein (eggs, chicken, turkey, or fish) with a grain such as rice or pasta at least 2 times a week.

WEIGHT LOSS:

- Eliminate sugar.
- Limit fats to 10-15% of caloric intake.
- Include 15% dense protein.
- Drink 64 oz. water daily.
- Exercise.

WEIGHT GAIN:

- Consume 30% of calories from dense protein.
- Increase fats to 20-30%.
- Include sugar (fruits).
- Drink 64 oz. water daily to flush kidneys.

VEGETARIAN DIET:

- Recommended when healthy, although up to 30% of calories may consist of dense protein.

FATS:

- 10-30% of caloric intake.
- Best sources are nuts (almonds, pine nuts, pecans, coconuts, cashews), seeds, protein (beef, chicken, turkey, lamb, fish, eggs), olive oil, and butter.

KEY

—all menus may be used by healthy persons
( ) around foods means that they're optional
L denotes weight loss menus
S denotes sensitive menus
G denotes weight gain menus

BREAKFAST:

7-8 a.m. Heavy, with protein, grain, nuts, seeds, dairy, fruit, legumes, and/or vegetables. 2 eggs 3 times per week, nuts 4 times per week – may be added to cereal.

SENSITIVE: Protein, grain, fruit, nuts and/or vegetables.

L	S	G	Menu
		G	Eggs, Jack or Cheddar cheese, and rye or 7-grain sprouted toast
	S		Eggs and rye or 7-grain sprouted toast
L			Eggs, rice, beans, and vegetables
L	S		Eggs, potatoes, and dark rye, sprouted rye, or raisin toast
		G	Eggs, cheese, potatoes, and dark rye, sprouted rye, or raisin toast
	S		Eggs, broccoli, and rye toast w/butter
L	S		Omelette w/basil, onions, and mushrooms
		G	Omelette w/Jack cheese, and basil (tomato and/or rye toast)
L	S		Omelette w/ onions and mushrooms
L			Omelette w/basil and Jack cheese
L			Scrambled eggs and broccoli
	S		Scrambled eggs, broccoli, and sprouted rye toast w/butter
		G	Scrambled eggs, broccoli, and sprouted rye toast w/butter (turkey sausage)
		G	Scrambled eggs w/cheddar cheese and ham or bacon (rye or 7-grain sprouted toast)
L			Poached eggs and Kashi®
	S		Eggs and potatoes
	S		Eggs and croissant
			Eggs and croissant (bacon)
	S		Eggs and sprouted spice bread
	S		Eggs and blueberry muffin w/butter
L			Cream of rice w/banana, peaches, or blueberries
	S		Cream of rice and eggs or chicken
	S	G	Oatmeal, eggs, and turkey or turkey sausage
	S		Oatmeal and soy milk (eggs or turkey)

Lung

	S	G	Oatmeal, plain kefir, and eggs or turkey
	S		Oatmeal and chopped pecans
			Oatmeal, soy milk, and banana (eggs or turkey)
		G	Oatmeal, plain kefir, banana, and eggs or turkey
			Oatmeal, chopped pecans, and banana
L			Oatmeal (Sun Rider®, stevia, or Re-Vita®)
	S		Oatmeal and raisins
			Oatmeal, raisins, and/or banana
L			Quinoa and steamed vegetables (sesame oil)
			White basmati rice
	S		Rice and miso soup (steamed greens or toast)
L			Curried rice
	S		Corn grits w/cheese (corn bread)
	S	G	Nutri Grain® w/banana and walnuts
	S		Granola w/almond milk
L			Couscous w/banana or strawberries and pine nuts
	S		Couscous and apples
	S	G	Turkey sausage and broccoli or brussels sprouts (rice)
L	S		Chicken and green beans
L	S		Chicken (rice – any variety)
	S		Chicken and pita bread
L	S		Chicken, spinach, and wild rice
L	S		Chicken, chinese pea pods, and oriental rice
	S		Chicken salad: romaine lettuce, tomatoes, onions, artichoke hearts, and grilled chicken
L	S		Tuna and broccoli, brussels sprouts, or cauliflower
L		G	Minute steak and broccoli, brussels sprouts, or cauliflower
		G	Steak (eggs)
		G	Lamb chops (eggs)
	S		Pine nuts
L	S		Raw almonds or pine nuts and apples, banana, pears, or figs (orange juice or apple juice)
	S		Almonds and cauliflower
	S		Almond butter on banana or toast
		G	Sunflower seeds and raisins
	S	G	Kefir – plain or flavored
			Plain nonfat yogurt and grape-nuts
	S		Cottage cheese, brown rice, and broccoli
L	S		Papaya and lowfat cottage cheese
	S	G	Cottage cheese, muffin made w/rice and oat flour, and banana
	S		Nonfat cottage cheese and rice cake (banana or apple)
	S	G	Apple sauce, walnuts, bread, and banana (orange juice)
	S	G	Berries or peaches w/cashews
	S		Swedish pancakes and bacon
	S	G	Blueberry, apple, or banana and walnut pancakes
	S		Blueberry pancakes, potatoes, and eggs
	S		Rye toast – no butter
	S		Sprouted rye or 7-grain toast w/almond or cashew butter
	S		Sourdough or sprouted rye toast w/avocado and pine nuts
			Toasted bagel w/cream cheese and grapefruit
		G	All-1 protein powder in juice, banana, and cottage cheese (bagel)
			All-1 in juice, flour tortilla, and cheese
			With meal:
	S		Hot water w/lemon juice or Soya coffee
			Capuccino w/pine nuts
			Decaf coffee w/Mocha Mix

MID-MORNING (10-11 a.m.) or **MID-AFTERNOON SNACK:** (4 p.m.) (Optional) Vegetables, protein, nuts, seeds, dairy, legumes, grain and/or fruit.

L	S		Carrots or bell pepper
L	S		Carrot, carrot/broccoli/spinach, carrot/spinach, or carrot/beet juice
	S		Chicken or pine nuts

Lung

S G Couscous and apples
S G Rice cake (almond or peanut butter and/or pine nuts)
S Popcorn (butter and Parmesan cheese)
S Sprouted rye bread (honey)
S G Sprouted spice bread
G Bagel w/cream cheese
S Almond milk

LUNCH:
12-2 p.m. Moderate, with grain, vegetables, legumes, dairy, nuts, seeds, protein, and/or fruit.
SENSITIVE: Avoid dense protein.

L Steamed cauliflower and broccoli (w/pine nuts or almonds)
Millet in chicken broth, peas, and pine nuts
Plain yogurt and pine nuts or pecans
S Burrito: Cheddar cheese, romaine lettuce, and refried pinto beans
S Tostada: corn tortilla, refried pinto or black beans, mozzarella or Cheddar cheese, lettuce, and salsa
S Cheese enchilada (guacamole)
S Nachos w/cheese, guacamole, and salad
L Tofuburgers
L Tofu and rice
G Chicken fajita, rice, and beans
Chicken tortilla soup
S Black bean soup w/rice, sourdough bread, and butter
Lasagna or spaghetti w/sauce and salad
S Semolina pasta w/garlic, tomatoes, basil, and Parmesan cheese (mushrooms)
S Pasta w/onion, celery, carrots, garlic, broccoli, zucchini, and cheese sauce
S G Pasta w/garlic, broccoli, mushrooms, onions, and French bread
L S Pasta and broccoli, brussels sprouts, or green peppers
L S Pasta, vegetables, herbs, garlic, and onions
L S Pasta, pine nuts, and raw spinach
S Tomato garlic pasta and broccoli
L S Pasta salad w/peppers, tomatoes, green onions, and cucumbers
Salad: mixed greens, dandelion greens, carrots, and sesame seeds w/vegeburger
L S Salad: lettuce, pears, cauliflower, walnuts, and/or pine nuts
L S Spinach salad w/pine nuts
S Caesar Salad
L Crab or shrimp salad
Provolone cheese on rye sourdough bread
G Turkey, cucumber, tomato, and lettuce on rye bread
G Chicken stir-fry
L Sushi/cucumber roll
L S Spinach, beet greens, beets, and brown rice
S Spinach souffle
S Baked potato w/flaxseed oil
L Baked potato w/salsa, vegetables w/Bragg® aminos, and green or black bean juice
L S Mixed vegetables and yams or brown rice
S G Dried pineapple, mango, papaya, and/or nuts (honey)
G Plums and bananas
S G Peanut butter w/bananas
S Juice: carrot (broccoli and/or spinach, celery, bell pepper, or Re-Vita®)
Carrot, celery, and apple juice

LUNCH or DINNER:

S Macaroni and cheese w/peas
S Spinach pasta w/pine nuts and pesto sauce
S Pasta, broccoli, and pine nuts
S Pasta w/broccoli sauce: pureed broccoli, basil, and dill (salmon)
S Pasta, mushrooms, onion, broccoli, green beans, and pine nuts
S Pasta w/pesto sauce and pine nuts

Lung

L S	Pasta w/mushroom sauce and salad
L S	Pasta w/eggplant
S	Pasta w/sundried or fresh tomatoes
S	Pasta w/tomato sauce and pine nuts
L S	Pasta w/tomato sauce, onion, broccoli, and mushrooms
S	Pasta, basil, and pine nuts (tomatoes)
S	Pasta, Parmesan cheese, basil, and tomato (butter)
S	Pasta and fish
L S	Lentil soup w/sprouted rye bread or rye crackers
S	Split pea soup (corn bread)
S	Carrot soup and salad: lettuce and pine nuts
S	Turkey soup w/corn bread
S	Vegetable soup
S	Lentil soup w/French bread
S	Spinach salad
S	Salad: romaine lettuce, peas, onions, and pecans
S	Salad: feta cheese, Yarlsburg cheese, bacon, walnuts, and romaine lettuce
S	Greek salad: feta cheese, lettuce, and pine nuts (olives and/or onions)
S	Lentil salad: wild and brown rice, lentils, corn, and spinach w/flaxseed oil and lemon dressing
L S	Yams, spinach, and brown rice
L S	Baked potato, Muenster cheese, and green peppers
L	Baked potato, broccoli, raw red bell peppers, and raw carrots
S	Baked potato w/butter, (salt and pepper), broccoli, and raw carrots (raw red peppers)
S	Baked potato w/butter, green onions, chopped tomato, Parmesan cheese, and steamed broccoli
S	Macadamia/cashew butter and Re-Vita®
S	Fish taco
S	Tempura shrimp, rice, water chestnuts, shitake mushrooms, and green onions
S	Bell peppers stuffed w/corn, rice, ground turkey, onion, and garlic

DINNER:
7-9 p.m. Light, with small portions of protein, legumes, vegetables and/or grain.

L	Snapper, halibut, cod, shark, or swordfish and mixed vegetables
S	Salmon or sea bass and pasta, basil, olive oil, and garlic
G	Salmon, baked potato, and beans
S	Pasta w/shrimp, garlic, parmesan cheese, parsley, and butter (oil)
S	Pasta w/chicken
S	Pasta, broccoli, and pine nuts
S	Pasta, zucchini, and mushrooms
G	Pasta, marinara sauce, and hamburger
	Lasagna
L S	Stir-fry: shrimp, rice, water chestnuts, shitake mushrooms, and green onions
L	Rice w/chicken taco
L	Spanish rice w/carne asada burrito and avocado
L G	Baked potato w/flaxseed oil, chicken or steak, and broccoli
	Potato, beans, peas, or lentil soup
L G	Fillet of sole, rice, and brussels sprouts
L G	Salmon w/rice and broccoli
S	Salmon, cauliflower, broccoli, and white rose potatoes
S	Salmon w/rice and broccoli (cauliflower)
S	Salmon loaf w/oatmeal and steamed broccoli
L	Salmon loaf and steamed vegetables
L S	Orange roughy, rice, and peas
S	Trout, spinach pasta w/pesto sauce, and carrots
L	Trout, marinara sauce, pasta, carrots, and Parmesan cheese
L	Swordfish, rice, and broccoli
S	Swordfish and corn on the cob
L	Sushi
L S G	Chicken and brown basmati rice or barley in chicken broth
L S G	Chicken, spinach, wild rice (peas and carrots, and yellow squash)

Lung

L			Chicken or fish and brown basmati rice
L	S		Chicken, chinese pea pods, and oriental or spanish rice
	S	G	Chicken, corn on the cob, and potato or potato salad
	S		Chicken breast and Caesar salad
L	S	G	Grilled chicken breast and marinated vegetables: cauliflower, cucumbers, and green onions
	S		Chicken salad: grilled chicken, romaine lettuce, tomatoes, onions, and artichoke hearts
	S		Thai chicken salad: chicken and wild rice
	S		Chicken quesadilla: flour tortilla, cheese, chicken, tomatoes, peppers, and onions
	S	G	Chicken enchilada w/beans and rice
	S		Turkey w/rice or pasta
L		G	Turkey w/rice or potatoes, peas and carrots, and yellow squash
	S		Turkey w/potatoes or rice, and brussels sprouts or spinach
			Turkey, mashed potatoes, and squash
	S		Turkey, mashed potatoes, and turkey gravy
	S	G	Turkey, brown rice, and stir-fry vegetables
	S		Turkey w/avocado on rye bread or crackers
L			Turkey, avocado, and sprouts on sprouted rye bread
	S	G	Turkey club sandwich w/bacon, tomato, lettuce, avocado, and dijon mustard on rye bread
L			Jack cheese, avocado, and sprouts on sprouted rye bread
	S		Bell peppers stuffed w/corn, rice, ground turkey, onion, and garlic
L			Hamburger, onion, tomato, lettuce, and cheese
L			Lamb or beef w/potatoes or rice
	S	G	Lamb and russet potatoes
			Lamb and russet potatoes (salad: romaine lettuce, tomato, onions, garbanzo and/or kidney beans or lettuce, tomato, and pine nuts)
L	S		Lamb w/rice and cooked celery
L	S		Lamb, summer squash, and swiss chard
	S	G	Lasagna w/French bread
L		G	Pinto beans w/red and yellow peppers, onions, and small beef tenderloin fillet
		G	Bean and beef burrito
	S		Lentils w/rice and spinach
		G	Oat bagel w/cream cheese and lox
			Plain bagel w/cream cheese and caviar
	S	G	Barbecued chicken pizza
	S		Shrimp pizza
L			Red port wine after dinner

EVENING SNACK:
(Optional) 10 p.m.-2 a.m. Fruit, sweets, dairy, grain, nuts, seeds, protein, legumes, and/or vegetables.

	S	G	Apple, peach, pear, cherries, grapes, or pineapple
			Nonfat yogurt
L	S		Peppermint tea
	S		Mints
		G	Chocolate candy
	S	G	Muffins
	S	G	Oatmeal cookies
		G	Chocolate chip cookies, chocolate truffles. or angel food cake
		G	Dreyer's or Swensen's® chocolate chip ice cream
		G	Swensen's® coffee ice cream
		G	Hot fudge sundae

NOTE: Eating sweets between 8 and 10 p.m. may result in waking up around 3 to 4 a.m. Eating cheese or cheese and crackers will often allow one to go back to sleep.

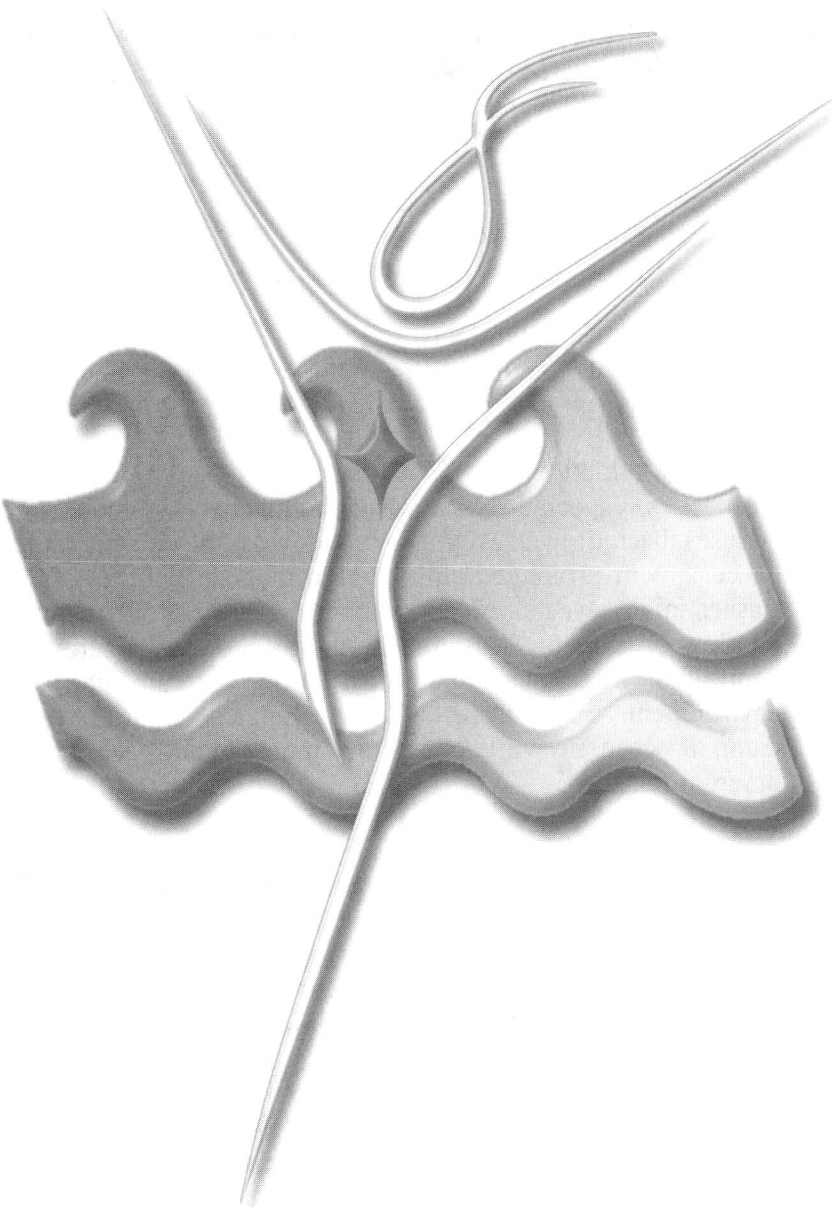

LYMPH

***The "Lymph Body Type"
is symbolized by ocean waves.
Constant movement, fluidity and
variety through physical or mental
activity provide the stimulation they
need to feel vibrant and alive.
Fun-loving and playful,
they are happiest when
they are active.***

Lymph

BODY TYPE PROFILE

LOCATION	Throughout body – large numbers of lymph nodes in groin, under arms, and in neck, chest, and behind knees.
FUNCTION	Lymphatic system collects lymph, which carries waste and contains lymphocytes (white blood cells) that fight infection.
POTENTIAL HEALTH PROBLEMS	Generally athletic with good stamina, muscular tone and development. Headaches, especially with weather changes. Immune system weakness (viruses, bacteria) and eventual breakdown (e.g., chronic fatigue syndrome or cancer), with prolonged stress. Hormonal difficulties (PMS, cramps, hot flashes, night sweats); ulcers or other digestive problems; kidney weakness; and low back pain. Muscle aching, stiffness, low energy, sluggishness, or depression when inactive or not getting enough sunlight. Sensitive to environment. Some do better in dry climates and are adversely affected by damp or ocean air, while others love moisture and feel uncomfortable in dry desert climates.
RECOMMENDED EXERCISE	Exercising at least 1 hour every other day is essential, as it activates the immune system. Lymphatic activation requires all-over movement, such as walking, although not necessarily vigorously, for 20 minutes, 5 times a week. Variety is important. Sufficient vigorous exercise may be obtained in 15 minutes, from activities such as hiking, bicycling, roller-blading, yoga, callanetics, dancing, aerobics, stair-stepping, tennis, racquetball, swimming, diving, running, or weight training. When sensitive, reduce exercise and emphasize bodily movement with music, such as walking, floor exercises, or dancing with musical accompaniment. Be aware of your body and stop when it begins to feel excessive. Running may be contraindicated if having difficulty maintaining weight.

WOMEN'S CHARACTERISTICS

DISTINGUISHING FEATURES	Physical exercise is essential. Usually athletic, with broad shoulders and well-proportioned, attractive face and body. To prevent stagnation, require regular physical or mental stimulation. Change, variety, and movement keep them happy. Generally playful, bright, and quick-witted. They thrive on excitement.
ADDITIONAL PHYSICAL CHARACTERISTICS	Buttocks rounded-to-prominent. Low back curvature average-to-swayed. Breasts small-to-average. Shoulders relatively even with, to broader than, hips. Waist straight-to-defined. Average to long-waisted. Height very petite

Lymph

to average. Bone structure small-to-medium. Average, elongated musculature. Strong abdominal muscles and thighs. Small, average, or long slender hands. Head rectangular and proportionate to body, but may have long appearance.

WEIGHT GAIN AREAS

Lower body with initial gain in entire upper 2/3rds of thighs, including upperinner thighs, buttocks, and possibly upper hips. Secondary weight gain in lower abdomen, waist, hips (predominantly upper or lower), thighs extendingto knees, middle back, and upper arms. May have difficulty gaining or maintaining weight.

DIETARY GUIDELINES

SCHEDULING MEALS:

"HEALTHY"

Breakfast: Light-to-moderate, with grain, nuts, seeds, vegetables, legumes, protein and/or dairy; eggs 2 times per week. Fruit or fruit juice alone 30 minutes before or 1 hour after breakfast, 2 meals per week. Mix grains with fat such as nuts or butter.

Lunch: Moderate-to-heavy, with grain, dairy, nuts, seeds, and/or protein (limited vegetables).

Dinner: Moderate-to-heavy, with grain, protein, dairy, nuts, seeds, legumes and/or vegetables.

"SENSITIVE"

Breakfast: Heavy, with protein, nuts, seeds, grain, and/or vegetables.

Lunch: Light, with grain and/or vegetables

Dinner: Moderate, with grain, vegetables and/or legumes.

DIETARY EMPHASIS

- Carrots, rice (white basmati if sensitive), and adequate protein.
- For weight loss, eliminate all dairy except butter, reduce breads, and include 20-25% of caloric intake as dense protein. Will gain weight if fat from appropriate sources falls below 20%.
- For weight gain, add dairy and increase fats to 25-35%. Include at least 15% of caloric intake from dense protein.
- Vegetarian diet recommended; or diet may consist of up to 30% dense chemical-free protein.
- Fats, 20-25% of caloric intake, should be from sunflower seeds, almonds, pecans, and avocados. When fats are increased to 25-35%, add butter, kefir, fish, and other dense protein.

Lymph

DIETARY EMPHASIS (Continued)	• When rebuilding the body (e.g., after chemotherapy), increase fats to 50% of caloric intake from fish (especially salmon), chicken, turkey, duck, game hen, goose, kefir and kefir cheese and increase dense protein to 30%.
KEY SUPPORTS FOR SYSTEM	Blue/green algae cleanses lymphatic system. It also supplies most amino acids, and is highest form of vegetable protein available – particularly important for vegetarians, as adequate protein is essential. Rotate foods. Spicy foods (Thai spices, salsa, or cayenne pepper) stimulate lymphatic movement.
COMPLEMENTARY GLANDULAR SUPPORT	Spleen, through connecting heart-felt emotions physically in supportive way, as in healing, helping, or massaging someone or through animal contact. Kidney, through building courage by doing something different at least 2 times a week.
FOODS CRAVED	*(When Energy is Low)* Sweets, such as chocolate, ice cream, pastries. Carbohydrates, like breads, rice, pasta, chips, potatoes. Spicy foods, such as Thai or Szechuan, salsa. Protein, such as yogurt and chicken. Generally don't care to eat when stressed.
FOODS TO AVOID	Chicken, turkey, and beef that have been fed hormones; fried foods. Dairy, as it can cause stomach aching or bloating, joint stiffness, menstrual cramps and clotting.
RECOMMENDED CUISINE	Frequently, Thai, Chinese, steamed vegetables; moderately, Mexican, Italian.

Lymph

PSYCHOLOGICAL PROFILE

ESSENCE

Just as the lymphatic system requires stimulation to move the waste away from the tissues, the Lymph body type needs continual stimulation in the form of movement and change. It's this constant movement that adds variety to life. Lymph types require a lot of variety through physical activity or mental stimulation to maintain mental clarity and a sense of vitality. They are happiest when they feel excitement. Fun loving and playful, activity allows them to feel vibrant and alive. Consequently, stimulation, either mental or physical, is essential.

CHARACTERISTIC TRAITS

Lymphs are physically strong and naturally well coordinated. Athletically inclined and usually health conscious, they often become professional athletes or personal trainers. Basically playful, they thrive on constant stimulation, variety and change. Mentally quick and alert, Lymph types are stimulated by learning, and will use this as another way of experiencing constant change and variety. Creative and artistic, they love to express themselves imaginatively, usually in areas associated with movement, such as dance, playing a musical instrument, or other forms of artistic or aesthetic expression.

As a type, Lymphs are extremely beautiful or handsome, and the most consistently physically attractive of all the 25 body types. Their bodies are characterized by fine, well-sculpted features, broad shoulders and easily definable muscles. Sensitive to outward appearances, they typically are quite conscientious about their dress and grooming, generally always maintaining a striking appearance. Since physical attractiveness is usually a high priority, Lymphs tend to put a lot of energy into youthfulness and the way things look.

Typically extroverted and sociable, Lymphs add stimulation and excitement to whatever they do. Romantically inclined, they tend to enter new relationships with great optimism. Sensitive and caring, charismatic and mentally focused, Lymphs can come on very strong, easily sweeping the object of their attention off their feet.

MOTIVATION

Highly optimistic, when attracted to a potential mate, Lymphs are likely to throw themselves totally into the relationship. They tend to come on very strong, focusing almost all their attention on the other person and outward appearances, rather than on what may actually be taking place below the surface. They can become so absorbed by idealized fantasies of the relationship's potential that they lose sight of what may be a much less promising reality. Also, wanting to be "up front," they're likely to reveal themselves more than may be appropriate during the earlier stages of a relationship.

In addition to putting themselves on the line, they're apt to put strain on the relationship by continually questioning the other person about their thoughts

Lymph

MOTIVATION

and feelings. For they desperately need to be reassured that they're cared for, loved, and appreciated. Without such reassurances, unresolved or buried feelings of self-doubt and inadequacy surface. Emotional pain is the Lymph's main motivation for change and personal growth, so relationships play an important role. Ultimately, Lymphs need to learn to love themselves, and the tendency is to seek validation that they are loveable from outside sources.

Lymphs tend to judge themselves by their accomplishments, so challenges provide opportunities for growth. Meeting and overcoming those that stifle their feelings of aliveness or creativity builds their sense of self-worth, while those challenges that are creative make them feel more alive.

Stagnation occurs when movement is missing, and this leads to depression. Variety and frequent changes, even if it's only minor sensory changes, such as the colors, smells, or textures of their immediate environment can keep them from getting bored. Lymphs like to keep things active and lively, and can experience a real lift when they change their place of residence, which they do much more often than most other types.

"AT WORST"

Lymphs are susceptible to boredom when they allow their lives, because of their fears and insecurities, to become too routine. Without stimulation and excitement, Lymphs become discouraged, lethargic, stagnant, or depressed. While they are generally quite adept at handling details and not given to procrastination, when an endeavor begins to bore them, they become distracted, inattentive or inefficient.

When unable to sufficiently express themselves, Lymph types feel tense and restricted, causing their underlying feelings of inadequacy and rejection to surface. In their need to feel secure, they give too much of themselves at the expense of their own needs. Needing reassurance, they will fish for what they want to hear, asking impelling questions about the other person's thoughts and feelings. Seeking approval and acceptance from others, and wishing to avoid criticism, they may suppress their own needs. It's this internalized suppression that produces feelings of tension and constriction, and triggers deep-seated feelings of rejection or personal inadequacy.

Without sufficient reassurances that they are loved, cared for, and appreciated in their significant relationship, their deep-seated feelings of distrust will be aroused. Such distrust or suspicion can end up becoming a self-fulfilling prophecy; for the urgency of their questioning may lead the other person to question the relationship's viability. The more Lymph types demand from their primary relationship, the harder it is for their partner to meet their expectations and they often end up feeling overwhelmed or "cornered," causing them to react negatively. Because relationships are so important, female Lymphs tend to work too hard, or long, on a relationship, doing their best to make it succeed even after its limited potential has become fairly obvious.

Lymph

With their partner in an emotional straight-jacket, the relationship is apt to lose its authenticity, and go downhill. Even when the suspiciousness that sparked the difficulties in the first place becomes a self-fulfilling prophecy, and the relationship for all practical purposes has failed, female Lymphs will often continue to do their best to maintain it. Men, on the other hand, have more of a tendency to get out as soon as a problem arises, as their fear of failure and need to excel in everything they do will not allow them to be the one who is rejected.

"AT BEST"

Lymph types are conscientious, capable, mentally quick, and self-motivated. They are attentive to details, can logically organize and quickly learn whatever they are studying. Since Lymphs like a lot of activity with variety, they are stimulated by being on the front line, and can handle the pressure of having a lot going on at once without feeling overloaded. With high personal expectations and their natural ability to excel at whatever they do, Lymph types are often entrepreneurs or heads of corporations. It's their openness to new ideas, change and variety, that puts Lymphs on the leading edge of technology.

Health oriented, Lymphs have a sense of well-being and relate well to the outside world. While they hold high expectations of themselves, they are rarely judgmental of others, generally accepting people for who and what they are. Having learned to truly love and accept themselves, Lymphs are free to love others unconditionally without judgement and expectations. This is when their personal relationships are rewarding and fulfilling. Sensitive and genuinely helpful, with good focus and sense of direction, Lymphs are excellent leaders and role-models.

Blessed with a naturally high energy level, Lymphs love to be active. In touch with their bodies, exercise connects them with their intuitive side and their true self. Feeling connected and sure of themselves, enables them to live in the moment, free to express their spontaneity and enthusiasm for life. They thrive on excitement, welcome change, and enjoy the opportunity to add variety to life.

Lymph

FOOD LISTS

HEALTHY FOOD LIST

FREQUENTLY FOODS	3-7 meals per week – refers to each food, rather than category.
DENSE PROTEIN	Chemical-free beef, beef broth, beef liver, bear, buffalo, rabbit, organ meats (heart, brain), venison; chemical-free turkey or chicken, chicken broth, chicken livers, duck, cornish game hen, quail, pheasant; rattlesnake; anchovy, catfish, cod, flounder, haddock, halibut, herring, mackerel, mahi-mahi, perch, roughy, sardines, shark, red snapper, sole; calamari (squid), clams, crab, eel, lobster, mussels, octopus, oysters, scallops
DAIRY	Kefir, butter
CHEESE	Cheddar, ricotta
NUTS and SEEDS	Coconuts, sunflower seeds
GRAINS	Popcorn, rice (all varieties), rice bran, rice cakes, cream of rice
VEGETABLES	Artichokes, asparagus, green beans, broccoli, carrots, celery, swiss chard, peas, spinach, yams
FRUITS	Bananas, strawberries, oranges
SWEETENERS	Re-Vita®, stevia
BEVERAGES	Green tea
MODERATELY FOODS	1-2 meals per week – refers to each food, rather than category.
DENSE PROTEIN	Lamb; bass, bonita, salmon, swordfish, trout, tuna; abalone, shrimp, escargo; eggs
DAIRY	Raw milk, goat milk, buttermilk, half & half, sweet cream, sour cream, plain or flavored yogurt, ice cream (Dreyer's, Ben & Jerry's®, Swensen's®)
CHEESE	American, blue, brie, Camembert, Colby, cottage, cream, Edam, feta, goat, Gouda, Jack, kefir, Limburger, mozzarella, Muenster, Parmesan, Romano, Swiss
NUTS and SEEDS	Almonds, almond butter, Brazils, cashews, cashew butter, water chestnuts, filberts, hazelnuts, macadamias, macadamia butter, peanuts, peanut butter, pecans, pine nuts, pistachios, walnuts (black, English), caraway seeds, sunflower seed butter
LEGUMES	Beans (adzuki, black, garbanzo, kidney, lima [butter], great northern, navy, pinto, red, soy), lentils, black-eyed peas, split peas, hummus, miso, soy milk, tofu
GRAINS	Amaranth, barley, buckwheat, corn, corn grits, corn bread, corn tortillas, hominy grits, millet, oats, oatmeal, quinoa, rye, triticale, wheat germ, refined wheat flour, flour tortillas, breads (French, Italian, garlic, 7-grain, multi-grain, oat, corn, corn/rye, rye, rice, sprouted grain, sourdough, white), bagels, croissants, English muffins, crackers (saltine, oat, rye), couscous, pasta, udon noodles, rice noodles, cream of rye, cream of wheat

Lymph

VEGETABLES	Avocado, bamboo shoots, basil, yellow wax beans, lima beans, beets, bok choy, brussels sprouts, cabbage (red, napa, green), cauliflower, cilantro, corn, cucumbers, eggplant, garlic, greens (beet, collard, mustard, turnip), jicama, kale, kohlrabi, leeks, lettuce (all varieties), mushrooms, okra, olives (green, ripe), onions (brown, chives, green, red, white, yellow, vidalia), parsley, parsnips, snow pea pods, bell peppers (green, red, yellow), chili peppers, pimentos, potatoes (red, russet, yukon gold), sweet potatoes, pumpkin, radishes, daikon radishes, rutabaga, sauerkraut, seaweed (arame, dulse, kelp, nori, wakame), shallots, sprouts (alfalfa, clover, mung bean, radish, sunflower), squash (acorn, banana, butternut, spaghetti, yellow [summer], zucchini), tomatoes (vine-ripened), turnips, watercress
VEGETABLE JUICES	Carrot, celery, carrot/celery, parsley, spinach, tomato, V-8®
FRUITS	Apples (all varieties), apricots, blackberries, blueberries, boysenberries, cranberries, gooseberries, raspberries, cherries, grapes (black, green, red), grapefruits, (red, white), guavas, kiwi, kumquats, lemons, limes, loquats, mangos, melons (cantaloupe, casaba, crenshaw, watermelon, honeydew), nectarines, papayas, peaches, pears, persimmons, pineapples, plums (black, purple, red), pomegranates, rhubarb, tangelos, tangerines, dates, figs, prunes, raisins
FRUIT JUICES	Apple, apple cider, apple/apricot, apricot, black cherry, red cherry, cranberry, cranapple, grape (purple, red, white), grapefruit, guava, lemon, orange, papaya, pear, pineapple, pineapple/coconut, prune, tangerine, watermelon
VEGETABLE OILS	All-blend, almond, avocado, canola, coconut, corn, flaxseed, olive, peanut, safflower, sesame, soy, sunflower
CONDIMENTS	Mustard, horseradish, mayonnaise, barbecue sauce, pesto sauce, soy sauce, salsa, tahini, vinegar, paprika, Bragg's aminos, salt, sea salt, Vege-Sal®
SALAD DRESSINGS	Blue cheese, French, ranch, creamy Italian, creamy avocado, thousand island, vinegar and oil, lemon juice and oil
DESSERTS	Chocolate, desserts containing chocolate, custards, tapioca, puddings, pies, cakes, orange or raspberry sherbet
CHIPS	Bean, corn (blue, white, yellow), potato
BEVERAGES	Herbal tea, black tea, Japanese tea, Chinese oolong tea; mineral water, sparkling water; sake, wine (red, white), beer, barley malt liquor, champagne, gin, Scotch, vodka, whiskey; ginger ale, root beer
RARELY FOODS	No more than once a month
DENSE PROTEIN	Chemical-fed beef, veal, pork, bacon, ham, sausage; chemical-fed chicken or turkey
DAIRY	Pasteurized milk, frozen yogurt, most ice creams
NUTS and SEEDS	Seeds (pumpkin, sesame), sesame seed butter
GRAINS	Whole wheat, wheat bran, wheat germ, whole wheat bread, whole wheat crackers

Lymph

VEGETABLES	Arugula, broccoflower, white rose potatoes, hot-house tomatoes
SWEETENERS	Honey, molasses, sorghum, brown sugar, date sugar, raw sugar, refined cane sugar, maple syrup, brown rice syrup, barley malt syrup, corn syrup, fructose, succonant, saccharin, aspertame, Equal®, Sweet'n Low®, NutraSweet®
CONDIMENTS	Catsup, margarine
BEVERAGES	Coffee; regular sodas, diet sodas, Sprite®, coke
FOOD GROUPS	Individual foods from the moderately foods list shouldn't be eaten more than 1-2 meals per week, although foods from such food groups as cheese or dairy, grains, and legumes may be consumed up to 4 meals per week – e.g., Colby cheese 2 meals, and Jack and Swiss cheese, 1 meal each. Foods from such food groups as dense protein, nuts and seeds, vegetables, and fruits may be consumed up to 2 meals per day, 7 days per week, as long as individual foods are eaten no more than 2 meals weekly.

SENSITIVE FOOD LIST

FREQUENTLY FOODS	3-7 meals per week – refers to each food, rather than category.
DAIRY	Kefir, butter
GRAINS	Popcorn, white basmati rice
VEGETABLES	Carrots, celery, swiss chard, peas
BEVERAGES	Green tea
MODERATELY FOODS	1-2 meals per week – refers to each food, rather than category.
DENSE PROTEIN	Chemical-free beef, beef broth, beef liver, veal; chemical-free turkey, cornish game hen, duck, goose, chemical-free chicken, chicken broth, chicken livers; anchovy, bass, bonita, catfish, cod, flounder, haddock, halibut, herring, mackerel, mahi-mahi, roughy, salmon, sardines, shark, red snapper, sole, swordfish, trout, tuna; abalone, clams, crab, eel, lobster, mussels, octopus, oysters, scallops; eggs
DAIRY	Raw milk, goat milk, buttermilk, half & half, sweet cream, sour cream
CHEESE	American, blue, brie, Camembert, Cheddar, Colby, cream, cottage, Edam feta, goat, Gouda, Jack, kefir, Limburger, mozzarella, Muenster, Parmesan, ricotta, Romano, Swiss

Lymph

NUTS and SEEDS	Brazils, water chestnuts, coconuts, filberts, hazelnuts, macadamias, macadamia butter, pecans, pine nuts, pistachios, seeds (caraway, sunflower), sunflower seed butter
LEGUMES	Beans (adzuki, black, garbanzo, kidney, lima [butter], great northern, pinto, red), lentils, split peas, hummus, miso, soy milk
GRAINS	Amaranth, barley, corn, corn bread, corn grits, corn tortillas, hominy grits, oats, oatmeal, quinoa, rice (brown basmati, long or short grain white or brown, Japanese, wild), rice bran, rice cakes, triticale, bulgur wheat, wheat germ, refined wheat flour, flour tortillas, breads (French, Italian, sourdough, garlic, 7-grain, multi-grain, oat, corn, sprouted grain, rice, white), bagels, croissants, English muffins, crackers (saltine, oat), couscous, pasta, Udon noodles, rice noodles, cream of rice, cream of wheat
VEGETABLES	Asparagus, artichokes, bamboo shoots, basil, green beans, yellow wax beans, lima beans, beets, bok choy, brussels sprouts, cabbage (green, napa, red), cilantro, corn, cucumbers, eggplant, garlic, greens (beet, collard, mustard, turnip), jicama, kale, kohlrabi, leeks, lettuce (all varieties), mushrooms, okra, olives (green, ripe), onions (brown, chives, green, red, white, yellow, vidalia), parsley, parsnips, snow pea pods, chili peppers, pimentos, potatoes (red, yukon gold), sweet potatoes, pumpkin, radishes, daikon radishes, rutabaga, sauerkraut, seaweed (arame, dulse, kelp, nori, wakame), shallots, sprouts (alfalfa, clover, mung bean, radish, sunflower), spinach, squash (acorn, banana, butternut, spaghetti, yellow [summer], cooked zucchini), turnips, watercress
VEGETABLE JUICES	Carrot, celery, carrot/celery, parsley, spinach, V-8®
FRUITS	Apples (all varieties), apricots, bananas, blackberries, blueberries, boysenberries, cranberries, gooseberries, raspberries, strawberries, cherries, grapes (black, green, red), grapefruits (red, white), guavas, kiwi, kumquats, lemons, limes, loquats, mangos, melons (cantaloupe, honeydew), nectarines, oranges, papayas, peaches, pears, persimmons, pineapples, plums (black, purple, red), pomegranates, rhubarb, tangelos, tangerines, dates, figs, prunes, raisins
FRUIT JUICES	Apple/apricot, apricot, black cherry, red cherry, cranberry, cranapple, grape (purple, red, white), grapefruit, guava, lemon, papaya, pear, pineapple, prune, pineapple/coconut, tangerine
VEGETABLE OILS	All-blend, avocado, coconut
SWEETENERS	Re-Vita®, stevia
CONDIMENTS	Salsa, tahini, vinegar, paprika, Bragg™ aminos, salt, sea salt, Vege-Sal®
SALAD DRESSINGS	Vinegar and oil, lemon juice and oil
BEVERAGES	Herbal tea, Japanese tea, Chinese oolong tea; mineral water, sparkling water

Lymph

RARELY FOODS	No more than once a month
DENSE PROTEIN	Chemical-fed beef, veal, venison, lamb, pork, bacon, ham, sausage; bear, buffalo, rabbit, rattlesnake, pheasant, quail; chemical-fed chicken, turkey, duck; perch; calamari (squid), shrimp
DAIRY	Pasteurized milk, plain or flavored yogurt, frozen yogurt, ice cream
NUTS and SEEDS	Almonds, almond butter, cashews, cashew butter, peanuts, peanut butter, walnuts (black, English), seeds (pumpkin, sesame), sesame seed butter
LEGUMES	Navy, black-eyed peas, soy beans, tofu
GRAINS	Buckwheat, millet, polished rice, rye, whole wheat, wheat bran, breads (rye, whole wheat), crackers (rye, whole wheat), cream of rye
VEGETABLES	Avocados, arugula, broccoli, broccoflower, cauliflower, bell peppers (green, red, yellow), potatoes (russet, white rose), tomatoes, yams, raw zucchini
VEGETABLE JUICE	Tomato
FRUITS	Melons (casaba, crenshaw, watermelon)
FRUIT JUICES	Apple, apple cider, orange, watermelon
VEGETABLE OILS	Almond, canola, corn, flaxseed, olive, peanut, safflower, sesame, soy, sunflower
CONDIMENTS	Horseradish, barbecue sauce, pesto sauce, catsup, mustard, mayonnaise, margarine, soy sauce, hot/spicy foods, MSG
SALAD DRESSINGS	Blue cheese, French, ranch, creamy Italian, creamy avocado, thousand island
SWEETENERS	Honey, molasses, sorghum, brown sugar, date sugar, raw sugar, refined cane sugar, maple syrup, brown rice syrup, barley malt syrup, corn syrup, fructose, succonant, saccharin, aspertame, Equal®, Sweet'n Low®, NutraSweet®
DESSERTS	Custards, tapioca, puddings, pies, cakes, orange or raspberry sherbert, chocolate, desserts containing chocolate
CHIPS	Bean, corn (blue, white, yellow) potato
BEVERAGES	Coffee; black tea; wine, sake, beer, barley malt liquor, margueritas, champagne, gin, Scotch, vodka, whiskey; ginger ale, root beer, Coke®, Sprite®, regular sodas, diet sodas

Lymph

MENUS

DIETARY EMPHASIS:

- Carrots, rice (white basmati if sensitive), and adequate protein.
- Blue/green algae cleanses lymphatic system while spicy foods (Thai spices, salsa, or cayenne pepper) stimulate lymphatic movement.
- Rotate foods.

WEIGHT LOSS:

- Eliminate all dairy except butter.
- Reduce breads.
- Include 20-25% of caloric intake as dense protein.
- Will gain weight if fat from appropriate sources falls below 20%.

WEIGHT GAIN:

- Add dairy; increase fats to 25-35%. Include at least 15% of caloric intake from dense protein.

VEGETARIAN DIET:

- Recommended, or diet may consist of up to 30% dense chemical-free protein.

FATS:

- 20-25% of caloric intake. Best sources are sunflower seeds, almonds, pecans, and avocados.
- For 25-35%, add butter, kefir, fish, and other dense protein.
- When rebuilding the body (e.g., after chemotherapy), increase fats to 50% of caloric intake from fish (especially salmon), chicken, turkey, duck, game hen, goose, kefir and kefir cheese; increase dense protein to 30%.

KEY

—all menus may be used by healthy persons
( ) around foods means that they're optional
L denotes weight loss menus
S denotes sensitive menus
G denotes weight gain menus

BREAKFAST:
6-7 am. Fruit or fruit juice only. Eat fruit alone, 30 min. before or 1 hour after meals, 2 meals per week.

7-8 a.m. Light-to-moderate, with grain, nuts, seeds, vegetables, legumes, protein and/or dairy; eggs 2 times per week. Mix grains with fat such as nuts or butter.

SENSITIVE: Heavy, with protein, nuts, seeds, grain, and/or vegetables.

L	S	G	Eggs and bagel
		G	Yogurt and almonds
L			Basmati or short grain brown rice (butter or tamari) and green beans
L			Rice (peas and/or butter) (almonds)
L			Rice and beans
		G	Cheese omelette and bagel w/cream cheese
			Brown rice (eggs and/or vegetables)
L			Cream of rice and almonds
L			Oatmeal w/ReVita® and/or butter
L			Oatmeal w/sunflower seeds
		G	Protein powder in milk and oatmeal w/butter
L			Corn grits w/butter (at least 15 min. later, papaya or pineapple)
L			Cream of rice or cream of wheat w/ReVita®
L			Cream of wheat w/rice milk (banana later)
L			Quinoa and sunflower seeds
L			Buckwheat and almonds
L			Cream of rye w/almonds and sunflower seeds
			English muffin and avocado or butter
		G	Onion bagel w/cream cheese (tomato)
L			Oatmeal crumble: oatmeal, oat flour, butter, and ReVita®
			Carrot, zucchini, or poppy seed muffin
L	S		Pasta and peas
L	S		Potato and green beans (squash)
L			Baked yukon gold potato or yam w/butter
L			Vegetable soup: carrot, onion, yam, cumin, coriander, pepper, and turmeric w/brown rice and raw cucumber

Lymph

L	S	G	
L			Peaches, pears, red apples, grapefruit, strawberries, banana, oranges, melons – early
L			Apple juice, banana, and ReVita®
L			Cranberry juice or concentrate and ReVita®
			Kiwi or apple; then barley
			Apple, papaya, or orange juice – 1 hr. after breakfast
			SENSITIVE: (For healthy, best eaten at dinner only.)
	S	G	Crab omelette, rice, and vegetable soup
	S		Tuna, noodles, and peas
	S		Game hen, rice, and yellow squash, or carrots and peas
	S		Chemical-free chicken, rice, and green beans, or asparagus
	S		Chemical-free chicken, white rice, and water chestnuts
	S		Chemical-free turkey, gravy, red potatoes, carrots and peas
	S		Chemical-free turkey patty, rice, and swiss chard
	S	G	Eggs and chemical-free ground turkey
			LUNCH: 12-2 p.m. Moderate-to-heavy, with grain, dairy, nuts, seeds, and/or protein (limited vegetables).
			SENSITIVE: Light, with grain and/or vegetables.
		G	Chemical-free chicken and rice or snow peas
L			Spinach pasta and chemical-free chicken w/hot or cold salad
		G	Chemical-free turkey w/stuffing, roll, and gravy
		G	Chemical-free turkey or grilled cheese sandwich
L		G	Salmon and/or crab, clams, or tuna w/pasta
L		G	Sea bass or sole w/rice pilaf and snow peas
			Tuna and pasta
L			Baked tuna, rice, and cooked celery in casserole
	S		Lentil soup and rice cake
			Water packed tuna sandwich on white or rye bread
L			Fish taco: flour tortilla, light fish fillet, slice of avocado, lemon, shredded green cabbage w/rice
		G	Tofu stroganoff w/mushrooms and cream sauce
L			Chicken soup: chicken broth, chicken, rice, celery, and carrots
L			Matza ball soup w/noodles and rice
	S		Vegetable soup: carrots, onions, cumin, coriander, pepper, and turmeric w/brown rice and raw cucumber
		G	Cheese enchiladas
		G	Cheddar cheese, flour tortilla, rice, and avocado
		G	Corn tamale w/black or pinto beans, cheese, and/or rice or barley
L		G	Beans, rice, and corn tortilla
L		G	Pinto beans and rice w/sliced black olives, corn tortilla, and sliced cucumber
		G	Brown rice, tamale, and beans or tofu
		G	Eggs, potatoes, mushrooms, and pumpernickle bread
			Baked yukon gold potato, butter, and broccoli
	S		Steamed red potato and green beans
	S		Mashed yukon gold potatoes
	S		Squash or pumpkin w/ReVita
L			Rice, eggs, and mushrooms (potatoes)
L		G	Crab omelette and rice
L			Rice cooked in chicken broth
L			Saffron rice (Indian rice curry)
		G	Tofu lasagna and rice crackers
		G	Ravioli, manicotti, or tofu lasagna and rice, rye cracker, pumpernickle, or rye bread
	S		Pasta w/garlic and butter
	S		Pasta or rice and vegetables
			Spinach or artichoke pasta w/diced vegetables and pesto sauce
			Millet w/Re-Vita®
		G	Pro-Gain® and oatmeal
		G	Bagel, cream cheese, lox, chives, and scallions

Lymph

MID-MORNING OR MID-AFTERNOON SNACK:
(Optional) Fruit, vegetables, protein, grain, nuts, seeds, dairy.

SENSITIVE: No fruit or dairy for mid-morning snack.

L			Raw carrots, tomatoes, red bell peppers, or celery
L	S		Raw carrots
			Carrot juice
L			Avocado (pepper)
		G	Rice cake w/almond butter
L	S		Grapes, banana, or apple
		G	Pretzels or popcorn
L		G	Scone – any variety; fruit, fruit juice, or vitamin drink 15 min. later
		G	Ice cream w/coconut and almonds

LUNCH or DINNER:

L		G	Chicken and rice (tortilla)
L		G	Game hen or sole and rice
L		G	Turkey and croissant
		G	Buffalo, corn tortilla, goat cheese, and salsa
L			Tuna and rice or noodles
L	S		Sushi – fish and rice
L			Eggs and rice
		G	Eggs, potatoes, and English muffin
		G	Pasta, ricotta cheese, spices, and garlic bread
		G	Pasta, ricotta cheese, and peas
	S		Pasta w/pesto sauce
L		G	Spaghetti w/ground turkey, tomatoes, tomato paste, basil, garlic, and spices
L	S		Rice and lima beans or peas
			Red potato and Caesar salad
			Rice cake w/almond butter
	S		Split pea soup and rice
		G	Split pea soup and rye cracker
L			Beans, corn tortilla, avocado, and salsa
	S		Beans, corn tortilla, and brown or white basmati rice (salsa)
L			Vegetarian or black bean and rice burrito

DINNER:
6-8 p.m. Moderate-to-heavy, with grain, protein, dairy, nuts, seeds, legumes, and/or vegetables.

SENSITIVE: Moderate with grain, vegetables and/or legumes.

L			Chemical-free chicken, rice, and green beans or asparagus
L		G	Chemical-free chicken, potato, and green beans
		G	Chicken, potato salad, corn, and corn tortillas
L		G	Cornish game hen, rice, and peas
L			Cornish game hen w/rice and vegetables
		G	Turkey, gravy, rice stuffing, carrots, and cranberries
L			Turkey patty and broccoli (asparagus)
L		G	Duck, rice or barley, green beans, and/or asparagus
L		G	Pheasant, carrots, peas, and rice
L			Pheasant wild rice, and red lettuce salad
L		G	Rabbit and white rose potatoes (carrots, broccoli and onions)
L		G	Rack of lamb, new red potatoes, and asparagus
L		G	Veal Parmesan, carrots, and peas
		G	Veal, potato, and salad (white wine)
		G	Cheeseburger and carrots
L			Scallops, pasta, and peas
L			Mahi-mahi, halibut, cod, or salmon, and pasta w/olive oil
L			Halibut, artichoke pasta, and spinach
L			Sole, rice, and romaine lettuce w/lemon juice, olive oil, and garlic
		G	Tuna and noodles w/mushroom soup and peas or Swiss chard
L			Tuna w/brown rice and peas
	S		Pasta and peas (carrots)
		G	Fettucini or angel hair pasta w/alfredo sauce
L			Vegetable manicotti w/tomato sauce
L			Lentils and/or carrots, peas, or rice — any combination

Lymph

L G Almonds, green beans, and rice

G Flour tortilla, cheese, avocado, or sour cream

Flour tortilla, soy cheese, broccoli, and carrots

L Regular or blue corn tortilla, pinto beans, rice, and avocado

G Brown basmati rice, nori, and cheese

White rice, broccoli, peanuts, and water chestnuts

S Rice (green beans, and/or artichoke hearts, and/or miso soup)

L Rice, asparagus, broccoli, and/or peas

S Rice, asparagus, carrots, and peas

G Rice, cheese, and peas

S Rice or couscous and peas (butter)

Rice and vegetables w/fresh basil and raw tomato

G Rice, Swiss cheese, cooked zucchini, and onions

S Salad: carrots, cucumber, butter leaf or Romaine lettuce w/ranch dressing, and 3-bean salad

G Shark, rice and casserole: green beans, onions, Worcestershire sauce, cream of mushroom soup, and topped w/crispy onion rings

G Baked potato w/sour cream and butter

L S Steamed red potatoes and green beans

Potato and sauerkraut

L S Red potatoes, carrots, and peas

G Potatoes w/broccoli and Cheddar cheese (sour cream and/or butter)

L Red potatoes and plain yogurt

L Potatoes and eggs

L Bell peppers stuffed w/rice and tomato sauce

L Rice w/steamed squash – yellow, acorn, crookneck, or banana – green beans, white onion, and dill weed

L Stir-fry vegetables and basmati rice w/low sodium soy sauce

L S Lentils w/carrots, peas, or rice – any combination

G Beef stew: chemical-free beef, beef broth, red potatoes, carrots, celery, onions, and Worcestershire sauce

L G Indian curry soup: carrots, peas, and rice

S Vegetable soup: carrot, onion, red potato, cumin, coriander, pepper, and turmeric w/brown rice and raw cucumber

S Vegetable stew and corn bread

L G Split pea soup and corn muffin or sourdough bread

L S Lentil soup and rice cakes

G Vegetarian thin crust pizza w/cheese

EVENING SNACK:
(Optional) 9 p.m.-2 a.m. Sweets, fruit, vegetables, protein, grain, dairy, nuts and seeds.

S G Garlic bread w/butter

L Grapes, banana, or apple

L Popcorn (butter)

Cracker w/peanut butter

G Ice cream (chocolate syrup and nuts)

G Banana pudding

G Sour cream raisin pie

G Pumpkin pie w/whipped cream

G Brownie w/cream

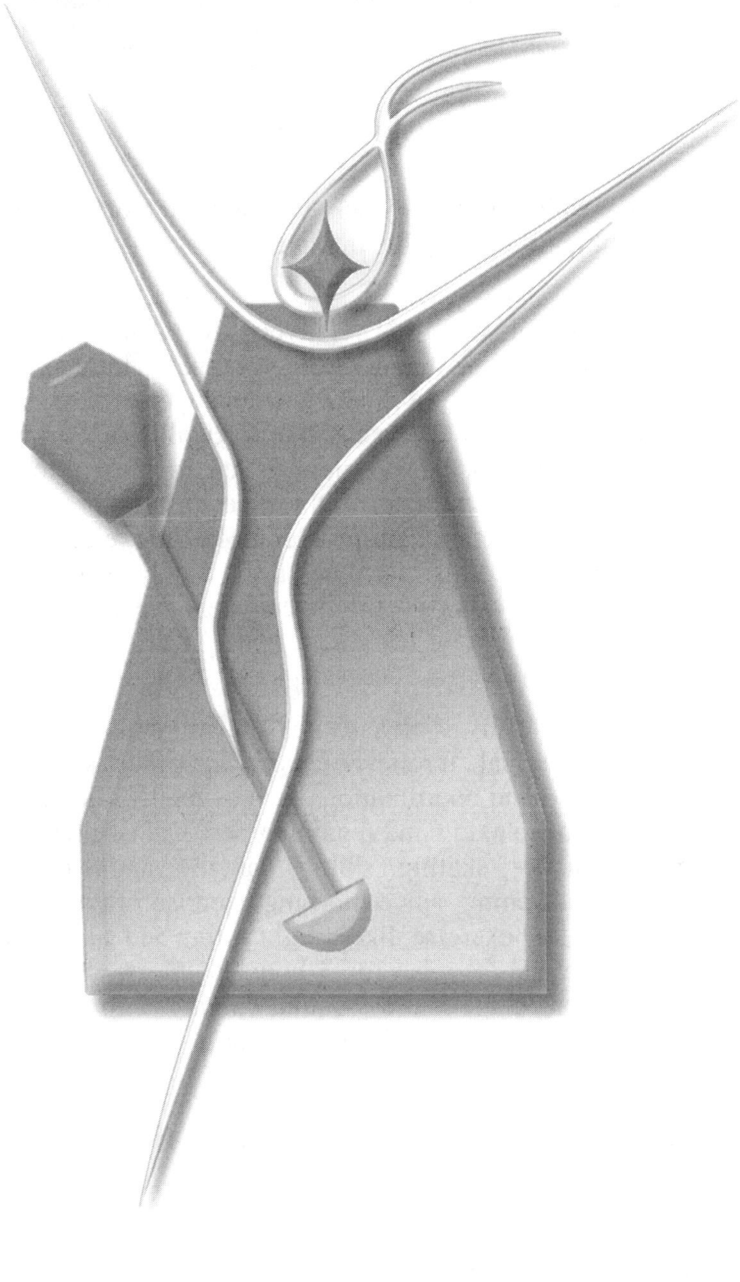

The "Medulla Body Type"
is symbolized by a metronome.
Steady and consistent, they will persevere,
unwavering in their activities and beliefs.
With an intense sense of responsibility,
they will remain loyal indefinitely
to a worthwhile cause.

MEDULLA

Medulla

BODY TYPE PROFILE

LOCATION	In brain stem between pons and spinal cord.
FUNCTION	Controls respiration and muscle function; area of brain that initiates muscle movement, putting thoughts into physical action.
POTENTIAL HEALTH PROBLEMS	Physically strong but tires relatively easily and requires adequate sleep. When energy is low, experiences weakness, fatigue, and lack of mental clarity. Tends to have high and low energy periods. Stiffness, muscle and joint problems, muscle spasms like torticollis or Parkinson-like condition. Eyes first indicator of problem. Sensitive to odors. Predisposed to environmental sensitivities. Digestive system problems, including food sensitivities, fat metabolism problems (leading, e.g., to psoriasis), and such complications as colitis. Face and neck may be prone to chronic acne, often with redness and lumps. Immune system weaknesses typical of sensitive system.
RECOMMENDED EXERCISE	Exercise is helpful, as it activates the immune system, but its benefit is primarily emotional. It relieves tension and moves stuck emotions. Activities requiring eye-hand coordination, such as tennis, racquetball, and volleyball. As a means of relaxing and regaining personal equilibrium, walking, biking, yoga, callanetics, skating, skiing, dancing, and stretching–particularly in afternoon or evening, since morning exercise often results in midafternoon fatigue. Regular exercise, like weight lifting and stairstepping, builds muscle mass. Sustained exercise for 3 hours or more, such as dancing, walking, hiking, backpacking, or cross-country skiing, 1 to 2 times per week, causes weight loss, as it acts to pull glucose out of muscles.

WOMEN'S CHARACTERISTICS

DISTINGUISHING FEATURES	Typically low forehead with heavy eyebrows, although can have high forehead. Hands may be large and broad, with rectangular or square palms and short, thick fingers, which sometimes have knobby knuckles. Easily build muscle mass with regular exercise, but require sustained exercise to lose weight. Steady, stable, and persistent. Generally known and appreciated for their perseverance.
ADDITIONAL PHYSICAL CHARACTERISTICS	Buttocks relatively flat-to-rounded. Low back curvature average. Breasts average. Waist straight-to-defined. Average to long-waisted. Shoulders relatively even with hips. Height average-to-tall. Bone structure small-to-medium. Average, elongated musculature. Feet average-to-wide. Hair average-to-thick. Face average oval, rectangular, or heart-shaped.

Medulla

WEIGHT GAIN AREAS

Lower body with initial gain in lower abdomen, entire upper 2/3rds of thighs including upper inner thighs, upper hips, waist, and middle back. Secondary weight gain in waist, entire abdomen and back, buttocks, upper arms, and face. Weight loss occurs first in face, then lower back.

DIETARY GUIDELINES

SCHEDULING MEALS

Breakfast: Moderate, with vegetables. May have protein, nuts, seeds, legumes, or grain if vegetables, even a few bites, are eaten first.

Lunch: Heavy, with protein, dairy, nuts, seeds, legumes, grain, vegetables, and/or fruit.

Dinner: Moderate, with vegetables, legumes, and/or grain.

Late dinner: (Optional) 9-11 p.m. Protein, nuts, seeds, dairy, legumes, vegetables, grain, fruit, and/or sweets.

DIETARY EMPHASIS

- Vegetables, especially at breakfast.
- For weight loss, eat from recommended food groups only at designated meals, limit fats to 20% of calories, and emphasize vegetables. May fast on apple juice and water up to 2 days per week, with walking or yoga to keep lymphatics moving. Working up a sweat for 3 hours or more activates weight loss.
- For weight gain, consume 20-30% of calories from dense protein, 35% from grains, and at least 15% from fats. Emphasize nuts, seeds, dairy (may include ice cream), and vegetables. Adhere to eating schedules for recommended food groups.
- Vegetarian diet recommended unless depleted or underweight, although up to 30% of calories may consist of dense protein.
- Fats, 15-20% of caloric intake, from dense protein (chicken, turkey, cornish game hen), and/or nuts; to increase fat intake to 20-30%, add to the above butter, ghee, kefir, yogurt, and cheese (including sheep cheese).

KEY SUPPORTS FOR SYSTEM

Vegetables at every meal, especially at breakfast, and eating at appropriate times. Green beans, celery, greens, peas, and soups. Rotation important.

Blue-green algae is good source of protein. Fruit, 2 pieces per day, will often keep bowels regular.

COMPLEMENTARY GLANDULAR SUPPORT

Intestines through consuming legumes, including such starchy vegetables as peas and green beans. Brain, by connecting feelings with intellect through physically nurturing self.

Medulla

FOODS CRAVED	*(When Energy is Low)* Fats, sweets, and carbohydrate such as pastries, cookies, cake, donuts, breads, crackers, ice cream, cheese, and fruit juices; alcohol.
FOODS TO AVOID	Strawberries, artificial sweeteners (including Equal® and Sweet'n Low®), margarine, whole wheat, skim milk, and chocolate.
RECOMMENDED CUISINE	Home-style cooking (e.g., fish, vegetables, meat, and potatoes), Continental; Thai, Chinese, Japanese, Vietnamese; Mexican – moderately.

PSYCHOLOGICAL PROFILE

ESSENCE

Just as the medulla or brain stem is responsible for controlling respiration and heart rate, functions that require steady perseverance, Medulla body types are known for their consistency and persistence. Undaunted by time or trends, Medulla types are unwavering in their activities and beliefs, staying with what they choose to be doing with unusual resolve. With an abundance of patience, Medullas possess an intense sense of responsibility and remain loyal indefinitely, especially when they have identified with the group or cause. It's their high sense of responsibility that makes them patient teachers, and the appreciation of their students, patients, or clients makes it all worthwhile.

CHARACTERISTIC TRAITS

Medullas are characteristically steady, stable, and persistent. They love structure, order, consistency and stability. Highly responsible, once they have committed to something they will generally follow through, keeping their promises and agreements. Loyal, patient and tenacious, they typically won't quit until the job is finished, particularly when it's for someone else.

Endowed with strong, inquiring minds, Medulla types are drawn to things that appeal to their creativity. While open to new ideas and philosophies, they are typically cautious about getting into new situations. Conscientious, conservative and generally conventional, they like to study subjects in depth, applying what they own and what they know to be true. Feeling more secure, they may at times swing to the opposite extreme of "flying by the seat of their pants."

Medulla types can readily build muscle mass. Since the function of the medulla gland is to control muscle activity, regular exercise acts as a stimulant. The medulla gland is the portion of the brain that links the brain to the body, or the mental to the physical. When this connection is sound, the result is balance, flexibility, and integration in thought and action. However, if the energy stays in the head and is not directed down into the body, there is a tendency to become physically lethargic or fatigued and psychologically stiff and rigid.

Medulla

Medullas possess a sensitivity that is expressed in their responsiveness to others or protected with a hard exterior. Tending to fall into one of two extremes, they will either be quite sensitive to people around them or closed and self-centered. Until their sensitivity has been fully integrated, they will protect it with a hardness that can vary from situation to situation. They may portray a soft exterior with a hard interior just waiting to surface or a hard exterior with a soft interior once the original barrier has been crossed. For men in particularly, the hard exterior is often expressed in the work place or around other male friends. When sensitive to people, Medullas have strong nurturing and/or healing qualities coupled with a depth of caring and compassion. Kind, gentle and helpful, they are altruistic, with a strong desire to help people individually and the human race in general.

MOTIVATION

Medullas generally start life with a strong physical energy that needs to be channeled. When it isn't, it reverses and illnesses or environmental sensitivities manifest. While their physical body is still strong, they are able to handle working long hours, smoking and alcohol. They are able to drive themselves, particularly with work. Because their bodies are basically strong, when they are stressed they go into overdrive and become hyper, resulting in a surplus of nervous energy. This can causes them to become scattered and run around in circles, expending energy without focus.

While physically strong, Medullas possess an inherent sensitivity that makes them especially sensitive to chemicals, antibiotics and pollutants. Many experience chronic health problems of a degenerative nature or environmental sensitivities after a period of prolonged chemical exposure or physical trauma. Typical examples are: chemical exposure as in a hairdresser using bleaches, dyes, etc.; digestive assault like intestinal parasites or food poisoning; or physical trauma like a whiplash type of injury. The neck tends to be a particularly vulnerable area, with stiffness, rigidity and muscle aching, followed by chronic illness or diseases that involve muscle rigidity, such as Parkinson-like muscle spasms.

Being sensitive to their environment, there is a need to control it to protect themselves. Control usually takes the form of mental exactness, wanting to know everything about an area before stepping into it. Being too detail-oriented can cause Medullas to become too rigid in their thought process and narrow-minded, afraid to step out into the world and let life take them where they need to go. Mental rigidity can lead to indecisiveness causing a disorganization that prevents them from getting anything done or bringing things to completion.

Change triggers old fears and feelings of inadequacy. Fear of failure or lack of acceptance is the main impetus for change, so there is a tendency to avoid it at all costs. With the security of structure and stability being so strong, change is difficult. It usually only occurs after all the options on the current path have been exhausted. If Medullas can't find a way of implementing change, life's challenges cause them to give up, accept defeat and become impotent – physically unable to move forward in life.

Medulla

"AT WORST"

Medullas can become too stiff and rigid. Insisting on being too precise, they can belabor a point, insisting that things be done a certain way. They can become narrow-minded and controlling by being too cautious and exacting. Afraid to make a move, they limit themselves and those around them, resulting in a lack of growth, spontaneity, and movement. It's easy for them to become too serious or too intense, restricting freedom and expansion. By being too cautious, they become hard, heavy, and boring. By being too analytical, they take the fun out of life. Medullas can be demanding, abrasive and authoritarian when trying to get things done or get things to work their way. This inflexibility can manifest as obsessiveness in behavior or relationships, and lead to food or substance addiction. When Medullas are stuck in their development, their sensitivity can be directed inward, causing them to overfocus on their own desires, and become self-centered and demanding. By being too dependent on structure and stability, Medullas resist change, staying too long in circumstances that are clearly draining or detrimental.

Armored and controlling, they can be skeptical and pessimistic about everything new. Intellectually exacting, it's easy for them to rationalize their skepticism. Prone to indecisiveness and disorganization, Medulla types can find it almost impossible to get anything done. They can get caught up in their fears and beliefs, causing them to frantically keep plugging dikes rather than addressing real issues, or otherwise manifest some form of impulsive or self-defeating behavior.

Medullas will be overly responsible for someone else, but fail to take personal responsibility for their own destinies. They will consciously or unconsciously manipulate others to take over for them. By not truly knowing themselves, they get caught in appearances, looking to the outside world for approval or to take care of them and tell them what is accepted. In an attempt to gain appreciation and acceptance, they try to fix things and others. By trying too hard to please others, Medullas push themselves too hard, neglecting their own needs and emotional welfare.

"AT BEST"

Steady, persistent, and imaginative, when Medullas are able to successfully integrate their mental capability with their physical energy, they can accomplish almost anything. Accomplishing their goals in life is relatively easy when their self-confidence has been developed to the point of letting go of their need to control. Their love of structure, order, consistency, and stability provides Medullas with the ability to be highly successful in both the business and professional worlds.

Medullas are naturally consistent, responsible and loyal. With their high level of perseverance and mental acuity, they can master any subject that peaks their interest. Patient, caring and committed, they will "go the extra mile" and methodically stay with a person until the student fully understands the subject, making them excellent teachers. Having connected with their own

Medulla

"AT BEST"
(Continued)

intuitive process, they have a great deal of insight and perception, which allows them to see the value in leading technology or interpersonal work. Not only do they have the ability to "understand things differently" or figure things out through other than the accepted channels, they are able to take the information and bring it or teach it to others.

Committed to excellence, Medullas are thorough and willing to do whatever it takes to do things right. Sensitive, caring, and committed, Medullas take their relationships seriously and will do what is in the highest and best interest for everyone. Willing to learn, they'll explore new areas and embrace change that reflects forward movement, integrating it into established structure.

Having integrated their emotional and spiritual or intuitive sides with their strong physical and mental aspects, Medullas are in step with life, changing and flowing with it, allowing it to change them. Flexible and self-confident, Medullas are self-reliant, validating and appreciating themselves, they excel in thought and action. Kind, gentle, helpful and compassionate, they effectively express their altruistic nature, helping people individually and the human race in general.

Medulla

FOOD LISTS

HEALTHY FOOD LIST

FREQUENTLY FOODS	3-7 meals a week – refers to each food, rather than category.
DENSE PROTEIN	Beef broth, buffalo, veal, pork, bacon, ham, sausage; chemical-free turkey or chicken, chicken broth; anchovy, bass, cod, flounder, halibut, herring, mackerel, mahi-mahi, perch, roughy, salmon, sardines, shark, red snapper, sole, swordfish, trout, tuna; calamari (squid), clams, crab, eel, lobster, mussels, octopus, oysters, scallops
DAIRY	Kefir (peach, apricot)
CHEESE	Blue, extra sharp Cheddar
NUTS and SEEDS	Almonds, cashew butter, coconuts, pine nuts, sesame seed butter, raw sunflower seeds
GRAINS	Corn tortillas, rice (white basmati, Japanese), rye, pasta, couscous
VEGETABLES	Carrots, cauliflower, celery, red chard, collard greens, green beans, acorn squash, yams
VEGETABLE JUICE	Carrot
FRUITS	Lemons, pears, persimmons, plums (black, purple, red), pomegranates, rhubarb, tangelos, tangerines, raisins
VEGETABLE OIL	Olive
SWEETENERS	Molasses, sorghum, Re-Vita®, stevia
SALAD DRESSINGS	Balsamic vinegar and olive oil
BEVERAGES	Herbal tea
MODERATELY FOODS	1-2 meals a week – refers to each food, rather than category.
DENSE PROTEIN	Beef, beef liver, lamb, venison, organ meats (heart, brain) wild game; Foster Farms® or Zacky® turkey or chicken, chicken livers, cornish game hen, duck; bonita, catfish, haddock; abalone, shrimp; eggs
DAIRY	Milk (2%, low fat, whole, raw), goat milk, buttermilk, half & half, sweet cream, sour cream, yogurt (plain or flavored), frozen yogurt, ice cream (Dreyer's, Ben & Jerry's®, Swensen's®), butter
CHEESE	American, brie, Camembert, Cheddar, Colby, cottage, cream, Edam, feta, goat, Gouda, Jack, kefir, Limburger, mozzarella, Muenster, Parmesan, ricotta, Romano, Swiss
NUTS and SEEDS	Almond butter, Brazils, cashews, water chestnuts, filberts, hazelnuts, macadamias, macadamia butter, peanuts, peanut butter, pecans, pistachios, walnuts (black, English), raw or roasted seeds (caraway, pumpkin, sesame), roasted sunflower seeds, sunflower seed butter

Medulla

LEGUMES	Beans (adzuki, black, garbanzo, kidney, lima [butter], navy, great northern, pinto, red, soy), lentils, split peas, black-eyed peas, hummus, miso, soy milk, tofu
GRAINS	Amaranth, barley, buckwheat, corn, corn bread, corn grits, hominy grits, millet, oats, popcorn, quinoa, rice (brown basmati, long or short grain brown, wild, polished), rice cakes, rice bran, triticale, wheat bran, wheat germ, sprouted wheat, refined wheat flour, flour tortillas, breads (French, Italian, corn, oat, corn/rye, rye, garlic, rice, multi-grain, sprouted grain, white, pumpernickel, sourdough), bagels, croissants, English muffins, crackers (saltines, oat, rye), udon noodles, rice noodles, cream of rice, cream of rye, cream of wheat
VEGETABLES	Artichokes, arugula, asparagus, avocados, bamboo shoots, lima beans, yellow wax beans, beets, bok choy, broccoli, broccoflower, brussels sprouts, cabbage (green, napa, red), chard, cilantro, corn, cucumbers, eggplant, garlic, greens (beet, mustard, turnip), jicama, kale, kohlrabi, leeks, lettuce (Boston, butter, endive, iceberg, red leaf, romaine), mushrooms, okra, olives (green, ripe), onions (chives, green, brown, red, white, yellow, vidalia), parsley, parsnips, peas, snow peas, bell peppers (green, red, yellow), chili peppers, pimentos, potatoes (red, russet, white rose, yukon gold), pumpkin, radishes, daikon radishes, rutabaga, seaweed (arame, dulse, kelp, nori, wakame), sauerkraut, shallots, spinach, sprouts (alfalfa, clover, mung bean, radish, sunflower), squash (banana, butternut), tomatoes, turnips, watercress
VEGETABLE JUICES	Carrot/celery, celery, spinach, parsley, lettuce, beet, tomato, V-8®
FRUITS	Apples (Red or Golden Delicious, Granny Smith, Jonathan, McIntosh, Pippin, Rome Beauty), apricots, bananas, blackberries, cranberries, gooseberries, raspberries, cherries, grapes (black, green, red), grapefruits (red, white), guavas, kiwi, kumquats, limes, loquats, mangos, melons (cantaloupe, crenshaw, honeydew, watermelon), nectarines, oranges, papayas, peaches, pineapples, dates, figs, prunes
FRUIT JUICES	Apple, apple cider, apple/apricot, apricot, black cherry, red cherry, cranapple, cranberry, grape (red, purple, white), guava, grapefruit, lemon, orange, papaya, pear, pineapple, pineapple/coconut, prune, tangerine, watermelon
VEGETABLE OILS	All-blend, almond, avocado, canola, coconut, corn, flaxseed, peanut, safflower, sesame, soy, sunflower
SWEETENERS	Honey, brown sugar, date sugar, raw sugar, refined cane sugar, maple syrup, brown rice syrup, barley malt syrup, corn syrup, fructose, succonant, saccharin
CONDIMENTS	Catsup, mustard, horseradish, mayonnaise, barbecue sauce, pesto sauce, soy sauce, salsa, tahini, vinegar, salt, sea salt, Vege-Sal®
SALAD DRESSINGS	Blue cheese, French, ranch, creamy Italian, creamy avocado, thousand island, lemon juice and oil

Medulla

DESSERTS	Custards, tapioca, puddings, pies, cakes, orange or raspberry sherbet
CHIPS	Bean, corn (blue, white, yellow), potato
BEVERAGES	Coffee; black tea, green tea, Japanese tea, Chinese oolong tea; mineral water, sparkling water; wine (red, white), sake, beer, barley malt liquor, champagne, gin, Scotch, vodka, whiskey; root beer, regular sodas
RARELY FOODS	No more than once a month
DENSE PROTEIN	Chemical-fed turkey or chicken
DAIRY	Nonfat milk, most ice creams
GRAINS	Whole wheat, whole wheat bread, 7-grain bread, whole wheat crackers
VEGETABLES	Sweet potatoes, squash (spaghetti, yellow [summer], zucchini)
FRUITS	Blueberries, boysenberries, strawberries, casaba melons
SWEETENERS	Aspertame, Equal®, Sweet'n Low®, NutraSweet®
CONDIMENTS	Margarine
DESSERTS	Chocolate, desserts containing chocolate
BEVERAGES	Diet sodas

SENSITIVE FOOD LIST

FREQUENTLY FOODS	3-7 meals a week – refers to each food, rather than category.
DENSE PROTEIN	Chemical-free chicken or turkey, chicken broth
GRAINS	White basmati rice, couscous, pasta (durum, semolina)
NUTS	Coconuts (fresh, milk)
FRUITS	Lemons
BEVERAGES	Herbal teas (Yogi®, Dr. Chang®)
MODERATELY FOODS	1-2 meals a week – refers to each food, rather than category.
DENSE PROTEIN	Beef, beef broth, buffalo, lamb, beef liver, pork, bacon, ham, sausage, venison, veal, organ meats (heart, brain); Foster Farms® or Zacky® turkey or chicken, chicken broth, chicken livers, duck, cornish game hen; anchovy, bass, bonita, cod, flounder, haddock, halibut, herring, mackerel, mahi-mahi, perch, roughy, salmon, sardines, shark, red snapper, sole, spelt, swordfish, trout, tuna; abalone, calamari (squid), clams, crab, eel, lobster, mussels, octopus, oysters, scallops, shrimp; eggs
DAIRY	Milk (whole, 2%, low fat, raw), goat milk, buttermilk, half & half, acidophilus, bifidus, sweet cream, sour cream, kefir (peach, apricot), plain yogurt, frozen yogurt

Medulla

CHEESE	American, blue, brie, Camembert, Cheddar, Colby, cottage, cream, Edam, feta, goat, Gouda, Jack, kefir, Limburger, mozzarella, Muenster, Parmesan, ricotta, Romano, Swiss
NUTS and SEEDS	Almonds, almond butter, Brazils, cashews, cashew butter, water chestnuts, filberts, hazelnuts, macadamias, macadamia butter, peanuts, peanut butter, pecans, pine nuts, pistachios, walnuts (black, English), seeds (caraway, pumpkin, sesame, roasted sunflower) sesame seed butter, sunflower seed butter
LEGUMES	Beans (adzuki, black, garbanzo, kidney, lima [butter], navy, great northern, pinto, red, soy), lentils, split peas, black-eyed peas, hummus, miso, soy milk, tofu
GRAINS	Amaranth, buckwheat, corn, corn bread, corn grits, corn tortillas, hominy grits, kamut, millet, oats, popcorn, quinoa, rice (brown basmati, long or short grain brown, Japanese, wild), rice bran, rice cakes, rye, triticale, whole wheat, wheat bran, wheat germ, refined wheat flour, flour tortillas, breads (French, Italian, sourdough, garlic, oat, corn, corn/rye, rye, rice, pumpernickel, white), bagels, croissants, English muffins, crackers (saltines, oat, rye), udon noodles, rice noodles, cream of rice, cream of rye, cream of wheat
VEGETABLES	Artichokes, asparagus, avocados, bamboo shoots, green beans, yellow wax beans, lima beans, beets, bok choy, broccoli, broccoflower, brussels sprouts, cabbage (green, napa, red), carrots, celery, chard, cilantro, cucumbers, corn, eggplant, garlic, greens (beet, collard, mustard, turnip), jicama, kale, kohlrabi, leeks, lettuce (Boston, butter, red leaf, endive, iceberg, romaine), mushrooms, okra, olives (green, ripe), onions (chives, green, brown, red, white, yellow, vidalia), parsley, parsnips, peas, snow pea pods, bell peppers (green, red, yellow), chili peppers, pimentos, potatoes (red, white rose, russet, yukon gold), pumpkin, radishes, daikon radishes, rutabaga, sauerkraut, seaweed (arame, dulse, kelp, nori, wakame), spinach, shallots, sprouts (alfalfa, clover, mung bean, radish, sunflower, squash (acorn, banana, butternut), tomatoes, turnips, yams
VEGETABLE JUICES	Celery, carrot, carrot/celery, parsley, spinach, tomato, V-8®
FRUITS	Apples (Red or Golden Delicious, Granny Smith, Jonathan, McIntosh, Pippin, Rome Beauty), apricots, bananas, blackberries, cranberries, gooseberries, raspberries, cherries, grapes (black, green, red), grapefruit, (white, red), guavas, kiwi, kumquats, limes, loquats, mangos, melons (cantaloupe, crenshaw, honeydew, watermelon), nectarines, unsprayed oranges, papayas, peaches, pears, persimmons, pineapples, plums (black, purple, red), pomegranates, rhubarb, tangelos, tangerines, dates, figs, prunes, raisins
FRUIT JUICES	Apple, apple cider, apple/apricot, apricot, black cherry, red cherry, cranapple, cranberry, grape (red, white, purple), grapefruit, guava, lemon, orange, pear, papaya, pineapple, pineapple/coconut, prune, tangerine, watermelon
VEGETABLE OILS	All-blend, avocado, coconut

Medulla

SWEETENERS	Re-Vita®, stevia
CONDIMENTS	Salsa, tahini, salt, sea salt, Vege-Sal®, ginger
SALAD DRESSINGS	Balsamic vinegar and olive oil, lemon juice and oil
BEVERAGES	Japanese tea, Chinese oolong tea; mineral water, sparkling water
RARELY FOODS	No more than once a month
DENSE PROTEIN	Catfish, chemical-fed turkey or chicken
DAIRY	Nonfat milk, kefir (blueberry, raspberry, strawberry), flavored yogurt, ice cream
GRAINS	Barley, rice (instant, polished), whole wheat, breads (multi-grain, 7-grain, sprouted grain, whole wheat), whole wheat crackers
VEGETABLES	Arugula, cauliflower, sweet potatoes, squash (spaghetti, yellow [summer], zucchini), watercress
FRUITS	Boysenberries, blueberries, strawberries, sprayed oranges, casaba melons
VEGETABLE OILS	Almond, canola, corn, flaxseed, olive, peanut, safflower, sesame, soy, sunflower
SWEETENERS	Honey, molasses, sorghum, refined cane sugar, brown sugar, date sugar, raw sugar, maple syrup, barley malt syrup, corn syrup, brown rice syrup, fructose, succonant, saccharin, aspertame, Equal®, Sweet'n Low®, NutraSweet®
CONDIMENTS	Catsup, mustard, horseradish, barbecue sauce, pesto sauce, soy sauce, mayonnaise, margarine, yeast, vinegar
SALAD DRESSINGS	Blue cheese, French, ranch, creamy Italian, creamy avocado, thousand island
DESSERTS	Custards, tapioca, puddings, pies, cakes, orange or raspberry sherbert, chocolate, desserts containing chocolate
CHIPS	Bean, corn (blue, white, yellow), potato
BEVERAGES	Coffee; black tea; wine (red, white), sake, beer, barley malt liquor, champagne, gin, Scotch, vodka, whiskey; root beer, diet sodas, regular sodas

FREQUENCY

When the body is extremely sensitive, even the number of times a food is eaten within a food group needs to be limited.

Beans as a group – 2 x/week	Cheeses – 1 x/week
Grains as a group – 3 x/week	Oils – 2 x/week
Potatoes as a group – 2 x/week	Sauces – 2 x/week
Carrots for breakfast – 4 x/week	Butter – 1 tsp 2 x/week
Beets for breakfast – 3 x/week	Fruit juices – unlimited. Rotate.

Nonfat frozen yogurt or dates after a restaurant or difficult meal aids digestion.

Medulla

MENUS

DIETARY EMPHASIS:

- Vegetables at every meal – especially breakfast – particularly green beans, celery, greens, peas, and soups.
- Follow food and time schedule.
- Rotation important.
- Fruit often helps regulate bowels. Green beans and peas strengthen intestines.

WEIGHT LOSS:

- Eat from recommended food groups only at designated meals.
- Limit fats to 20% of calories.
- Emphasize vegetables.
- May fast on apple juice and water up to 2 days per week, with walking or yoga to keep lymphatics moving.
- Working up a sweat for 3 hours or more activates weight loss.

WEIGHT GAIN:

- Consume 20-30% of calories from dense protein, 35% from grains, and at least 15% from fats.
- Emphasize nuts, seeds, dairy (may include ice cream), and vegetables.
- Adhere to eating schedules for recommended food groups.

VEGETARIAN DIET:

- Recommended when healthy, although up to 30% of calories may consist of dense protein.

FATS:

- 15-20% of caloric intake.
- Best sources are dense protein (chicken, turkey, cornish game hen), and/or nuts.
- To increase fat intake to 20%-30%, add butter, ghee, kefir, yogurt, and cheese (including sheep cheese).

KEY

—all menus may be used by healthy persons

( ) around foods means that they're optional

L denotes weight loss menus

S denotes sensitive menus

G denotes weight gain menus

BREAKFAST:
7-9 a.m. Moderate, with vegetables: May have potatoes 5 meals/week, carrots or carrot juice 7 meals/week. May have protein, nuts, seeds, legumes, or grain if vegetables, even a few bites, are eaten first.

		G	Avocado – then oatmeal
			Cucumber, carrots, carrot juice, or V-8® juice, and pancakes
		G	Broccoli or carrots – raw or steamed (chicken and/or rice)
L			Raw or steamed broccoli (carrots)
L	S		Raw or cooked carrots, peas, or green beans
		G	Raw carrot, millet, and Ezekiel bread
		G	Carrots or beets, Ezekiel bread, and millet w/chicken broth, raisins, wheat germ, sunflower seeds, and blanched almonds
			Carrots, broccoli, beets, and millet (bread)
L	S		Steamed artichoke
L	S		Green beans, then rice
		G	Mung beans and eggs
L			Mixed vegetables: peas, carrots, and corn
L	S		Yam (green peas)
		G	Potatoes, eggs, and bread
	S		Russet baked potato w/chicken broth
L			Boiled potato or hash browns and Raisin Bran® w/low fat or 2% milk
			Potato salad (sourdough toast)
L	S		Baked potato, yam, or acorn squash w/butter
			Hash browns (eggs and/or turkey)

Medulla

L			Spinach and eggs
L			Carrots – raw or steamed (eggs or chicken)
			Carrots and sourdough toast
			Carrots, Cheerios®, honey, and milk
L	S		Carrot juice, then peas and broccoli
L	S		Carrot juice, then oatmeal
L	S		Carrot and chard juice (oatmeal)
	S		Carrot and kale juice (buckwheat groats)
L	S		Celery and romaine lettuce juice, then lima beans
L	S		Celery and romaine lettuce juice (beets)
L	S		Celery, parsley, and carrot juice (rice)
			V-8® or carrot juice (sourdough toast)
	S		Tomato juice, then lima beans and green beans
		G	Kale soup: kale, water, beans, vegetables, rice, and spaghetti (pancakes, eggs, or cereal)
L			Potato soup
		G	Beef vegetable soup
L			Vegetable soup

MIDMORNING SNACK:

(Optional) Fruit.

Red Delicious apple

LUNCH:
10:30 a.m.-3 p.m. Heavy, with protein, dairy, nuts, seeds, legumes, grain, vegetables, and/or fruit.

L		G	Salmon, rice, and cauliflower (butter)
	S		Salmon w/plain yogurt (raw tomatoes)
L	S	G	Salmon or swordfish and rice (peas)
L	S	G	Swordfish (garlic and/or green beans)
L			Red snapper and broccoli (raw purple cabbage)
L			Tuna and rice (corn)
L	S		Mussels (rice, and/or butter, and/or kale)
L	S	G	Calamari or scallops and pasta (butter)
L	S		Oysters and pasta (collard greens)
L	S	G	Shrimp, pasta, and peas (butter)
	S	G	Spaghetti w/meat balls (garlic toast)
L	S	G	Pork chops and raw or cooked spinach
L	S	G	Beef and green beans or mustard greens
L		G	Steak and tomatoes (potato or rice)
		G	Steak, potato, and gravy (green beans)
L	S		Corned beef and cabbage
	S	G	Corned beef on rye (sauerkraut)
		G	Roast beef and avocado sandwich
		G	Ham sandwich on sourdough and carrots
	S		Chicken enchiladas
		G	Lasagna (garlic bread and/or salad)
L	S		Liver and onions w/mustard greens, beet greens, or kale
L	S	G	Chicken, rice, and broccoli
L		G	Chicken, rice, and green beans, carrots, or broccoli
			Chicken chow mein (rice or egg roll)
	S	G	Almond chicken w/Chinese rice
L	S	G	Cornish game hen, rice, and asparagus
L		G	Cornish game hen and rice (spinach, kale, or mustard greens)
L			Turkey and broccoli
		G	Turkey and rice, pasta, or couscous (broccoli, carrots, and onions)
L			Eggs and spinach
L	S		Boiled or scrambled egg and potato
		G	Eggs, brown rice, and refried beans
L		G	Eggs and rice (turkey)
		G	Eggs, potatoes, and bread
	S	G	Potato, cottage cheese, and butter, then apple
			Tofu, vegetable, and rice
		G	Cheese, tortilla, and tomato or corn
L	S	G	Beans, corn tortilla, and avocado
L	S		Pinto beans, white basmati rice (plain yogurt)
		G	Chili and cheese (crackers and/or salsa)
L	S		Vegetable beef soup and mushrooms
L			Miso soup w/broccoli, carrots, or squash
L	S		Adzuki beans and rice
	S		Rye bread and cucumbers

Medulla

MIDAFTERNOON SNACK:
(Optional) 3-5 p.m. Fruit, seeds, nuts, dairy, vegetables, grain.

S G Cheese and celery

G Vanilla yogurt w/pecans

L Red Delicious apple (raisins and blanched almonds)

G Raw or roasted almonds or raw sunflower seeds

Popcorn (cheese)

G Cinnamon raisin bagel (cream cheese)

DINNER:
6-8 p.m. Moderate, with vegetables, legumes, and/or grain. May have pasta 4 times a week.

L S Salad: romaine lettuce, green onions, celery, and peas w/Hain™ Creamy Avocado dressing

Caesar salad

L G Broccoli and rice, pasta, or mashed potato

L Miso soup w/broccoli, carrots, or squash

S G Adzuki beans and rice

S Rye bread and cucumbers

L S G Broccoli and rice

L G Carrots, peas, and rice or pasta

G Corn tortilla, beans, avocado, and butter

L S Brown basmati rice and string beans

G Basmati rice w/Bragg™ aminos and steamed green beans

L G Basmati rice and mung bean sprouts

L G Rice or pasta (butter, broccoli, carrots, eggplant, and/or tomato sauce)

L Couscous, carrots, green beans, and Bragg™ aminos

L G Pasta with peas or tomato sauce

L S Vegetable soup

L S Soup: russet or red potatoes, celery, mustard greens, kale, carrots, olive oil, and sea salt, boiled in water

L G Soup: split peas, carrots, and onions in chicken broth

L G Soup: carrots, onions, broccoli, and barley in chicken broth

L G Pinto beans, rice, and/or corn tortilla

S G Corn bread and pinto, lima, navy, kidney, or red beans

L S Yams and peas (butter)

L Yukon gold potato and green beans

G Baked potato (butter, sour cream, and/or sprouts)

L S White rose potato (raw or steamed spinach)

S Russet potato (butter)

L Pumpernickel toast and carrot, celery, or raw broccoli

S Popcorn

EVENING SNACK
(Optional) 1 hour after dinner. Fruit.

S Banana

S Coor's® beer

BEDTIME SNACK or LATE DINNER: (Optional) 9-11 p.m. Protein, nuts, seeds, dairy, legumes, vegetables, grain, fruit, sweets.

S G Kefir – plain, cherry, or peach

G Yogurt – plain, cherry, peach, or apple

S G Banana and plain yogurt

S G Ice cream (Dryer's, Ben & Jerry's,® or Swensen's®)

L S Berry Re-Vita® in cranberry concentrate w/water

S Dates

S Orange

G Cinnamon rolls

G Oatmeal raisin cookies

L Popcorn

Pizza

LARGE MEAL MAY BE EATEN IF DESIRED

L S Steamed butternut squash and apples

G Steak (potato and or carrots)

Fish and rice

G Chili w/beans (meat sauce and/or salsa)

L G Chicken, potato or rice, and broccoli

NERVOUS SYSTEM

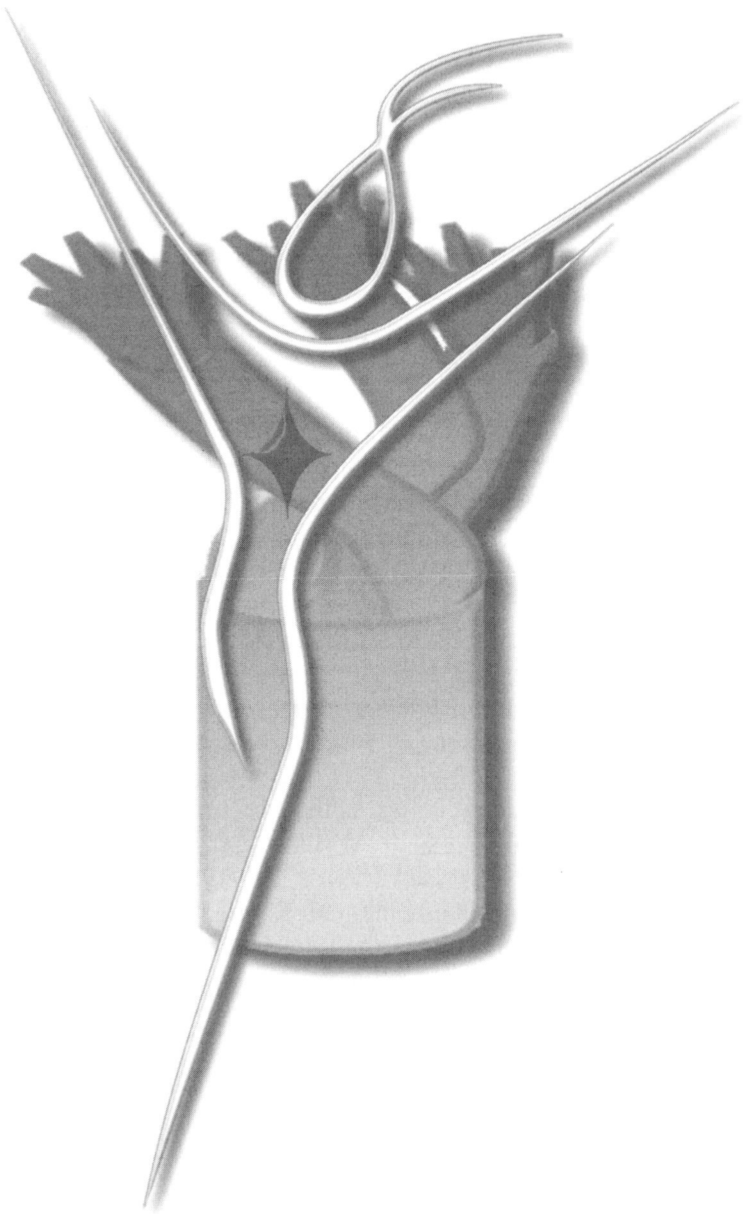

The "Nervous System Body Type" is symbolized by wires. Nerves are the "wires" that connect all parts of the body and keep the brain informed. Practical and efficient, they are happiest when connecting with people and ideas.

Nervous System

BODY TYPE PROFILE

LOCATION	Brain, spinal cord, and all nerves.
FUNCTION	Communication network – conveys nerve impulses from one part of body to another.
POTENTIAL HEALTH PROBLEMS	High energy, with good stamina and drive; good physical and mental integration. Generally have strong, solid physical bodies, so problems are frequently structural and injury related. May be prone to fluid retention, especially in legs, calves, and thighs. Digestive distress, constipation, bloating, and menstrual problems – including difficulty with conception, often related to emotional stress. Sensitive to emotions (can be "emotional sponges"), so will often build hard exterior for survival. Highly susceptible to anxiety and nervous tension, frequently triggered by frustration or unresolved stress. Memory loss and depression may follow.
RECOMMENDED EXERCISE	Exercise is essential, as it activates the immune system. It is also effective in releasing emotional stress. At least 20 minutes every other day is recommended. Best exercise varies as life-style changes. Common activities include all over body movement, such as yoga or swimming; aerobic activity, such as running, biking, racquetball, or dance. Need interaction with people, so any exercise meeting this criteria is supportive.

WOMEN'S CHARACTERISTICS

DISTINGUISHING FEATURES	Integrated, strong, solid body. Generally, quite verbal with good integration and common sense. Enjoy introducing and connecting people. High energy, excellent stamina and determination. Practical and efficient, they are known for accomplishing what they set out to do.
ADDITIONAL PHYSICAL CHARACTERISTICS	Buttocks relatively flat-to-rounded. Low back curvature average-to-swayed. Breasts average. Shoulders relatively even with hips. Waist straight-to-defined. Average to long-waisted. Height petite to very tall. Bone structure small-to-medium. Average, elongated musculature. Broad, square, or proportional hands and feet. High forehead. Average-to-large head with long, oval, or rectangular face, which often comes forward at the chin. Frequently have square or firm jaw, indicative of strong determination.

Nervous System

WEIGHT GAIN AREAS	Lower body with initial gain in lower abdomen, entire upper 2/3rds of thighs, including upper inner thighs, upper hips, middle back, and waist, or all over. Secondary gain extending into entire abdomen, entire back, upper arms, buttocks, thighs, breasts, face, and under chin. Capable of putting on and losing large amounts of weight, or may have difficulty gaining weight.

DIETARY GUIDELINES

SCHEDULING MEALS:

"HEALTHY"

Breakfast: Heavy, with protein, nuts, seeds, dairy, legumes, grain, vegetables, and/or fruit.

Lunch: Light-to-moderate, with grain, legumes, dairy, nuts, seeds, raw vegetables, and/or fruit.

Dinner: Moderate-to-heavy, with protein, nuts, seeds, dairy, legumes, cooked or steamed vegetables, and/or grain.

"SENSITIVE"

Breakfast: Light, with fruit.

Lunch: Heavy, with protein, nuts, seeds, dairy, legumes, grain, steamed vegetables (may also be raw for weight loss), and (occasionally) fruit.

Dinner: Moderate, with protein, dairy, legumes, raw vegetables, and (occasionally) nuts and seeds.

DIETARY EMPHASIS

- For weight loss, consume 20-30% of calories from dense protein. Consume 20-25% of calories from fats. Will gain weight if below 15%. Follow Sensitive meal schedule. Eat majority of food by 2 p.m.
- For weight gain, consume 30% of calories from dense protein and 30% from fats. Follow Healthy meal schedule and eat four equally spaced meals per day.
- For rebuilding the body, follow Healthy or Weight Gain meal schedule with heavy breakfast, Weight Loss schedule with heavy lunch and moderate dinner.
- Vegetarian diets inadequate, since require 10-30% of calories from dense protein sources.
- Fats, 20% of caloric intake, from dense protein, dairy, and butter, For fats over 20%, include flaxseed, olive, and sesame oils, nuts, and seeds.

Nervous System

KEY SUPPORTS FOR SYSTEM	Dense protein, at least 2 oz. 5 meals per week, and fats (sesame oil, and butter). Olive oil relieves constipation; potatoes support the lungs; Kombucha tea aids digestion; and whey aids carbohydrate digestion. Physical contact with animals has calming effect. Baking soda baths and hot sweats soothe nerves.
COMPLEMENTARY GLANDULAR SUPPORT	Thyroid, through consuming at least 2 oz. of dense protein (eggs, chicken, turkey, or fish) with a grain, such as rice or pasta, 5 meals a week. Thymus, through consuming dense protein.
FOODS CRAVED	*When Energy is Low)* Sweets such as ginger snaps, soups, salty and/or spicy foods.
FOODS TO AVOID	Artificial sweeteners; regular and diet sodas (but sparkling waters good); fried foods; caffeine.
RECOMMENDED CUISINE	Mexican, Italian, Thai, Chinese, Japanese.

Nervous System

PSYCHOLOGICAL PROFILE

ESSENCE

Just as the nervous system connects all parts of the body and keeps the brain informed of what is happening, Nervous System body types connect all parts on all levels. They enjoy listening to others and connecting people according to their needs, desires, or interests. Practical and efficient, they are happiest when they are connecting people and ideas. Nervous System types tend to have an abundance of nervous energy, and manifest it through a myriad of activities. For the Nervous System, listening to others is an adventure.

CHARACTERISTIC TRAITS

With their strong physical presence and mental focus, Nervous Systems are characterized and easily recognized by their direct, intense (often forceful), take-charge manner. It's very easy for them to come into a situation and verbally take over. They thrive on a lot of activity and love to get things moving, so they tend to go around connecting people. This gives them a great sense of joy and fulfillment, since they derive most of their knowledge and stimulation from others and their interactions with them.

Although Nervous Systems can at times be fairly reserved, when they feel free to be themselves they're typically gregarious and outgoing. Naturally curious, with excellent analytical abilities, they are interested in learning what other people know and how they do things. While they are quite conscientious about learning all that is necessary to effectively utilize and integrate the information, they don't need to know every detail. They just need to be able to use it and explain it to someone else.

Nervous Systems are happiest when they can collect knowledge from one person and bring it to another, like a bee going from flower to flower gathering its' essence getting to know each one and bringing each one what it needs. Consequently, they are most effective when they have a good overview of a lot of things. Practical and efficient, Nervous Systems initially prefer the physical or concrete to the theoretical. Highly selective in what they like, most of their choices are ones that add meaning to their lives.

While they often appear to have a hard exterior, Nervous Systems are quite sentimental. They are service oriented, sensitive to the energies around people and things, and enjoy helping people. They are particularly good at helping or providing emotional support and encouragement to others. Well organized, logical, and persistent, Nervous Systems have the ability to determine what needs to be done in any situation and the physical stamina to follow the project through to completion, meeting their goals. Altruistically oriented, they will often find a noble cause to serve sometimes identifying with being a benefactor to the human race.

Nervous System

MOTIVATION

Typically quite verbal with good integration and a grounded perspective, Nervous Systems tend to forcefully assert their viewpoints. Strong-willed and determined, they can easily get too intense as their energy builds and they get excited or stressed. Their emotions are expressed in their tone of voice which, unfortunately, often comes across as being abrasive to the receiver. Not surprisingly, they were often raised in an environment where they had to forcefully speak up in order to be heard. This forcefulness then, often becomes their normal matter-of-fact manner making it easy for them to enter a situation, quickly size things up, and more or less take over.

They tend to be perfectionists and over do, expending all their energy on duty and responsibility with little left for themselves. Because of their inherent strength, stamina and clarity of direction, they tend to do things themselves rather than delegate, often taking on too much and spreading themselves too thin. The belief is, "I'm strong, I can handle it. It needs to be done, so I'll do it." People around them often feel intimidated by the Nervous Systems' expertise. Their intention is never to intimidate, but simply to demonstrate that others can also do the task.

Movement is vital to their sense of well-being, so they thrive on a lot of activity and being constantly on the go. Since the nervous system is their strongest system, the nerves are able to carry large quantities of energy and this energy needs to be moved. If not, nervousness, sluggishness or low energy occurs. Moving the energy through activities or exercise increases their sense of well-being. Because of their strong mental and physical connections, their energy is easily channeled productively. They abhor chaos, and have even been known to clean someone else's house whom they have come to visit.

Adventure will stimulate change, and adventure is defined as learning or gaining knowledge, which is usually acquired through people. People often constitute the adventure, so they will travel simply to experience the people. They like activity, particularly that which provides mental and emotional stimulation, motivating them to participate in an activity just because it's a new experience. Nervous System types don't like the restriction of rules and regulations, so they will do things differently to cause change. Learning takes them to a new place and nature is a welcome teacher.

There is a fear of expressing their emotions because of their strength, depth and intensity. The fear is that the expression of the emotion, because of its strength, will upset things, threatening survival for the Nervous System. This fear is reinforced by the frequent experience of others not being able to handle the intensity of the Nervous System and consequently leaving them, giving rise to a sense of loss. Consequently, they will use their strong mental energies to block out or separate themselves from their feelings, and redirect their attention to external things, such as physical activities or intellectual pursuits.

Nervous System

"AT WORST"

Blunt, outspoken and abrasive, Nervous Systems control their environment and everyone around them. Intolerant, rigid and inflexible, they demand that others follow their rules. Harsh, negative and judgmental, they judge others by how well they follow their direction. Seeing everyone as less than them, Nervous Systems believe that others are here to serve them, justifying their using and draining others. Regardless of what others do, it's never enough.

When their abundance of energy is not properly channeled, Nervous Systems become nervous themselves, and/or make other people nervous. Being defensive, they often come across as offensive. Without sufficient emotional connection, their judgement is impaired, causing them to be too assertive in some situations, and not assertive enough in others. Trying to protect their ego, Nervous Systems will defend their rationalized viewpoints with a stubborn ferocity; yet needing to feel connected to others, they may hesitate to assert their legitimate interests, fearing it might jeopardize the relationship. Unable to deal with their own emotions and effectively shift their anger without hurting those around them, they can't stand for others to express their emotions. When unable to resolve their negative feelings, they often become either moody or withdrawn.

By placing their values on external appearances and making the outside world their reality, they try to control, becoming too mental and consequently, too rigid. Their way is best, and everything has to be according to their schedule, in a systematic fashion. Their net-working and interactions with others is based on their self-serving, ulterior motives. Manipulative, they will have a well calculated agenda, before they ask for what they want and make everyone miserable until they get it.

The more sensitive, responsible Nervous System types will overextend themselves and take on too much, rather than give adequate consideration to their own needs and limitations. Insisting on being totally informed and a perfectionist, they often overdo things, getting too picky or exacting. By spending so much time and energy on duty and responsibility, they find they have little left for personal needs and become angry and resentful.

Imbalances occur when they become too mental, fail to listen and get caught up in themselves. Constant talking, or chatter, is a way to scatter energy. Building a smoke screen is a means of confusing the issue by bringing in all kinds of additional energy or things, directing the focus outside of themselves. Becoming very busy, so they don't have to think about the problem or situation is a way of disconnecting or blocking personal feelings.

Nervous System

"AT BEST"

The basic nature of Nervous System body types is to connect things on all levels, making them excellent communicators, both verbally and in writing. With their genuine interest in people, they know what others want and what motivates them. Socially adept, they are gracious, polite, and charming. They will perfectly set the stage, and make sure every detail is carried out with precision in its proper order. Elegant and meticulous about appearances, they love social situations and are exceptional at organizing them.

Gregarious and outgoing, Nervous Systems are in their element in social gatherings where they can circulate and introduce people to one another. They love being the force that gets things moving. Motivated by their deep desire to help humanity, they will tirelessly gather information and bring it to those who need it. Sensitive to the needs of other people, they are good at providing emotional support to friends and family. Giving compliments, reassurances, and encouragement comes naturally for Nervous Systems.

Born leaders, Nervous Systems are energetic, determined and achievement oriented, as well as logical, practical and efficient. While mentally focused, they are flexible and spontaneous enough to let life flow. Accessing their creativity allows them to balance their strong masculine traits with the gentle, receptive feminine side that is best expressed through service. Since listening and service are synonymous for the Nervous System, and creativity is best expressed when it involves other people, doing things for them such as organizing social events or doing social volunteer work makes their lives fulfilling.

Having found their inner peace and tranquility by centering themselves and developing their spiritual connection, Nervous Systems are highly intuitive and instinctive. Coupling their physical strengths of practicality and efficiency with their intuition allows them to truly express their full potential and purpose. Listening to the emotions, their's as well as those of others, allows them to link emotions with the experience, and relay the lesson or message. Not only can they focus their energy productively, they can effectively communicate the message. By being a channel, or a messenger, they can be of great service to humanity.

Nervous System

FOOD LISTS

HEALTHY FOOD LIST

FREQUENTLY FOODS	3-7 meals a week – refers to each food, rather than category.
DENSE PROTEIN	Beef, beef broth, beef liver, buffalo, lamb; chicken livers, cornish game hen; bass, bonita, catfish, cod, flounder, haddock, halibut, herring, mackerel, mahi-mahi, perch, roughy, salmon, sardines, shark, red snapper, sole, swordfish, trout, tuna; calamari (squid), clams, eel, lobster, mussels, octopus, oysters, scallops, shrimp
VEGETABLES	Asparagus, avocado, broccoli, carrots, cauliflower, corn, cucumbers, eggplant, potatoes (all varieties), seaweed (dulse, kelp, nori, wakame), spinach, zucchini
VEGETABLE JUICE	Carrot
FRUITS	Oranges
FRUIT JUICE	Orange
SWEETENERS	ReVita®, stevia
BEVERAGES	Coffee with whipped cream or half & half; Perrier® water
MODERATELY FOODS	1-2 meals a week – refers to each food, rather than category.
DENSE PROTEIN	Veal, venison, organ meats (heart, brain), bacon; chicken, chicken broth, turkey, duck; anchovy, lox; abalone, crab; eggs
DAIRY	Milk (whole, 2%, low fat, nonfat, raw), goat milk, half & half, sour cream, sweet cream, kefir, plain or strawberry yogurt, frozen yogurt, ice cream (Ben & Jerry's®, Dreyer's, Swensen's®) butter
CHEESE	American, blue, brie, Camembert, Cheddar, Colby, cottage, cream, Edam, feta, goat, Gouda, Jack, kefir, Limburger, mozzarella, Muenster, Parmesan, ricotta, Romano, Swiss
NUTS and SEEDS	Almonds, almond butter, Brazils, cashews, cashew butter, water chestnuts, coconuts, filberts, hazelnuts, macadamias, macadamia butter, peanuts, peanut butter, pecans, pine nuts, pistachios, walnuts (English, black), seeds (caraway, pumpkin, sesame, sunflower), sesame seed butter, sunflower seed butter
LEGUMES	Beans (adzuki, black, garbanzo, kidney, navy, great northern, lima [butter], pinto, red, soy), lentils, black-eyed peas, split peas, soy milk, tofu, hummus, miso
GRAINS	Amaranth, barley, buckwheat, corn, corn bread, corn grits, corn tortilla, hominy grits, millet, oats, popcorn, quinoa, rice (brown or white basmati, long or short grain brown, Japanese, wild), rice bran, rice cakes, rye, triticale, whole wheat, wheat bran, wheat germ, refined wheat flour, flour tortillas, breads (French, Italian, garlic, sourdough, 7-grain, multi-grain, oat, corn, rice, corn/rye, rye, sprouted grain, white, whole wheat), croissants, bagels,

Nervous System

GRAINS (Continued)	English muffins, crackers (saltines, wheat, oat, rye), couscous, pasta, udon noodles, Chinese rice noodles, cream of rice, cream of rye, cream of wheat
VEGETABLES	Artichokes, arugula, bamboo shoots, green beans, yellow wax beans, lima beans, beets, bok choy, broccoflower, brussels sprouts, cabbage (green, napa, red), celery, chard, cilantro, garlic, greens (beet, collard, mustard, turnip), jicama, kale, kohlrabi, leeks, lettuce (Boston, butter, endive, iceberg, red leaf, romaine), mushrooms, okra, olives (green, ripe), onions (chives, green, brown, red, white, yellow, vidalia), parsley, parsnips, peas, snow pea pods, bell peppers (green, yellow, red), chili peppers, pimentos, sweet potatoes, pumpkin, radishes, daikon radishes, rutabaga, sauerkraut, seaweed (arame), shallots, spinach, sprouts (alfalfa, clover, mung bean, radish, sunflower), squash (acorn, banana, butternut, yellow [summer], spaghetti), tomatoes, turnips, watercress, yams
JUICES	Carrot/celery, celery, parsley, spinach, tomato, V-8®
FRUITS	Apples (Golden or Red Delicious, Granny Smith, Jonathan, McIntosh, Pippin, Rome Beauty), apricots, bananas, blackberries, blueberries, boysenberries, cranberries, gooseberries, raspberries, strawberries, cherries, grapes (black, green, red), guavas, kiwi, kumquats, lemons, limes, loquats, mangos, melons (cantaloupe, casaba, crenshaw, honeydew, watermelon), nectarines, papayas, peaches, pears, persimmons, pineapples, plums (black, purple, red), pomegranates, rhubarb, tangelos, tangerines, dates, figs, prunes, raisins
FRUIT JUICES	Apple, apple cider, apple/apricot, apricot, red cherry, black cherry, cranapple, cranberry, grape (red, white, purple), grapefruit, guava, lemon, papaya, pear, pineapple, pineapple/coconut, prune, tangerine, watermelon
VEGETABLE OILS	All-blend, almond, avocado, canola, corn, flaxseed, peanut, olive, safflower, sesame, soy, sunflower
SWEETENERS	Honey, molasses, sorghum, brown sugar, date sugar, raw sugar, refined cane sugar, maple syrup, brown rice syrup, barley malt syrup, corn syrup, fructose, succonant
CONDIMENTS	Horseradish, barbecue sauce, pesto sauce, salsa, tahini, salt, sea salt, Vege-Sal, red wine vinegar
SALAD DRESSINGS	Blue cheese, French, ranch, creamy Italian, creamy avocado, thousand island, vinegar and oil, lemon juice and oil. Good substitute for mayonnaise: Hain™ Creamy Italian dressing
DESSERTS	Custards, tapioca, puddings, pies, cakes, white chocolate, raspberry or orange sherbet
CHIPS	Bean, corn (blue, white, yellow), potato
BEVERAGES	Coffee; herbal tea, black tea, green tea, Japanese tea, Chinese oolong tea; mineral water, sparkling water; wine (red, white), sake, beer, barley malt liquor, hot apple cider and brandy, fruit juice and vodka, champagne, Scotch, gin, vodka, whiskey; root beer

Nervous System

RARELY FOODS	No more than once a month
DENSE PROTEIN	Pork, ham, sausage
DAIRY	Smoked cheese, buttermilk, most ice creams
GRAINS	Polished rice
FRUIT	Grapefruits
SWEETENERS	Saccharin, aspertame, Equal®, Sweet'n Low®, NutraSweet®
CONDIMENTS	Catsup, mayonnaise, mustard, soy sauce, margarine
DESSERTS	Dark chocolate, desserts containing chocolate
BEVERAGES	Diet sodas, regular sodas

SENSITIVE FOOD LIST

FREQUENTLY FOODS	3-7 meals per week – refers to each food, rather than category.
VEGETABLES	Carrots, corn, eggplant, seaweed (dulse, kelp, nori, wakame), spinach
MODERATELY FOODS	1-2 meals per week – refers to each food, rather than category.
DENSE PROTEIN	Beef, beef broth, beef liver, buffalo, lamb, bacon. veal, venison, organ meats(heart, brain); chicken broth, chicken livers, chicken, cornish hen, duck, turkey; anchovy, bass, bonita, catfish, cod, flounder, haddock, halibut, herring, lox, mackerel, mahi-mahi, perch, roughy, salmon, sardines, shark, red snapper, sole, swordfish, trout, tuna; abalone, calamari (squid), clams, crab, eel, lobster, mussels, octopus, oysters, scallops, shrimp; eggs
DAIRY	Milk (whole, 2%, low fat, nonfat, raw), goat milk, half & half, sour cream, sweet cream, kefir, frozen yogurt, ice cream, plain or strawberry yogurt, butter
CHEESE	American, blue, brie, Camembert, Cheddar, Colby, cottage, cream, Edam, feta, goat, Gouda, Jack, kefir, Limburger, mozzarella, Muenster, Parmesan, ricotta, Romano, Swiss
NUTS and SEEDS	Almonds, almond butter, Brazils, cashews, cashew butter, water chestnuts, coconuts, filberts, hazelnuts, macadamias, macadamia butter, peanuts, pecans, pine nuts, pistachios, walnuts (black, English), seeds (pumpkin, caraway, sesame, sunflower), sesame seed butter, sunflower seed butter
LEGUMES	Beans (adzuki, black, garbanzo, kidney, navy, great northern, lima, [butter]pinto, red, soy), black-eyed peas, split peas, lentils, soy milk, tofu, hummus, miso

Nervous System

GRAINS	Amaranth, barley, buckwheat, corn, corn bread, corn grits, corn tortillas, hominy grits, millet, oats, popcorn, quinoa, rice (brown or white basmati, brown long or short grain, Japanese, wild), rice bran, rice cakes, rye, triticale, whole wheat, wheat bran, wheat germ, refined wheat flour, flour tortillas, breads (French, Italian, garlic, sourdough, 7-grain, multi-grain, oat, corn, rice, corn/rye, rye, white, sprouted grain, whole wheat), croissants, bagels, English muffins, crackers (saltines, wheat, oat, rye), pasta, couscous, udon noodles, Chinese rice noodles, cream of rice, cream of rye, cream of wheat
VEGETABLES	Artichokes, asparagus, bamboo shoots, green beans, yellow wax beans, lima beans, beets, bok choy, brussels sprouts, cabbage (green, napa, red), cauliflower, celery, chard, cilantro, cucumber, garlic, greens (beet, collard, mustard, turnip), jicama, kale, kohlrabi, leeks, lettuce (Boston, butter, iceberg, red leaf, romaine, endive), mushrooms, okra, olives (green, ripe), onions (chives, green, brown, red, white, yellow, vidalia), parsley, parsnips, peas, snow pea pods, bell peppers (green, yellow, red), chili peppers, pimentos, potatoes (all varieties), pumpkin, radishes, daikon radishes, rutabaga, sauerkraut, seaweed (arame), shallots, sprouts (alfalfa, clover, mung bean, radish, sunflower), squash (acorn, banana, butternut, yellow [summer], spaghetti), sweet potatoes, tomatoes, turnips, yams
VEGETABLE JUICES	Celery, carrot, carrot/celery, parsley, spinach, tomato, V-8®
FRUITS	Apples (all varieties), apricots, bananas, blackberries, blueberries, boysenberries, cranberries, gooseberries, raspberries, strawberries, cherries, grapes (black, green, red), guavas, kiwi, kumquats, lemons, limes, loquats, mangos, melons (cantaloupe, casaba, crenshaw, honeydew, watermelon), nectarines, oranges, papayas, peaches, pears, persimmons, pineapples, plums (black, purple, red), pomegranates, rhubarb, tangelos, tangerines, dates, figs, prunes
FRUIT JUICES	Apple, apple cider, apple/apricot, apricot, black cherry, red cherry, cranapple, cranberry, grape, (purple, red, white), grapefruit, guava, lemon, orange, papaya, pear, pineapple, pineapple/coconut, prune, tangerine, watermelon
VEGETABLE OILS	All-blend, avocado, coconut, flaxseed, olive, sesame
SWEETENERS	ReVita®, stevia
CONDIMENTS	Salsa, tahini, salt, sea salt, Vege-Sal®, red wine vinegar
SALAD DRESSINGS	Creamy Italian, vinegar and oil, lemon juice and oil
BEVERAGES	Coffee with ReVita®; herbal tea, Japanese tea, Chinese oolong tea; mineral water, sparkling water
RARELY FOODS	No more than once a month
DENSE PROTEIN	Pork, ham, sausage
DAIRY	Smoked cheese, buttermilk, ice cream
NUTS	Peanut butter

System

Polished rice

Arugula, avocados, broccoli, broccoflower, watercress, zucchini

Grapefruits, raisins

Almond, canola, corn, peanut, safflower, soy, sunflower

Honey, molasses, sorghum, brown sugar, date sugar, raw sugar, refined cane sugar, maple syrup, brown rice syrup, barley malt syrup, corn syrup, fructose, succonant, saccharin, aspertame, Equal®, Sweet'n Low®, NutraSweet®

Horseradish, barbecue sauce, pesto sauce, catsup, mayonnaise, mustard, soy sauce, margarine

Blue cheese, French, ranch, creamy avocado, thousand island

Custards, tapioca, puddings, pies, cakes, dark or white chocolate, desserts containing chocolate, raspberry or orange sherbert

Bean, corn (blue, white, yellow), potato

Coffee; black tea; Perrier® water; wine (red, white), sake, beer, barley malt liquor, hot apple cider and brandy, champagne, fruit juice and vodka, gin, Scotch, vodka, whiskey; root beer, regular sodas, diet sodas

Fried foods

MENUS

...ASIS:

- ... 2 oz. dense protein 5x/week ...rkey, or fish) with a grain ...sta, and fats: sesame oil, and
- ...es constipation, potatoes support the lungs, Kombucha tea aids digestion, and , whey aids digestion of carbohydrates.

WEIGHT LOSS:

- 20-30% of caloric intake from dense protein.
- 20-25% fats, will gain weight if below 15%.
- Consume majority of food by 2 p.m.
- Follow Sensitive meal schedule of light breakfast, heavy lunch with protein, and moderate dinner avoiding grains. Grains may be eaten for lunch, vegetables may be raw or steamed.

WEIGHT GAIN:

- 30% of caloric intake from dense protein and 30% from fats.
- Follow Healthy meal schedule.
- Eat four equally spaced meals per day.

REBUILDING BODY:

- Follow healthy or weight gain meal schedule with heavy breakfast, weight loss meal schedule with heavy lunch and moderate dinner.

VEGETARIAN DIET:

- Inadequate, since require 10-30% of calories from dense protein sources.

FATS:

- 20% of caloric intake for maintenence, up to 30% for weight gain.
- Best sources are dense protein, dairy, and butter. For fats over 20%, add flaxseed, olive, and sesame oils, nuts, and seeds.

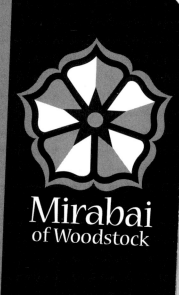

Nervous System

KEY

—all menus may be used by healthy persons

( ) around foods means that they're optional

L denotes weight loss menus

S denotes sensitive menus

G denotes weight gain menus

BREAKFAST:
6-8 a.m. Heavy, with protein, nuts, seeds, dairy, legumes, grain, vegetables, and/or fruit.

SENSITIVE: Light, with fruit.

G Pot roast or roast beef, potatoes, turnips, rutabagas, and peas

G Steak (egg, toast, and/or potatoes)

G Steak, eggs (up to 4) and oatmeal

G Lamb chops, scalloped potatoes, and asparagus

G Lamb and red potatoes

G Lamb, potato, cauliflower, and cheese

G Chicken, rice, and zucchini

G Chicken, potatoes, and orange juice

G Chicken w/blueberries, strawberries, or banana and orange

G Turkey and orange

G Tuna, rice, and carrot w/lettuce salad

G Eggs, potatoes, green onions, and orange juice

Eggs, wheat toast, and jam (potatoes)

G Eggs, chicken, wheat toast, and jam (potatoes)

G Egg and English muffin w/peanut butter

Eggs and raisin nut bread w/butter

G English muffin, eggs, cheese, and turkey or bacon

G Eggs and pancakes (berries)

G Pancakes or waffles (maple syrup) w/blueberries, peaches, strawberries, or apples

Waffles w/berries and skim milk

G Waffles w/berries and whole milk

Waffles w/butter and berries

Raisin bagel w/butter

Bagel and cream cheese

Flour or corn tortilla and lowfat Jack cheese

Flour or corn tortilla, lowfat cream cheese, and blueberries or strawberries

Tortilla w/lowfat melted cheese

Tortilla w/cream cheese (fruit)

G Burrito: refried beans, Jack cheese, lettuce, and flour tortilla

G Burrito: refried beans and rice w/flour tortilla

Couscous or barley w/skim milk, blueberries, and orange

Granola, fruit, and skim or whole milk

Granola w/nectarine

Whole wheat Total® w/slivered almonds, oat flakes, and milk

Corn and oat flakes, raisins, and milk

For weight loss or sensitive, eat up to 2 x/week, any of:

L S Nectarines, mangos, plums, or green or red grapes

L S Bananas

L S Apples such as Gala or Delicious

L S Pears – any variety

L S Mangos

L S Nectarines

L S Plums

L S Grapes

L S Papaya

Raspberry zinger tea, orange pekoe tea, Roast-A-Roma®, or Take A Break

MID-MORNING SNACK:
(Optional) Fruit, grain, protein, nuts, seeds, dairy, legumes, vegetables.

G Raisins and almonds

G Blackberries and yogurt

G Protein powder w/orange juice or milk and banana

Nervous System

LUNCH:
12-2 p.m. Light-to-moderate, with grain, legumes, dairy, nuts, seeds, raw vegetables, and/or fruit.

SENSITIVE: Heavy, with protein, nuts, seeds, dairy, legumes, grain, steamed vegetables (may also be raw for weight loss) and (occasionally) fruit.

L S Chicken or bean burrito

G Enchilada

G Corn tortilla, refried pinto beans w/lettuce and cucumber salad (slivered almonds and/or kumquat)

G Pasta, bell peppers, zucchini (marinara or tomato sauce), and strawberries

G Pasta w/spaghetti or tomato sauce (salad)

G Salad: zucchini, cauliflower, and broccoli w/ranch dressing

G Salad: romaine lettuce, 3-bean salad, carrots, cucumbers, and banana

G Cob salad and fruit

G Barley, lentils, and raw spinach

G Carrot juice or mixed vegetable juice (apple)

L S Chicken, beef, lamb, or shellfish w/vegetables, such as, peas, green beans, cauliflower, or eggplant

L S Chicken, rice and peas, green beans, cauliflower, or eggplant

L Almond chicken, rice and peas, or potato, cauliflower, and broccoli

L S Chicken, pasta, and cooked tomato

L S Lamb chops, asparagus, and rice (salad)

L S Smoked salmon, bread, brie cheese and apple

L Fish, rice, and green beans or broccoli and carrots

L S Sea bass, potato, and beets

L Turkey, rice, and vegetables, such as, peas, green beans, cauliflower, eggplant, or steamed broccoli and carrots

L S Pot roast or roast beef, potatoes, turnips, rutabagas, and peas

L Beef or turkey, linguini, and white cheese sauce (raw vegetable)

L S Shrimp, linguini, and asparagus

L S Pasta primevera and peas, green beans, cauliflower, eggplant, or asparagus

L Beef or lamb, barley, and lentils (cooked spinach, green beans, broccoli, or peas)

L S Beef or lamb and green beans (potato)

L S Beef, pasta, and tomato sauce (garlic bread)

L S Hamburger w/pasta and peas, green beans, cauliflower or eggplant

L S Corn tortilla, refried pinto beans, and guacamole or cooked tomato

L S Hard-boiled egg, tuna, and cooked tomato (bread)

L S Pizza w/cooked tomatoes

MID-AFTERNOON SNACK:
(Optional) Fruit, grain, nuts, seeds, dairy, vegetables, legumes, protein.

G Dried fruit

G Raisins and almonds

G Apple or orange

G Blackberries and yogurt

G Carrot juice or mixed vegetable juice (apple)

G Cashews, cheese, or potato chips

DINNER: 7-9 p.m. Moderate-to-heavy, with protein, nuts, seeds, dairy, legumes, vegetables (cooked/steamed), and/or grain.

SENSITIVE: Moderate, with protein, dairy, legumes, raw vegetables, and (occasionally) nuts and seeds.

L S Calamari or mahi-mahi, potatoes, and green salad

L S Salmon w/celery, green onions, and lettuce

L S Sea bass, baked potato, and raw asparagus, or raw vegetable salad

L S Orange roughy, rice, and raw salad

L S Tuna w/broccoli or cucumber and green salad

L S Tuna w/millet and lettuce salad

L S Tuna, salmon, or chicken w/lettuce and Hain™ Creamy Italian dressing

Nervous System

L S	Shellfish and salad
L S	Shrimp salad
G	Shrimp stir-fry and rice
L S	Turkey salad w/romaine lettuce, 3-bean salad, carrots, and cucumbers
G	Spaghetti w/red sauce and turkey
L S	Chicken salad
G	(Almond) chicken, rice or potato, and cauliflower and broccoli (cheese)
G	Chicken, fish, or steak, baked potato, or rice (Scotch)
G	Chicken, rice, and zucchini
	Chicken and rice (bell pepper and/or carrots)
G	Beef or turkey, linguini, white cheese sauce, and broccoli
G	Pot roast or roast beef, potatoes, turnips, rutabagas, and broccoli or peas
L S	Beef and salad
G	Beef or chicken chili (kidney beans)
G	Lamb w/broccoli and turnips
G	Lamb chops, scalloped potatoes, and asparagus
L S	Lamb chops and raw vegetables
G	Lamb and red potatoes (cauliflower and cheese)
L S	Hard-boiled egg and salad
L S	Hard-boiled egg, tuna, and raw tomato (bread)
L S	Yogurt, cucumber, and raw vegetables
L	Salad: lettuce, sprouts, celery, cucumber, zucchini or summer squash, cabbage, spinach, and broccoli w/olive or canola oil and tofu, eggs, or cottage cheese
G	Pizza topped w/cheese, mushrooms, chicken, and vegetables w/steamed carrots and broccoli
	Bean and cheese burrito
L S	Corn tortilla, refried pinto beans, and guacamole or raw tomato
L	Rice w/raw broccoli and carrots
L S	Raw vegetable salad w/oil and vinegar
L	Nonfat cottage cheese and salad: watercress, endive, garlic, spinach, radishes, tomatoes, cucumbers, onions, and sprouts w/olive oil, lemon, fresh pepper, and garlic dressing
L S	Beef vegetable soup (bread)
L S	Barley lentil soup and spinach
	Cream of broccoli soup (bran, oat or whole wheat bread)
G	Beef broth w/lentils and mixed vegetables

EVENING SNACK:
(Optional) 8 p.m.-2 a.m. Protein, vegetables, nuts, seeds, grain, legumes, dairy, fruit, sweets.

WEIGHT GAIN: 4th meal may include selections from dinner.

G	Dried fruit
G	Raisins and almonds
G	Cashews
L S G	Applesauce
L S G	Fruit or fruit juice
G	Cheese
G	Frozen yogurt w/nuts
G	Plain yogurt w/nuts (maple syrup)
G	Air-popped popcorn w/butter and/or parmesan cheese
L S	Air-popped popcorn – plain
G	Celery and almond butter
G	Rice cakes (jelly)
G	Fig bar
G	Graham crackers

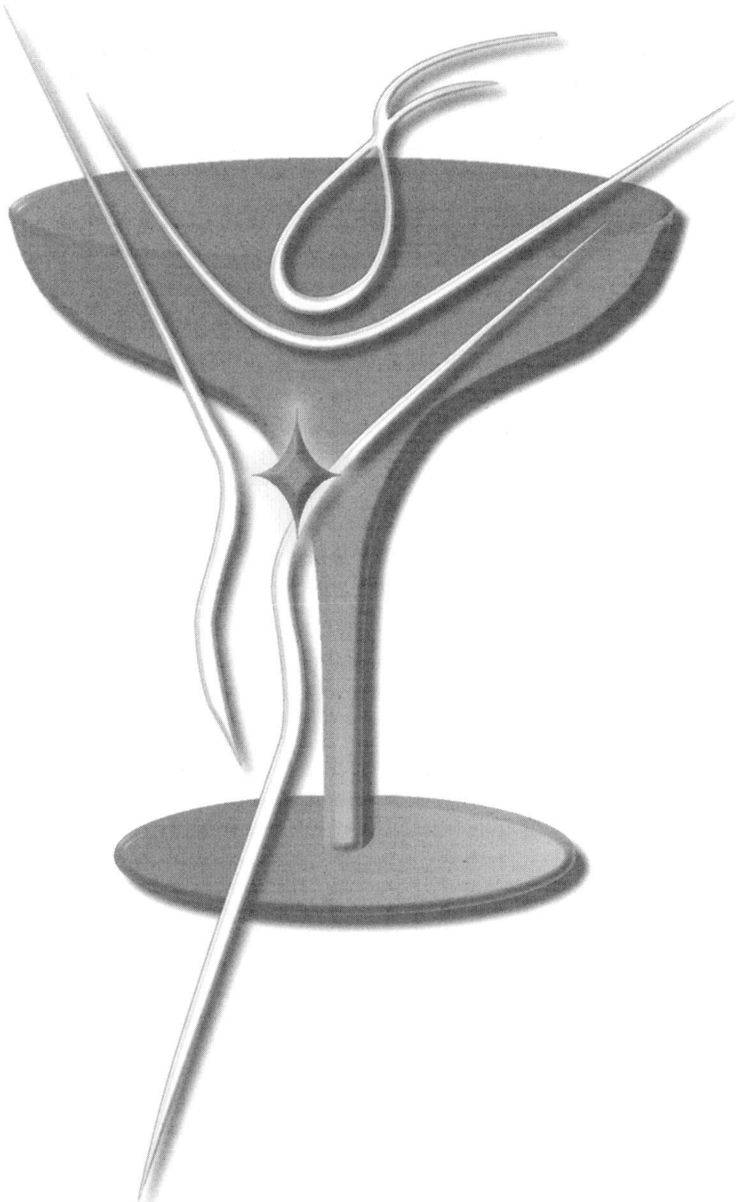

*The "Pancreas Body Type"
is symbolized by a champagne
glass. Bubbly and joyful, they love
socializing, especially around food.
With their genuine concern for people
and their ability to use laughter to burst
out of the most uncomfortable
situations, they bring joy to
their environment.*

PANCREAS

Pancreas

BODY TYPE PROFILE

LOCATION	Left upper abdomen behind stomach, next to spleen and duodenum.
FUNCTION	Secretes enzymes that aid in digestion of proteins, carbohydrates, and fats; and secretes insulin, which helps to control carbohydrate (sugar) metabolism.
POTENTIAL HEALTH PROBLEMS	Body utilizes or stores nearly everything consumed, and food generally high priority, so show strong tendency toward obesity (30 or more pounds overweight) throughout life. Frequently has family history of overweight, and possibly diabetes. Often has structural injuries due to weight (neck, shoulder, hip, ankle, foot pain). Tends to eat very rapidly; often emotional eater. Problems with digestion and proper utilization of fats and certain proteins. Vascular weakness, leading to fluid retention and headaches.
RECOMMENDED EXERCISE	Exercise is helpful, as it speeds up metabolism. Benefit is initially emotional. To maintain or reduce weight, exercising 6 days per week for 1 hour is required. Most effective times are morning or afternoon Do exercises that are enjoyable, such as brisk walking, low impact aerobics, dancing, callanetics, biking, swimming, or hiking.

WOMEN'S CHARACTERISTICS

DISTINGUISHING FEATURES	Tendency toward "rut" eating – eating same food 3 to 4 days in a row. Predominantly rounded appearance – particularly noticeable from behind in upper hips and buttocks. Small hands and often small feet, with little weight gain from knees to feet or elbows to hands. Known for bringing joy.
ADDITIONAL PHYSICAL CHARACTERISTICS	Buttocks rounded, with rounded upper hips. Excess fat initially firm, not flabby. Low back curvature straight-to-average. Breasts average-to-large. Shoulders narrower than, to relatively even with, hips. Waist defined to well-defined. Average to short-waisted. Height generally short-to-average. Bone structure small-to-medium. Average, elongated musculature. Hands generally small, unless large bone structure. Hair frequently thin or fine. Long rectangular, or average-to-long oval-shaped face.

Pancreas

WEIGHT GAIN AREA

Lower body with initial gain in lower abdomen, upper hips, upper inner thighs, inner knees, middle back, and waist in firm rolls. Excess fat initially firm, not flabby. Secondary gain in entire abdomen, upper hips, entire back, upper arms, breasts, entire inner and possibly entire thighs extending to knees, buttocks, face, and under chin. Alternative secondary weight gain pattern: lower buttocks, lower hips and entire upper 2/3rds of thighs, outer thighs, extending throughout entire thighs – with cellulite predominantly on buttocks and thighs.

Unless severely restrict food intake, gain weight easily when not exercising. Can put on large amounts of weight and have great difficulty losing and keeping it off. Often have suffered from weight problems most of life, with at least one overweight parent. May, however, have been thin earlier in life until having undergone period of stress.

DIETARY GUIDELINES

"HEALTHY"

SCHEDULING MEALS:

Breakfast: Moderate, with grain, legumes, nuts, seeds, dairy, eggs, vegetables, and/or fruit.

Lunch: Heavy, with protein, legumes, nuts, seeds, dairy, vegetables, and/or grain.

Dinner: Moderate, early, with vegetables, protein, legumes, nuts, seeds, dairy, and/or grain.

"SENSITIVE"

Avoid protein at breakfast and dinner. Fruit is recommended as evening snack only.

DIETARY EMPHASIS

- Vegetables (mainly root type); complex carbohydrates, like rice, potatoes, beans, and popcorn; fruit, such as grapefruit, cherries, papaya, and pineapple; and protein, from such sources as fish or turkey (up to 10% of diet as dense protein) or, if vegetarian, from such sources as yogurt and cottage cheese. Rotation – ideally, 4-day, reduces pancreatic stress.
- For weight loss, caloric intake of 10-20% protein and 10-15% fat recommended. Will gain weight if fats fall below 10%. Rotate foods and vary them as much as possible; exercise for at least 1 hour 6 days per week; get ample emotional support; make lunch your main meal; avoid alcohol, caffeine, artificial sweeteners, and carbonated beverages.; reduce salt, fats, breads, sugar, dairy, and quantity of food consumed; undertake detoxification program on seasonal basis; emphasize vegetables (particularly root); eat only at specified times; and employ variety. Consuming 10% dense protein helps maintain energy levels.
- Best to consume 60% of total food by 2 p.m. and, ideally, 100% by 7 p.m. Often easier to lose weight in summer than winter.

Pancreas

DIETARY EMPHASIS	• For weight gain, eat regularly (avoid tendency to get so involved with something that you end up skipping meals). • Vegetarian diet recommended for maintenance, since adequate protein can be obtained from vegetables and grains; although, may have up to 20% dense protein. • Fats, 10-15% for weight loss, 25% for maintenance. Best sources are olive oil, nuts, seeds, butter, cheese, and dense protein (chicken, turkey, fish).
KEY SUPPORTS FOR SYSTEM	Rotation of foods, as it reduces pancreatic stress. Eat recommended foods only at specified times; exercise; emotional support.
COMPLEMENTARY GLANDULAR SUPPORT	Adrenals, through consuming dense protein (eggs, poultry, and fish), fruits, and vegetables. Liver, through emotional support (such as support groups – particularly helpful with weight loss).
FOODS CRAVED	*(When Energy is Low)* Like most foods. Tend to crave same food (out of any food group) 3 to 4 days consecutively. Especially drawn toward sweets, such as chocolate chip cookies, peanut butter cookies and milk; creamy foods, such as ice cream; carbohydrates, especially potato chips, almonds, or mixed nuts; spicy foods.
FOODS TO AVOID	Alcohol, as it upsets blood sugar balance; caffeine, as it overloads kidneys; carbonated beverages, because they decrease oxygen in tissues resulting in fatigue; and artificial sweeteners, as they cause liver stress.
RECOMMENDED CUISINE	Chinese, Mongolian, Japanese, Middle Eastern, Moroccan, Thai, Italian, Mexican (delete the cheese); Soup and Salad bars.

Pancreas

PSYCHOLOGICAL PROFILE

ESSENCE	Just as the pancreas, by breaking down carbohydrates or sugars, releases energy, Pancreas body types release energy, bringing joy. They love socializing, especially around food, and are usually the life of a party. Food, particularly sugar, produces energy. Likewise, Pancreases, in their exuberance, produce joy. Conscientious and reliable, when their energy is channeled into a particular area, Pancreases can be quite dynamic. They are the ones that continually release the energy that keeps an organization running. With their genuine concern for people and their ability to use laughter to burst out of the most uncomfortable situations, they are known for bringing joy to their environment.
CHARACTERISTIC TRAITS	By nature, Pancreas types are highly sociable, caring, considerate, and compassionate. They tend to be able to maintain a certain joyous childlike quality that gives them a positive nature, full of laughter, joy, and lightness. With their delightful attitude, Pancreas types energetically transmit joy to those around them. Food is a major issue for Pancreases and is connected with having fun. Since food is usually present in positive social experiences, it's easy for them to become "pleasure eaters." Going out to eat is generally the basis of getting together with friends. So when they're alone, Pancreas types tend to be "emotional eaters," using food to fill the void when they're feeling stressed, bored, or lonely. While Pancreases love to eat, they generally don't like to cook, so they tend to fall into a pattern of eating the same thing for several consecutive days. This "rut" eating stimulates their pancreas but also depletes it. Consequently, it's very easy for them to put on excess weight, particularly when they've stopped a physically active lifestyle. Pancreases like being with people, and enjoy bringing delight to their surroundings. Physically expressive, they like to touch, nurture, and help others. With an air of lightness about them, they are good at using humor to alleviate stressful circumstances. While the last thing they want to do is offend, being highly emotional, Pancreases are so enthusiastic that their spirited outbursts sometimes come across as pushy or overbearing.
MOTIVATION	While Pancreas types are socially oriented and genuinely like people, they often experience problems in their relationships due to limitations in their communication skills. Focusing on accomplishing their agenda, they often comes across as being short or abrasive. Pancreases tend to need to talk a lot, to use others as sounding boards to sort through their thoughts and feelings in order to clarify them and get necessary feedback. This is usually stream-of-consciousness speaking, editing and refining as they talk aloud. Because of their inability to edit before they speak and in their haste to get the thoughts and feelings out, they may make a request sound more like an order or demand.

Pancreas

MOTIVATION

The tendency is to give orders, instead of asking, then to become hurt and upset when their interaction doesn't work. Being extremely zealous or emotionally excitable, they tend to speak about things with such animation and force that they come across as curt, manipulative, abrasive, or controlling. Then they can't understand why the other person seems upset or angry. Once they learn to communicate effectively, they're very considerate and caring of others.

The childlike trusting nature of Pancreases often sets them up for a rude awakening when someone they've put their faith in betrays their confidence. Because of their general innocence and lack of discernment, they may have difficulty evaluating the integrity of others, assuming honesty in another that's just not there. Not wanting to speak, act or express their own truth for fear of rejection or hurting someone else's feelings, truth and honesty become major issues. Unfortunately, when they are taken advantage of by others they believe in, Pancreases often experience deep hurt and disappointment that can cause them to close down and refuse to trust anyone.

Pancreases have a belief in lack and scarcity which is reflected in the way their body processes food. It will hang on to everything, getting the maximum benefit from every morsel. If the body is unable to process something it has taken in, it will store it as fat. This attitude of scarcity is reflected in the way Pancreas types need to have food around and keep their cupboards full. Because of the belief that there isn't enough, Pancreases take maximum advantage of every situation and store it up. They tend to hold on to things, getting locked into or attached to patterns, including eating the same food for 3 or 4 days, and resist change. Since food represents security, they often have a tendency to eat until their stomach hurts, especially as a child. Excess weight is a way of holding on to energy which represents security.

"AT WORST"

Needy and insecure, Pancreas types will play the victim by living off anyone who will give them a handout, or staying in co-dependent relationships and getting locked into being a caretaker for someone else. In their desire for security in their relationships, they may neglect their own self-care. When they become overly stressed, they often withdraw into sleeping, burying themselves in a project, or go into hiding. Reluctant to make changes, they will set up and perpetuate a failure pattern, particularly when their significant initial effort was unsuccessful. Pancreases get locked into patterns of behavior that keep them from realizing the successes and fulfillment of desires that they seek. Feeling insecure is the same as feeling powerless.

There is often a fear of growing up, which may be associated with the fear of not being able to make it on their own. There is a feeling that too much is expected of them and a fear of not being successful. This is particularly true when their initial attempts to excel or achieve have failed so further attempts to strike out their own are often delayed due to a fear of repeating the past. Men often get caught in the Peter Pan syndrome of not wanting to grow up, wanting to stay in the safe spot of being taken care of forever. They will stay

Pancreas

"AT WORST"

in co-dependent relationships until they evolve and find their truth, accepting themselves. The fear of stepping out on their own will often keep them in bad situations too long. The tendency is to internalize problems.

When insecurity levels are high, Pancreases generally have no sense of control, so they need to have boundaries and rules, particularly around food. They can easily become emotional eaters, putting on a lot of extra weight, particularly when there is insufficient joy or a feeling of insecurity. For men, the extra weight is often a way of saying, "I'm a big man and I have power." Their excess weight is generally an insulation for an inferiority complex due to not fully realizing or implementing what they know to be true. This inferiority complex is often instilled at an early age and the extra weight further instills it.

In areas where there have been past failures, the need for boundaries and rules is particularly high. Until Pancreases feel secure, they don't like grey areas, so they prefer to have everything black and white because it minimizes the chance of failure. They feel most comfortable when their jobs consist of tasks that are straightforward or well laid out for them. Projects that are ambiguous or overly complicated stir up feelings of inadequacy and fears of failure, bringing up past memories of personal defeat.

Highly sociable, Pancreases are at their best with others. Nothing gives them greater pleasure than bringing joy to their environment, which makes them extremely popular at social gatherings. Givers by nature, Pancreases are genuinely concerned with the welfare of others, and are among the most altruistic of the 25 body types.

"AT BEST"

Meticulous about learning new things, Pancreases take great pleasure in teaching others what they have learned. Often acquiring knowledge through experience, they can be quite resourceful when it comes to applying their newly discovered information. Enthusiastic and dependable, they work well with others and are good team players. Having a responsible and "take-charge" attitude, they will conscientiously see a project through from start to finish.

Loyal, steadfast, and dependable, Pancreases are good at routine or repetitive duties, successfully completing tasks that others may have abandoned as too tedious or hum-drum. They generally excel in areas where their work is well-defined. When a situation is clear-cut, they can apply new information and reliably complete the job.

With a positive, vivacious nature, one that is full of laughter and lightness, Pancreases bring joy to everyone they're around. They love life and are interested in a lot of subjects, with their main focus being the people and their feelings.

Pancreas

FOOD LISTS

HEALTHY FOOD LIST

FREQUENTLY FOODS	3-7 meals per week – refers to each food, rather than category.
DENSE PROTEIN	Anchovy, catfish, cod, halibut, herring, mackerel, perch, redsnapper, trout, water pack tuna; calamari (squid), crab, eel, lobster, octopus, scallops
DAIRY	Buttermilk, pineapple kefir, plain yogurt, butter
CHEESE	Feta, Jack, mozzarella, Muenster, Parmesan, low fat ricotta, Romano, Swiss
NUTS and SEEDS	Water chestnuts, almond milk, raw or roasted sesame seeds
LEGUMES	Beans (garbanzo, great northern, pinto)
GRAINS	Corn, corn tortillas, corn grits, corn bread, hominy grits, popcorn, brown orwhite basmati rice, Japanese rice, rice cakes, rye, durum wheat, pasta (all varieties), ramen noodles, bread (corn/rye, rye, pumpernickel, sesame pita bread), rye or sesame crackers, cream of rice, cream of rye
VEGETABLES	Basil, cooked celery, corn, cucumbers, hominy, jicama, snow pea pods, potatoes (red, white rose), sweet potatoes, radishes, sea vegetables (dulse, kelp), squash (acorn, banana, butternut), raw tomatoes, yams
FRUITS	Apricots, cherries, grapefruits (red, white), guavas, papayas, nectarines, persimmons, pineapples (canned, sugar loaf)
FRUIT JUICES	Apricot, cranberry, grape (purple, red, white), pineapple
VEGETABLE OIL	Olive oil
SWEETENERS	Maple syrup, molasses, sorghum, honey, Re-Vita®, stevia
CONDIMENTS	Sea salt w/kelp, ginger
SALAD DRESSING	Dill salad dressing
BEVERAGES	Green tea; Calistoga® berry water
MODERATELY FOODS	1-2 meals per week – refers to each food, rather than category.
DENSE PROTEIN	Beef, beef broth, beef liver, buffalo, lamb, veal, venison, organ meats (heart, brain); turkey, chicken, chicken broth, chicken livers, cornish hen, duck; ahi, abalone, sea bass, bonita, flounder, haddock, mahi mahi, orange roughy, salmon, sardines, thresher shark, sole, swordfish, yellowtail tuna; clams,imitation crab, mussels, oysters, shrimp; eggs
CHEESE	American, blue, brie, Camembert, Cheddar, Colby, low fat or regular cottage cheese, cream, Edam, Gouda, goat, kefir, Limburger, regular ricotta, all yellow cheeses

Pancreas

DAIRY	Low fat or whole milk, raw milk, half & half, goat milk, sweet cream, sour cream, kefir (plain, peach, or strawberry), fruit flavored yogurt, ice cream (Dreyer's, Swensen's®), Ice Bean® (brown salt)
NUTS and SEEDS	Almonds, almond butter, Brazils, roasted cashews, raw cashews, cashew butter, cashew milk, coconut, filberts, hazelnuts, macadamias, macadamia butter, peanuts, peanut butter, pecans, pine nuts, pistachios, black or English walnuts, seeds (caraway, poppy, pumpkin, sunflower), sesame butter, sunflower seed butter
LEGUMES	Beans (adzuki, black, butter [lima], kidney, red, soy), lentils, black-eyed peas, split peas, soy milk, tofu, hummus, miso
GRAINS	Amaranth, barley, buckwheat, millet, oats, quinoa, rice (brown short or long grain, wild), rice bran, triticale, refined wheat flour, sprouted wheat, wheat germ, wheat bran, flour tortillas, cream of wheat, breads (Italian, French, oat, potato, sourdough, white), croissants, egg bagels, English muffins, couscous, macaroni, udon noodles, oat or saltine crackers, pita bread (plain, rye, or whole wheat), tabouli
VEGETABLES	Artichokes, arugula, asparagus, avocados, bamboo shoots, green beans, lima beans, yellow wax beans, beets, bok choy, broccoli, broccoflower, brussels sprouts, raw cabbage (green, napa, red), carrots, cauliflower, raw celery, chard, cilantro, eggplant, garlic, greens (beet, collard, mustard, turnip), kale, kohlrabi, leeks, lettuce (Boston, butter, endive, iceberg, red leaf, romaine), mushrooms, okra, olives (green, ripe), onions (chives, brown, green, red, vidalia, white, parsley, parsnips, peas, bell peppers (green, red, yellow), chili peppers, pimentos, potatoes (russet, yukon gold), pumpkin, daikon radishes, rutabaga, sauerkraut, sea vegetables (arame, nori, wakame), shallots, spinach, sprouts (alfalfa, clover, mung bean, radish, sunflower), squash (spaghetti, yellow [summer], zucchini), cooked tomatoes, turnips, watercress
VEGETABLES JUICES	Carrot, carrot/celery, celery, parsley, spinach, tomato, V-8 ®
FRUITS	Apples (Red and Golden Delicious, Granny Smith, Jonathan, McIntosh, Pippin, Rome Beauty), bananas, blackberries, blueberries, boysenberries, cranberries, gooseberries, raspberries, strawberries, frozen cherries, grapes (green, black, red), kiwi, kumquats, lemons, limes, loquats, mangos, melons (cantaloupe, honeydew, watermelon), oranges, peaches, pears, plums (black, purple, red), pomegranates, rhubarb, tangelos, tangerines, dates, figs, prunes, raisins
FRUIT JUICES	Apple, apple cider, apple/apricot, black cherry, cherry, cranapple, grapefruit, guava, lemon, orange, papaya, pear, pineapple/coconut, prune, tangerine
VEGETABLE OILS	All-blend, almond, avocado, canola, corn, flaxseed, peanut, safflower, sesame, soy, sunflower
SWEETENERS	Date sugar, raw sugar, refined cane sugar, brown rice syrup, barley malt syrup, corn syrup, succonant
CONDIMENTS	Dijon mustard, soy sauce, barbecue sauce, pesto sauce, salsa, tahini, horseradish, vinegar, eggless mayonnaise, soy margarine, chocolate, Morton® salt substitute, sea salt

Pancreas

SALAD DRESSINGS	Marie's® Blue Cheese, Hain™ Creamy Italian, Hain™ Avocado, French, ranch, thousand island
DESSERTS	Custards, tapioca, puddings, chocolate, desserts containing chocolate, raspberry sherbet, orange sherbet
CHIPS	Bean, corn (blue, white, yellow)
BEVERAGES	Raspberry tea, mint tea, herbal tea, black tea, Chinese oolong tea; mineral water, sparkling water; wine (red, white), beer, barley malt liquor, champagne, gin, liqueurs, Scotch, vodka, whiskey; regular sodas

RARELY FOODS	No more than once a month
DENSE PROTEIN	Pork, ham, sausage, bacon
DAIRY	Nonfat frozen yogurt, most ice creams
GRAINS	Polished rice, whole wheat, cracked wheat, breads (7-grain, multi-grain, whole wheat), whole wheat crackers, whole wheat pasta
FRUITS	Casaba or crenshaw melons
SWEETENERS	Fructose, brown sugar, saccharin, aspertame, Equal®, NutraSweet®, Sweet'n Low®
CONDIMENTS	Catsup, yellow mustard, mayonnaise, margarine, potato chips
BEVERAGES	Coffee; Japanese tea; root beer, Pepsi®, diet sodas

SENSITIVE FOOD LIST

FREQUENTLY FOODS	3-7 meals per week – refers to each food, rather than category.
DENSE PROTEIN	Water pack tuna
DAIRY	Butter (sweet or light salt)
NUTS and SEEDS	Water chestnuts, cashew butter, macadamia butter, sesame seeds (raw or roasted)
LEGUMES	Pinto beans
GRAINS	Corn, corn tortillas, corn bread, corn grits, popcorn, Japanese rice, rye, pasta (all varieties), ramen noodles, breads (corn, corn/rye, sesame pita, rye, pumpernickle), durum wheat, sesame crackers
VEGETABLES	Basil, cooked celery, potatoes (red, white rose), daikon radishes, squash (acorn, butternut), turnips
FRUITS	Dates, raisins
VEGETABLE OIL	Extra virgin olive oil
SALAD DRESSINGS	Dill, Hain™ Creamy Italian or Avocado
BEVERAGES	Constant Comment® tea; Calistoga® berry water

Pancreas

MODERATELY FOODS	1-2 meals per week – refers to each food, rather than category.
DENSE PROTEIN	Beef, beef broth, beef liver, buffalo, lamb, veal, organ meats (heart, brain); chicken, chicken livers, chicken broth, cornish hens, duck; abalone, anchovy, sea bass, cod, bonita, flounder, haddock, halibut, herring, mackerel, mahi-mahi, perch, orange roughy, salmon, sardines, shark, red snapper, sole, swordfish, trout, yellowtail tuna; calamari (squid), clams, crab, eel, lobster, mussels, octopus, oysters, scallops, shrimp; eggs
DAIRY	Low fat or whole milk, raw milk, half & half, plain yogurt, Dannon® fruit flavored yogurt, pineapple kefir, Ice Bean®
CHEESE	American, blue, brie, Camembert, Cheddar, Colby, low fat cottage, cream, Edam, feta, goat, Gouda, Jack, kefir, Limburger, mozzarella, Muenster, Parmesan, low fat ricotta, Romano, Swiss
NUTS and SEEDS	Brazils, coconut, filberts, hazelnuts, macadamias, peanut butter, pecans, pine nuts, pistachios, walnuts (black, English), pumpkin, caraway, poppy seeds, sesame seed butter
LEGUMES	Beans (adzuki, black, butter [lima], garbanzo, great northern, kidney, red, soy), lentils, split peas, black-eyed peas, soy milk, tofu, hummus, miso
GRAINS	Amaranth, barley, buckwheat, hominy grits, millet, oats, quinoa, white basmati rice, rice bran, rice cakes, white flour, wheat germ, wheat bran, white flour tortillas, triticale, breads (brown rice, French, Italian, potato, rye, sourdough, white), croissants, egg bagels, English muffins, macaroni, couscous, udon noodles, oat and rye crackers, cream of rice, cream of rye, cream of wheat
VEGETABLES	Artichokes, asparagus, avocados, bamboo shoots, green beans, lima beans, yellow wax beans, beets, bok choy, broccoli, broccoflower, brussels sprouts, raw cabbage (green, napa, red), carrots, cauliflower, raw celery, chard, cilantro, corn, cucumbers, eggplant, garlic, greens (beet, collard, mustard, turnip), hominy, jicama, kale, kohlrabi, leeks, lettuce (Boston, butter, endive, red leaf, romaine), mushrooms, okra, onions (chives, brown, green, red, white, vidalia), parsley, parsnips, peas, snow pea pods, bell peppers (green, red, yellow), chili peppers, pimentos, yukon gold potatoes, pumpkin, radishes, rutabaga, sauerkraut, sea vegetables (arame, dulse, kelp, nori, wakame), shallots, spinach, sprouts (alfalfa, clover, mung bean, radish, sunflower), squash (spaghetti, yellow [summer], zucchini), sweet potatoes, yams
VEGETABLE JUICES	Carrot, celery, carrot/celery, parsley, spinach, tomato, V-8®
FRUITS	Apples (Golden and Red Delicious, Granny Smith, Jonathan, McIntosh, Pippin, Rome Beauty), apricots, bananas, blackberries, blueberries, boysenberries, cranberries, gooseberries, raspberries, strawberries, cherries, grapes (black, green, red), grapefruits (red, white), guavas, kiwi, lemons, limes, loquats, mangos, melons (cantaloupe, honeydew, watermelon), oranges, papayas, peaches, pears, persimmons, pineapples, plums (black, purple, red), pomegranates, rhubarb, tangerines, figs, prunes

Pancreas

FRUIT JUICES	Apple, apple cider, apple/apricot, apricot, black cherry, cherry, cranberry, cranapple, grape (purple, red, white), grapefruit, guava, lemon, orange, papaya, pear, pineapple, pineapple/coconut, prune, tangerine
VEGETABLE OILS	Olive
SWEETENERS	Honey, molasses, sorghum, date sugar, refined cane sugar, brown rice syrup, maple syrup, barley malt syrup, corn syrup, succonant
CONDIMENTS	Black or white pepper, sea salt, chili pepper, tahini, salsa, vinegar, ginger
SALAD DRESSINGS	Blue cheese, French
BEVERAGES	Mint tea, herbal tea, green tea, Chinese oolong tea; mineral water, sparkling water
RARELY FOODS	No more than once a month
DENSE PROTEIN	Pork, ham, bacon, sausage, turkey; catfish, thresher shark
DAIRY	Buttermilk, goat milk, cream, sour cream, kefir, nonfat milk, nonfat frozen yogurt, lemon yogurt, most ice creams
NUTS and SEEDS	Almonds, almond butter, cashews, peanuts, sunflower seeds, sunflower seed butter
GRAINS	Rice (brown short or long grain, brown basmati, polished, wild), whole wheat, breads (whole wheat, sprouted wheat, 7-grain, multi-grain), saltine crackers, wheat thins
VEGETABLES	Arugula, iceberg lettuce, olives (green, ripe), russet potatoes, banana squash, tomatoes, watercress
FRUITS	Casaba or crenshaw melons, nectarines, tangelos
VEGETABLE OILS	Almond, all-blend, avocado, canola, corn, flaxseed, peanut, safflower, sesame, sunflower, soy
SWEETENERS	Fructose, brown sugar, raw sugar, saccharin, aspertame, Equal®, NutraSweet®, Sweet'n Low®
CONDIMENTS	Soy margarine, margarine, catsup, mustard, mayonnaise, soy sauce, barbecue sauce, pesto sauce, horseradish, eggless mayonnaise, dijon mustard, Morton® salt substitute, baker's or brewer's yeast, chocolate, ranch salad dressing
DESSERTS	Custards, tapioca, raspberry sherbet, orange sherbet, chocolate, desserts containing chocolate
CHIPS	Bean, corn (blue, white, yellow), potato
BEVERAGES	Coffee; sugar-free hot chocolate; black tea, Japanese tea; wine, beer, barley malt liquor, champagne, gin, Scotch, vodka, whisky; root beer, regular sodas, diet sodas, Pepsi

Pancreas

MENUS

DIETARY EMPHASIS:

- Rotation of foods, ideally 4-day, reduces pancreatic stress.
- Eat recommended foods only at specified times.
- Vegetables (mainly root type).
- Complex carbohydrates, like rice, potatoes, beans, and popcorn.
- Fruit, such as grapefruit, cherries, papaya and pineapple.
- Protein, particularly from fish and turkey, or yogurt and cottage cheese.

WEIGHT LOSS:

- Best to consume 60% of total food by 2 p.m. and, ideally, 100% by 7 p.m.
- Caloric intake of 10-20% protein and 10-15% of fat is recommended. Will gain weight if fats fall below 10%.
- Rotate foods and vary them much as possible.
- Exercise for at least 1 hour 6 days per week.
- Get ample emotional support.
- Make lunch your main meal.
- Avoid alcohol, caffeine, artificial sweeteners, and carbonated beverages; reduce salt, fats, breads, sugar, dairy, and quantity of food consumed.
- Undertake detoxification program on seasonal basis.
- Emphasize vegetables (particularly root).
- Employ variety.
- Consuming 10% dense protein helps maintain energy levels.
- Eat only at specified times.

WEIGHT GAIN:

- Eat regularly (avoid tendency to get so involved with something that you end up skipping meals).

VEGETARIAN DIET:

- Recommended for maintenance, since adequate protein can be obtained from vegetables and grains; although, may have up to 20% dense protein.

FATS:

- 10-15% for weight loss, 25% for maintenance.
- Best sources are olive oil, nuts, seeds, butter, cheese, and dense protein (chicken, turkey, fish).

KEY

—all menus may be used by healthy persons
( ) around foods means that they're optional
L denotes weight loss menus
S denotes sensitive menus
G denotes weight gain menus

BREAKFAST:
8-9 a.m. Moderate, with grain, legumes, nuts, seeds, dairy, eggs, vegetables, and/or fruit.
SENSITIVE: Avoid fruit.

L	S	G	Menu
	S		Oatmeal w/Re-Vita®
		G	Oatmeal or rice w/raisins, walnuts, or almonds, and plain nonfat yogurt
L			Oatmeal w/banana
L			Oatmeal, Rice Dream®, and straw-berries
			Cream of rice w/rice syrup, apricots, or cherries
	S		Cream of rice or cream of rye
			Cream of rye w/Re-Vita®
	S		Corn grits or white basmati rice (small amount of butter)
L			Grits w/berry Re-Vita®
	S		Couscous (butter)
	S		Millet in chicken broth
		G	Rice w/raisins, almonds, or walnuts, and plain yogurt
L			Rice w/green peas or green beans
L			Cream of wheat and pink grapefruit
			Rice cakes w/sesame or almond butter, or sesame seeds
		G	Rice bread or rye toast, w/almond butter and banana
	S		Rice bread toast w/sesame butter or seeds
		G	Rye toast and raisins
L			Plain bagel and pear w/cinnamon
	S	G	Bagel w/cream cheese and Re-Vita®
L			Raisin bread w/butter and cinnamon (pear or walnuts)
		G	Blueberry pancakes w/butter

Pancreas

			Apple pancakes
			Oatmeal/apple pancakes
		G	Pancakes w/Re-Vita® or jam
L			Poached eggs, rye bread, and grapefruit
L	S		Eggs and mushrooms
		G	Scrambled eggs w/mushrooms and red peppers, cooked in olive oil, and pumpernickle bread
L			Low fat yogurt w/Re-Vita®
L	S		Refried beans and corn tortilla
L	S		Baked acorn or butternut squash (butter)
L	S		Green peas (white basmati rice)
L	S		Yukon gold or purple potato, w/butter
L	S		Sweet potato (peas and/or butter)
L	S		Yam (butter)
			Raw or roasted almonds w/apple
		G	Dried mangos, dates, or figs, and sunflower seeds
L			Pineapple and dry-roasted cashews or Brazil nuts
		G	Dates, nectarines, grapefruit, tangerines, or apples
L			Re-Vita® or spirulina w/fruit juice and banana or pineapple
			Blue/green algae w/apricot juice, banana, raspberries, or strawberries
L			Papaya filled w/pineapple chunks
L			Papaya, nectarines, tangerines, or apples
L			Papaya and raw sunflower seeds
L			Dates, papaya, or strawberries
L			Banana or mango and sunflower seeds
L			Apple and raw or toasted almonds
L			Pear and plain bagel w/cinnamon
L			Grapes and almonds
L			Red grapefruit w/almonds
L			Pineapple juice

BREAKFAST or DINNER:

With meal:

L			Cranberry concentrate, berry Re-Vita®, and water
L			Good Earth® tea (Re-Vita®)
L			Apple sun tea, red clover tea, or lemon mist tea– no honey
L			Raspberry patch or chamomile tea
			Mint herbal tea
			Note: Use lemon juice in tea to neutralize acid.

ANYTIME SNACK:
(Optional)

L			Wild berry zinger, Cafe Vienna, or orange cappuccino

MID-MORNING SNACK:
(Optional) Grain, vegetables, nuts, seeds, protein, fruit.

L			California roll w/Bragg™ aminos
L			Trail mix
			Flour tortilla w/butter and orange spice herbal tea
	S	G	Fruit – such as dates, raisins, or pineapple
		G	Papaya (pineapple)
L			Cranberry or raspberry Calistoga®
L			Mandarin orange spice tea or almond orange tea

LUNCH:
12-2 p.m. Heavy, with protein, dairy, legumes, nuts, seeds, vegetables and/or grain.

L		G	Sea bass or sole w/rice, carrots, and broccoli
L	S	G	Sea bass or sole w/white basmati rice or rice pilaf, and snow peas
L	S		Sea bass or red snapper, white basmati rice, asparagus, or green beans
L	S		Halibut or red snapper w/white basmati rice and yellow squash
L			Red snapper w/lemon pepper and spinach
L			Mahi-mahi and stir-fry vegetables w/rice and low sodium soy sauce
		G	Broiled scallops w/butter, garlic, and green beans
L			Scallops, rice, carrots, and broccoli
	S	G	Tuna w/noodles, zucchini, or green beans

Pancreas

	S		Stir-fry: chicken breast, celery, onions, carrots, acorn squash, broccoli, and cauliflower
L	S		Chicken sukiyaki
L		G	Chicken terriyaki, basmati white rice, and butternut squash
L		G	Chicken fajita, basmati rice, and steamed broccoli, cauliflower, and carrots
	S	G	Japanese spicy chicken and white basmati rice with tempura cabbage, broccoli, carrots, onions, and soy sauce
	S	G	Chicken and dumplings w/gravy
L	S		Garlic chicken
L			Chicken, rice, and cole slaw
L		G	Baked chicken w/Thai peanut sauce and vegetables
	S		Chicken w/broccoli and carrots
	S		Chicken (corn and/or red potatoes)
L			Turkey, cranberries, and carrots
L			Turkey sausage, brown rice, and green beans
		G	Turkey, mashed potatoes, cranberry sauce, and gravy (peas)
			Beef and green beans
	S	G	Beef, red potato, and peas (onions)
	S	G	Monterey Jack cheese, alfalfa sprouts, and avocado on French bread
L			Eggs and potatoes (tossed salad)
L			Stir-fry vegetables w/basmati rice and soy sauce
L			Spinach w/Spike® and corn w/Bragg™ aminos
		G	Baked russet potatoes w/Monterey Jack cheese, and shredded cabbage and carrot salad w/creamy Italian dressing
L			Hubbard squash w/butter and butternut Re-Vita®
L			Lentils and brown rice
L		G	Red beans and rice
L			Minestrone or bean and rice soup
	S	G	Bagel, cream cheese, and Re-Vita®
L			Hummus w/rice or sesame crackers
L		G	Carne asada burrito (rice)
	S	G	Hummus, sunflower sprouts, and rye pita bread

MID-AFTERNOON SNACK:
(Optional) 4 p.m. Grain, vegetables (no fruit for weight loss).

	S		Rice cakes or sesame crackers (butter)
		G	Squaw bread w/butter and butternut Re-Vita®
L	S		Popcorn
L			Carrots, celery, or jicama
			Salad: shrimp, cucumber, tomatoes, and red onion w/lime juice
	S		Fruit, such as strawberries or watermelon
L			Mandarin orange spice, almond orange, or raspberry patch tea w/lemon juice

LUNCH or DINNER:

L		G	Mexican omelette
		G	Beef, white basmati rice, and spinach
L		G	Chicken burrito: flour tortilla, refried pinto beans, and salsa (rice)
		G	Turkey croissant sandwich w/turkey, lettuce, cheese, and avocado
L			Turkey, rice, and cranberry sauce
L			Fish w/rice and corn, green beans, or peas
	S	G	Pasta, mushrooms, and Parmesan cheese
L			Pasta w/tuna and 1 Tbs Hain™ Creamy Italian or 1/2 Tbs Hain™ Poppy Seed Ranch Dressing
L			Pasta and zucchini or green beans
L			Noodles w/broccoli, carrots, peas, and onions
L	S		White basmati rice, broccoli, and butter
L	S		Broccoli and white basmati rice cooked in chicken broth
L	S		White basmati rice, butternut squash, and carrots, or peas
	S		Red, yellow, and green peppers sauteed w/onions and garlic over white rice
L	S		Sweet potato (butter)
L			Mushrooms sauteed in butter and potato
L	S	G	Pinto beans and white basmati rice, corn bread, or corn tortilla
L	S		Hummus w/rice cakes, carrots, and string beans

Pancreas

L G Baked falafel w/hummus and tomato (rye, or sesame pita)

L S G Split pea, black bean, or lentil soup w/corn muffin

DINNER:
5-7 p.m. Early, moderate, with vegetables, protein, grain, legumes, nuts, seeds and/or dairy.

SENSITIVE: Avoid protein.

L Steamed potatoes, mushrooms, onions, and carrots

L Baked potato, butter, green beans, Spike®, and Bragg™ aminos

L Butternut squash

L Split pea soup and carrot salad w/Hain™ Creamy Italian Dressing

L Rice and steamed zucchini, onions, and dill weed

L G Steak w/steak sauce and broccoli or green beans

L G Barbecued chicken, peas, rice, butter, and Spike®

L G Grilled chicken w/peas and yams

L S Chicken or chicken broth w/white basmati rice

L G Sushi (peas)

L G Turkey or turkey ham, grits, butter, and black pepper

G Meat loaf w/tomato sauce, mushrooms, celery, onions, and peppers

L Tuna w/spinach and red onion

G Eggs, white cheese, and Italian bread

L Hard-boiled egg w/rice cake, green beans, and Spike®

L S Vegetable pasta w/butter

L Pasta w/Romano cheese and sundried tomatoes (tomato sauce)

G Macaroni and cheese, and green beans

L S Rice and steamed zucchini, onions, and dill weed

L Spinach, avocado, and shrimp salad w/ vinegar & oil, or Italian dressing

L Caesar salad

G Spinach salad w/ creamy Italian dressing and cheese

S G Pinto beans, white basmati rice, black olives, corn tortilla, and cucumber

L S Sweet potatoes and cranberries

L S Sleepy Time tea

L Mandarin orange spice tea

EVENING SNACK:
(Optional) 9 p.m.-2 a.m. Sweets, fruit, vegetables, nuts, seeds, grain, protein, dairy.

Note: Only time when alcohol, sweets, or rich desserts can be used in moderation with minimal negative effects.

L Watermelon or nectarine

Orange juice

Fruit, such as pineapples, dates, or raisins

S Fruit, such as apples, tangerines, strawberries, or watermelon

S Frozen cherries

Lemon Sorbet

G Ice cream (chocolate syrup, cherries, and/or macadamias)

G Vanilla ice cream w/pineapple and cherries

G Cookies and ice cream w/cherries

G Honey roasted macadamia nuts

G Raw pistachios

L Sunflower seeds (raw carrot)

S Seeds, such as pumpkin or sesame

S Popcorn

S Cookies

L Toast and honey

S Wheat Thins®, Keebler® Club Crackers,

S Sesame crackers (butter)

Pretzels

G Cheese streudel

G Cherry pie and Sleepy Time tea

Almond or lemon pound cake

Protein drink

The "Pineal Body Type"
is symbolized by the sun.
Representative of the intuition,
the sun supplies light and awareness.
More so than with any other type,
sunlight positively affects
their emotional state.

Pineal

BODY TYPE PROFILE

LOCATION	In center of brain, above brain stem and behind thalamus.
FUNCTION	Synthesizes and releases melatonin. Activated by sunlight. Body's "receiver" for intuition. Key regulating factor in PMS irritability and mood swings.
POTENTIAL HEALTH PROBLEMS	Tendencies toward anxiety/depression, constipation/irregularity, hormonal imbalances (such as PMS), cysts, painful or irregular periods. Poor calcium utilization, fluctuating energy levels, immune system weakness, digestive distress, vascular weakness. Gums may be sensitive. Prone to depression and may need supplemental vitamin D if sunlight inadequate.
RECOMMENDED EXERCISE	Exercise is optional. Its benefit is emotional, as it stops mind chatter and helps overcome depression. Frequency: 5 times per week, ideally before 3 p.m. Most beneficial: biking, callanetics, walking. Also helpful: swimming, weights, aerobics, stairmaster, or rebounder.

WOMEN'S CHARACTERISTICS

DISTINGUISHING CHARACTERISTICS	Have physical need for sunlight. Prone to depression (from a transient "blue mood" to more abiding feelings of depression) when sunlight is unavailable. Small head in relationship to body. Known for talking to collect or focus their thoughts.
ADDITIONAL PHYSICAL FEATURES	Buttocks relatively flat-to-prominent. Low back curvature average-to-swayed. Shoulders narrower than, to relatively even with, hips. Defined waist. Relatively long-waisted with small breasts, or short-waisted with large breasts. Upper body may be smaller than lower body. Height ranges from petite-to-tall. Bone structure small-to-medium. Average, elongated musculature. Hands long, slender, and delicate; or average, with short fingers making hands appear small. Feet may be narrow. May have fine hair and hair loss resulting in thinning or balding. Average-to-long oval or rectangular face with thin lips.
WEIGHT GAIN AREAS	Lower body with initial gain in lower abdomen, buttocks, waist, upper hips, upper inner thighs, and entire upper 2/3rds of thighs. Alternative weight gain pattern: lower hips, buttocks and entire thighs. Cellulite below buttocks (possibly since childhood). Secondary gain on upper arms, entire back, breasts, and eventually extending into entire abdomen, face, and under chin. Alternative secondary weight gain in upper and lower hips. May be chronically underweight or have difficulty maintaining weight.

Pineal

DIETARY GUIDELINES

SCHEDULING MEALS:

"HEALTHY"

Breakfast: Moderate, with grain, dairy, nuts, seeds, vegetables, fruit, and/or protein.

Lunch: Moderate-to-heavy, with protein, dairy, nuts, seeds, grain, vegetables, legumes, and/or limited fruit. Need starch/grain with salad. Emphasize dense protein.

Dinner: Light, early with grain, vegetables, nuts, seeds, legumes, and/or dairy.

"SENSITIVE"

Breakfast: Moderate, with protein, grain, vegetables, and/or fruit.

Lunch: Moderate-to-heavy, with protein, grain, and/or vegetables.

Dinner: Light, early, with grain, legumes or light protein, and/or vegetables.

DIETARY EMPHASIS

- Vegetables, particularly carrots, butter or red leaf lettuce; fresh fruits; fish, especially salmon; chicken; soups; and pasta with light sauce. Majority of vegetables, steamed or cooked. May have difficulty digesting raw vegetables, which are best eaten at lunch. May have potatoes every day, but limit each variety to 2 meals a week. Rotation is important – no more than 2 days per food per week, ideally every other week. Frequent small meals are often better than large.
- May have up to 3 eggs, 3 meals per week. Breakfast important. Need at least 8 oz. of protein per day. May eat part of protein for breakfast, especially when stores are low. Eat majority of protein at lunch between 11:30 a.m. and 2 p.m., although fish may be included at dinner, especially if protein-deficient.
- For weight loss, consume majority of food, before 2 p.m., with 20-30% of calories from dense protein.
- For weight gain, consume 25-40% of calories from dense protein before 2 p.m. May experience weight loss if not getting sufficient protein. Protein deficiencies are common when under prolonged stress.
- Vegetarian diets inadequate, since require at least 10-20%, up to 40% of calories from dense protein. For sensitive, increase protein, including at breakfast, and eliminate fruit at lunch.
- Fats, 20-25% of caloric intake. Best sources are olive and canola oils, nuts (roasted cashews or filberts), seeds (sunflower and pumpkin), dense protein (fish, eggs, chicken, turkey), and cheese.

Pineal

KEY SUPPORTS FOR SYSTEM	Sunlight, not necessary actually to be in sun, but exposure to natural light is essential. Foods high in Vitamin D and carrots. Pasta with light sauces, salmon, and chicken. Butter lettuce and/or red leaf lettuce supports pineal. Rotate foods.
COMPLEMENTARY GLANDULAR SUPPORT	Pituitary, through developing greater understanding of self and others through life experiences. Pancreas, through rotation of foods.
FOODS CRAVED	(*When Energy is Low*) Sweets, especially, ice cream and chocolate. Carbohydrates. Stimulants containing caffeine (coffee, colas). Carbonated fruit drinks, like Sundance.
FOODS TO AVOID	Caffeine, pork, almonds, dried fruits.
RECOMMENDED CUISINE	Oriental, Chinese, Thai, Japanese, Seafood. Pasta with light sauce (may include chicken or fish).

Pineal

PSYCHOLOGICAL PROFILE

ESSENCE

Just as the pineal is sensitive to light and regulates the sleep cycle, Pineal body types listen to their intuition. The pineal gland is derived from a third eye that begins to develop early in the embryo and later degenerates. Likewise, our intuition is present early in life and can be developed or suppressed. Pineals tend to retain their intuition longer and stronger than most types. Generally sensitive on all levels, their challenge is to learn to accurately listen to their intuition and balance it with their mental acuity. Being highly susceptible to a barrage of internal information, talking is a way of collecting or focusing, as well as a means of sorting out what is most appropriate.

CHARACTERISTIC TRAITS

With their quick wit, strong active minds and gift of verbal expression, Pineals often find they have trouble balancing their mental acuity with their intuition. Some will shut down their intuition, ignoring their insights and try to live their lives purely from a mental perspective. While they may get by with it for a short time, closing down a part of themselves leads to problems because self-realization is essential to their well-being. Denial of any aspect usually results in their experiencing difficulty manifesting or in developing health, emotional or relationship problems.

Pineals sense the emotional states of others. They may even absorb these emotions without realizing the feelings are not their own. Natural givers, they have a strong tendency to be caretakers. In their desire to maintain a pleasant environment, it's easy for them to blend in with the habits and patterns of those around them. Highly sensitive to their environment, beauty and nature are frequently essential to their obtaining a quiet, peaceful state.

Sensitive and intuitive, Pineal types, consciously or unconsciously, must sift through a multitude of random thoughts to get a meaningful message. Until they learn to selectively tune into what they want to hear, Pineals receive information from many avenues, including what they see, hear, feel, and sense from their immediate vicinity, as well as beyond. The easiest way to organize this information is to articulate their thoughts, which can take several minutes – or several listeners – before the essence of their message becomes clear.

Having an abundance of valuable ideas, Pineals often don't record or even remember them, and unless they can be communicated to someone else, the fruits of their imagination are lost forever. The challenge is to sort through and bring their essence down into practical, earth terms. Being able to understand and grasp concepts that often take them into other realms, Pineals frequently experience difficulty communicating ideas, particularly since they are often new to many of their listeners. Consequently, Pineals tend to experience a feeling of being different and misunderstood.

Pineal

MOTIVATION

Personal intimacy is usually a challenge for Pineals because their intellect tends to take precedence over their feelings, and keeps them separated or segregated and alone. While they may be loved by many and have many friends, true intimacy in a relationship can be elusive. Emotional issues are generally a challenge, as they will often deny their own feelings to avoid feeling weak or stupid. They then tend to emphasize their mental abilities and overwork, particularly when they don't trust others to know as much as they do and feel they need to handle everything, or, lacking a pragmatic approach to life, swing to the opposite extreme of doing nothing.

While they expect a lot from others, they expect superior abilities from themselves and are constantly striving to do greater and greater things in life. Creative, expressive and compassionate, Pineals often have difficulty dealing with the harshness and practicalities of the physical world. They are independent thinkers and except to direct and counsel others, Pineals like to work alone so they can focus on the task and let their intuition guide them.

Since Pineals readily perceive things that are not apparent to others, they become impatient when others don't acknowledge or respond to their reality. Because they often have the ability to receive from other realms and very few humans measure up to their standards, they generally find it difficult to take orders or submit to others' leadership. If they're unhappy working within some conventional, hierarchical structure, they may, usually unconsciously, act so as to sabotage the system that stifles them. They prefer to plan, oversee, or supervise a project rather than actually do the work themselves. Since their expertise often exists only in theory, their lack of practical experience and know how can sometimes cause problems.

"AT WORST'

Pineals tend to be nervous and high-strung and can get so caught up in thinking about what they want to accomplish that they have a hard time getting started on a project. They can get trapped in their mental process and fail to accomplish or make significant progress, spending their time setting up rules and policies. With their strong mental focus, they can be very intense, staying with a subject until it's exhausted, getting caught in a mental loop or spacing out. Generally more of a dreamer than realist, they often have difficulty bringing their ideas to practical reality and can be very critical of themselves and others when things don't manifest according to their time frame. Other Pineals will take the opposite approach and become too impulsive and impatient, jumping in before they look or know what they are getting into.

Possessing a superiority attitude, they like to be in control, and feel they have all the answers. The tendency is to always try to teach without recognizing when it's time to listen or be the student. In spite of their feelings of superiority, Pineals are prone to having an inferiority complex, and will try to avoid feeling weak or incompetent through denial. Being insecure, they are easily triggered and readily jump to conclusions. Sensitive to subtle humor, Pineal types sometimes find sarcasm where it was not intended. Though

Pineal

"AT WORST" (Continued)

generally accommodating and considerate, they will become assertive when they feel they are being belittled.

When stressed, Pineals become highly emotional, hyperactive and scattered, which can lead to an aggressive emotional reaction. Their lack of focus and clarity tends to be expressed as verbose verbiage in abstract terms. Emotionally insecure, females will often acquiesce to a male. Another tendency is to panic, space out, or shift into fantasy which may manifest as spending long periods of time staring off into space.

Impulsive behavior is often the underlying cause of their financial problems. Since beauty is a means of connecting with their spiritual center, Pineals tend to look for beautiful things to enhance their environment. When their desire for beauty is coupled with impulsive behavior, Pineals will go on frivolous shopping sprees to lift their spirits.

"AT BEST"

Being open-minded, quick and bright, Pineals are usually on the leading edge of new thought and psychology. With their intuitive awareness and clear mental focus, they are able to see how life's challenges allow them to find their own depth and abilities to understand life more fully. Acutely aware of the importance the mind and emotional states play in determining a person's reality, Pineals are particularly effective counseling others. Combining their own experience, intuitive awareness, and intense interest in people, they can successfully communicate their insights to others and become innovators in their chosen fields.

The Pineals' greatest strength lies in their personal quest to find meaning and understanding, in other words, reaching self-realization and experiencing ultimate freedom. Inquisitive, free-thinking, and creative, they are idealists with high personal standards of excellence.

Once Pineals learn to go inside and connect their thoughts with their feelings, their intuition is free to come through, enabling them to express from a centered place. It's from here that they can connect with the physical world and bring their thoughts into practical terms. Having reached a certain level of awareness and achievement, they are able to access the receiving side of their nature so support seems to come forward more from their beingness than their doingness. At this point, expressing their truth and sharing with others in a calm, relaxed manner is easy.

Pineals' greatest gift is their deep, intuitive Universal connection. This allows them to directly access information from other dimensions, such as the collective unconscious or higher realms. They are then able to express these Universal truths and bring this creative energy into physical form or practical manifestation. Listening to their intuition offers Pineals a unique sense of freedom. While they still maintain and use their strong ability to analyze and understand deep or abstract concepts, it isn't necessary for them to have all possible information on a subject, because they can act or respond according to their own internal messages.

Pineal

FOOD LISTS

HEALTHY FOOD LIST

FREQUENTLY FOODS	3-7 meals per week – refers to each food, rather than category.
DENSE PROTEIN	Beef; chicken (white), chicken broth, cornish game hen; cod, halibut, mahi-mahi, roughy, salmon, sardines, shark, red snapper, swordfish, trout, tongle tuna; calamari (squid), clams, eel, lobster, scallops, shrimp
DAIRY	Half & half, sweet cream, sour cream, butter
NUTS and SEEDS	Cashews, cashew butter, coconuts, seeds (caraway, pumpkin, sesame, raw sunflower)
LEGUMES	Beans (adzuki, garbanzo), split peas, hummus
GRAINS	Barley, oats, oat bran, quinoa, white or brown basmati rice, rye, flour tortillas, breads (corn, corn/rye), pasta
VEGETABLES	Artichokes, asparagus, yellow wax beans, beets, red cabbage, capers, carrots, celery, chard, cilantro, corn, cucumbers, garlic, beet greens, jicama, lettuce (butter, red leaf, romaine), green onions, peas, bell peppers (green, red, yellow), radishes (daikon, red, white), rutabaga, seaweed (arame, dulse, kelp, nori, wakame), alfalfa sprouts, squash (acorn, banana, butternut, spaghetti, yellow [summer], zucchini), taro root, yams
FRUITS	Bananas, blueberries, raspberries, lemons, melons (cantaloupe, honeydew, watermelon)
SWEETENERS	Honey, date sugar, brown rice syrup, Re-Vita®, stevia
CONDIMENTS	Basil, vanilla
BEVERAGES	Good Earth® tea, decaffeinated tea
MODERATELY FOODS:	1-2 meals per week – refers to each food, rather than category.
DENSE PROTEIN	Beef broth, beef liver, buffalo, lamb, veal, venison, ham, organ meats (heart, brain); chicken (dark), chicken livers, turkey, duck; anchovy, bass, bonita, catfish, flounder, haddock, herring, mackerel, perch, sole, tuna (light chunk, yellow tail); abalone, crab, mussels, octopus, oysters; eggs
DAIRY	Milk (raw, whole, 2%, low fat, nonfat), goat milk, buttermilk, kefir, lowfat or nonfat plain or flavored yogurt, frozen yogurt, ice cream (Ben & Jerry's®, Dreyer's, Swensen's®)
CHEESE	American, blue, brie, Camembert, Cheddar, Colby, cottage, cream, Edam, feta, goat, Gouda, Jack, kefir, Limburger, mozzarella, Muenster, Parmesan, ricotta, Romano, Swiss
NUTS and SEEDS	Brazils, water chestnuts, filberts, hazelnuts, macadamias (raw, roasted), macadamia butter, pecans, pistachios, walnuts (black, English), flaxseed, sesame seed butter, sunflower seed butter

Pineal

LEGUMES	Beans (black, lima [butter], kidney, great northern, pinto, red), lentils, black-eyed peas, miso, soy milk, tofu
GRAINS	Amaranth, corn, blue corn, corn grits, corn tortillas, hominy grits, millet, popcorn, rice (brown or white long or short grain, wild, Japanese), rice cakes, popcorn/rice cakes, rice bran, whole wheat, wheat bran, wheat germ, refined wheat flour, breads (French, Italian, sourdough, garlic, oat, rice, rye, raisin-nut, sprouted grain, pita, white, whole wheat), bagels, croissants, English muffins, crackers (oat, rye, saltines, wheat thins), couscous, udon noodles, rice noodles, cream of rice, cream of rye, cream of wheat
VEGETABLES	Arugula, avocados, bamboo shoots, green beans, lima beans, bok choy, broccoli, broccoflower, brussels sprouts, cabbage (green, napa), cauliflower, eggplant, greens (collard, mustard, turnip) kale, kohlrabi, leeks, lettuce (Boston, endive), mushrooms, okra, olives (green, ripe), onions (chives, brown, red, white, yellow, vidalia), parsley, parsnips, snow peas, chili peppers, pimentos, potatoes (red, white rose, russet, yukon gold), pumpkin, sweet potatoes, sauerkraut, shallots, spinach, sprouts (clover, mung bean, radish, sunflower), tomatoes, turnips, watercress
VEGETABLE JUICES	Carrot, celery, carrot/celery, parsley, spinach, tomato, V-8®
FRUITS	Apples (all varieties), apricots (fresh or canned), blackberries, boysenberries, cranberries, gooseberries, strawberries, cherries, fresh figs, black grapes, grapefruits, guavas, kiwi, kumquats, loquats, mangos, melons (casaba, crenshaw), nectarines, oranges, papayas, peaches, pears, persimmons, canned pineapples, plums (black, red, purple), rhubarb, tangelos, tangerines
FRUIT JUICES	Apple, apple cider, apple/apricot, apricot, black cherry, red cherry, cranapple, cranberry, cranberry concentrate, grape (purple, red, white), guava, lemon, orange, pear, pineapple/coconut, tangerine, watermelon
VEGETABLE OILS	All-blend, almond, avocado, canola, cashew, coconut, corn, flaxseed, olive, peanut, safflower, sesame, soy, sunflower
SWEETENERS	Fructose, succonant, brown sugar, raw sugar, refined cane sugar, barley malt syrup, corn syrup, maple syrup
CONDIMENTS	Mustard, mayonnaise, barbecue sauce, pesto sauce, soy sauce, brewer's yeast, tahini, carob, Spike®, Veg-It®, Vege-Sal®, sea salt, Bragg™ aminos, cinnamon, vinegar
SALAD DRESSINGS	Blue cheese, French, ranch, creamy Italian, creamy avocado, thousand island, vinegar and oil, lemon juice and oil
DESSERTS	Custards, tapioca, puddings, pies, cakes, orange or raspberry sherbet
CHIPS	Bean, corn (blue, white, yellow), potato
BEVERAGES	Herbal tea, peppermint tea, black tea, green tea, Japanese tea, Chinese oolong tea; mineral water, sparkling water; wine (red, white), sake, beer, barley malt liquor, champagne, gin, Scotch, vodka, whiskey; root beer, regular sodas

Pineal

RARELY FOODS	No more than once a month
DENSE PROTEIN	Pork, bacon, sausage
DAIRY	Most ice creams
NUTS and SEEDS	Almonds, almond butter, peanuts, peanut butter, pine nuts, roasted sunflower seeds
LEGUMES	Navy beans, soy beans
GRAINS	Buckwheat, triticale, multi-grains, breads (7-grain, multi-grain), stoneground wheat crackers, 7-grain cereal
FRUITS	Red or green grapes, limes, pomegranates, dried apples, apricots, dates, pineapples, black Mission figs, prunes, raisins
FRUIT JUICES	Grapefruit, papaya, pineapple, prune
SWEETENERS	Molasses, sorghum, aspertame, saccharin, Equal®, Sweet'n Low®, NutraSweet®
CONDIMENTS	Catsup, horseradish, margarine, salt
DESSERTS	Chocolate, desserts containing chocolate
BEVERAGES	Coffee; diet sodas

SENSITIVE FOOD LIST

FREQUENTLY FOODS	3-7 meals per week – refers to each food, rather than category.
DAIRY	Unsalted butter
LEGUMES	Adzuki beans
GRAINS	Oats, white or brown basmati rice
SEEDS	Sesame seeds (toasted)
VEGETABLES	Steamed carrots, chard, jicama, green onions, peas, rutabaga, squash (acorn, banana, butternut, yellow [summer], spaghetti), yams
FRUITS	Raspberries
CONDIMENTS	Basil
MODERATELY FOODS	1-2 meals per week – refers to each food, rather than category.
DENSE PROTEIN	Beef broth, beef liver, buffalo, veal, venison, organ meats (brain, heart); chicken (white), chicken broth, chicken livers, cornish game hen, turkey, duck; anchovy, bass, bonita, catfish, cod, flounder, haddock, perch, halibut, herring, mackerel, mahi-mahi, roughy, sole, salmon, snapper, tongle or light chunk tuna; abalone, octopus; eggs
DAIRY	Nonfat milk, sweet cream, sour cream, kefir, low fat or nonfat plain yogurt

Pineal

CHEESE	American, brie, Camembert, Cheddar, Colby, cottage, cream, Edam, feta, Gouda, Jack, kefir, Limburger, mozzerella, ricotta, Romano
NUTS and SEEDS	Brazils, cashews, cashew butter, cashew milk, water chestnuts, filberts, hazelnuts, macadamias, macadamia butter, pecans, unsalted pistachios, seeds (caraway, flaxseed, raw or roasted pumpkin, raw sesame, raw sunflower), sesame seed butter, sunflower seed butter
LEGUMES	Beans (black, garbanzo, lima [butter], great northern, pinto, red), lentils, black-eyed peas, split peas (with cashews), hummus, miso, soy milk
GRAINS	Barley, corn, blue corn, corn bread, corn grits, corn tortillas, hominy grits, popcorn, quinoa, Japanese rice, rice bran, unsalted rice cakes, wheat germ, refined wheat flour, breads (French, Italian, sourdough, garlic, corn, corn/rye, pita, raisin-nut, white), bagels, croissants, English muffins, oat bran muffins, crackers (saltines, oat), couscous, pasta, udon noodles, rice noodles, cream of rice, cream of rye, cream of wheat
VEGETABLES	Asparagus, bamboo shoots, green beans, yellow wax beans, lima beans, beets, bok choy, broccoli, broccoflower, brussels sprouts, capers, raw carrots, cauliflower, cilantro, eggplant, garlic, greens (collard, mustard, turnip), kale, kohlrabi, leeks, shitake mushrooms, mushrooms, okra, olives (green, ripe), onions (chives, brown, red, white, yellow, vidalia), parsley, parsnips, snow peas, bell peppers (green, red, yellow), chili peppers, pimentos, potatoes (white rose, yukon gold), sweet potatoes, pumpkin, radishes, daikon radishes, sauerkraut, shallots, spinach, sprouts (alfalfa, clover, mung bean, radish, sunflower), tomatoes, turnips
VEGETABLE JUICES	Carrot, celery, carrot/celery, parsley, spinach, tomato, V-8®
FRUITS	Fresh or canned apricots, blueberries, blackberries, cranberries, gooseberries, fresh figs, black grapes, grapefruits, guavas, kiwi, kumquats, loquats, mangos, melons (casaba, crenshaw), nectarines, oranges, papayas, peaches, persimmons, pineapples, rhubarb, tangelos, soaked prunes
FRUIT JUICES	Apricot, grape, guava
VEGETABLE OILS	Canola, olive
SWEETENERS	Re-Vita®, stevia
CONDIMENTS	Soy sauce, salsa, carob, vanilla, Bragg™ aminos, sea salt, Veg-It®, Vege-Sal®, kelp, apple cider vinegar
SALAD DRESSINGS	Vinegar and oil, lemon juice and oil
BEVERAGES	Herbal tea, Good Earth® tea, decaf tea, Japanese tea, Chinese oolong tea; mineral water, sparkling water
RARELY FOODS	No more than once a month
DENSE PROTEIN	Beef, lamb, pork, bacon, ham, sausage; dark chicken; sardines, shark, swordfish, trout; calamari (squid), clams, crab, eel, lobster, mussels, oysters, scallops, shrimp

Pineal

DAIRY	Milk (raw, whole, low fat, 2%), goat milk, buttermilk, half & half, frozen yogurt, ice cream
CHEESE	Blue, goat, Muenster, Parmesan, Swiss
NUTS and SEEDS	Almonds, almond butter, coconuts, peanuts, peanut butter, pine nuts, pistachios (roasted, salted), walnuts (black, English), sunflower seeds (roasted)
LEGUMES	Beans (kidney, navy, soy), split peas (alone), tofu
GRAINS	Amaranth, buckwheat, millet, brown or wild rice, salted rice cakes, popcorn/rice cakes, rice milk, rye, triticale, whole wheat, wheat bran, flour tortillas, breads (oat, rice, rye, sprouted wheat, 7-grain, multi-grain), raisin bran muffins, crackers (wheat thins, stoneground wheat, rye)
VEGETABLES	Artichokes, arugula, avocado, cabbage (green, napa, red), celery, corn, cucumbers, beet greens, lettuce (Boston, butter, endive, iceberg, red leaf, romaine), potatoes (red, russet), seaweed (arame, dulse, kelp, nori, wakame), watercress, zucchini
FRUITS	Apples (all varieties), bananas, boysenberries, strawberries, cherries, grapes(green, red), lemons, limes, melons (cantaloupe, honeydew, watermelon), pears, plums (black, red, purple), pomegranates, tangerines
DRIED FRUITS	Apples, dates, black Mission figs, pears, apricots, pineapple, prunes, raisins
FRUIT JUICES	Apple, apple cider, cranapple, black cherry, red cherry, cranberry, cranberry concentrate, grapefruit, lemon, orange, papaya, pear, pineapple, prune, tangerine
VEGETABLE OILS	All-blend, almond, avocado, cashew, coconut, corn, flaxseed, peanut, sesame, soy, safflower, sunflower
SWEETENERS	Honey, molasses, sorghum, brown sugar, date sugar, raw sugar, refined cane sugar, barley malt syrup, brown rice syrup, corn syrup, maple syrup, fructose, succonant, saccharin, aspertame, Equal®, Sweet'n Low®, NutraSweet®
CONDIMENTS	Catsup, mustard, barbecue sauce, pesto sauce, horseradish, margarine, mayonnaise, canola mayonnaise, tahini, brewer's yeast, salt, Spike®, cinnamon, red wine vinegar
SALAD DRESSINGS	Blue cheese, French, ranch, creamy Italian, creamy avocado, thousand island
DESSERTS	Custards, tapioca, puddings, pies, cakes, orange or raspberry sherbert, chocolate, desserts containing chocolate
CHIPS	Bean, corn (blue, white, yellow), potato
BEVERAGES	Coffee; peppermint tea, black tea, green tea; wine (red, white) sake, beer, barley malt liquor, champagne, gin, Scotch, vodka, whiskey; root beer, regular sodas, diet sodas

Pineal

MENUS

DIETARY EMPHASIS:

- Need at least 8 oz. of protein per day. May eat part of protein for breakfast, especially when low.
- Breakfast is important meal.
- May have up to 3 eggs, 3 meals per week.
- Eat majority of protein at lunch between 11:30 a.m. and 2 p.m., although fish may be included at dinner, especially if protein-deficient.
- Rotation important – no more than 2 days per food per week, ideally every other week.
- May have potatoes every day, but limit each variety to 2 meals per week.
- Vegetables, particularly carrots, butter or red leaf lettuce; fresh fruits; fish, especially salmon; chicken; soups; and pasta with light sauce.
- Majority of vegetables, steamed or cooked. May have difficulty digesting raw vegetables, which are best eaten at lunch.
- Frequent small meals are often better than large.

WEIGHT LOSS:

- Consume majority of food before 2 p.m., with 20-30% of calories from dense protein.

WEIGHT GAIN:

- Consume 25-40% of calories from dense protein before 2 p.m. May experience weight loss if not getting sufficient protein. Protein deficiencies are common when under prolonged stress.

VEGETARIAN DIET:

- Inadequate, since require at least 10-20%, and up to 40% of calories from dense protein.

SENSITIVE:

- Increase protein, including at breakfast, and eliminate fruit at lunch.

FATS:

- 20-25% of caloric intake.
- Best sources are olive and canola oils, nuts (roasted cashews, filberts), seeds (sunflower and pumpkin), dense protein (fish, eggs, chicken, turkey), and cheese.

KEY

—all menus may be used by healthy persons
( ) around foods means that they're optional
L denotes weight loss menus
S denotes sensitive menus
S* denotes extremely sensitive menus
G denotes weight gain menus

BREAKFAST:
7-8 a.m. Moderate, with grain, dairy, nuts, seeds, vegetables, fruit, and/or protein.

SENSITIVE: Moderate, with protein, grain, vegetables, and/or fruit.

G	Oatmeal w/whole milk and banana or blueberries (raw sunflower seeds)
L S	Oatmeal w/low fat or nonfat plain yogurt or unsalted butter
G	Oatmeal w/plain yogurt or half & half
L S G	Oatmeal treat: oatmeal, oat flour, and butternut Re-Vita® (butter)
S	Oatmeal, then grapefruit
S	Oatmeal and peaches – fresh, frozen, or canned w/out sugar
G	Oatmeal w/raisins, or fresh figs
L S*	Oatmeal and Re-Vita®
G	Oatmeal w/Re-Vita®, coconut, or pistachios
S*G	Regular plain kefir (Re-Vita®), then oatmeal
L	Corn grits w/egg – no butter
S G	Corn grits w/butter (eggs)
L S*	Corn grits w/peas
G	Corn flakes, half & half, raw sunflower seeds, and Re-Vita®
L	Millet and raisins
L G	Millet in chicken broth
G	Cream of rice and brown rice syrup (butter)
G	Cream of rye and peaches or banana
L S*	Basmati rice w/carrots and snow peas
L	Basmati rice w/blueberries

Pineal

L S* Basmati rice, peas, and/or green beans (parsley)

G English muffin w/cashew butter and banana

S Blue corn, oat, or flour pancakes w/Re-Vita® (unsalted butter)

G Buttermilk pancakes w/maple syrup and cashews (Re-Vita®)

G Blueberry bagel w/cream cheese

S G Kefir cheese and Re-Vita®

L G Yogurt w/almonds or cashews

L G Protein drink w/fruit or vegetable juice

L S G Eggs, basmati rice, and peas (parsley)

S G Eggs and rye toast (butter)

L Eggs, toast, and jelly, or marmalade

L S Scrambled eggs and broccoli

G Omelette: eggs, mushrooms, light Cheddar cheese, and whole milk w/Re-Vita®

L S Turkey and carrots

S G Turkey or chicken breast, white rose potato, and mixed vegetables

L S G Chicken breast, basmati rice, carrots, and red peppers

L S G Mahi-mahi and rice

L S G Salmon, basmati rice, and broccoli

L S White rose baked potato (unsalted butter)

L Baked potato, carrots, snow peas, and celery

L S* Peas (yukon gold potatoes)

L Carrots and broccoli

S Lima beans

L Rice and squash

L S* Squash (Re-Vita®)

Blueberries, raspberries, or grapefruit

S Papaya or cashews

MID-MORNING SNACK:
(Optional) 10 a.m. Fruit, nuts, seeds, dairy, grain, or vegetables.

S G Chocolate or butternut Re-Vita®, oatmeal, and butter

G Frozen strawberries w/half & half

L S Peach

S G Unsalted rice cakes and cashew butter (blueberry jam)

G Rice cake w/avocado or hummus

G Rice bread, cashew butter, and blueberry jam

G All-Bran,® oat bran, or sourdough muffin and half & half

L Purple grape juice

LUNCH:
11:30 a.m.-2 p.m. Moderate-to-heavy, with protein, dairy, nuts, seeds, grain, vegetables, legumes, fruit - moderately. Need starch/grain with salad. Emphasize dense protein.

SENSITIVE: Moderate-to-heavy, with protein, grain, and/or vegetables.

L G Chicken, rice, and cashews (vegetables)

L G Chicken, rice, and salad: red or green leaf lettuce, cucumber, avocado, carrots, celery, red pepper, and onion w/oil and vinegar or garlic dressing

S G Chicken breast, corn tortilla, and refried beans (carrots)

L Chicken or turkey tacos w/lettuce and tomatoes

G Chicken tacos w/lettuce, tomatoes, and avocado

L S G Stir-fry: chicken breast, broccoli, snow peas, carrots, or celery (cashews) over rice

G Chicken, sweet potato, lettuce, avocado, and cabbage

G Turkey or tuna on rye roll, avocado, and sparkling apple juice

L S G Stir-fry: turkey, carrots, chard, peppers, and sprouts over rice

L S G Turkey, peas, and cashews

L S G Turkey, rice, carrots, and bell peppers (sprouts)

L S*G Turkey, broccoli, and cauliflower

S G Turkey, beans, and rice (raw carrots)

L S G Turkey, white rose potatoes, gravy, and broccoli

L S G Ground turkey, mashed yukon gold potatoes, and green beans

L S*G White turkey, yams, and broccoli or cauliflower

Pineal

- L G — Beef and bean chili
- L G — Pot roast, carrots, potatoes, and mushroom gravy
- L G — Roughy, wild rice, and turnip greens
- L G — Salmon and rice (green salad and/or yellow squash)
- L S G — Tuna and sweet potato
- L S G — Tuna, basmati rice, and squash, or green beans
- G — Tuna, celery, and Hain™ Creamy Italian dressing on rye
- L S G — Halibut, basmati rice, and peas
- L S G — Mahi-mahi, basmati rice, and broccoli
- G — Sardines in olive oil and rye or oat bread
- L G — Water chestnuts, bamboo shoots, shrimp, snow pea pods, and rice
- L S G — Fish, rice, water chestnuts, bamboo shoots, and snow pea pods
- L S — Basmati rice, carrots, green peppers, and garlic
- L G — Shrimp and pasta
- L G — Eggs and flour tortillas (salsa)
- G — Eggs, mushroom, and light Cheddar cheese omelette (whole milk w/Re-Vita®)
- G — Flour tortilla, spanish rice, pinto beans, and green onions
- S G — Corn tortilla, beans, and basmati rice
- G — Linguini pasta w/butter, sesame seeds, and Parmesan cheese
- S* — White rose potato, broccoli, and chard
- S G — Chicken rice soup
- S — Chicken vegetable soup
- S G — Beef vegetable soup

MID-AFTERNOON SNACK:
(Optional) 3-4 p.m. Fruit, nuts, seeds, dairy, grain, or vegetables.

- Apple juice, apple, or blueberries
- S G — Toasted bagel and butter
- G — Sourdough English muffin (butter or jelly)
- S — Sesame seed cookies
- L S — Popcorn
- S G — Cashews
- G — Pineapple/coconut juice
- L S G — Berry Re-Vita® w/cranberry concentrate and water

DINNER:
5-7 p.m. Light, early with grain, vegetables, nuts, seeds, legumes , and/or dairy.

SENSITIVE: Light, early, with grain, legumes or light protein, and/or vegetables.

- L S G — Pearl barley, carrots, peas, and unsalted butter
- L — Potato and steamed broccoli
- L S G — Baked yukon gold potato and asparagus (white Cheddar cheese), (butter)
- L S G — Baked yukon gold potato w/unsalted butter, cheese and/or peas, and/or broccoli
- L S G — Baked white rose potato, squash, hummus, and unsalted rice cakes
- S G — White rose potatoes, cheese, and asparagus
- L S — Yams or sweet potatoes, and peas, or chard
- L S G — Sweet potato, basmati rice, and carrots
- L S G — Butternut, acorn, spaghetti, or yellow squash, and Re-Vita® w/basmati rice (tamari)
- L S G — Squash, basmati rice, and hummus on unsalted rice cakes
- L S — Squash, basmati rice, and carrots, or onions
- L S G — Basmati rice with stir-fry vegetables
- L S — Basmati rice and green beans
- S G — Lentils, basmati rice, and garlic
- L S — Couscous, carrots, and parsnips
- S G — Asparagus, white rose potatoes, and white Cheddar cheese
- L G — Beets, millet, and rice cakes
- L S G — Pinto or adzuki beans and basmati rice w/broccoli and/or carrots

Pineal

L S*G Lima beans (carrots and garlic)
L S* Lentils (basmati rice)
L S*G Black beans (carrots)
S G Refried beans and corn tortilla
L S Wanton soup
L S G Lentil soup w/cashews (corn muffin)
S Barley soup: barley, turkey broth, carrots, and parsley
L G Turkey soup: turkey broth, carrots, white rose potato, corn, and lima beans
L G Mushroom barley soup w/rice and carrots
G Cheddar cheese soup
G Vegetable soup: red potatoes, celery, carrots, parsley, cilantro, olive oil, and Vege-Sal® w/sourdough toast and butter
L S G Black bean soup
S G Split pea soup and cashews (corn muffin)
L G Artichoke pasta, broccoli, and olive oil or butter, and Vege-Sal®
L S G Pasta and tomato sauce (basmati rice)
L S G Pasta, peas, parsley, and olive oil, or butter (carrots)
G Spinach pasta and cauliflower w/medium to light Cheddar cheese
G Pasta w/Parmesan cheese and steamed artichoke hearts (butter)
L G Tofu, rice, broccoli, and carrots w/soy sauce or tamari
L S G Rice noodles, peas, and feta cheese
L S G Spaghetti w/butter and broccoli (tomato sauce)
S G Oat bran muffin and broccoli, onions, and carrots
G Bagels and cheese, then fruit
S G Protein powder w/Re-Vita®
G Peanut butter and apple butter on rice cakes

EVENING SNACK:
(Optional) At least 1 hour after dinner 9 p.m.-2 a.m. Sweets, grain, legumes, vegetables, protein, nuts, seeds, dairy, fruit.

S G Pumpkin pie
G Ice cream
S G Cheese cake
S G Granola bar
L S Peaches, blueberries, casaba, or crenshaw melons
S G Cashews
L S G Raspberry or blueberry yogurt
S G Unsalted rice cake and hummus
G Rice cake w/peanut butter and apple butter
G Rice cake w/macadamia/cashew butter and banana
S*G Oat bran muffin
S Oat bran cereal
G Pumpkin bread
L S Oatmeal and butternut Re-Vita® (butter)
L S Nonfat milk w/Re-Vita®

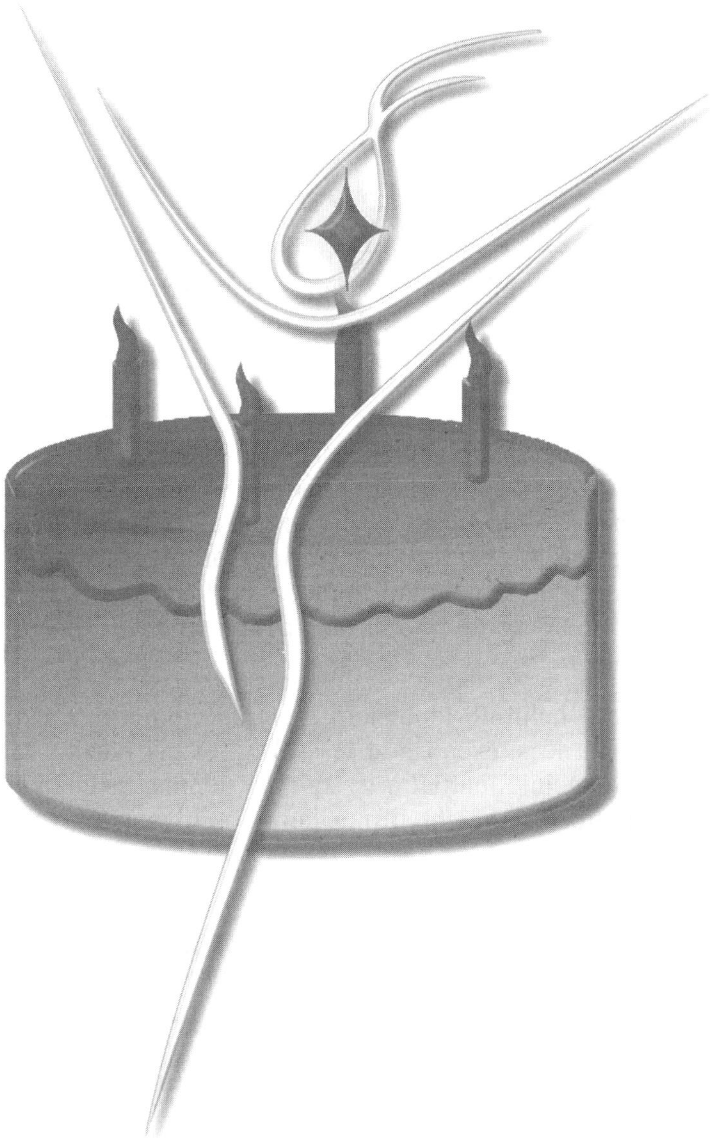

The "Pituitary Body Type"
is symbolized by a birthday cake.
Happy and light, they approach life
with a childlike openness and wide-eyed
innocence. Capable and responsible,
they are stimulated by new
ideas and concepts.

Pituitary

BODY TYPE PROFILE

LOCATION	Center of forehead, 1/2 inch above eyebrows and 2-3 inches into head.
FUNCTION	Governs endocrine system, as directed by hypothalamus; anterior lobe secretes hormones regulating function of thyroid, gonads, and adrenal cortex (consequently, of vital importance to growth, maturation, and reproduction); posterior lobe regulates kidneys through antidiuretic hormone and activates cholesterol production to increase hormone levels.
POTENTIAL HEALTH PROBLEMS	Generally very healthy and, because body is basically strong, it holds toxins in fluid between cells rather than storing them in organs – so weight maintenance, unfortunately, tends to be chronic problem. Also prone to edema (fluid retention) and asthma. Various problems relating to digestive system, including digestive disturbances and/or food allergies, bloating, gas, constipation or loose bowels, and development of ulcers.
RECOMMENDED EXERCISE	Exercise is helpful. Its benefit is initially emotional as it relieves stagnation. For weight loss, exercise at least 3 times per week. Mind/body integration, aerobic dancing, martial arts, Tai Chi, tennis, racquetball, hiking, or walking are beneficial. Weight lifting helps build muscle. Stretching assists body awareness.

WOMEN'S CHARACTERISTICS

DISTINGUISHING CHARACTERISTICS	Large head in proportion to rest of body and generally positioned in front of shoulders. Generally retain baby fat over entire body throughout life – giving soft, underdeveloped look. Stomach may be rounded like child's. Weight gain all over (like baby fat), especially around knees, which tend to be pudgy; or carried predominantly in abdomen. Prefer mental to physical activity. Known for making life fun.
ADDITIONAL PHYSICAL FEATURES	Buttocks relatively flat-to-prominent. Low back curvature straight-to-swayed. Breasts average–to-large. Shoulders relatively even with hips. Waist straight-to-defined. Average to short-waisted. Height petite-to-tall. Bone structure medium-to-large. Layer of softness covering muscles or average elongated musculature. Even when short, however, general appearance is often large. Well-defined, shapely calves. Hands and feet proportionate-to-large. Feet frequently wide. Often high forehead, wider than cheekbones by 1/4 inch or more. Ears centered toward back of head with more space above ears than behind. Face round, oval, or long oval. Soft, pliable skin, usually without blemishes.

Pituitary

WEIGHT GAIN AREAS	Entire body with initial gain evenly in soft rolls, or predominantly in lower abdomen, waist, upper hips, upper inner or entire thighs, inner knees, arms, hands, and legs (including knees). Secondary gain in entire abdomen, upper to entire back, upper arms, breasts, face, hands, feet, under chin, entire inner thighs or entire thighs to knees, and buttocks. Alternative weight gain pattern is predominantly in upper body on abdomen with small buttocks and little, if any, gain in thighs. Frequently have had weight problems since childhood or were very thin as children with weight gain afterwards. Occasionally have difficulty gaining weight.

DIETARY GUIDELINES

SCHEDULING MEALS

Breakfast: Heavy, with main emphasis on protein, vegetables, grain, nuts, seeds, legumes, and/or fruit. Rotate varieties.

Lunch: Moderate-to-heavy, with protein, vegetables, grain, nuts, seeds, legumes, dairy, and/or fruit. Salad is best after meat and grain.

Dinner: Light-to-moderate, with vegetables, legumes, and/or fruit.

DIETARY EMPHASIS

Adequate protein – either from concentrated plant sources, such as red algae, bee pollen, and Sunrider® herbs, or from animal protein prepared with as little fat as possible (beef, organ meat, chicken, fish); carbohydrates in moderation cooked and raw, with more cooked than raw when sensitive. Protein at breakfast supplies more energy and decreases appetite later in day: too little protein creates craving for sweets later on. Red meat and/or exercise stimulate adrenals.

- May include cheese as a group up to 2 times a week.
- May include nuts as a group up to 5 times a week.
- For weight loss, eliminate all dairy except butter, avoid breads, and reduce quantity of food. Eat substantial breakfast, including meat or fish, then wait 4-5 hours before having moderate lunch and another 6 hours before having very light dinner. May have evening snack. Can safely use appetite suppressants.
- For weight gain, simply increase food intake and include snacks.
- Vegetarian diet recommended as long as adequate protein is assimilated, although may consume up to 30% of caloric intake from dense protein.
- Fats, 20-25% from dense protein (all), butter, coconut milk, coconuts.

KEY SUPPORTS FOR SYSTEM

Best supporting foods include rice, chicken, and turkey. Include variety and rotate menus, particularly at breakfast. Insufficient protein consumption early in day will cause need to eat at night, with prominent desire being for sweets, particularly ice cream.

Pituitary

COMPLEMENTARY GLANDULAR SUPPORT	Thyroid, through consuming at least 3 oz. of dense protein (fish, eggs, chicken, or turkey) with a grain such as rice or pasta 5 times a week. Build adrenals through consuming vitamin C found in fruits and vegetables and dense protein (fish, eggs, chicken, or turkey), and stimulate adrenals with red meat and/or exercise.
FOODS CRAVED	*(When Energy is Low)* Creamy sweets and fats such as ice cream, pudding, cream pie, cream cheese, cheeses generally, and yogurt (including frozen yogurt); also, pastries, cookies, chocolate candy, dried fruit, fresh fruit, and sweet foods in general.
FOODS TO AVOID	Dairy products, refined carbohydrates, sugar, honey, white flour, caffeine, MSG. Avoid late night snacking.
RECOMMENDED CUISINE	Chinese, Mexican, Thai, Greek, Italian.

PSYCHOLOGICAL PROFILE

ESSENCE	Just as the pituitary gland controls growth hormones necessary for a child to grow, Pituitary body types manifest the childhood quality of making life fun. They approach life with a childlike openness and wide–eyed innocence that makes them fun to be around. As the master gland in charge of directing the entire body, the pituitary gland has to be extremely responsible. Likewise, Pituitaries are naturally capable, responsible people. Lighthearted and creative, Pituitaries are stimulated by new ideas and concepts which they use to bring happiness.
CHARACTERISTIC TRAITS	Pituitary types are characterized by a childlike openness, curiosity, and creativity. Their bodies tend to have a certain soft, childlike look – large head with a kind of soft cushion of fat over the body, predominantly on the abdomen. Just as a baby learns more in the first six months than at any other time during its life, the Pituitary type exemplifies a grown-up version of that amazing mental acuity, curiosity, and stimulation, as well as the basic joy and love of life of a young child. Pituitaries can and must constantly learn and be stimulated by fresh, new ideas and concepts to bring more joy and happiness into their environment and the world in general. Their basic nature is kind, considerate, and compassionate. They easily connect with people and enjoy them. With good verbal skills, Pituitaries readily communicate their thoughts and feelings. Sensitive to the feelings of others, Pituitaries are extremely tactful and diplomatic, excelling at "people skills".

Pituitary

CHARACTERISTIC TRAITS

Pituitaries tend to take things in stride. They are not likely to get upset about circumstances beyond their control. Even in a tense situation, they can assume a certain philosophical detachment rather than reacting with anger or frustration. They are able to accept things as they are without feeling a strong need to manipulate or change them. Although analytical, they are rarely judgmental or critical of others, and can see both sides of most situations.

Pituitaries have a high degree of mental acuity and clarity, which they balance through trusting their intuition. They are logical, analytical, and systematic with a natural aptitude for computers, including the mental programming of the mind. There is a flexibility to their intellectual precision. Their soft, gentle exterior and cheerfulness, often conceals a resiliance and inner strength that generally only becomes apparent over time.

Most of the Pituitaries' energy is in their head, which is apparent by its physical size and their intellect. Balance through physical expression, including weight management, requires moving energy down into the body. Physical exercise is a definite challenge for Pituitaries and requires much personal discipline. Even though activities that promote mind/body integration are effective, Pituitaries rarely make these activities spontaneous occurences.

MOTIVATION

External stimulation provides the motivation for Pituitaries to grow and change, while feeling happy gives them their greatest sense of satisfaction. Imaginative with good reasoning abilities, they're stimulated by learning new things and have an excellent aptitude for concepts and ideas. While mentally precise and adept at handling abstract details, Pituitaries bring a lightness into learning by approaching life with a childlike openness, curiosity, and creativity.

Their respect of others and of life in general is reflected in their altruistic attitude of helpfulness and harmony. Generous and giving, they will take on more than they can realistically handle. Pituitaries tend to spread themselves too thin until they've learned to set appropriate limits as to what others can expect of them. By being sociable and receptive, Pituitary types foster an attitude of cooperation and agreement, making them quite successful in getting others to agree to what they want.

Dependable and reliable, Pituitaries will keep their promises and do what they say to the best of their ability. They will stay with a problem or project until they have successfully completed it. This persistence also applies to people and situations. They are very forgiving in relationships until they have reached the point where they are finished. Once they have learned what they need to learn and feel complete with a relationship, it's over. Mentally focused and internally motivated, Pituitaries are good at setting goals for themselves and then doing whatever is necessary to reach them.

Conflict makes Pituitaries feel vulnerable or uneasy, so they delay discussing things that may provoke others. Instead, they are inclined to smooth things over or "fix" things in order to postpone confrontation. Even when they know that an unresolved conflict must eventually be faced, they will still let a problem build up until it explodes or they are otherwise forced to deal with it.

Pituitary

"AT WORST'

When the mental becomes unbalanced, the power of their determination can take on a headstrong or obstinate quality. Fearful, they can become domineering and controlling. They may develop a skeptical attitude or swing to the opposite extreme of becoming weak or wishy-washy. In their desire to help or protect, they can become so focused on what they feel is right that they will become picky, overly concerned with details.

Procrastination is common when Pituitaries have to make a decision or tackle something about which they are ambivalent. They tend to avoid doing things they perceive as unpleasant or difficult. Instead, they'll go for something fun such as eating creamy foods like ice cream that stimulate the pituitary gland.

Feeling vulnerable or uneasy, Pituitaries will censor their emotions and block them out of their minds. Highly developed mentally, there is a tendency to live in their heads and escape into fantasy – living in a world of make-believe, books, movies, television, or the computer. They may also use sleep, meditation, drugs, or alcohol as forms of escape.

Needing to experience the physical world, but often lacking stamina, Pituitaries are apt to experiment with recreational drugs. Sexual addictions or fantasies, when there is a lack of social skills, are common. Food can also be a source of comfort and there is a strong tendency toward obesity.

With low self-esteem, they can become trapped in addictive, co-dependent, or physically abusive relationships that keep them stifled. They can lose touch with reality and become irresponsible or self-centered, doing only what makes them feel happy in the moment. Using their innocence to play on other people's sympathies to support a habit, Pituitaries can resort to lying, making promises they have no intention of keeping, or being a "fair-weather" friend.

"AT BEST"

Pituitaries are happy and bring happiness to everyone they encounter. Their whole orientation to life is characterized by a childlike openness, curiosity, and creativity. People love infants because of their connection with Spirit, and Pituitaries are able to retain this connection, bringing happiness into the adult world.

Maintaining their connection with their spiritual nature enables Pituitaries to express their divinity through their mind and body in the physical realm. They know they have the power to change and can accomplish whatever they desire, even though it may be difficult. They also know that others can achieve the same goals and are able to effectively communicate this awareness.

Pituitaries have a positive attitude toward themselves and life in general, enabling them to bounce back from adversity. Displaying a basic joy and love of life, they are outgoing and gregarious, relaxed, and easygoing. They have learned to balance their mental development with practical knowledge or common sense through physical activity and play. Relying on their intuition

Pituitary

"AT BEST"
(Continued)

when dealing with unfamiliar information allows them to make the right decisions without lengthy deliberation.

Open to new concepts and ideas, Pituitaries possess a gentle quality, a freshness and receptivity, yet are also prudent and practical. Reliable and dependable with a good aptitude for detail and high integrity, Pituitaries accomplish what they commit to do. Self-motivated by their strong sense of wonder and curiosity, or finding new and challenging aspects of a situation, project, or relationship, Pituitaries are able to fulfill their mission of bringing happiness to the world.

Pituitary

FOOD LISTS

HEALTHY FOOD LIST

FREQUENTLY FOODS	3-7 meals per week – refers to each food, rather than category.
DENSE PROTEIN	Beef with visible fat removed, beef broth, beef liver, organ meats (heart, brain), buffalo; chicken, chicken broth, chicken livers, turkey; halibut
DAIRY	Butter
CHEESE	Swiss, regular cottage
LEGUMES	Hummus
GRAINS	Corn, corn bread, corn grits, corn tortillas, oats, rice (all varieties), rice bran, rice cakes, cream of rice
VEGETABLES	Green beans, carrots, grape leaves, jicama, sweet potatoes
FRUITS	Tart apples (Pippin, Granny Smith), bananas, cherries, green grapes, cantaloupes
SWEETENERS	Re-Vita®, stevia
CONDIMENTS	Lite salt, tahini
BEVERAGES	Herbal teas (peppermint, camomile, rose hips, Good Earth® herb blend), Green Magma®
MODERATELY FOODS	1-2 meals per week – refers to each food, rather than category.
DENSE PROTEIN	Lamb, pork, ham, bacon, sausage, veal, venison; cornish game hen, duck; anchovy, bass, bonita, catfish, cod, flounder, haddock, herring, mahi-mahi, mackerel, perch, orange roughy, salmon, sardines, shark, red snapper, sole, swordfish, trout, tuna; abalone, calamari (squid), clams, crab, eel, lobster, mussels, octopus, oysters, scallops, shrimp; eggs
DAIRY	Milk (whole, 2%, low fat, nonfat, raw), flavored yogurt
CHEESE	American, blue, brie, Camembert, Cheddar, Colby, cream, Edam, feta, Gouda, Jack, kefir, Limburger, mozzarella, Muenster, Parmesan, ricotta, Romano
NUTS and SEEDS	Almonds (raw, roasted), almond butter, Brazils, cashews (raw, roasted), cashew butter, water chestnuts, coconuts, filberts, hazelnuts, macadamias (raw,roasted), macadamia butter, peanuts (raw, roasted), peanut butter, pecans, pine nuts (raw, roasted), pistachios, walnuts (black, English), raw or roasted seeds (caraway, pumpkin, sesame, sunflower), sesame seed butter, sunflower seed butter
LEGUMES	Beans (adzuki, black, garbanzo, kidney, lima [butter], navy, great northern, pinto, red, soy), lentils, black-eyed peas, split peas, miso, soy milk, tofu

Pituitary

GRAINS	Amaranth, barley, buckwheat, hominy grits, millet, popcorn, quinoa, rye, triticale, breads (sourdough, garlic, oat, corn, corn/rye, rye, sesame pita, rice), flour tortillas, crackers (saltines, wheat, oat, rye), pasta, couscous, udon noodles, rice noodles, fried rice, cream of rye
VEGETABLES	Asparagus, artichokes, avocados, bamboo shoots, yellow wax beans, lima beans, beets, bok choy, broccoli, broccoflower, brussels sprouts, cooked cabbage (green, napa, red), cauliflower, celery, chard, cilantro, corn, cucumbers, eggplant, garlic, greens (beet, collard, mustard, turnip), hominy, kale, kohlrabi, leeks, lettuce (Boston, butter, endive, iceberg, red leaf, romaine), mushrooms, okra, olives (green, ripe), onions (chives, green, brown, red, white, yellow, vidalia), parsnips, parsley, peas, snow pea pods, bell peppers (green, red, yellow), chili peppers, pimentos, pumpkin, potatoes (all varieties), radishes, daikon radishes, rutabaga, sauerkraut, seaweed (arame, dulse, kelp, nori, wakame), shallots, spinach, sprouts (alfalfa, clover, mung bean, radish, sunflower), squash (acorn, banana, butternut, spaghetti, yellow [summer], zucchini), cooked tomatoes (canned, hot–house, vine–ripened), turnips, watercress, yams
FRUITS	Apples (Golden or Red Delicious, Jonathan, McIntosh, Rome Beauty), apricots, blackberries, blueberries, boysenberries, cranberries, gooseberries, raspberries, strawberries, grapes (black, red), grapefruits (white, red), guavas, kiwi, kumquats, lemons, loquats, limes, mangos, nectarines, oranges, papayas, peaches, pears, persimmons, plums (black, purple, red), pomegranates, rhubarb, tangelos, tangerines, dates, figs (fresh, dried), prunes, raisins
FRUIT JUICES	Apple, apple cider, apple/apricot, apricot, black cherry, red cherry, cranapple, cranberry, grape (purple, red, white), orange, grapefruit, guava, lemon, papaya, pear, pineapple, pineapple/coconut, prune, raspberry, tangerine, watermelon
VEGETABLE OILS	All-blend, almond, avocado, canola, corn, flaxseed, peanut, olive, safflower, sesame, soy, sunflower
SWEETENERS	Honey, molasses, sorghum, brown sugar, date sugar, raw sugar, maple syrup, brown rice syrup, barley malt syrup, corn syrup, fructose, succonant, saccharin
CONDIMENTS	Curry, cinnamon, chili powder, horseradish, barbecue sauce, pesto sauce, salsa, tempeh, vinegar, salt, sea salt, Vege-Sal®
SALAD DRESSINGS	Blue cheese, French, ranch, creamy Italian, creamy avocado, thousand island, vinegar and oil, lemon juice and oil
DESSERTS	Custards, tapioca, puddings, pies, cakes, raspberry sherbet, orange sherbet
CHIPS	Bean, corn (blue, white, yellow), potato
BEVERAGES	Decaffeinated coffee; decaffeinated tea; Cafix®; Perrier® water, Arrowhead® carbonated water, mineral water; wine (red, white), sake, beer, barley malt liquor, champagne, brandy, gin, Scotch, vodka, whiskey

Pituitary

RARELY FOODS	No more than once a month
DAIRY	Goat milk, buttermilk, half & half, sweet cream, sour cream, kefir, plain yogurt, frozen yogurt, ice cream
CHEESE	Low fat cottage, goat
GRAINS	Whole wheat, wheat bran, wheat germ, sprouted wheat, refined wheat flour, breads (French, Italian, white, 7-grain, multi-grain, sprouted grain, whole wheat), bagels (plain, sesame seed), croissants, English muffins, cream of wheat
VEGETABLES	Arugula, raw cabbage (green, napa, red), raw tomatoes (canned, hot house, vine-ripened)
VEGETABLE JUICES	Celery, carrot, carrot/celery, parsley, spinach, tomato, V8®
FRUITS	Melons (casaba, crenshaw, honeydew, watermelon), pineapples
SWEETENERS	Refined cane sugar, aspartame, Equal®, Sweet'n Low®, NutraSweet®
CONDIMENTS	Catsup, mayonnaise, margarine, mustard, soy sauce
DESSERTS	Chocolate, desserts containing chocolate
BEVERAGES	Coffee; black tea, green tea, Japanese tea, Chinese oolong tea; root beer, diet sodas, regular sodas

SENSITIVE FOOD LIST

FREQUENTLY FOODS	3–7 meals per week – refers to each food, rather than category.
DENSE PROTEIN	Beef with visible fat removed, beef broth, beef liver, organ meats (heart, brain), buffalo; turkey, chicken, chicken broth, chicken livers
GRAINS	Corn tortillas, rice (all varieties), rice bran, rice cakes, cream of rice
VEGETABLES	Green beans, carrots, grape leaves, sweet potatoes
FRUITS	Tart apples (Pippin, Granny Smith), bananas, cherries, green grapes
BEVERAGES	Herbal teas (peppermint, camomile, rose hips, Good Earth® herb blend), Green Magma®
MODERATELY FOODS	1–2 meals per week – refers to each food, rather than category.
DENSE PROTEIN	Lamb, pork, ham, bacon, sausage, veal, venison; cornish game hen, duck; anchovy, bass, bonita, catfish, cod, flounder, haddock, halibut, herring, mahi-mahi, mackerel, perch, orange roughy, salmon, sardines, shark, red snapper, sole, swordfish, trout, tuna; abalone, calamari (squid), clams, crab, eel, lobster, mussels, octopus, oysters, scallops, shrimp; eggs

Pituitary

DAIRY	Butter
CHEESE	American, blue, brie, Camembert, Cheddar, Colby, regular cottage, cream, Edam, feta, Gouda, kefir, Limburger, mozzarella, Muenster, Parmesan, ricotta, Romano, Swiss
NUTS and SEEDS	Almonds (raw, roasted), almond butter, Brazils, cashews (raw, roasted), cashew butter, water chestnuts, filberts, hazelnuts, macadamias (raw, roasted), macadamia butter, peanuts (raw, roasted), peanut butter, pecans, pine nuts (raw, roasted), pistachios, walnuts (black, English), raw or roasted seeds (caraway, pumpkin, sesame, sunflower), sesame seed butter, sunflower seed butter
LEGUMES	Beans (adzuki, black, garbanzo, kidney, lima [butter], navy, great northern, pinto, red, soy), lentils, black-eyed peas, split peas, hummus, miso, soy milk, tofu
GRAINS	Amaranth, barley, buckwheat, corn, corn bread, corn grits, hominy grits, millet, oats, popcorn, quinoa, rye, triticale, flour tortillas, breads (sourdough, garlic, oat, corn, corn/rye, rye, sesame pita, rice), crackers (saltines, wheat, oat, rye), rice noodles, fried rice, cream of rye
VEGETABLES	Asparagus, artichokes, avocados, bamboo shoots, yellow wax beans, lima beans, beets, bok choy, broccoli, broccoflower, brussels sprouts, cooked cabbage (green, napa, red), steamed cauliflower, celery, chard, cilantro, corn, cucumbers, eggplant, garlic, greens (beet, collard, mustard, turnip), hominy, jicama, kale, kohlrabi, leeks, lettuce (Boston, butter, endive, iceberg, red leaf, romaine), mushrooms, okra, olives (green, ripe), onions (chives, green, brown, red, white, yellow, vidalia), parsley, parsnips, peas, snow pea pods, bell peppers (green, red, yellow), chili peppers, pimentos, potatoes (red, white rose, russet, yukon gold, purple), pumpkin, radishes, daikon radishes, rutabaga, sauerkraut, seaweed (arame, dulse, kelp, nori, wakame), shallots, spinach, sprouts (alfalfa, clover, mung bean, radish, sunflower), squash (acorn, banana, butternut, spaghetti, yellow [summer], zucchini), cooked tomatoes (canned, hot house, vine-ripened), turnips, yams
FRUITS	Apples (Golden or Red Delicious, Jonathan, McIntosh, Rome Beauty), apricots, blackberries, blueberries, boysenberries, cranberries, gooseberries, raspberries, strawberries, cantaloupes, grapes (black, red), grapefruits (white, red), guavas, kiwi, kumquats, lemons, limes, loquats, mangos, nectarines, oranges, papayas, peaches, pears, persimmons, plums (black, purple, red), pomegranates, rhubarb, tangelos, tangerines, dates, figs (fresh, dried), prunes, raisins
FRUIT JUICES	Apple, apple cider, apple/apricot, apricot, black cherry, red cherry, cranapple, cranberry, grape (purple, red, white), grapefruit, guava, lemon, orange, papaya, pear, pineapple, pineapple/coconut, prune, raspberry, tangerine, watermelon
VEGETABLE OILS	All-blend
SWEETENERS	Re-Vita®, stevia

Pituitary

CONDIMENTS	Salt, sea salt, Vege-Sal®
SALAD DRESSINGS	Lemon juice and oil
BEVERAGES	Mineral water, sparkling water
RARELY FOODS	No more than once a month
DAIRY	Milk (whole, 2%, low fat, nonfat, raw), goat milk, buttermilk, half & half, sweet cream, sour cream, kefir, plain or flavored yogurt, frozen yogurt, ice cream
CHEESE	Low fat cottage, Jack, goat
NUTS and SEEDS	Coconuts
GRAINS	Whole wheat, wheat bran, wheat germ, sprouted wheat, refined wheat flour, breads (French, Italian, 7-grain, multi-grain, sprouted grain, white, whole wheat), croissants, bagels, English muffins, pasta, couscous, udon noodles, cream of wheat
VEGETABLES	Arugula, raw cabbage (green, napa, red), raw tomatoes (hot house, vine-ripened), watercress
SALAD DRESSINGS	Blue cheese, French, ranch, creamy Italian, creamy avocado, thousand island, vinegar and oil
VEGETABLE JUICES	Celery, carrot, carrot/celery, parsley, spinach, tomato, V8®
VEGETABLE OILS	Almond, avocado, canola, corn, flaxseed, olive, peanut, safflower, sesame, soy, sunflower
FRUITS	Melons (casaba, crenshaw, honeydew, watermelon), pineapples
SWEETENERS	Honey, molasses, sorghum, raw sugar, refined cane sugar, brown sugar, fructose, date sugar, maple syrup, brown rice syrup, barley malt syrup, corn syrup, saccharin, succonant, aspartame, Equal®, Sweet'n Low®, NutraSweet®
CONDIMENTS	Catsup, mustard, mayonnaise, margarine, soy sauce, tempeh, horseradish, barbecue sauce, pesto sauce, salsa, tahini, vinegar, curry, cinnamon, chili powder
CHIPS	Bean, corn (blue, white, yellow), potato
DESSERTS	Chocolate, desserts containing chocolate, custards, tapioca, puddings, pies, cakes, raspberry sherbet, orange sherbet
BEVERAGES	Decaffeinated coffee, regular coffee, coffee with Re-Vita®; black tea, green tea, Japanese tea, Chinese oolong tea, regular tea; Cafix®; wine (red, white), beer, barley malt liquor, champagne, brandy, gin, Scotch, vodka, whiskey; root beer, diet sodas, regular sodas

Pituitary

MENUS

DIETARY EMPHASIS:

- Adequate protein – either from concentrated plant sources such as red algae, bee pollen, and Sunrider® herbs, or from animal protein prepared with as little fat as possible (beef, organ meat, chicken, fish).
- Protein at breakfast supplies more energy and decreases appetite later in day; too little protein creates craving for sweets later on.
- Red meat and/or exercise to stimulate adrenals.
- Carbohydrates in moderation (preferably whole grains).
- Abundant fruits and vegetables. Balance between cooked and raw, with more cooked than raw when sensitive.
- Best supporting foods include rice, chicken, and turkey.
- Include variety, and rotate menus, particularly at breakfast.
- May include cheese as group up to 2 times a week.
- May include nuts as group up to 5 times a week.

WEIGHT LOSS:

- Reduce quantity of food.
- Avoid breads.
- Eliminate all dairy except butter.
- Fats 20-25%. If below 15%, will gain weight.
- Follow meal schedule by eating a substantial breakfast including meat or fish, wait 4-5 hours, then have a moderate lunch, wait 6 hours, then have a very light dinner. May have evening snack.
- Can safely use appetite suppressants.

WEIGHT GAIN:

- Simply increase food intake.
- Include snacks.

VEGETARIAN DIET:

- Recommended as long as adequate protein is assimilated, although may consume up to 30% of caloric intake from dense protein.

FATS:

- 20-25%of caloric intake.
- Best sources are dense protein (all), butter, coconut milk, coconuts.

KEY

—all menus may be used by healthy persons

( ) around foods means that they're optional

L denotes weight loss menus

S denotes sensitive menus

G denotes weight gain menus

BREAKFAST:
7-8 a.m. Heavy, with main emphasis on protein, vegetables, grain, nuts, seeds, legumes, and/or fruit. Rotate varieties.

	S	G	Eggs, potatoes or rice, and sourdough bread
L	S	G	Eggs or turkey and rice
L		G	Scrambled egg and turkey sausage (fruit)
		G	Egg, chicken, and English muffin
		G	Egg and sausage burrito
L		G	Eggs and protein drink w/apple or cranberry juice and water
L		G	Orange juice, then turkey and eggs
L		G	Bacon or beef, eggs, potatoes, and corn tortilla
L	S	G	Steak and eggs or potatoes
L		G	Corned beef hash and eggs
L		G	Ham and scrambled eggs or potatoes
L		G	Ham and black beans
L		G	Ham, Brazil nuts, and stir-fry: zucchini, onions, squash, and mushrooms (orange juice)
L		G	Beef stew w/potatoes
L		G	Lean hamburger, potato, onions, and green beans
L		G	Sausage and pancakes
		G	Turkey sausage, toast, and orange
L		G	Turkey ham and Rye Krisp®
			Fruit, then turkey and brown basmati or Japanese rice
L	S		Shrimp or chicken, rice, and mixed vegetables
		G	Tuna, lettuce or avocado, and oat bread
L			Protein powder w/banana, cherries, strawberries, or soy milk

Pituitary

L	Sweet potato and 1/2 tsp butter
L	Potato (couscous)
L S	Acorn squash – baked or steamed – w/rice
L	Steamed broccoli, lima beans, and corn
	California roll and miso soup
L	Oat bread toast and sugarless jam
L	Fruit juice w/Re-Vita®

BREAKFAST or LUNCH:

L G	Turkey and sweet potatoes (peas)
L G	Chicken, rice, and corn
L G	Chicken breast, potato, and green beans
G	Chicken enchiladas
L G	Deviled egg, chicken breast, and potato salad
L G	Pork chops or sausage, peas, rice or potato, and onions, chilies, or garlic
L G	Beef vegetable stew
L G	Swordfish and sweet potatoes
L S G	Broiled sea bass, salmon, halibut, or shark, w/lemon and rice
L S G	Tuna, pasta, and peas, or green beans
L S G	Halibut, rice, and asparagus, or green beans
L G	Shark, sea bass, halibut, or salmon, baked potato, butter, and chives (steamed carrots)
L S G	Shark, rice, mixed vegetables, and asparagus or broccoli
L S G	Lamb chop, potato, asparagus and/or beets, or beets and beet greens
G	Potato, Cheddar cheese, and broccoli

MID-MORNING SNACK:
(Optional) 10 a.m. Grain, vegetables.

G	Granola
S G	Popcorn
	Decaffeinated coffee
	Herbal tea

LUNCH:
12-2 p.m. Moderate-to-heavy, with protein, vegetables, grain, nuts, seeds, legumes, dairy and/or fruit. Salad is best after meat and grain.

L S	Egg, rice, and broccoli
L S	Rice, broccoli, carrots, cauliflower, and onions
S G	Rice, beans, and Swiss cheese
S G	Rice or potatoes and lentils
L S	Basmati rice and carrots or green peas
L S G	Squash, rice, and pumpkin seeds
L S G	Lentils, rice, and mushrooms, or black beans
L G	Vegetable curry w/rice (beef or chicken)
L S G	2 scrambled eggs and rice w/parsley (cilantro)
L G	Beef sandwich on rye or sourdough, then salad: bell pepper or cucumber, carrots, jicama, and spinach
G	Tacos w/meat and cheese
L G	Sirloin tips, carrots, string beans, gravy, apple sauce, and green salad
L G	Lean roast beef, rice, then salad: lettuce and carrots
L G	Broiled lamb chops and rice, then salad: romaine lettuce, grated carrots, parsley, green onion, celery, and red wine vinegar
L G	Lamb gyro sandwich – no sauce – and avocado or apple (vegetables)
L G	Lamb sandwich on oat, rye, or sourdough bread
L S G	Chicken and rice (peas)
G	Chicken breast, pasta, mushrooms, and Parmesan cheese
L S G	Chicken, chinese vegetables, and rice (egg drop soup)
G	Chicken, noodles, and mixed vegetables
L G	Chicken burrito: flour tortilla, vegetables, chicken, and lettuce w/rice and beans
L G	Chicken tostada: corn tortilla, chicken, lettuce, corn, and red onion
L G	Chicken tostada w/beans and rice
L G	Turkey and raw broccoli

Pituitary

L G Tostada: corn tortilla, shredded turkey, and lettuce

L G Cornish game hen stuffed w/long grain and wild rice, then cucumber and cold pea salad or mixed salad

L G Tuna, and any variety rice, then bell peppers, and jicama

L G Tuna on sourdough bread, raw broccoli, red peppers, carrots, and/or celery

L S G Salmon, rice, green beans, and broccoli

L S G Sole, baked potato, and broccoli

L S G Halibut, rice, and corn

L S G Shrimp and stir-fry vegetables w/soy sauce

L S G Shrimp or lobster, corn, lima beans, and broccoli

S G Swordfish and rice

S G Swordfish, salmon or tuna, and potatoes

L G Egg salad on sourdough bread

L G Fish, pasta, and mixed vegetables: squash, green beans, peas, and corn

S G Pinto beans and rice

S Vegetables, such as broccoli, carrots, cauliflower, onions, green onions, and/or yellow squash w/soy sauce

L G Pasta and salad: romaine or leaf lettuce, carrots, cucumber, parsley, and garbanzo beans w/oil and vinegar or lite Italian dressing

L G Chicken noodle soup

L G Hot and sour soup w/rice (chicken and snow peas)

L S G Beef soup: beef, carrots, celery, parsley, and onion

MID-AFTERNOON SNACK:
(Optional) 4 p.m. Fruit.

G Apple, orange, or banana

DINNER:
5:30-6 p.m. (7 p.m. is okay if after a 4 p.m. fruit snack.) Light-to-moderate, with vegetables, legumes, and/or fruit.

L S G Red potatoes, steamed broccoli, and carrots

L G Squash w/butternut Re-Vita®

G Peas and potatoes

L G Sweet potato and green beans

L G Beets and cucumber salad w/Italian dressing

L S G Salad: romaine lettuce, finely diced cauliflower, broccoli, and cucumbers w/vinegar and olive oil

L G Salad: lettuce, garbanzo beans, green pepper, red pepper, and raw zucchini w/Caesar dressing

L G Green salad w/non-creamy dressing

S G Romaine lettuce salad w/Italian salad dressing

S G Artichokes, butter, and tarragon or dill

L G Spinach salad (grapes)

L G Artichoke and raw carrot, or steamed or raw cauliflower

S G Split pea soup w/rice

L G Cream of mushroom soup w/lentils

L G Wonton soup

L G Vegetable soup cooked in chicken broth, and green salad

L G Vegetable curry

L G Stewed apples w/cinnamon (sourdough bread)

L G Apple, banana, cherries, or green grapes

S G Strawberries

S G Papaya juice, banana, and mango smoothie

L G Diced orange and banana or dried cherries

EVENING SNACK:
(Optional) 10-11 p.m. Fruit, vegetables, grain, nuts, seeds, sweets.

S G Corn flakes and almond milk

S G Popcorn (w/soy sauce)

G Rice cake

L G Oatmeal treat: oat flour, oatmeal, butter, and Re-Vita®

G Bran muffin w/apple butter or cherry jam

S G Plain rice w/cherries or blueberries

L S G Smoothie w/ice, banana, cherries, or berries

L S G Cantaloupe (blueberries)

G Oatmeal or peanut butter cookies

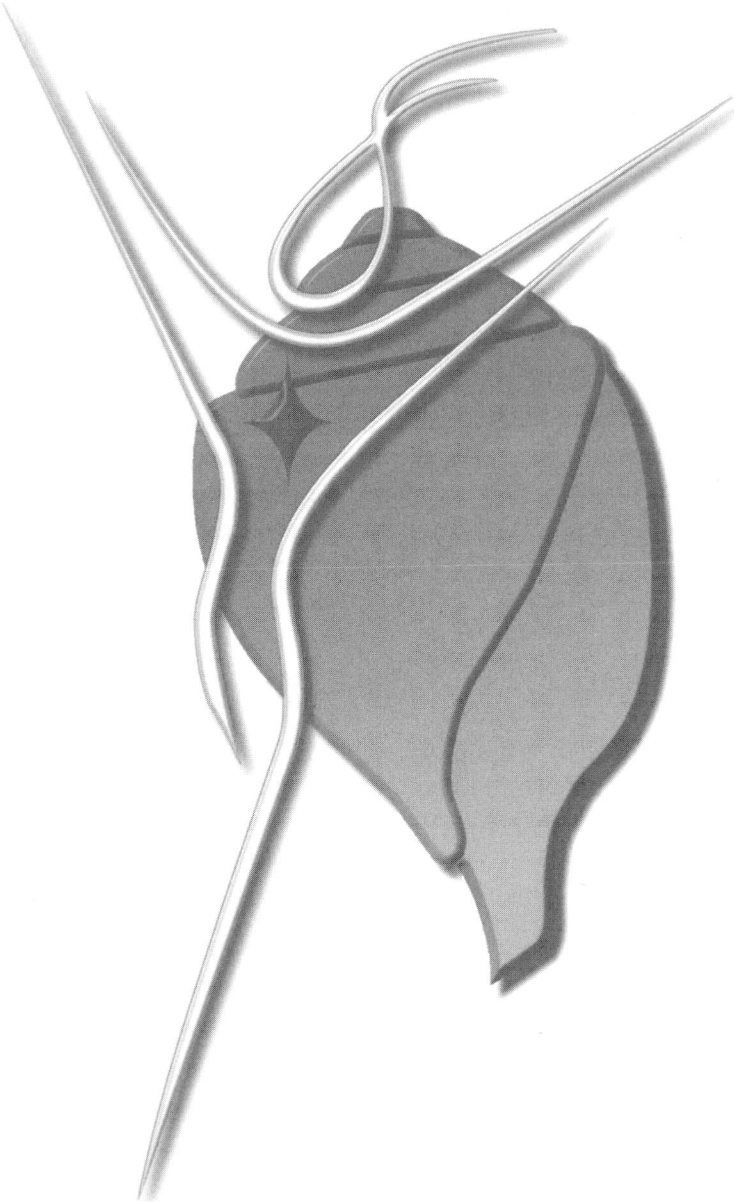

The "Skin Body Type" is symbolized by a conch shell. The skin forms the outer shell that connects with the outside world. Sensitive to emotions, subtle energies and vibrations, they communicate largely through their expanded sense of touch.

SKIN

Skin

BODY TYPE PROFILE

LOCATION	Covers entire body.
FUNCTION	Sensory organ of touch and second largest elimination organ. Provides body with its borders and boundaries.
POTENTIAL HEALTH PROBLEMS	Skin either very good, particularly when dark, or, when fair, frequently sensitive or prone to skin rashes or blemishes. Subject to vascular weakness, especially affecting head, and to lung, bronchial, or respiratory infections. May have difficulty digesting animal protein. Body highly reactive to foods – e.g., stimulants, depressants, additives. Can easily become addicted to foods, such as chocolate or cola (caffeine), particularly when used to alleviate pain (whether physical or emotional).
RECOMMENDED EXERCISE	Exercise is optional. Its benefit is emotional. It is a way of connecting with people and expressing emotions. Stretching, even for few minutes each day (ideally, 15) is by far the most beneficial way of supporting the body. Daily activities and general bodily movement along with stretching is generally sufficient. Additional exercise needs to be fun, such as walking, swimming, Tai Chi, and dancing. Avoid repetitive movement exercise, such as weight-lifting or aerobics, since it causes excessive muscle fatigue. Change program at least every 3 months.

WOMEN'S CHARACTERISTICS

DISTINGUISHING FEATURES	Soft, gentle appearance. Full face, which gets fuller with weight gain. Puffiness in hands and feet to extent that tendons in back of hands not visible, even at ideal weight. Hands (with ring size going up and down) and feet good barometers of weight gain and fluid retention. Prone to excess weight gain, particularly after puberty, childbirth, injury, illness, or emotional stress. Communicate through feeling.
ADDITIONAL PHYSICAL CHARACTERISTICS	Rounded-to-prominent buttocks, generally firm and shapely, occasionally flat. Low back curvature can range from straight-to-swayed. Breasts small-to-large. Shoulders relatively even with hips. Square, flat upper back extending across shoulders and shoulder blades with relatively straight torso extending to waist. Average to short-waisted. Straight-to-defined waist. Layer of softness covering muscles, or average elongated musculature. Height very petite (less than 5 ft.) to tall. Usually medium-to-large bone structure, but with small-to-average hands and often wide feet. Average-to-long oval or round face. Mouth either wide with full lips, or small (often rosebud-shaped).

Skin

WEIGHT GAIN AREAS	Lower body with initial gain in lower abdomen, upper hips, waist, middle back, face, and entire upper 2/3rds of thighs, including upper inner, thighs. Secondary gain in buttocks, back, then all over – including upper arms, hands, and feet. Alternative weight gain pattern: entire abdomen, upper hips, waist, face, and inner thighs with little, if any, on outer thighs. Being sensitive to physical and emotional energies around them, will often use weight to buffer or protect themselves from unpleasant vibrations. Majority of weight carried in torso – either predominantly in front of body, or balanced between abdomen and buttocks.

DIETARY GUIDELINES

SCHEDULING MEALS

"HEALTHY"

Breakfast: Light, with grain, vegetables, nuts, seeds, and/or fruit.

Lunch: Moderate-to-heavy, with vegetables, grain, nuts, seeds, legumes, protein, fruit, and/or dairy.

Dinner: Light-to-moderate, early (by 6 p.m.), with protein, grains vegetables, nuts, seeds, and/or legumes.

"SENSITIVE"

Same as "Healthy", but may include protein at breakfast.

DIETARY EMPHASIS

- Vegetables, brown or wild rice with vegetables. Keep meals and foods simple. Follow basic food-combining rules: avoid combining protein and grains (sandwiches), protein and fruit, protein and citrus or acids (meat and tomato sauce), two proteins (meat and milk or cream sauce), or acids and starches (vinegar and rice). Most vegetables combine well with protein and with starches. Milk may be used with other foods, including cereal, or may be taken after a meal as a moderate food. Sunrider herbs often effective in rebuilding body. Eat melons alone. Avoid refined cane sugar, as can cause muscle degeneration and weight gain. Dairy foods often interfere with memory.
- For weight loss, eliminate refined sugar, alcohol, dairy, breads (because of yeast and sweetener), and reduce salt; consume 15-30% of calories from dense protein, or use Sunrider herbs along with vegetarian diet; reduce quantity of food; rotate and use variety; and limit fats to 25% of total calories. However, if dietary fat falls below 10% from appropriate sources (see "fats" below) weight loss will not occur. Stretch at least 15 minutes per day.
- For weight gain, simply increase food consumption.
- Vegetarian diet recommended when healthy, although up to 35% of caloric intake may consist of dense protein.

Skin

DIETARY EMPHASIS

• Fats, 10-30% of caloric intake. Best sources are almonds, sunflower and sesame seeds, tahini, avocados, olive oil, fish, meat, and poultry. May use Hain Creamy Italian or Avocado dressing instead of mayonnaise.

KEY SUPPORTS FOR SYSTEM

Brown or wild rice with vegetables, whole grains, and cashews. Follow basic food-combining rules. Meals and foods should be kept simple. Watermelon, as well as other melons, best eaten alone. Sweets, if eaten at all, best consumed after dinner, as dessert. As way of checking foods before eating, useful to employ muscle testing or, eventually, to "sense" what body may require (i.e., filter out extraneous stimuli and simply listen to your body). Sunrider herbs often effective in rebuilding body.

COMPLEMENTARY GLANDULAR SUPPORT

Lungs, through nurturing self and/or others; kidneys, through building courage (by experiencing that it's safe to do things differently – something as minor as varying daily routine or adding something new 2 times a week may be sufficient).

FOODS CRAVED

(When Energy is Low) Chocolate (can easily become addictive), carbohydrates, like chocolate with nuts, cookies, candy, ice cream, bagels, or rice. Protein, such as shrimp, chicken, beef, and fish. When system is balanced, rice and vegetables, beans, and almonds.

FOODS TO AVOID

Refined cane sugar, as it depletes glucose stores in muscles, resulting in muscle degeneration and also robs body of its mineral stores, leading to weight gain (often excessive). Alcohol consumption because the liver can't detoxify. Most dairy foods as they can interfere with memory.

RECOMMENDED CUISINE

Mandarin Chinese, Cantonese, Sushi, Japanese (soups and noodle dishes). Moderately, Mexican, Filipino, Seafood. Simple foods, like soups, potatoes, and roasted meats.

Skin

PSYCHOLOGICAL PROFILE

ESSENCE

Just as the skin communicates with the outside world, Skin body types communicate through feeling. Feelings are used as a way of receiving information. While they are generally very open to others and their environment, when stressed, Skins will retreat by detaching, disassociating, or essentially closing down and turning their focus inward. Strongly attached to and affected by their environment, Skins have a strong connection with the earth, nature, and animals which allows them to naturally recharge. Highly visual, they generally see, remember and learn through pictures. Many are extremely sensitive, easily "picking up on" subtle energies and vibrations including sounds and voice inflections.

CHARACTERISTIC TRAITS

The skin is a heightened sense organ that sends and receives feeling messages, making Skin types extremely sensitive to vibrations and subtle energies. Being physically orientated, they have a strong, solid connection with the earth and nature, including the weather, which can often affect their moods. Many have an innate affinity for the Native American culture.

Sensual and romantic and with an enviable lust for life, Skins like to fully experience their senses. They find satisfaction in natural, simple pleasures like the taste of foods, the sound of music, or the visual stimulation of bright colors and the intrigue of designs. Highly attuned to their sense of touch, they like the feel of things, particularly enjoying fabrics that have a pleasant texture, like silk, cashmere, or flannel. With a good sense of humor and strong play element, they're typically able to "flow" with what life presents. The greatest sense of fulfillment for Skins comes from being able to discover and reveal aspects of life generally unknown

Skins are perceptive and visual. Some even have a photographic memory, enabling them to see and absorb all that is presented. They will often get a feel for something, as they tend to assimilate new information through their feelings. School work or formal learning is most appealing when they experience it in a visual picture. They learn best when discovering the material directly, or through multiple sensory perceptions. For example, being very receptive, simply watching the instructor helps them to understand a lecture.

Open and receptive, Skin types create a warm, nurturing environment where others feel safe and appreciated. Sociable in nature and extremely sensitive to other people, they are usually happiest when involved with others in a mutual undertaking. While they are committed and dependable in whatever they accept, to be most rewarding, work needs to be creative, productive and fun. With their strong nurturing qualities, Skins are exceptionally good with children, and particularly effective in service professions.

Their love and respect for life and all its creatures is often reflected in their selflessness or altruism. With their heightened empathic feeling energy, they have a tendency to take in and retain all they experience. If they're not careful, simply witnessing others' emotional suffering can cause their own spirits to sink.

Skin

MOTIVATION

Being so affected by, and responsive to, the moods and feelings of those around them, as well as to their environment, Skins will often put on large amounts of weight to act as a protective barrier or buffer. Weight gain typically occurs following an accident, illness, personal violation, or situation where energies are less than harmonious. Diet can also cause weight gain due to the Skin's inability to process refined sugar, and the resulting loss of muscle mass.

Being inordinately sensitive, they tend to take the responses of others too seriously. This sensitivity can often leave them feeling vulnerable with a need to defend. Skins will then disconnect, directing their attention elsewhere. The energy shift can be so dramatic that the recipient can feel abandoned or that the Skin is mad at them.

By being so sensitive to others' disapproval and rejection, Skins are often overly reluctant to share their knowledge and ideas. Unfortunately, not only are others deprived of the Skins' insights, but since discovery and social interaction are so important to them, they severely limit themselves when they don't share their awareness.

While they are good at receiving ideas, even known as dreamers, they can have difficulty following through on their ideas and plans. Anything that is overly mundane, mechanical, or conventional, can leave them feeling bored or frustrated. When the project no longer requires creativity, lacks excitement or becomes routine, they need to move on as their life path is to experience and stretch, moving physically and/or mentally. Consequently, they can have difficulty consistently manifesting money. They frequently lack direction in life and are often late bloomers, not discovering their true life's work until after age 40.

"AT WORST"

Skins can be very reluctant or "picky" about sharing information and knowledge when their environment doesn't feel safe, usually due to someone's disapproval, rejection or anger. They can also swing to the opposite extreme and express themselves in an aggressive manner. Some are able to see pictures and receive insights that they shared when it wasn't appropriate, only to painfully experience the repercussions of their lack of discretion.

When dealing with emotional situations, Skins will either deny their existence or immerse themselves in it. Once they get involved, if they can't solve the problem, they don't know how to let it go. They have a tendency to take on the problems of those around them to the degree that it can interfere with their own need to adequately nurture themselves. A form of control is feeling they need to fix what is wrong. In so doing, they take in and hold others' negative emotional energy. Feeling more secure when they know what will happen, Skins will attempt to control circumstances and situations by becoming care-takers and taking on others' responsibilities.

Their desire to hide can come from not wanting to stand out or be noticed. They may abruptly retreat from relationships and become inaccessible leaving others feeling offended or abandoned. When stressed, Skins will close down, become lazy, depressed, disconnect mentally, and feel sorry for

Skin

"AT WORST"

themselves. They can get into such a negative space that all they want to do is sit. Even getting up to water a plant is too much effort. The problem arises when they become indulgent, using food as a stimulant. Overeating then causes a loss of self-esteem and self-acceptance, which triggers the cycle of using food, particularly sweets, for self-nurturing. Other common methods of escape include alcohol or drugs. Since their bodies do not process refined sugar well, it is easy for them to become addicted to alcohol or chocolate.

Skins have an inherent fear of projecting something that they don't own, so they will set unrealistic expectations for themselves. They will then move into a pattern of self-doubt where they do not accept themselves, and follow it by setting unrealistic expectations for others. Their self-doubt continues to build until it becomes critical and hinders every other aspect of their lives. To break the barrier, they simply need to get in and get started; actually doing it feels good and helps them move through the fear of not doing it right and the need to be perfect.

"AT BEST"

With a flair for life, Skins are light and romantic, open to new experiences and discovery. Artistic and imaginative, clever original ideas easily come to them. Skins are very intuitive, yet well grounded. Being especially visual, they tend to see images which can then be transposed into usable information. Highly social, they enjoy people and life in general. They approach life with respect and a sense of selfless altruism.

Extremely receptive, Skins are able to sense what is going on, and allow the energy to flow around and through them without absorbing it. Physical activity that doesn't require thought such as stretching, gardening, or going for a walk will move blocked energy. Emotionally detaching allows them to go with the flow, and accept whatever is happening. They are then able to use their sensitivity to feel safe in the world. Nature helps them rebalance and get re-connected with God. The key is to connect with spirit by going through the body, such as in an active meditation or going inside and taking time to be by themselves.

Receptive and intuitive, their special strength lies in receiving information rather than directing or controlling it. This is when new discoveries are made. The first step is to release the need to control the outcome and be truly comfortable regardless of which way it goes. Once they get their direction, they can proceed in a practical, competent, and reliable manner.

Having developed their self-confidence and self-worth, they are able to express their inner truth and essence without fear of rejection. They are able to share when appropriate without taking other people's responses personally. They can feel safe, even in a harsh or insensitive world. When connected with their spiritual side, they often receive information and can be excellent channels, using the information for counseling or healing.

Skin

FOOD LISTS

HEALTHY FOOD LIST

FREQUENTLY FOODS	3-7 meals per week – refers to each food, rather than category.
DENSE PROTEIN	Game meats (buffalo, pheasant, rabbit, venison); cornish game hen, duck; flounder, haddock, halibut, herring, mackerel, mahi-mahi, perch, red snapper
DAIRY	Butter
NUTS and SEEDS	Almonds (raw, roasted), almond butter, cashews (roasted), cashew butter, raw or roasted seeds (caraway, pumpkin, sesame, sunflower), sesame seed butter, sunflower seed butter
LEGUMES	Garbanzo beans, miso
GRAINS	Corn, corn grits, oats, rice (all varieties), rice bran, rice cakes, Swedish Rye Krisp®, pasta (durum, semolina), udon noodles, rice noodles, cream of rice
VEGETABLES	Asparagus, avocados, green beans, lima beans, beets, broccoli, napa cabbage, carrots, cauliflower, celery, cilantro, corn, garlic, mustard greens, shitake mushrooms, onions (all varieties), peas, bell peppers (green, red, yellow), chili peppers, potatoes (all varieties), sweet potatoes, pumpkin, daikon radishes, spinach, sprouts (alfalfa, clover, radish, sunflower), banana squash, yellow (summer) squash, turnips, yams
FRUITS	Bananas, blackberries, blueberries, boysenberries, cranberries, gooseberries, strawberries, green grapes, melons (cantaloupe, honeydew, watermelon), oranges, figs (fresh, dried)
SWEETENERS	Re-Vita®, stevia
CONDIMENTS	Salsa, tahini
BEVERAGES	Arrowhead® flavored carbonated water (cherry, lemon, lime, orange)
MODERATELY FOODS	1-2 meals per week – refers to each food, rather than category.
DENSE PROTEIN	Beef, beef broth, beef liver, lamb, pork, bacon, ham, sausage, veal, organ meats (heart, brain); chicken, chicken broth, chicken livers, turkey; anchovy, bass, bonita, catfish, cod, orange roughy, salmon, sardines, shark, sole, swordfish, trout, tuna; abalone, calamari (squid), clams, crab, eel, lobsters, mussels, octopus, oysters, scallops, shrimp; eggs in foods (i.e. rice, broccoli)
DAIRY	Half & half, sweet cream, sour cream, regular and low fat plain yogurt, nonfat plain and flavored yogurt, ice cream (Ben & Jerry's®, Dreyer's, Swensen's®, Baskin-Robbins™)
CHEESE	American, blue, brie, Camembert, Cheddar, Colby, cottage, cream, Edam, feta, Gouda, Jack, kefir, Limburger, mozzarella, Muenster, Parmesan, ricotta, Romano, Swiss

Skin

NUTS and SEEDS	Brazils, raw cashews, water chestnuts, coconuts, filberts, hazelnuts, macadamias (raw, roasted), macadamia butter, peanuts (raw, roasted), peanut butter, pecans, pine nuts (raw, roasted), pistachios, walnuts (black, English)
LEGUMES	Beans (adzuki, black, kidney, lima [butter], mung, navy, great northern, pinto, red, soy), lentils, black-eyed peas, split peas, hummus, soy milk, tofu
GRAINS	Amaranth, barley, buckwheat, corn bread, corn tortillas, hominy grits, millet, popcorn, quinoa, rye, triticale, whole wheat, wheat bran, wheat germ, refined wheat flour, flour tortillas, breads (French, Italian, sourdough, garlic, 7-grain, multi-grain, oat, corn, corn/rye, rye, rice, sprouted grain, white, whole wheat), bagels, croissants, English muffins, crackers (saltines, oat, rye, wheat), unsalted pretzels, couscous, cream of rye, cream of wheat
VEGETABLES	Artichokes, arugula, yellow wax beans, bamboo shoots, bok choy, broccoflower, brussels sprouts, cabbage (green, red), chard, cucumbers, eggplant, greens (beet, collard, turnip), hominy, jicama, kale, kohlrabi, leeks, lettuce (Boston, butter, endive, iceberg, red leaf, romaine), mushrooms, okra, olives (green, ripe), parsley, parsnips, snow pea pods, pimentos, radishes (red, white), rutabaga, sauerkraut, seaweed (arame, dulse, kelp, nori, wakame), shallots, squash (acorn, butternut, spaghetti, zucchini), mung bean sprouts, tomatoes (canned, hot-house, vine-ripened), watercress
VEGETABLE JUICES	Celery, carrot, carrot/celery, parsley, spinach, tomato, V-8®
FRUITS	Apples (Golden or Red Delicious, Granny Smith, Jonathan, McIntosh, Pippin, Rome Beauty), apricots, raspberries, cherries, grapes (Concord, black, red), guavas, kiwi, kumquats, lemons, limes, loquats, melons (casaba, crenshaw), mangos, nectarines, papayas, peaches, pears, persimmons, pineapples, plums (black, purple, red), pomegranates, rhubarb, tangerines, tangelos, dates, prunes, raisins
FRUIT JUICES	Apple, apple cider, apple/apricot, apricot, black cherry, red cherry, cranapple, cranberry, grape (purple, red, white), grapefruit, guava, lemon, orange, papaya, pear, pineapple, pineapple/coconut, prune, tangerine, watermelon
VEGETABLE OILS	All-blend, almond, avocado, canola, corn, flaxseed, olive, peanut, safflower, sesame, soy, sunflower
SWEETENERS	Molasses, sorghum, date sugar, barley malt syrup, corn syrup, maple syrup, brown rice syrup, fructose, succonant
CONDIMENTS	Catsup, horseradish, mustard, barbecue sauce, pesto sauce, soy sauce, vinegar, regular salt, sea salt, Vege-Sal®, Spike®, Bragg™ aminos, dill pickles, pickle relish
SALAD DRESSINGS	Blue cheese, French, ranch, creamy Italian, creamy avocado, thousand island, vinegar and oil, lemon juice and oil
DESSERTS	Custards, tapioca, puddings, pies, cakes, orange or raspberry sherbet, carob squares

Skin

CHIPS	Bean, corn (blue, white, yellow), potato
BEVERAGES	Coffee with Re-Vita®; herbal tea, cammomile tea, Ignatia tea, black tea, green tea, Japanese tea, Chinese oolong tea; mineral water, sparkling water; wine (red, white), sake, beer, barley malt liquor, champagne, gin, Scotch, vodka, whiskey; root beer, regular sodas
RARELY FOODS	No more than once a month
DENSE PROTEIN	Eggs (alone)
DAIRY	Milk (whole, 2%, low fat, nonfat, raw), goat milk, buttermilk, kefir, frozen yogurt, goat cheese, ice cream
FRUITS	Grapefruits (white, red)
SWEETENERS	Honey, brown sugar, raw sugar, refined cane sugar, saccharin, aspertame, Equal®, Sweet'n Low®, NutraSweet®
CONDIMENTS	Margarine, mayonnaise
DESSERTS	Chocolate, desserts containing chocolate
BEVERAGES	Caffeinated beverages (coffee, diet sodas)

SENSITIVE FOOD LIST

FREQUENTLY FOODS	3-7 meals per week – refers to each food, rather than category.
DAIRY	Butter
NUTS and SEEDS	Almonds (raw, roasted), almond butter, cashews (roasted), cashew butter, raw or roasted seeds (sunflower, pumpkin), sunflower seed butter
GRAINS	Corn, corn grits, corn tortillas, oats, rice (all varieties), rice bran, rice cakes, pasta (durum, semolina), udon noodles, rice noodles, cream of rice
VEGETABLES	Asparagus, green beans, beets, napa cabbage, carrots, mustard greens, daikon radishes, yellow (summer) squash
BEVERAGES	Arrowhead® flavored carbonated water (cherry, lemon, lime, orange)
MODERATELY FOODS	1-2 meals per week – refers to each food, rather than category.
DENSE PROTEIN	Beef broth, beef liver, lamb, pork, bacon, ham, sausage, veal, organ meats (heart, brain), game meats (buffalo, pheasant, rabbit, venison); chicken, chicken broth, chicken livers, turkey, cornish game hen, duck; anchovy, bass, bonita, catfish, flounder, haddock, halibut, herring, mackerel, mahi-mahi, perch, orange roughy, salmon, sardines, shark, red snapper, sole, swordfish, trout, tuna; abalone, calamari (squid), clams, crab, eel, lobster, mussels, octopus, oysters, scallops, shrimp

Skin

DAIRY	Half & half, sweet cream, sour cream, strawberry yogurt
CHEESE	American, blue, brie, Camembert, Cheddar, Colby, Edam, feta, Gouda, Jack, kefir, Limburger, mozzarella, Muenster, Parmesan, ricotta, Romano, Swiss
NUTS and SEEDS	Brazils, cashews (raw), water chestnuts, coconuts, filberts, hazelnuts, macadamias (raw, roasted), macadamia butter, peanuts (raw, roasted), peanut butter, pecans, pine nuts (raw, roasted), pistachios, walnuts (black, English), raw or roasted seeds (caraway, sesame), sesame seed butter
LEGUMES	Beans (adzuki, black, kidney, lima [butter], mung, navy, great northern, pinto, red, soy), lentils, black-eyed peas, split peas, hummus, soy milk, miso
GRAINS	Amaranth, barley, corn bread, hominy grits, millet, popcorn, quinoa, rye, triticale, wheat bran, wheat germ, refined wheat flour, flour tortillas, breads (French, Italian, sourdough, garlic, 7-grain, multi-grain, oat, corn, corn/rye, rice, sprouted grain, white, whole wheat), bagels, croissants, English muffins, crackers (saltines, oat, rye, wheat), couscous, cream of rye
VEGETABLES	Artichokes, avocados, yellow wax beans, bamboo shoots, bok choy, broccoli, broccoflower, brussels sprouts, cabbage (green, red), cauliflower, celery, chard, cilantro, corn, cucumbers, eggplant, garlic, greens (beet, collard, turnip), hominy, jicama, kale, kohlrabi, leeks, lettuce (Boston, butter, endive, red leaf, romaine), mushrooms, okra, olives, (green, ripe), onions (all varieties), parsley, parsnips, peas, snow pea pods, chili peppers, pimentos, sweet potatoes, pumpkin, rutabaga, sauerkraut, seaweed (arame, dulse, kelp, nori, wakame), shallots, spinach, sprouts (alfalfa, clover, mung bean, radish, sunflower), squash (acorn, banana, butternut, spaghetti), turnips
VEGETABLE JUICES	Celery, carrot, carrot/celery, parsley, spinach, tomato, V-8®
FRUITS	Apples (Golden or Red Delicious, Jonathan, McIntosh, Rome Beauty), bananas, blackberries, blueberries, boysenberries, cranberries, gooseberries, raspberries, strawberries, cherries, grapes (Concord, black, green, red), guavas, kumquats, lemons, limes, loquats, mangos, melons (cantaloupe, casaba, crenshaw, honeydew, watermelon), nectarines, oranges, papayas, peaches, pears, persimmons, pineapples, plums (black, purple, red), pomegranates, rhubarb, tangerines, tangelos, dates, figs (fresh, dried), prunes, raisins
FRUIT JUICES	Apple, apple cider, apple/apricot, apricot, black cherry, red cherry, cranapple, cranberry, grape (purple, red, white), guava, lemon, orange, papaya, pear, pineapple, pineapple/coconut, prune, tangerine, watermelon
VEGETABLE OIL	Olive
SWEETENERS	Re-Vita®, stevia
CONDIMENTS	Soy sauce, tahini, vinegar, salt, sea salt, Vege Sal®, Spike®, Bragg™ aminos
SALAD DRESSINGS	Vinegar and oil, lemon juice and oil
BEVERAGES	Coffee w/Re-Vita®; herbal tea, cammomile tea, Japanese tea, Chinese oolong tea; mineral water, sparkling water

Skin

RARELY FOODS	No more than once a month
DENSE PROTEIN	Beef; codfish; eggs
DAIRY	Milk (whole, 2%, low fat, nonfat, raw), goat milk, buttermilk, kefir, plain or favored yogurt, frozen yogurt, most ice creams
CHEESE	Cottage, cream, goat
LEGUMES	Garbanzo beans, tofu
GRAINS	Buckwheat, whole wheat, cream of wheat
VEGETABLES	Arugula, iceberg lettuce, bell peppers (green, red, yellow), potatoes (all varieties), radishes (red, white), tomatoes (canned, hot-house, vine-ripened), zucchini, watercress, yams
FRUITS	Apples (Granny Smith, Pippin), apricots, grapefruits (red, white), kiwi
FRUIT JUICES	Grapefruit
VEGETABLE OILS	All-blend, almond, avocado, canola, corn, flaxseed, peanut, safflower, sesame, soy, sunflower
SWEETENERS	Honey, molasses, brown sugar, date sugar, raw sugar, refined cane sugar, maple syrup, fructose, sorghum, barley malt syrup, corn syrup, brown rice syrup, succonant, saccharin, aspertame, Equal®, Sweet'n Low®, NutraSweet®
CONDIMENTS	Catsup, mustard, horseradish, barbecue sauce, pesto sauce, margarine, mayonnaise, salsa
SALAD DRESSINGS	Blue cheese, French, ranch, creamy Italian, creamy avocado, thousand island
DESSERTS	Custards, tapioca, puddings, pies, cakes, orange or raspberry sherbet, chocolate, desserts containing chocolate
CHIPS	Bean, corn (blue, white, yellow), potato
BEVERAGES	Caffeinated beverages (coffee, diet sodas); black tea, green tea; wine (red, white), sake, beer, barley malt liquor, champagne, Scotch, gin, vodka, whiskey; diet sodas, root beer, regular sodas

Skin

MENUS

DIETARY EMPHASIS:

- Vegetables.
- Brown or wild rice with vegetables.
- Keep meals and foods simple. Follow basic food-combining rules: avoid combining protein and grains (sandwiches), protein and fruit, protein and citrus or acids (meat and tomato sauce), two proteins (meat and milk or cream sauce), and acids and starches (vinegar on rice).
- Eat melons alone.
- Most vegetables combine well with protein and with starches.
- Sunrider® herbs often effective in rebuilding body.
- Avoid refined cane sugar, as can cause muscle degeneration and weight gain.
- Dairy foods often interfere with memory.
- Milk may be used with other foods, including cereal, or after a meal as a moderate food.

WEIGHT LOSS:

- Eliminate refined sugar, alcohol, dairy, breads, and reduce salt.
- Consume 15-30% of calories from dense protein, or use Sunrider® herbs along with vegetarian diet.
- Reduce quantity of food; use variety and rotate.
- Avoid snacks.
- Limit fats to 25% of total calories. However, if dietary fat falls below 10% from appropriate sources (see below) weight loss will not occur.
- Stretch at least 15 minutes per day.

WEIGHT GAIN:

- Increase food consumption.

SENSITIVE:

- May include dense protein at breakfast.

VEGETARIAN DIET:

- Recommended when healthy, although up to 35% of caloric intake may consist of dense protein.

FATS:

- 10-30% of caloric intake. Best sources are almonds, sunflower and sesame seeds, tahini, avocados, olive oil, fish, meat, and poultry.
- May use Hain™ Creamy Italian or Avocado salad dressing instead of mayonnaise.

KEY

—all menus may be used by healthy persons
( ) around foods means that they're optional
L denotes weight loss menus
S denotes sensitive menus
G denotes weight gain menus

BREAKFAST:
7-8 a.m. Light, with grain, vegetables, nuts, seeds, and/or fruit.
(melons – alone)

SENSITIVE: May include dense protein.

L	S	G	Menu
	S		Brown rice (carrots, and/or garlic, and daikon radish)
L		G	Brown rice w/garlic, daikon radish, carrots, and Sunrider® Sunpak™ w/stevia
L			Sunrider® Sunpak™ w/stevia and Fortune Delight™
L		G	Brown rice bread w/sweet or brown rice miso, umeboshi plum, and tahini
L	S		Cream of rice
L	S	G	Rice w/almonds
L			Puffed rice, corn or rye w/apple juice, applesauce or almond milk
	S	G	Corn tortilla w/avocado
L		G	Oatmeal (Re-Vita® and/or banana)
L		G	Oatmeal w/rice milk
	S	G	Cream of rice w/prunes
L	S	G	Roasted cashews, unsalted
		G	Toast, peanut butter, and banana
L		G	Rice cakes w/cashew, almond, or peanut butter
		G	Bagel, almond butter, and apple
		G	Bagel, pine nuts, and pear
L		G	Pancakes w/applesauce
L			Tortilla and avocado
		G	Baked potato (butter)
L			Acorn or spaghetti squash and Re-Vita®
	S		Peas

Skin

L	Broccoli or peas
L G	Banana and almonds, or sunflower seeds
L S	Banana
L G	Apple and peanut butter or almonds
S G	Peanut butter on Red Delicious apple
L G	Orange and roasted, unsalted pumpkin seeds
L	Honeydew melon or watermelon
G	Cantaloupe
L S	Papaya
L G	Re-Vita® and cranberry concentrate (oatmeal)

MID-MORNING SNACK:
(Optional) Grain, alone or with nut butter, and/or fruit.

L	Frozen mango
S	Rice cakes
L G	Rice cake w/almond or peanut butter
S G	Almond butter and banana on Wasa™ Crispbread or Rye Krisp®
S G	Peanut butter and banana on rice cake

LUNCH:
12-2 p.m. Moderate-to-heavy, with vegetables, grain, nuts, seeds, legumes, protein, fruit and/or dairy.

L S G	Rice and stir-fry: squash, carrots, celery, chinese cabbage, onion, water chestnuts, bean sprouts, cauliflower, broccoli, and seeds or nuts
L S	Rice and broccoli
L	Brown rice bread w/sweet or brown rice miso, umeboshi plum, tahini, Sunrider® NuPlus™ w/stevia and Fortune Delight™
L	Sunrider® NuPlus™ w/stevia and Fortune Delight
L G	Bean tostada w/onion, lettuce, and cilantro, Sunrider® NuPlus™ w/stevia and Fortune Delight™
L	Miso soup w/scallions, udon noodles, tahini, and lemon sauce w/squash, daikon radish, carrots, onions, and scallions
L	Miso soup w/scallions, brown rice, and vegetables
L	Noodles and broccoli
L G	Bean burrito (salsa and/or lettuce)
G	Bacon, lettuce, and tomato sandwich
S G	Vegetarian taco
L S	Udon noodles w/carrots, broccoli, cauliflower, and squash
S	Udon noodles w/tahini and lemon sauce
	Caesar salad
S	3-bean salad w/pickles, cucumbers, and celery
S G	Lentil salad w/Hain™ Creamy Italian dressing
L S G	Beans and rice (chicken)
G	Beans, corn tortillas, guacamole, cheese, and lettuce
S G	Bean burrito
S G	Beans w/barbecue sauce and celery or cucumber
L S G	Tuna and avocado (rice cake)
S	Tuna salad (Hain™ Creamy Avocado dressing) and/or romaine lettuce
S G	Tuna w/Hain™ Creamy Italian dressing on Italian bread or bagel
S G	Turkey and mustard on French roll or bagel
L S G	Turkey or fish and rice
L S G	Chicken and rice or pasta
L	Egg, rice, and broccoli
G	Eggs, ham, and toast
L G	Pork, chicken, or shrimp fajita w/vegetables (rice)

LUNCH or DINNER:

L S	Rice w/vegetables: broccoli, bok choy, greens, onions, celery, carrots, scallions
L S	Rice, broccoli, and carrots
L S G	Rice and stir-fry: squash, carrots, celery, chinese cabbage, onion, water chestnuts, bean sprouts, cauliflower, broccoli, seeds or nuts, and chicken
G	Split pea soup and chicken on rye sandwich
L S G	Corn tortilla w/avocado and alfalfa sprouts (chicken and/or vegetables)

Skin

G Flour tortilla, beans, avocado, and salsa

G Baked potato w/butter or salsa (chicken)

S G Ramen noodles, chicken, broccoli, and carrots

G Pasta w/meat balls (green beans)

G Fettucini, pesto, garlic, and romano cheese

S G Bagel and lox (carrots)

L S G Black bean soup

L G Eggs and rice or broccoli

S G Yellow or green squash, w/Parmesan cheese (rice)

L S G Cornish game hen and wild rice (corn)

L S G Chicken, rice, and asparagus

L S G Chicken, corn tortilla, cilantro, beans, and rice

S G Turkey, cranberry sauce, bread stuffing, and spinach salad

L S G Turkey breast, rice, and yellow squash

L S G Sole, rice, carrots, and broccoli

L S G Shark, swordfish, or mahi-mahi, w/rice, cauliflower, and broccoli

L G Scallops w/pasta

G Roast beef, potatoes, gravy, and beets (carrots)

L G Beef or lamb w/dill, herbs, and rice or potatoes (carrots, green beans, eggplant, and/or salad)

MIDAFTERNOON SNACK:
(Optional) Nuts, seeds, grain, vegetables.

L G Water crackers

L G Graham crackers

S G Almonds or roasted cashews

S G Unsalted sunflower or pumpkin seeds – raw or roasted

L S Carrots or carrot juice

L S Celery, raw broccoli, or jicama

G Peanut butter or almond cookie w/green tea

DINNER:
Early, by 6 p.m. Light-to-moderate, with protein, vegetables, grain, nuts, seeds and/or legumes.

L S Beets w/salad

L S Salad w/out lettuce or salad dressing: cucumber, broccoli, and celery (carrots, spinach, pumpkin seeds)

L G Salad: sprouts and red cabbage w/Italian salad dressing, oil and vinegar, or wine vinegar, olive oil, garlic, and parsley dressing

G Salad: iceberg lettuce and red cabbage (carrots, celery, cucumber, red onion, garbanzo beans, and/or cucumber dressing or lemon juice, olive oil and oregano)

L G Greek chicken salad and vegetables

L G Cornish game hen, chicken or beef w/vegetables: carrots, celery, bell peppers, broccoli, cauliflower, peas, green beans and/or asparagus

L S G Chicken noodle soup (steamed broccoli or salad)

L G Fish taco

L S G Sea bass, rice, and broccoli

L G Bean tostada w/onion, lettuce and cilantro, Sunrider® NuPlus™ w/stevia and Fortune Delight, and Sports Caps

L Miso soup w/scallions and rice w/vegetables, such as broccoli, bok choy, greens, onions, celery, and/or carrots

L G Sushi (ginger)

L Squash (Re-Vita®)

L G Peas (baked potato or yams)

L Vegetable soup

L G Beans and salad

L G Rice or oatmeal

L Sun Bar® w/Sunrider® NuPlus™ and stevia

Skin

EVENING or BEFORE BED:
(Optional) 10 p.m.-12 midnight.
Protein, vegetables, grain, fruit, nuts, seeds

L S Red Delicious apples, peaches, or plums

L S G Tortilla chips

L S G Popcorn

L G Fruit juice (popcorn)

L Sun Bar®

S Raw or steamed vegetables, such as carrots, celery, and/or broccoli

G Potato or yam

S Carrot juice

S G Cottage cheese and peaches

S Strawberries

G Dates (cream cheese and/or walnuts)

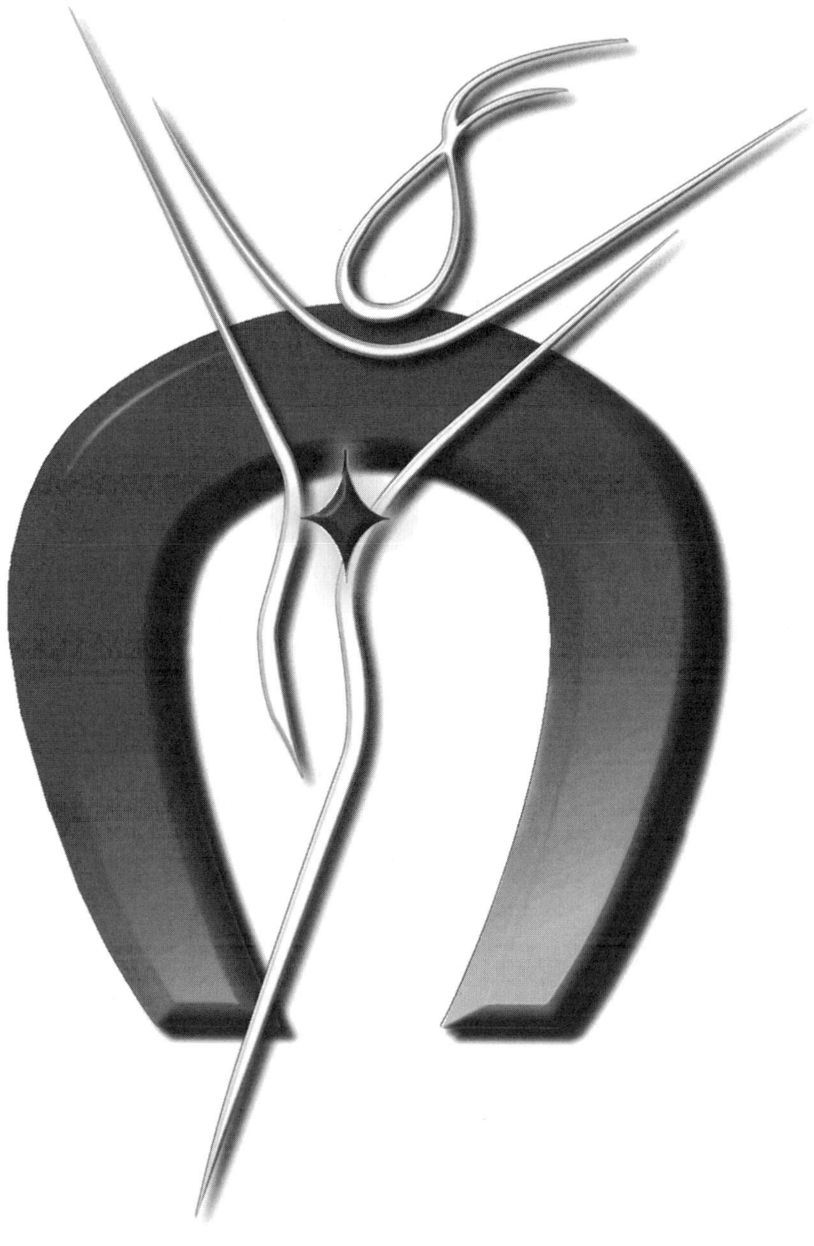

The "Spleen Body Type" is symbolized by a horseshoe magnet. The spleen reclaims the iron from red blood cells and disseminates energy as needed. Tenacious, they will stay with and provide the sustaining energy needed to get a job done right.

Spleen

BODY TYPE PROFILE

LOCATION	Upper left of abdomen, between stomach and diaphragm.
FUNCTION	As largest organ in lymphatic system (major part of immune system), serves several important functions – including removal of iron from old red blood cells.
POTENTIAL HEALTH PROBLEMS	Generally very healthy, with strong immune system. Slow metabolism. Tendency toward nervous tension and anxiety. Sometimes given to compulsive/addictive behavior, e.g., eating disorders. Solid body, with muscular or heavy/chunky legs. Friendly, down-to-earth personality, and/or intense, tenacious, determined, strong-willed. Known for making things happen by disseminating energy.
RECOMMENDED EXERCISE	Exercise is helpful, as it releases stress. While exercise is not necessary to lose weight, it is good for muscle tone. Mornings best. Ideally, 1 hour before breakfast, 4 times a week, getting heart rate up to 120 for a minimum of 30 minutes. Exercise that provides mental, physical, and emotional integration is best. Examples include: low impact aerobics, walking, callanetics, dance – swing, jitterbug, etc.

WOMEN'S CHARACTERISTICS

DISTINGUISHING FEATURES	Solid body, with muscular or heavy/chunky legs. Friendly, down-to-earth personality, and/or intense, tenacious, determined, strong-willed. Known for making things happen by disseminating energy.
ADDITIONAL PHYSICAL CHARACTERISTICS	Buttocks rounded-to-prominent. Low back curvature straight-to-swayed. Breasts average. Shoulders narrower than, to relatively even with, hips. Average torso. Defined to well-defined waist. Height petite-to-tall. Bone structure medium. Average, elongated to dense, solid musculature. Lower body often at least full size larger than upper body, with hips generally more wide than thick. Thighs and calves often heavy with solid, dense appearance. Hands small-to-average, often with short fingers. Average oval-shaped head which may appear large for body size, although will appear small if much excess weight is gained.
WEIGHT GAIN AREAS	Lower body with initial gain in lower abdomen, entire upper 2/3rds of thighs, including upper inner thighs, buttocks, upper and lower hips, waist, and middle back. Often carry bulk of weight and cellulite in legs, which can then

Spleen

WEIGHT GAIN (Continued)	appear chunky. Secondary weight gain in entire abdomen, breasts, upper and entire back, entire inner thighs to knees, face, and upper arms. First place weight is lost is in face.

DIETARY GUIDELINES

SCHEDULING MEALS	Breakfast: Light-to-moderate, with protein, vegetables, grain, fruit, nuts, seeds, legumes, and or dairy. May have coffee with grain twice a week. Lunch: Moderate-to-heavy, with protein, vegetables, grain, fruit, nuts, seeds, legumes, and/or dairy. Dinner: Light, with protein, vegetables, grain, fruit, nuts, seeds, legumes, and/or dairy.
DIETARY EMPHASIS	• Rotate foods. • Consume 10-25% of caloric intake from dense protein; include 25-30% from fats; and vegetables, especially green beans. Blueberries strengthen white blood cells (but for weight loss, need to limit to 3 to 5 times a week). Spices, especially curry, up to 4 times a week, as curry strengthens the red and white blood cells and capillaries. Cayenne pepper stimulates lymphatics. • For weight loss, limit sugar (including fruit) to 2 times a week; limit bread to 3 times a week. • For weight gain, consume 20-25% of caloric intake from dense protein. • Vegetarian diets are nutritionally inadequate; require 10-25% of calories from dense protein. • Fats, 25-30% of caloric intake from nuts, seeds and oils, especially sunflower seed oil, and low fat yogurt.
KEY SUPPORTS FOR SYSTEM	Because of tendency to become overly tenacious or obsessive, need to relax self (e.g., through nurturing others or connecting with nature) to restore mental/emotional equilibrium. Music or animal contact may also aid relaxation.
COMPLEMENTARY GLANDULAR SUPPORT	Liver, through emotional validation from others; thymus, through consuming 3 oz. dense protein daily.
FOODS CRAVED	*(When Energy is Low)* Sweets, particularly ice cream and chocolate, often with nuts. Sugar of any kind, including fruit. Carbohydrates, such as peanut butter, bread with butter or mayonnaise, sandwiches, and bagels with cream cheese, muffins, and pastries. Spicy foods (e.g., Indian curry). Pizza.

Spleen

FOODS TO AVOID Artificial sweeteners (e.g., Equal® or Sweet'n Low®); grapefruit; and pork, including ham.

RECOMMENDED Indian, Greek, Middle Eastern, Japanese, Chinese, Thai, Sushi; salad bars.

PSYCHOLOGICAL PROFILE

ESSENCE

Just as the spleen stores blood and the spleen acupuncture point draws energy into the body to be disseminated through the blood as needed, Spleen body types disseminate energy. They have a strong ability to organize and delegate, making sure projects get done, many of which often involve food and social or group interaction. Noted for their tenacity, Spleens will stay with a subject until they get the results they want. They are most comfortable when they can solve a problem in a logical step-by-step fashion, and are noted for providing the sustaining energy needed to get a job done right.

CHARACTERISTIC TRAITS

Basically social and naturally outgoing, Spleens are personable and thrive on helping others. Social interaction gives them a sense of fulfillment, particularly when they can be the authority or center of attention. Spleen types are generally good organizers, and like to do things in a big way, such as being involved in organizing huge social events. Good at doing things on an enormous scale, they will often undertake and succeed in enterprises of major proportions. They like businesses where they can duplicate themselves and are often physically large, which assists them in taking in, holding, and disseminating large amounts of energy on a sustained basis.

Intense and forceful by nature, they tend to be passionate in their ideas and convictions. Their enthusiasm can be expressed so forcefully that they easily overwhelm people and may be perceived as aggressive. They love to present new ideas or viewpoints, Especially rewarding is introducing others to non-traditional or alternative ways of seeing or doing things. So passionate are they about their ideas regarding change and reform, that they often express them with such emotional fervor that other people feel uncomfortable.

Spleens are tenacious. Whatever their focus, they will stay with it until they get the results they desire, whether it be a point they want clarity on, a job they want done, or a concept they want someone to see. They can get so focused on a particular detail that they keep the conversation or project at a standstill until it is resolved.

Spleens derive a sense of security from having detail clarification and a solid, organized structure. Being easily distracted in areas where immediate direction is unclear or where they have strong personal attachments, structure and precise guidelines provide them with a tangible point of reference.

Spleen

MOTIVATION

Spleens love being the "achiever," regardless of the area, and will persist in a task, giving it their best. Not succeeding in everything they set out to do, however, causes them to feel like total failures. So, if there is any doubt in their ability to succeed, they will procrastinate, finding excuses and diversions. Spleen types will try or start a lot of new things, but if success doesn't come as quickly as they would like, procrastination begins, and provides an acceptable means of avoidance. When they don't succeed, they blame themselves, and think something is wrong with them because they couldn't accomplish the task.

Spleen types love to eat, and are often excellent cooks. It's easy for them to put on and carry excess weight because their bodies are so strong that they rarely get indigestion or feelings of being too full from over-indulgence or dietary indiscretions. Deriving a great deal of sensual pleasure from food, it's easy for them to rationalize and bend the rules when it comes to getting the treats they want. Consequently, food and diet suggestions need to be very clear, down to specific quantities or they will interpret moderation to fit their desires, which for them can mean unlimited quantities. While losing weight may be important, the sacrifice is often too hard, unless there is sufficient social support.

More people than task oriented, Spleens are better initially working with someone rather than independently. Working with someone provides the motivation that is difficult to find on their own, particularly for activities, such as exercise. Unless they have evolved to the point of being self-motivated, they will put off activities that require discipline unless they can find a partner. Personal motivation is inherently low, so emotional support and structure is essential for follow-through in areas that require consistency.

“AT WORST”

Their tenacity can be a liability when it comes to resolving conflict. Being exceedingly fixed and dogmatic in their beliefs, once their minds are made up, that is the end of the subject, and there is little, if any, flexibility. Domineering, bossy, and controlling, they tend to think that their way is the only way, and are not open to listening to or learning from others.

Defensive, stubborn and inflexible, Spleen types can be deadly when confronted with an opposing point of view, particularly when their personal interest is at stake. They may "go after" the person with the opposing view, rather than just the view, and overpower the opposition through personal harassment and character assassination. Direct and to the point, their written words can be lethal. Verbally adept, Spleens will cut rather than bite, or kill rather than argue using very well picked words. Persistent and tenacious, Spleens often display an adversary attitude and will try to win at all costs.

The need for security, both financial and emotional, motivates Spleens. It's easy for them to overfocus on career, at the expense of their family or own health. When aggressive, they can be ruthless in their business dealings. They can charm and seduce people, in an effort to create definition or

Spleen

"AT WORST"

enhance their image. To insure that people stay around, Spleens will become indispensable in some way or set themselves up in controlling positions to make others dependent upon them. They will often make big promises, playing on a person's hopes and dreams, but then never quite follow through.

Feeling insecure, Spleens will often resort to food for comfort and put on large amounts of excess weight. Just as they tend to hang on to their dogmatic beliefs, they tend to hang on to their weight until they learn to let go and be flexible in other areas of their lieves. Prone to obsessive/compulsive behavior, they can swing to the opposite extreme of losing weight when their security is threatened or they feel abandoned.

"AT BEST"

The Spleens' tenacity allows them to see a job through, staying with a problem until they have reached a viable solution. With a strong mental focus, they are good at figuring things out and resolving challenging tasks, especially when the task is viewed by others as being impossible or next to it. Spleens enjoy helping their friends and will consistently be there, whenever the need arises. By truly giving from their hearts, they connect with their spiritual side, and experience a true sense of security.

Spleens are most effective when they first gain a good mental understanding, whether it be how something is physically put together, what motivates others, the various aspects of themselves, or of life in general. Having established a solid, physical connection, they are able to let go. Allowing themselves to be flexible by detaching their focus on structure and detail, they are free to see the greater picture. Feeling secure, they are comfortable opening their hearts and sharing their emotions, integrating all aspects of themselves.

Once they have learned to integrate their feelings by connecting their head and heart through their spiritual nature, Spleens are able to embody the energy and powerfully disseminate it into the world. Being able to see the big picture, they can accurately forecast change, including market trends, allowing them to succeed in enterprises of major proportions. Spleens are highly effective in spearheading social reforms, bringing new awarenesses to the forefront of humanity's focus, and staying with the project, continually supplying the necessary energy, until the change is fully integrated.

Spleen

FOOD LISTS

HEALTHY FOOD LIST

FREQUENTLY FOODS	3-7 meals per week – refers to each food, rather than category.
DENSE PROTEIN	Beef broth, beef liver, buffalo, veal; chicken, chicken broth, chicken livers, cornish game hen, duck, turkey; bass, orange roughy, trout
DAIRY	Low fat or nonfat plain or flavored yogurt, butter
CHEESE	Raw feta, ricotta
NUTS and SEEDS	Natural peanut butter, walnuts (black, English), roasted, unsalted seeds (pumpkin, sesame, sunflower), caraway seeds
LEGUMES	Beans (black, garbanzo, lima [butter], pinto, red, soy), black-eyed peas, split peas, hummus
GRAINS	Amaranth, barley, buckwheat, corn tortillas, oats, oat bran, oatmeal, popcorn, white basmati rice, rye, breads (oat, rye), crackers (oat, rye)
VEGETABLES	Artichokes, asparagus, avocados, bamboo shoots, green beans, Italian green beans, yellow wax beans, lima beans, beets, bok choy, broccoli, broccoflower, brussels sprouts, cabbage (green, napa, red), carrots, cauliflower, chard, cilantro, corn, cucumbers, eggplant, garlic, lettuce (endive, red leaf, romaine), pumpkin, spinach
FRUITS	Apples (Golden or Red Delicious, Granny Smith, Jonathan, McIntosh, Pippin), apricots, blackberries, blueberries, boysenberries, cranberries, gooseberries, raspberries, grapes (green, red), melons (casaba, crenshaw, honeydew, watermelon), dates, raisins
FRUIT JUICES	Lime juice in water, orange juice
VEGETABLE OILS	All-blend, almond, avocado, canola, corn, flaxseed, olive, peanut, safflower, sesame, soy, sunflower
SWEETENERS	Honey, barley malt syrup, fructose, succonant, Re-Vita®, stevia
CONDIMENTS	Salsa, spices, Spike®, nutmeg
BEVERAGES	Teas (i.e., Take-A-Break, Roastaroma®, Orange Spice, licorice)
MODERATELY FOODS	1-2 meals per week – refers to each food, rather than category.
DENSE PROTEIN	Beef, bacon, lamb, venison, organ meats (heart, brain); anchovy, bonita, catfish, cod, flounder, haddock, halibut, herring, mackerel, mahi-mahi, perch, salmon, sardines, shark, snapper, sole, swordfish, tuna; abalone, calamari (squid), clams, crab, eel, lobsters, mussels, octopus, oysters, scallops, shrimp; eggs. Fish (2 meals per week – rotate type)

Spleen

DAIRY	Milk (whole, 2%, low fat, nonfat, raw), goat milk, buttermilk, half & half, sweet cream, sour cream, kefir, regular yogurt, Dreyer's imitation yogurt, ice cream (Dreyer's, Ben & Jerry's®, Swensen's ®)
CHEESE	American, blue, brie, Camembert, Cheddar, Colby, cottage, cream, Edam, pasteurized feta, goat, Gouda, low fat Jack, kefir, Limburger, mozzarella, Muenster, Parmesan, Romano, Swiss
NUTS	Almonds, almond butter, Brazils, cashews, cashew butter, steamed or cooked water chestnuts, coconuts, filberts, hazelnuts, macadamias, macadamia butter, peanuts, pecans, pine nuts, pistachios, sesame seed butter, sunflower seed butter
LEGUMES	Beans (adzuki, kidney, navy, great northern), lentils, miso, soy milk, soy protein, tofu
GRAINS	Corn, corn bread, corn grits, hominy grits, millet, quinoa, rice (brown basmati, long or short grain brown, Japanese, wild), rice bran, rice cakes, triticale, whole wheat, wheat bran, wheat germ, refined wheat flour, flour tortillas, breads (French, Italian, sourdough, garlic, 7-grain, multi-grain, corn, corn/rye, rice, pita, sprouted grain, white, whole wheat), bagels, croissants, English muffins, crackers (saltines, whole wheat), couscous, pasta, udon noodles, rice noodles, cream of rice, cream of rye, cream of wheat
VEGETABLES	Arugula, celery, greens (beet, collard, mustard, turnip), hominy, jicama, kale, kohlrabi, leeks, lettuce (Boston, butter, iceberg), mushrooms, okra, olives (green, ripe), onions (chives, green, red, white, brown, yellow, vidalia), parsley, parsnips, peas, snow pea pods, bell peppers (green, red, yellow), chili peppers, pimentos, potatoes (all varieties), radishes, daikon radishes, rutabaga, sauerkraut, seaweed (arame, dulse, kelp, nori, wakame), shallots, sprouts (alfalfa, clover, mung bean, radish, sunflower), squash (acorn, banana, butternut, spaghetti, yellow [summer], zucchini), sweet potatoes, tomatoes, turnips, watercress, yams
VEGETABLE JUICES	Carrot, celery, carrot/celery, parsley, spinach, tomato, V-8®
FRUITS	Rome Beauty apples, bananas, strawberries, cherries, black grapes, guava, kiwi, kumquats, lemons, limes, loquats, mangos, cantaloupe, nectarines, oranges, papayas, peaches, pears, persimmons, pineapples, plums (black, red, purple), pomegranates, rhubarb, tangelos, tangerines, figs, prunes
FRUIT JUICES	Apple, apple cider, apple/apricot, apricot, black cherry, red cherry, cranapple, cranberry, grape (red, purple, white), grapefruit, guava, lemon, papaya, pear, pineapple, pineapple/coconut, prune, raspberry, tangerine, watermelon
SWEETENERS	Molasses, sorghum, brown sugar, date sugar, raw sugar, refined cane sugar, barley malt syrup, corn syrup, maple syrup, brown rice syrup, fructose, succonant, saccharin
CONDIMENTS	Horseradish, barbecue sauce, pesto sauce, soy sauce, spaghetti sauce, tomato sauce, tahini, halva, carob, salt, sea salt, Vege-Sal®, vinegar

Spleen

SALAD DRESSINGS	Blue cheese, French, ranch, creamy Italian, creamy avocado, thousand island, vinegar and oil, lemon juice and oil
DESSERTS	Custards, tapioca, puddings. pies, cakes, chocolate, desserts containing chocolate, raspberry sherbet
CHIPS	Bean, corn (blue, white, yellow), potato
BEVERAGES	Calli tea with stevia, herbal tea, black tea, green tea, Japanese tea, Chinese oolong tea; mineral water, sparkling water; wine (red, white), sake, beer, barley malt liquor, champagne, gin, Scotch, vodka, whiskey; root beer, regular sodas

RARELY FOODS	No more than once a month
DENSE PROTEIN	Pork, ham, sausage
DAIRY	Frozen yogurt, most ice creams
NUTS	Commercial peanut butter
GRAINS	Polished rice
FRUITS	Grapefruits
SWEETENERS	Saccharin, aspertame, Equal®, Sweet'n Low®, NutraSweet®
CONDIMENTS	Catsup, mustard, mayonnaise, margarine
BEVERAGES	Coffee, any drink with caffeine; diet sodas

SENSITIVE FOOD LIST

FREQUENTLY FOODS	3-7 meals per week – refers to each food, rather than category.
DENSE PROTEIN	Beef broth, buffalo; chicken broth, chicken livers, cornish game hen
DAIRY	Low fat or nonfat plain yogurt
CHEESE	Raw feta, ricotta
NUTS	Natural peanut butter, walnuts (black, English)
GRAINS	Oats, oatmeal, oat bran, corn tortillas
VEGETABLES	Bamboo shoots, green beans, Italian green beans, yellow wax beans, beets, bok choy, brussels sprouts, cabbage (green, napa, red), carrots, chard, pumpkin
FRUITS	Blueberries, dates
FRUIT JUICE	Orange
VEGETABLE OILS	All-blend, almond, avocado, corn, safflower, soy, sunflower
SWEETENER	Honey
CONDIMENTS	Salsa, spices, Spike®

Spleen

MODERATELY FOODS	1-2 times per week – refers to each food, rather than category.
DENSE PROTEIN	Beef, beef liver, bacon, lamb, veal, venison, organ meats (heart, brain); chicken, turkey, duck; anchovy, bass, bonita, catfish, cod, flounder, haddock, halibut, herring, mackerel, mahi-mahi, perch, orange roughy, sardines, shark, sole, swordfish, trout, tuna; abalone, calamari (squid), clams, crab, eel, lobster, mussels, octopus, oysters, scallops, shrimp; eggs. Fish (2 meals per week – rotate type)
DAIRY	Milk (whole, 2%, low fat, nonfat, raw), goat milk, buttermilk, half & half, sweet cream, sour cream, kefir, plain or flavored regular yogurt
CHEESE	American, blue, brie, Camembert, Cheddar, Colby, cottage, cream, Edam, pasteurized feta, goat, Gouda, low fat Jack, kefir, Limburger, mozzarella, Muenster, Parmesan, Romano, Swiss
NUTS and SEEDS	Almonds, almond butter, Brazils, cashew butter, water chestnuts (steamed or cooked), coconuts, filberts, hazelnuts, macadamias, macadamia butter, peanuts, pecans, pine nuts, pistachios, seeds (caraway, pumpkin, sesame, sunflower), sesame seed butter, sunflower seed butter
LEGUMES	Beans (adzuki, black, garbanzo, kidney, lima [butter], navy, great northern, pinto, red, soy), lentils, black-eyed peas, split peas, hummus, miso, soy milk, soy protein, tofu
GRAINS	Amaranth, barley, buckwheat, hominy grits, millet, popcorn, quinoa, rice (basmati brown or white, brown long or short grain, wild, Japanese), rice bran, rice cakes, rye, triticale, whole wheat, wheat germ, wheat bran, refined wheat flour, flour tortillas, breads (French, Italian, sourdough, garlic, 7-grain, multi-grain, oat, rice, rye, corn, corn/rye, sprouted grain, whole wheat, white), bagels, croissants, English muffins, crackers (saltines, oat, rye, whole wheat), couscous, pasta, udon noodles, rice noodles, cream of rice, cream of rye, cream of wheat
VEGETABLES	Artichokes, asparagus, avocados, lima beans, broccoli, broccoflower, cauliflower, cilantro, corn, cucumbers, greens (beet, collard, mustard, turnip), hominy, jicama, kale, kohlrabi, leeks, lettuce (Boston, butter, endive, iceberg, red leaf, romaine), mushrooms, okra, olives (green, ripe), onions (chives, green, brown, red, white, yellow, vidalia), parsley, parsnips, peas, snow pea pods, bell peppers (green, red, yellow), chili peppers, pimentos, potatoes (all varieties), radishes, daikon radishes, rutabaga, sauerkraut, seaweed (arame, dulse, kelp, nori, wakame), shallots, spinach, sprouts (alfalfa, clover, mung bean, radish, sunflower), squash (acorn, banana, butternut, spaghetti, yellow [summer], zucchini), sweet potatoes, tomatoes, turnips, yams
FRUITS	Apples (Golden or Red Delicious, Granny Smith, Jonathan, McIntosh, Pippin, Rome Beauty), apricots, bananas, blackberries, boysenberries, cranberries, gooseberries, raspberries, strawberries, cherries, grapes (black, green, red), guava, kiwi, kumquats, lemons, limes, loquats, mangos, melons (cantaloupe, casaba, crenshaw, honeydew, watermelon), nectarines, oranges,

Spleen

FRUITS (Continued)	papaya, peaches, pears, persimmons, pineapples, plums (black, purple, red), pomegranates, rhubarb, tangelos, tangerines, figs, prunes, raisins
SWEETENERS	Re-Vita®, stevia
CONDIMENTS	Tahini, salt, sea salt, Vege-Sal®, vinegar
SALAD DRESSINGS	Vinegar and oil, lemon juice and oil
BEVERAGES	Calli tea with stevia, herbal tea, Japanese tea, Chinese oolong tea; mineral water, sparkling water
RARELY FOODS	No more than once a month.
DENSE PROTEIN	Pork, ham, sausage; salmon, snapper
DAIRY	Frozen yogurt, ice cream
GRAINS	Corn, corn bread, corn grits, polished rice
NUTS	Cashews, commercial peanut butter
VEGETABLES	Arugula, celery, eggplant, garlic, watercress
VEGETABLE JUICES	Carrot, celery, carrot/celery, parsley, spinach, tomato, V-8®
FRUITS	Strawberries, grapefruits
FRUIT JUICES	Apple, apple cider, apple/apricot, apricot, black cherry, red cherry, cranapple, cranberry, grape (red, purple, white), grapefruit, guava, lemon, lime juice w/water, papaya, pear, pineapple, pineapple/coconut, prune, raspberry, tangerine, watermelon
VEGETABLE OILS	Canola, flaxseed, olive, peanut, sesame
SWEETENERS	Molasses, sorghum, brown sugar, date sugar, raw sugar, refined cane sugar, barley malt syrup, corn syrup, maple syrup, brown rice syrup, fructose, succonant, saccharin, aspertame, Equal®, Sweet'n Low®, NutraSweet®
CONDIMENTS	Horseradish, barbecue sauce, pesto sauce, spaghetti sauce, tomato sauce, halva, carob, catsup, mustard, mayonnaise, soy sauce, margarine
SALAD DRESSINGS	Blue cheese, French, ranch, creamy Italian, creamy avocado, thousand island
DESSERTS	Custards, tapioca, puddings, pies, cakes, chocolate, desserts containing chocolate, orange or raspberry sherbet
CHIPS	Bean, corn (blue, white, yellow), potato
BEVERAGES	Coffee, any drinks with caffeine; black tea, green tea; wine (white, red), sake, beer, barley malt liquor, champagne, vodka, Scotch, gin, whiskey; root beer, regular sodas, diet sodas

Spleen

MENUS

DIETARY EMPHASIS:

- Rotate foods.
- Consume at least 10-25% of calories from dense protein.
- Vegetables, especially green beans.
- Blueberries strengthen white blood cells.
- Spices, especially curry, up to 4 times per week, as curry strengthens red and white blood cells, and capillaries. Cayenne pepper stimulates lymphatics.

WEIGHT LOSS:

- Limit sugar (including fruit) to 2 times a week. Limit bread to 3 times a week.

WEIGHT GAIN:

- 20-25% of caloric intake from dense protein.

VEGETARIAN DIET:

- Inadequate, since require 10-25% of calories from dense protein.

FATS:

- 25-30% of caloric intake. Best sources are nuts, seeds and oils, especially sunflower seed oil, and low fat yogurt.

KEY

—all menus may be used by healthy persons

( ) around foods means that they're optional

L denotes weight loss menus

L* denotes sensitive weight loss menus

S denotes sensitive menus

G denotes weight gain menus

BREAKFAST:
7-9 a.m. Light-to-moderate, with protein, vegetables, grain, fruit, nuts, seeds, legumes, and/or dairy. May have coffee with grain twice a week.

L	S	G	Blueberries
L		G	Apple, orange, banana, or blueberries
L		G	Melons: honeydew, watermelon, or crenshaw (oatmeal)
L	S	G	Peanut butter and apple or banana
L		G	Plain yogurt (banana or apple)
		G	Yogurt and banana, apple, mango, or papaya – in blender, if desired
L			Cottage cheese and pineapple
L		G	Cottage cheese and sunflower seeds and/or raisins (blueberries and oat bread)
	S	G	Cottage cheese and sunflower seeds
L		G	Oat bread toast and banana
		G	Blueberry muffin, pancakes, or waffles (butter and syrup)
L		G	Peanut butter and rice cake
L		G	Oatmeal w/banana and sunflower seeds, or apple
		G	Oatmeal, yogurt, and Re-Vita®
L			Oatmeal or Wheat Chex® w/blueberries and skim milk
L			Shredded wheat w/milk
		G	Cheerios® w/milk and raisins
		G	Rice Chex® w/milk and dates
L*			Rice and broccoli
L	S		Lentils and broccoli
	S	G	Potatoes w/butter
L	S		Baked potato and nonfat yogurt
L*		G	Baked potato, chicken, and red onions
L*		G	Eggs (Canadian bacon)
L	S	G	Eggs w/low fat Jack cheese
L	S		Cranberry juice and ReVita®
L		G	Orange juice w/corn bread (butter)
L*			Herbal tea before – not with – breakfast

BREAKFAST, LUNCH, or **DINNER**:

L		G	Potatoes w/butter and artichoke (asparagus)
L		G	Eggs w/salsa, broccoli, and rice
		G	Oatmeal (raisins or banana)

LUNCH:
12-2 p.m. Moderate-to-heavy, with protein, vegetables, grain, fruit, nuts, seeds, legumes and/or dairy.

		G	Plain yogurt w/raw almonds and dates (apple)
L		G	Tuna salad: tuna, onion, celery, eggs, and creamy Italian dressing on pumpernickel

Spleen

L S G	Shrimp, pasta, and spinach/tomato salad w/sesame oil
L G	Shrimp fried rice w/egg, mixed vegetables, and soy sauce
L G	Trout, fried eggplant, olive oil, and garlic
L G	Cornish game hen, rice, squash, eggplant, or spinach
L G	Turkey, potatoes (gravy), broccoli, and cauliflower
L S G	Turkey and scalloped potatoes
G	Turkey on rye w/avocado
G	Turkey sandwich w/tomato on oat, rice, or potato bread (cheese), (fruit – apple, pear or banana)
G	Chicken or turkey burrito: flour tortilla, lettuce, tomato, and white cheese (avocado)
L S G	Chicken breast and spaghetti
L G	Chicken breast, broccoli, and cauliflower w/salt & pepper, cooked in chicken stock
L S G	Chicken, rice, and green beans
L* G	Chicken, potatoes, and green beans w/almonds
L*	Chicken and romaine lettuce w/vinegar and lemon
L S G	Chicken burrito: flour tortilla, chicken, lettuce, and tomato
L S G	Salad: crumbled feta cheese, shredded carrot, and chopped chicken on romaine or Boston lettuce
L	Chef salad w/chicken – no dressing
L S G	Lamb, carrots, and green beans
L G	Gyro in whole wheat pita bread, onion, tomatoes, and tziki Greek yogurt sauce
G	Beef, cheese, or bean burrito
L S G	Spaghetti, ground turkey, spaghetti sauce, and leeks
L	Pasta w/olive oil and broccoli
L S G	Lasagna – w/ricotta cheese only – and Italian green beans
G	Grilled Cheddar cheese sandwich and tomato soup
L*	Rice cakes w/almond butter and cucumber slices
L	Crusty roll, nonfat cottage cheese w/red onion, cucumber, basil, cilantro, and parsley
L	Sourdough roll, nonfat cream cheese, and raw squash, broccoli, bok choy, spinach, red onion, and fresh basil w/balsamic vinegar
L	Spinach w/lemon and rice
L*	Cucumber slices and sunflower seeds
L	Fish chowder: white fish, tomato, and basil
S G	Black bean soup w/chicken
L	Squash soup

LUNCH or DINNER:
No coffee w/lunch or dinner.

L G	Orange roughy, baked potato and butter, or green beans and corn
G	Tuna, artichoke pasta, peas, and Parmesan cheese
G	Tuna, pickle relish, w/creamy avocado or Italian dressing, and romaine or iceberg lettuce, or spinach w/corn chowder or vegetable beef soup; apple
G	Shrimp, pasta, peas, and Caesar salad; blueberries
L G	Salmon, water chestnuts, green beans, and rice
G	Salmon w/macaroni and cheese (lettuce salad, w/creamy Italian or vinegar or lemon dressing; pear
L S	Fish tacos
L* G	Chicken, baked potato, and red onions
L G	Chicken marinated in white wine, garlic, ginger, pepper, and onion w/bok choy, squash, and onions
L G	Stir-fry: chicken, snow peas, ginger, and garlic over rice
G	Chicken and rice salad (onions, mushrooms, and curry)
G	Tostada: corn tortilla w/chicken, pinto (refried) beans, onion, lettuce, salsa, or cilantro
L	Salad: lettuce, mushroom, hard boiled egg, chicken breast, cajun spices, and oil or herb dressing (apple for dessert)
L	Salad: tomato, vidalia onion, cucumber, fresh basil, and vinaigrette dressing
L	Salad: shrimp, leaf lettuce, carrots, onions, and bok choy w/low fat ranch or low fat Italian dressing
G	Taco salad: iceberg lettuce, ground beef, kidney beans, Cheddar cheese, tomatoes, onions, salsa, and corn chips

Spleen

		G	Turkey, cheese, lettuce, tomato, mushrooms, and carrots; pear
		G	Turkey, cranberry sauce, mashed potatoes, gravy, corn, and dressing; berries
		G	Ground beef, cheddar cheese, potatoes, and tomato sauce
		G	Beef lasagna
		G	Vegetable and cheese lasagna
L	S		Pasta w/pesto sauce
L	S		Eggs w/low fat Jack cheese and rice
		G	Bacon, tomato, vidalia onion, and Hain™ mayonnaise on whole wheat bread
		G	Hummus in pita bread and tziki – Greek yogurt sauce
		G	Corn tortillas w/ricotta cheese; apple
		G	Quesadillas: flour tortilla w/cheese (chilis and chopped tomato or beans); apple
		G	Red beans over white rice and mixed vegetables; peaches
L	S		Steamed yellow crook-neck squash w/butter
		G	Cheese quiche and broccoli
		G	Clam chowder – white or red
L	S	G	Beef noodle soup
L		G	Lamb stew and potatoes
		G	Vegetable soup w/crusty French bread
		G	Lima bean soup w/chicken broth, salt, pepper, and milk
		G	Potato soup

DINNER:
5-6 p.m. Light, with protein, grain, vegetables, fruit, nuts, seeds, legumes and/or dairy.

		G	Tuna on oat bread, sprouts, and yogurt (pickle relish)
L		G	Tuna, celery, romaine lettuce, and rice
L	S	G	Fillet of halibut w/rice and broccoli
L	S	G	Fillet of sole or trout w/sesame seeds, couscous, and broccoli
L		G	California roll: crab, avocado, and rice wrapped in sea weed
L		G	Turkey, pasta with butter, green beans, and carrots
		G	Chicken tacos and peaches
L	S	G	Turkey and peas (rice)
L		G	Chicken or turkey, oriental rice noodles, and mixed vegetables
L		G	Chicken or turkey breast w/plain yogurt
L	S	G	Sesame chicken, rice, and broccoli
L		G	Beef, broccoli, and rice
L			Beef, squash, and beets
		G	Steak, corn on the cob, and potato salad
L		G	Lamb and rice wrapped in grape leaves w/lemon, onions, parsley, and olive oil (mint leaves)
L	S		Sweet potatoes and peas
L	S	G	Mashed sweet potato w/orange juice (cinnamon)
L*			Baked sweet potato, yam, or potato
L			Yam w/Bragg™ aminos (lemon pepper)
L			Steamed crook-neck squash w/Bragg™ aminos (turkey)
L		G	Lentils w/rice and broccoli (artichoke hearts)
	S		Chicken noodle soup
L*			Chicken broth w/lemon pepper and Bragg™ aminos
L	S		Vegetable beef soup w/rice cakes
		G	Chili w/ground beef
L*	S	G	Vegetable stew: potatoes, tomatoes, and onions in beef broth

EVENING SNACK:
(Optional) 9 to 10 p.m. (4 hours after dinner). Light, with fruit, vegetables, grain, protein, nuts, seeds, legumes, dairy, and/or sweets.

L		G	Apple, banana, blueberries, or other fresh fruit
L	S	G	Blueberries
L		G	Lemon yogurt
L	S	G	Blueberry yogurt
L	S	G	Unsalted popcorn (garlic powder, Parmesan cheese)
		G	Raw almonds
L		G	Corn tortilla chips baked w/out oil (salsa, guacamole)
L			Celery

The "Stomach Body Type" is symbolized by fire. Digestion requires heat, which is focused energy. Focusing their attention on what's at hand allows them to ignite their passion, enjoy the moment, and accomplish their goals.

Stomach

BODY TYPE PROFILE

LOCATION	Upper abdomen on left, immediately below diaphragm between liver and spleen.
FUNCTION	Digestion, particularly protein.
POTENTIAL HEALTH PROBLEMS	Predominantly structural (muscle, ligaments, nerves), usually the result of an injury. Heartburn, mid-thoracic pain, stomach – esophagus, ulcers. Digestive distress. Tendency to love hot weather and may feel fatigue in cold weather. Problems with feet.
RECOMMENDED EXERCISE	Exercise is helpful. Its benefit is emotional as it lifts depression, releases stress, and is a means of personal expression. Best when routine, however can easily get out of the habit. Water skiing, surfing, swimming, roller blading, bicycling, walking, callanetics, rebounding, and weight lifting are good for activating vascular system. Builds muscle easily. Feels best when some form of aerobic exercise is done regularly.

WOMEN'S CHARACTERISTICS

DISTINGUISHING FEATURES	Their passion, coupled with an intense mental focus enables them to accomplish their goals. Exceptional ability to come in and take charge. Average-to-large, dominant, striking head and face with prominent chin. Characteristic head posture is lifting the chin and tilting the head backward, particularly when looking up at someone.
ADDITIONAL PHYSICAL CHARACTERISTICS	Buttocks relatively flat-to-rounded. Low back curvature straight-to-average. Breasts average. Strong body with good stamina. Shoulders relatively even with, to broader than, hips. Waist straight-to-defined. Average to long-waisted. Height petite-to-tall. Bone structure small-to-medium. Average, elongated musculature. Slender, long, or delicate to average hands. May have narrow feet. Average-to-long, oval or long, rectangular head, proportional to upper body. Square, strong jaw, often with thin-to-average upper lip or lips. Body may be at least a full size larger above waist than below.
WEIGHT GAIN AREAS	Lower body with initial gain in lower abdomen, waist, upper hips, upper back, under arms to middle back, and entire upper 2/3rds of, including upper inner thighs. Secondary gain is fairly even over body including entire back, upper arms, breasts, thighs, face, and under chin. Alternative weight gain pattern: upper to entire abdomen, upper hips, waist, and possibly breasts.

Stomach

DIETARY GUIDELINES

SCHEDULING MEALS	Breakfast: Light-to-moderate, with protein and/or grain. May include dairy, nuts, seeds, legumes, and/or vegetables. No fruit. Lunch: Moderate-to-heavy, with protein, grain, vegetables, legumes, dairy, nuts, seeds, and/or fruit. Dinner: Moderate-to-heavy, with protein, grain, vegetables, legumes, dairy, nuts, seeds, and/or fruit. Weight Loss and Sensitive: *May have sugar with large meal that includes quality protein at either lunch or dinner, but not both meals in same day. Can handle sugar twice a week, but not for evening snack. Avoid fruits.*
DIETARY EMPHASIS	• Protein and vegetables. • For weight loss, reduce fat to 15-25% of calories; consume 25-30% of total calories from dense protein per day; reduce dairy products; restrict breads; eliminate caffeine as it affects the liver; avoid alcohol and snacking between meals; and do some form of exercise every day. May use appetite suppressant to reduce food quantities. • For weight gain, 25-35% of caloric intake from dense protein. Increase fats and food quantity. • Vegetarian diets inadequate since require 25-35% of calories from dense protein. • Fats, 15-25% of calories for weight loss, 25-35% for maintenance, 25% for sensitive. Best sources are dense protein (all), eggs, butter, fish. To reduce fats, emphasize white chicken and turkey, eliminating dark meat and butter.
KEY SUPPORTS FOR SYSTEM	Adequate dense protein, Sunrider® foods. Kombucha tea aids digestion, assimilation, regulation of bowels, helps relieve joint stiffness, and increases energy levels.
COMPLEMENTARY GLANDULAR SUPPORT	Lungs, through nurturing self and others; pituitary, through understanding self, others, and life experiences.
FOODS CRAVED	*(When Energy is Low)* Carbohydrates like pasta, potatoes, dark chocolate pieces, salty popcorn, and salty foods. Strong appetite. Can eat a large quantity at once, particularly when stressed or has missed meals. Can become uncomfortable if skipping meals or a meal is delayed, or when busy can easily skip meals without repercussions.

Stomach

FOODS TO AVOID

Spicy foods when digestive system is sensitive.

RECOMMENDED CUISINE

Home-style cooking, Italian, Mexican, Moroccan, Chinese, Irish, Hungarian.

PSYCHOLOGICAL PROFILE

ESSENCE

Just as the stomach focuses all its attention on the food it's digesting, Stomach body types focus on what's in front of them, allowing them to ignite their passion and truly live in the present moment. It's their focus, passion, and physical stamina that enables them to accomplish their goals. When dealing with a problem, they will often talk it out, either alone or with someone else, chewing the data until they have sufficiently digested it. They make their best decisions after they have thoroughly processed the material. Igniting their passion brings an aliveness to everything they undertake, which is especially apparent when expressed through music and dance.

CHARACTERISTIC TRAITS

Stomachs have a strong mental orientation to reality and often find that whatever they focus on, they create. While they prefer to develop an intellectual grasp of a situation before taking action, they can be impulsive, relying on their heart or gut feelings. It's their head and heart connection that allows them to live in the moment. While they are social and often gregarious, there is also a conscientious side that will internalize all aspects of an issue. Once they have assimilated significant material, they'll simplify and organize it in a manner that is clear, easy to teach, and understand.

In their communication, Stomach types are quite articulate and precise and project strength by the way they express themselves, causing people to listen when they speak. Trusting their intellect over their feelings and their own opinions over someone else's can make them quite skeptical of new ideas and opposing beliefs. Balance comes once they have learned to listen and trust their intuition.

Stomachs have a unique way of dealing with people, tasks, and situations. They completely focus their total attention on them as though they are engulfing them within their energy field. This allows them to ignite their own passion and experience things more intensely, causing them to manifest their desires. This approach is particularly apparent in the way they make love.

Fun and creativity are integral parts of the Stomach's makeup. No matter how difficult or routine the task, Stomachs will figure out a way to make it light and enjoyable.

Stomach

MOTIVATION

Meeting a challenge brings a sense of ultimate success and accomplishment like nothing else. So, a challenge will often serve to motivate them to succeed at difficult or seemingly impossible tasks. Being basically social in nature, Stomach types enjoy the public recognition that their accomplish-ments can bring.

Stomachs have a strong desire to please others as the responses of those around them are crucial to their sense of self-worth. They'll pay close attention to their behavior and will often push themselves to do something because of how they think others will respond. Women will often link and measure their personal identity and value with their physical attractiveness.

Men, generally, truly love women. They are inherently attracted to them, but don't know how to deal with them when conflict arises. Many would prefer to leave, then come back when the stress has dissipated. Women are generally much better at learning how to handle conflict. Men often have the need to experience many women, as a way of learning about their own feminine side, particularly if they have a strong "macho" pattern. Women are more likely than men to commit to a relationship and stay committed as family and particularly children are a high priority for them. While family is also a high priority for men, unless it's their main focus, they will not allow family to interfere with their current goal.

"AT WORST"

Stomachs need to be in control, which can even include controlling a situation to prevent anyone from being upset. The more insecure they are, the stronger the need. When others don't follow their wishes, they can become impatient, irritable, or angry. Insecurity can lead to behavior that is self-centered and manipulative or to the need to always be right. Strong-minded, with a strong will and definite beliefs, they can easily be forceful, stubborn, or dogmatic, even skeptical of change or new ideas that can't be physically proven or verified.

In an attempt to lighten or release their suppressed feelings, they are apt to rely on humor or play the role of a trickster. Unresolved emotional issues are often underneath their poking fun at people or excessive teasing.

Dealing with conflict is difficult as they will either blame themselves or deny any responsibility whatsoever. The tendency is to avoid the issues by becoming evasive, burying themselves in work, leaving the relationship, or going where they can be alone, often comforting or nurturing themselves in a destructive manner. They are prone to filling themselves with food, drugs, or alcohol to insulate against feelings of emptiness and deprivation. Not being able to "stomach it," they will nurture themselves with food, linking emotional fulfillment with feeling empty or full.

Stomach

"AT WORST"

Being passionate by nature, Stomachs will often use sex as a way of validating themselves, associating their ability to attract the opposite sex with their self-worth. Their insecurities often lead to problems with jealousy.

When low self-esteem is an issue, Stomach types can be quite critical of themselves and will often rate their performance lower than deserved. Being perfectionists, they are never satisfied with their own achievements, particularly when their sense of self-worth is dependent on how they think others perceive them.

"AT BEST "

Stomachs have a unique ability to totally encompass someone when speaking or focusing attention on them. Being the absolute center of their attention gives the feeling of being completely engulfed and unconditionally loved. Coupled with their sensitivity and desire to please, Stomachs can be an ideal friend or lover. With a good sense of humor and gregarious nature, they can be fun to be around.

When they direct their strong will, determination, practical application, and hard work, along with their passion, they have a winning combination. This is particularly apparent when expressed on stage in music or dance. Since they also have the ability to activate others' passion and appreciation, they make excellent speakers or performers.

Experiencing life physically provides a feeling of connectedness and meeting challenges is a way of adding meaning to life. While wholeheartedly devoting themselves to their endeavors, they can be imaginative and enterprising. When this feeling of being universally supported is present, there's an openness to new experiences, ideas, and emotions along with an adaptability to whatever life brings. This is particularly evident when dealing with confrontation, as it is handled in a positive, constructive manner, especially with the opposite sex, through discussion and respect.

Once they have learned to truly listen to everything around them, including their own inner voice, God, their feelings, their body, and their feminine side, they develop their own inner strength, validate themselves, and become secure within themselves. From here, they can evaluate a situation according to their inner truth rather than relying on outside appearances, partial information, or assumptions. This is when they are able to completely enjoy the moment, giving it their all while staying in balance, enabling them to give without sacrificing themselves. This is the essence of abundance.

Stomach

FOOD LISTS

HEALTHY FOOD LIST

FREQUENTLY FOODS	3-7 meals per week – refers to each food, rather than category.
DENSE PROTEIN	Beef, beef broth, beef liver, buffalo, lamb, pork, bacon, ham, sausage; chicken, chicken broth, chicken livers, cornish game hen, turkey, duck; anchovy, bass, bonita, cod, flounder, haddock, halibut, herring, mahi-mahi, perch, roughy, salmon, sardines, shark, red snapper, sole, swordfish, tuna; abalone, eel, lobster, mussels, octopus, scallops, shrimp; eggs
DAIRY	Milk (whole, 2%, low fat, nonfat, raw), butter
CHEESE	Ricotta
GRAINS	Barley, corn, corn bread, corn grits, corn tortillas, popcorn, wild rice, whole wheat, wheat bran, wheat germ, shredded wheat, breads (corn, whole wheat), whole wheat crackers, couscous, pasta, udon noodles, rice noodles, cream of wheat
VEGETABLES	Artichokes, avocados, cilantro, peas, snow pea pods, radishes (red, white), spinach, tomatoes, zucchini
FRUITS	Bananas, raspberries, grapes (black, green, red), watermelons, papayas, pineapples, plums (black, purple, red)
SWEETENERS	Re-Vita®, stevia
CONDIMENTS	Mustard, salt, sea salt
BEVERAGES	Tea (caffeine once a day), herbal tea, black tea, green tea, Japanese tea, Chinese oolong tea, mineral water, sparkling water, root beer
MODERATELY FOODS	1-2 meals per week – refers to each food, rather than category.
DENSE PROTEIN	Veal, venison, organ meats (heart, brain); catfish, mackerel, trout; calamari (squid), clams, crab, oysters
DAIRY	Goat milk, half & half, sweet cream, sour cream, kefir, plain or flavored yogurt, frozen yogurt, ice cream (Dreyer's, Ben & Jerry's®, Swensen's®)
CHEESE	American, blue, brie, Camembert, Cheddar, Colby, cottage, cream, Edam, feta, goat, Gouda, Jack, kefir, Limburger, mozzarella, Muenster, Parmesan, Romano, Swiss
NUTS and SEEDS	Almonds, almond butter, Brazils, cashews, cashew butter, water chestnuts, filberts, hazelnuts, macadamias, macadamia butter, peanuts, peanut butter, pecans, pine nuts, pistachios, walnuts (black, English), seeds (caraway, pumpkin, sesame, sunflower), sesame seed butter, sunflower seed butter
LEGUMES	Beans (adzuki, black, garbanzo, kidney, navy, great northern, lima [butter], pinto, red, soy), lentils, black-eyed peas, split peas, hummus, miso, soy milk, tofu

Stomach

GRAINS	Amaranth, buckwheat, hominy grits, millet, oats, oat bran, oat bran flakes, quinoa, rice (brown or white basmati, long or short grain brown, Japanese), rice bran, rice cakes, triticale, rye, refined wheat flour, flour tortillas, breads (French, Italian, sourdough, garlic, 7-grain, multi-grain, oat, rice, corn/rye, rye, sprouted grain, white), bagels, croissants, English muffins, crackers (saltines, oat, rye), cream of rice, cream of rye
VEGETABLES	Arugula, asparagus, bamboo shoots, green beans, yellow wax beans, lima beans, beets, bok choy, broccoli, broccoflower, brussels sprouts, cabbage (green, napa, red), carrots, cauliflower, celery, chard, corn, cucumbers, eggplant, garlic, greens (beet, collard, mustard, turnip), hominy, jicama, kale, kohlrabi, leeks, lettuce (Boston, butter, endive, iceberg, red leaf, romaine), mushrooms, okra, olives, onions (chives, green. brown, red, white, yellow, vidalia), parsnips, bell peppers, chili peppers, pimentos, potatoes (red, russet, white rose, yukon gold, purple), sweet potatoes, pumpkin, daikon radishes, rutabaga, sauerkraut, seaweed (arame, dulse, nori, wakame), shallots, sprouts (alfalfa, clover, mung bean, radish, sunflower), squash (acorn, banana, butternut, yellow [summer], spaghetti), turnips, watercress, yams
VEGETABLE JUICES	Celery, carrot, carrot/celery, spinach, tomato, V-8®
FRUITS	Apples (Golden or Red Delicious, Granny Smith, Jonathan, McIntosh, Pippin, Rome Beauty), apricots, blackberries, blueberries, boysenberries, cranberries, gooseberries, strawberries, grapefruits (white, red), guavas, kiwi, kumquats, lemons, limes, loquats, mangos, melons (cantaloupe, casaba, crenshaw, honeydew), nectarines, oranges, peaches, pears, persimmons, pomegranates, rhubarb, tangelos, tangerines, dates, figs, prunes, raisins
FRUIT JUICES	Apple, apple cider, apple/apricot, apricot, black cherry, red cherry, cranapple, cranberry, grape (red, purple, white), grapefruit, guava, lemon, orange, papaya, pear, pineapple, pineapple/coconut, prune, tangerine, watermelon
VEGETABLE OILS	All-blend, almond, avocado, corn, flaxseed, olive, peanut, safflower, sesame, sunflower
SWEETENERS	Honey, molasses, sorghum, brown sugar, date sugar, raw sugar, refined cane sugar, barley malt syrup, corn syrup, maple syrup, brown rice syrup, fructose, succonant, saccharin
CONDIMENTS	Catsup, cinnamon, spices, Vege-Sal®, mint, horseradish, barbecue sauce, pesto sauce, soy sauce, salsa, tahini, vinegar
SALAD DRESSINGS	Blue cheese, French, ranch, creamy Italian, creamy avocado, thousand island, vinegar and oil, lemon juice and oil
DESSERTS	Custards, tapioca, puddings, pies, cakes, chocolate, desserts containing chocolate, orange or raspberry sherbet
CHIPS	Bean, corn (blue, white, yellow), potato
BEVERAGES	Coffee (decaf), regular coffee, coffee with Re-vita®; wine (red, white), sake, beer, barley malt liquor, champagne, gin, Scotch, vodka, whiskey; regular sodas

Stomach

RARELY FOODS	No more than once a month
DAIRY	Buttermilk, most ice creams
NUTS	Coconuts
VEGETABLES	Kelp, parsley
VEGETABLE JUICE	Parsley
FRUITS	Cherries
VEGETABLE OILS	Canola, soy
SWEETENERS	Aspartame, Equal®, Sweet'n Low®, NutraSweet®
CONDIMENTS	Margarine, mayonnaise
BEVERAGES	Diet sodas

SENSITIVE FOOD LIST

FREQUENTLY FOODS	3-7 meals per week – refers to each food, rather than category.
DENSE PROTEIN	Beef, lamb; chicken, turkey; halibut, salmon, tuna; eggs
DAIRY	Whole milk, raw milk
CHEESE	Ricotta
VEGETABLES	Avocado, cilantro
MODERATELY FOODS	1-2 meals per week – refers to each food, rather than category.
DENSE PROTEIN	Bacon, beef broth, beef liver, buffalo, veal, venison, organ meats (heart, brain); chicken broth, chicken livers, cornish game hen, duck; anchovy, bass, bonita catfish, cod, flounder, haddock, herring, mackerel, mahi-mahi, perch, roughy, sardines, shark, red snapper, sole, swordfish, trout; abalone, calamari (squid), clams, crab, eel, lobster, mussels, octopus, oysters, scallops, shrimp
DAIRY	Low fat or nonfat milk, goat milk, half & half, sweet cream, sour cream, kefir, butter
CHEESE	American, blue, brie, Camembert, Cheddar, Colby, cottage, cream, Edam, feta, goat, Gouda, Jack, kefir, Limburger, mozzarella, Muenster, Parmesan, Romano, Swiss
NUTS and SEEDS	Almonds (dry roasted, unsalted), almond butter, Brazils, cashews, cashew butter, water chestnuts, filberts, hazelnuts, macadamias, macadamia butter, peanuts, peanut butter, pecans, pine nuts, pistachios, walnuts (black, English), seeds (caraway, pumpkin, sesame, sunflower), sesame seed butter, sunflower seed butter

Stomach

LEGUMES	Beans (adzuki, black, garbanzo, kidney, navy, great northern, lima [butter], pinto, red, soy), lentils, black-eyed peas, split peas, hummus, miso, soy milk, tofu
GRAINS	Amaranth, barley, buckwheat, corn, corn bread, corn grits, corn tortillas, hominy grits, millet, popcorn, quinoa, rice (brown or white basmati, long or short grain brown, Japanese, wild), rice bran, rice cakes, rye, triticale, refined wheat flour, flour tortillas, breads (French, Italian, sourdough, garlic, corn, corn/rye, rye, rice, sprouted grain, white), bagels, croissants, English muffins, crackers (saltines, rye), couscous, pasta, udon noodles, rice noodles, cream of rice, cream of rye
VEGETABLES	Bamboo shoots, green beans, yellow wax beans, lima beans, beets, bok choy, broccoli, broccoflower, brussels sprouts, cabbage (green, napa, red), carrots, cauliflower, celery, chard, corn, cucumbers, eggplant, greens (beet, collard, mustard, turnip), hominy, jicama, kale, kohlrabi, leeks, lettuce (Boston, butter, endive, iceberg, red leaf, romaine), mushrooms, okra, olives (green, ripe), onions (chives, green, brown, red, white, yellow, vidalia), parsnips, peas, snow pea pods, bell peppers (green, red, yellow), chili peppers, pimentos, potatoes (red, russet, white rose, yukon gold, purple), sweet potatoes, pumpkin, radishes, daikon radishes, rutabaga, sauerkraut, seaweed (arame, dulse, nori, wakame), shallots, spinach, sprouts (alfalfa, clover, mung bean, radish, sunflower), squash (acorn, banana, butternut, spaghetti, yellow[summer], zucchini), tomatoes, turnips, yams
VEGETABLE JUICES	Carrot, celery, carrot/celery, spinach, tomato, V-8®
FRUIT	Apples (Golden or Red Delicious, Granny Smith, Jonathan, McIntosh, Pippin, Rome Beauty), apricots, blackberries, blueberries, boysenberries, cranberries, gooseberries, raspberries, strawberries, grapes (black, green, red), grapefruits (white, red), guavas, kiwi, kumquats, lemons, limes, loquats, mangos, melons (cantaloupe, watermelon), nectarines, oranges, papayas, peaches, pears, persimmons, pineapples, plums (black, purple, red), pomegranates, rhubarb,tangelos, tangerines, dried apricots, dates, figs, prunes, raisins
FRUIT JUICES	Apple, apple cider, apple/apricot, apricot, black cherry, red cherry, cranapple, cranberry, grape (red, purple, white), grapefruit, guava, lemon, orange, papaya,pear, pineapple, pineapple/coconut, prune, tangerine, watermelon
VEGETABLE OILS	Coconut, sesame, soy
SWEETENERS	Re-vita®, stevia
CONDIMENTS	Salsa, tahini, salt, sea salt, Vege-Sal®
SALAD DRESSINGS	Vinegar and oil, lemon juice and oil
BEVERAGES	Herbal tea, Japanese tea, Chinese oolong tea; mineral water, sparkling water

Stomach

RARELY FOODS	No more than once a month
DENSE PROTEIN	Pork, ham, sausage
DAIRY	Buttermilk, yogurt, frozen yogurt, ice cream
NUTS	Coconuts
GRAINS	Oats, oat bran, oat bran flakes, whole wheat, wheat germ, wheat bran, breads (7-grain, multi-grain, oat, whole wheat), crackers (oat, whole wheat), taco shells, cream of wheat
VEGETABLES	Artichokes, arugula, asparagus, garlic, kelp, parsley, watercress
VEGETABLE JUICE	Parsley
FRUITS	Bananas, cherries, melons (casaba, crenshaw, honeydew)
VEGETABLE OILS	All-blend, almond, avocado, canola, corn, flaxseed, olive, peanut, safflower, sunflower
SWEETENERS	Honey, molasses, sorghum, brown sugar, date sugar, raw sugar, refined cane sugar, barley malt syrup, corn syrup, maple syrup, brown rice syrup, fructose, succonant, saccharin, aspartame, Equal®, Sweet'n Low®, NutraSweet®
CONDIMENTS	Catsup, cinnamon, spices, mustard, horseradish, mint, barbecue sauce, pesto sauce, soy sauce, margarine, mayonnaise, vinegar
SALAD DRESSINGS	Blue cheese, French, ranch, creamy Italian, creamy avocado, thousand island
DESSERTS	Custards, tapioca, puddings, pies, cakes, orange or raspberry sherbet, chocolate, desserts containing chocolate
CHIPS	Bean, corn (blue, white, yellow), potato
BEVERAGES	Coffee (decaffeinated), regular coffee, black tea, green tea; beer, sake, wine (red, white), champagne, vodka, Scotch, gin, whiskey, barley malt liquor; root beer, regular sodas, diet sodas

Stomach

MENUS

DIETARY EMPHASIS:

- Protein and vegetables.
- Kombucha tea, as it aids digestion, assimilation, regulation of bowels, helps relieve joint stiffness, and increases energy levels.
- Avoid spicy foods when digestive system is stressed or sensitive.

WEIGHT LOSS:

- Reduce fat to 15-25% of calories, less than 10% inhibits weight loss.
- 25-30% of caloric intake from dense protein.
- Restrict bread.
- Avoid fruit.
- Reduce dairy products, but may use low fat milk with cereal.
- Eliminate caffeine as it affects liver.
- Avoid alcohol, as it inhibits weight loss.
- Avoid snacking between meals.
- Do some form of exercise daily.
- Reduce food quantities, may use appetite suppressant.

WEIGHT GAIN:

- 25-35% of caloric intake from dense protein.
- Increase fats and food quantity.

VEGETARIAN DIET:

- Inadequate, since require 20-35% of calories from dense protein.

FATS:

- 15-25% of caloric intake for weight loss, 25-35% for maintenance, and 25% for sensitive.
- Best sources are dense protein (all), 2 eggs 3x/wk, butter, fish and tuna.
  To reduce fats, emphasize white chicken and turkey, eliminating butter.

KEY

—all menus may be used by healthy persons
( ) around foods means that they're optional
L denotes weight loss menus
S denotes sensitive menus
G denotes weight gain menus

BREAKFAST:

5-9 a.m. Light-to-moderate, with protein, and/or grain May include dairy, nuts, seeds, legumes, and/or vegetables. No fruit.

L		G	Total® wheat flakes or shredded wheat w/low fat milk
L		G	Oat groats w/skim milk
		G	Granola w/whole or raw milk
L			Cream of rice and nonfat milk
L	S		Cream of rice w/Amazaki™
L			Kashi® or Nutri-Grain® w/low fat or nonfat milk
L	S		Corn flakes w/soy milk
L	S		Amaranth and corn flakes or quinoa
L			Rye and rice cereal w/maple syrup and ground flaxseed
L			All-Bran® w/nonfat milk
L			Oat bran muffin w/wheat flakes and low fat milk
			Whole wheat toast w/butter and honey
			Brown rice and beans
L		G	Rice and chicken
		G	Bacon and biscuit w/butter (egg)
		G	Eggs w/bagel
	S*	G	Eggs and sprouted rye
	S*	G	Essene® bread (almond butter)
L		G	Eggs and whole wheat toast (flaxseed oil)
L	S		Eggs scrambled w/spinach

MID-MORNING SNACK:

(Optional) 10:30 a.m. Protein, grain, vegetables.

		G	Kamut bread
	S	G	Potatoes and Spike®
		G	Beef jerky, turkey, or fish, such as halibut or shark
		G	Sun bar® or protein bar

Stomach

	LUNCH: 11 a.m.-2 p.m. Moderate-to-heavy, with protein, grain, vegetables, legumes, dairy, nuts, seeds, and/or fruit. SENSITIVE: Avoid fruit.
L S G	Amaranth spaghetti w/ground turkey, veal, or lamb, tomato paste, garlic, green onion, and cilantro
G	Lasagna: ricotta cheese, spinach pasta, tomato sauce, and tomato paste
L	Chinese stir-fry (cashews)
S*	Eggs and potatoes (rye toast)
G	Eggs, potatoes, steak, and toast
L S*	Eggs and green beans
L S	Eggs and broccoli
L S	Eggs, cilantro, corn, and tomatoes
L	Eggs, cilantro, blue corn tortilla, and tomatoes
L S	Lentils, rice, spinach, and onions
S*	Lentils, rice, and onions
L S*	Steamed clams, kale, basmati rice, and cooked spinach
G	Tuna and mushroom quiche
S*	Tuna and avocado (rye toast or crackers)
L S	Lamb and cooked or raw carrots
G	Roast beef on pumpernickel bread w/lettuce and mustard (iced tea)
L S G	Beef and zucchini
L	Beef or chicken tostada w/small amount sour cream or avocado
L S G	Ground turkey and cauliflower
G	Turkey on whole wheat bread w/mustard and lettuce
L	Lean chicken, sauteed in water, herbs, lemon, and barley or rice
L G	Roasted chicken, baked potato, and salad (roll)
L G	Chicken breast w/steamed carrots, broccoli, or potato
L G	Chicken burrito
L	Steamed greens and broccoli w/lettuce salad and flaxseed oil
L	Rice, broccoli, and zucchini
L	Carrot/apple salad
L	Turkey vegetable soup
G	Minestrone soup w/tomatoes and lima beans
L G	Beef stew

LUNCH OR DINNER:

L G	Nori roll, haddock, and brown rice
L	Crab on romaine lettuce, parsley, and white basmati rice
L G	Mackerel, wild rice, cucumber, and green peas
L G	Tuna, rice, and carrots
S G	Tuna on kamut bread, watercress, and avocado
L	Tuna, tossed salad, and Caesar salad dressing
L S*	Tuna, pasta, and peas
S G	Tuna, pasta, peas, Cheddar cheese, and milk
L S	Tuna and spinach salad: tuna, spinach, onion, egg, and celery
L G	Salmon and asparagus
L S*G	Halibut, rice, and turnip greens or spinach
L G	Fillet of sole, and artichokes (corn)
L S*G	Snapper, swordfish, or cod, broccoli, and rice (cauliflower)
L S*	Trout, broccoli, and carrots
L S*	White fish, rice, lima beans, and carrots
L S*G	Fish, game hen, or chicken, wild rice, and green peas
L	Fish tacos: mackerel or whitefish, onions, tomatoes, and romaine lettuce w/balsamic vinegar and flaxseed oil
G	Cheese enchiladas
S*G	Chicken enchiladas w/rice
L S*	Chicken w/carrots and celery
L S G	Chicken, pasta, and raw or cooked spinach
L S*G	Chicken and pasta
L G	Chicken, russet potatoes w/nonfat yogurt, asparagus or broccoli, and carrots
L S*	Turkey, chicken, or beef, tomato sauce, and garlic

Stomach

- S*G Turkey, potato, and green beans (cranberry sauce)
- G Turkey sandwich on whole wheat bread, alfalfa sprouts, and avocado
- L S*G Turkey meat loaf and peas
- L S*G Pasta and turkey meat balls
- L S*G Steak or fish and potato (corn)
- G Beef tacos (tomatoes, romaine lettuce, onions, and black olives) and/or (Spanish rice)
- L S G Beef and baked potato (carrots)
- L S G Beef, veal, or lamb stew, potatoes, and salad
- G Sauteed mushrooms w/butter over hamburger steak and green peas or carrots
- L S G Rack of lamb or lamb roast, potato, carrots, and broccoli
- L S*G Lamb and potatoes
- L G Lamb chops, yams, and salad: green leaf lettuce, mushrooms, green onions, bean sprouts, and tomatoes
- G Ham hocks and beans w/cornbread
- L S*G Ham and sweet potato
- L Liver and onions
- L Brown basmati rice and asparagus w/raw carrots
- L Stir-fry: onions, garlic, mushrooms, eggplant, carrots, celery, red bell pepper, zucchini, and sesame oil or lite soy oil
- L Salad: beets, red leaf lettuce, radishes, cucumbers, green bell peppers, carrots, hard-boiled egg, and lite Italian dressing or vinegar and olive oil
- L S Spinach salad w/eggs
- G Spinach salad w/tuna, onion, hard-boiled egg, and celery
- S G Three bean salad: garbanzo, kidney, and green beans, and pasta w/Parmesan cheese
- Garbanzo beans and spinach
- L Baked potato w/pesto sauce and flaxseed oil
- L S* Millet in chicken broth (black bean soup)
- L S*G Lentil soup
- L S*G Black bean soup w/turkey
- L S*G Split pea w/ham soup
- L S G Spaghetti w/ground turkey, veal, lamb, or beef, tomato paste, garlic, green onion, and cilantro
- S Lasagna: ricotta cheese, spinach and lasagna noodles, tomato sauce and paste (salad of romaine lettuce, carrots, avocado, and celery w/o salad dressing)
- S*G Lasagna: lasagna noodles, tomato sauce, chicken, turkey, or beef, and Parmesan cheese w/salad: romaine lettuce, carrots, avocado, and celery (w/o salad dressing)
- S G Amaranth spaghetti w/ground turkey, pasta sauce, and Parmesan cheese
- S Tofu, vegetables, and rice
- L S Brown rice and vegetables

AFTERNOON SNACK:

(Optional) Fruit, vegetables, grain, protein, dairy, nuts, seeds, sweets.

- Popcorn (butter)
- Fruit juices
- Fruit such as oranges, pears, red Delicious apples, nectarines, peaches, mangos, raspberries, strawberries, blueberries, or bananas
- G Oatmeal w/Re-Vita®
- S G Plain nonfat yogurt w/berry Re-Vita®

DINNER:

5-9 p.m. Moderate-to-heavy, with protein, grain, vegetables, legumes, dairy, nuts, seeds, and/or fruit.

SENSITIVE: Avoid fruit.

- L S*G Salmon, lima beans, and carrots
- L G White fish, lima beans and carrots, and artichoke pasta
- L S* Halibut, red snapper, or white fish and green beans
- L G Halibut, tabouli, turnip greens, and pesto sauce
- L S* Halibut, kale, and collards
- L S* Fillet of sole, carrots, and broccoli
- S*G Trout (oysters on the half shell), scalloped potatoes, and broccoli
- G Crab cakes w/vegetables and butter
- L S*G Chicken, broccoli, and cauliflower

Stomach

S*	Almond chicken (rice)
L	Almond chicken
L S*G	Turkey and sweet potato
L S G	Turkey, sweet potato, kale, and collards
L G	Turkey, chicken, or fish w/green beans, zucchini, and/or mushrooms
L G	Beef tamales
L G	Roast beef, potatoes, and broccoli (green beans and/or squash, and/or cauliflower)
L S*G	Rack of lamb or lamb roast, beet greens, and sweet potatoes
L G	Broiled lamb chops, potatoes, and tomatoes
L S*G	Millet in chicken broth, black bean chili, and cooked celery
L G	Spaghetti and meat balls
S	Pasta primavera w/tomato sauce – no meat
L S	Pasta w/tomato sauce and broccoli, zucchini, and/or peppers
L	Couscous w/pesto sauce
G	Total® cereal, milk, and banana
L	Garbanzo beans, beets, tomato, cucumber, lettuce, and wine vinegar lo-cal dressing
L	Bananas or peaches
L S*G	Lamb stew w/potatoes
G	Seafood stew w/bread
	Wine w/dinner
G	Nonfat strawberry yogurt after dinner
L	Camomile tea

1 HOUR AFTER DINNER:
(Optional)

G	Hershey's® chocolate w/almonds
G	Chocolate chip cookies
G	Oreo cookies

Sweets are appropriate after lunch or dinner, or afternoon or evening snack, 1 or 2 x/week, no more than 1 x/day. Bourbon and water after dinner or before bed. If before a meal, foods such as carrots or celery are needed with it.

SNACK:
(Optional) 10 p.m.-2 a.m. Fruit, grain, vegetables, protein, nuts, seeds, dairy, sweets.

S	Rye/pumpernickel crackers
S*G	Rye bread
S*G	Sprouted rye Essene® bread
S*	Essene® bread w/raisins and dates
S	Rice cakes
S G	Dried apricots, prunes, peaches, pears, or figs
S*G	Dates
L S G	Popcorn
L S*G	Raw soaked almonds
L S*G	Sun Rider®Sun Bar® or NuPlus™
G	Plain yogurt w/berry Re-Vita®
	Oatmeal w/Re-Vita®

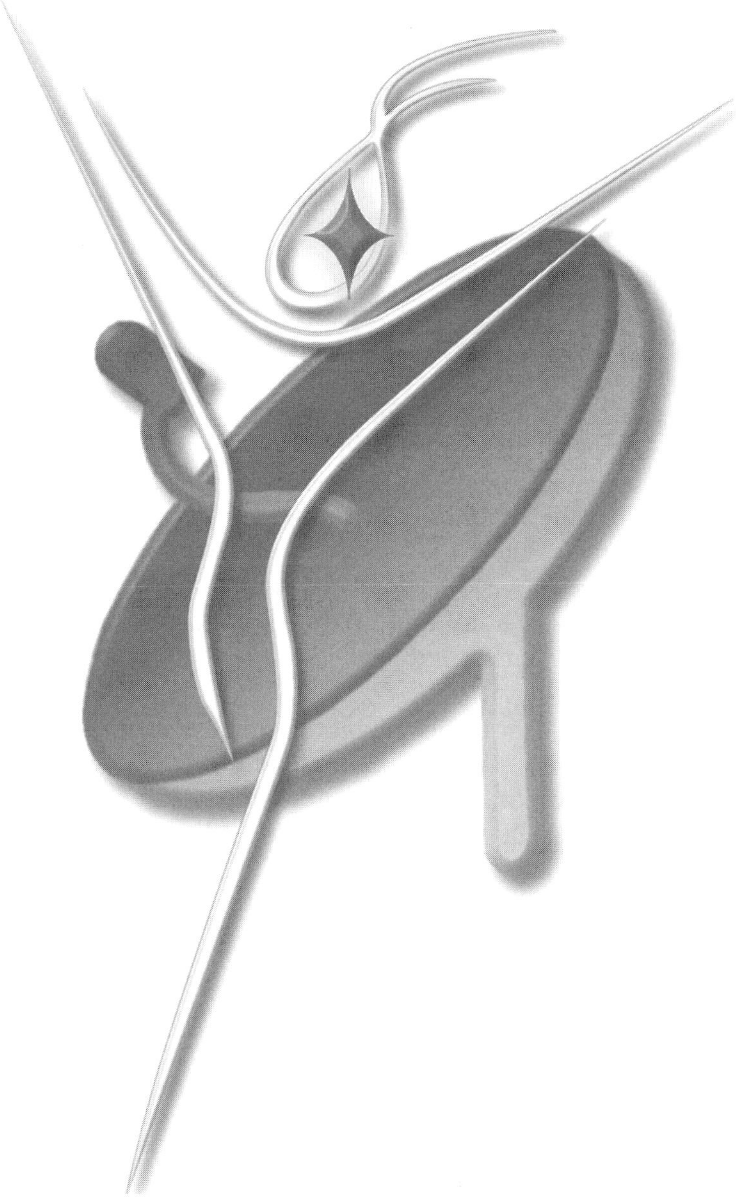

The "Thalamus Body Type"
is symbolized by a satellite dish.
Collecting and evaluating information
before passing it on, they are open to
new ideas. Sensitive to vibrations,
music is essential and will
readily shift their moods.

Thalamus

BODY TYPE PROFILE

LOCATION	Center of brain base, between hypothalamus and pineal glands.
FUNCTION	Main relay center for sensory impulses to cerebral cortex.
POTENTIAL HEALTH PROBLEMS	Mentally tense; difficulty in quieting mind; anxiety. Carry tension in shoulders. Digestive distress; constipation. Fear can cause sinus congestion. Headaches (vascular) affected by temperature, especially cold and moist, like air-conditioning, high humidity or atmospheric pressure changes. May be susceptible to high bacterial levels found in moist air. Often gets cold easily. Problems with eyes or vision. Needs sunlight or feels depressed. Affected by weather changes like high humidity or alterations in atmospheric pressure. Often feels better when close to ocean.
RECOMMENDED EXERCISE	Exercise is helpful, as it calms the mind. Ideally, do something daily, even if only for a few minutes scattered throughout the day, regardless of time. Best activities include walking, tennis, swimming, callanetics, and using an EMS machine. Almost all other exercise, including dance, racquetball, and volleyball are acceptable. Jogging and running are poor choices.

WOMEN'S CHARACTERISTICS

DISTINGUISHING CHARACTERISTICS	High, wide and/or dominant forehead, with long, slender oval face, or long-to-average rectangular face. Typically slender, delicate appearance, even with weight gain. Energy focus is predominantly in head, as they are noted for collecting and evaluating information that comes their way.
ADDITIONAL PHYSICAL FEATURES	Buttocks relatively flat-to-rounded. Low back curvature average-to-swayed. Continuous arching abdominal musculature with lower abdominal protrusion. Breasts small-to-average. Shoulders relatively even with hips. Defined waist. Average to long-waisted. Height generally average-to-tall. Bone structure small-to-medium. Average, elongated musculature. Hips generally more wide than thick. Average, muscular thighs and calves. Average to long, slender hands. Head proportionate to body, small-to-average eyes. May have protruding ears in childhood. Body often a full size smaller above waist than below.

Thalamus

WEIGHT GAIN AREAS	Lower body with initial gain in lower abdomen, face, entire upper 2/3rds of thighs including upper inner, and upper hips. Secondary gain in waist, entire abdomen, middle-to-entire back, upper arms, buttocks, lower hips, thighs, calves, and breasts. May have difficulty gaining or maintaining weight.

DIETARY GUIDELINES

SCHEDULING MEALS

Breakfast: Light-to-moderate, with light protein, such as eggs, fruit, grain, nuts, seeds, dairy, vegetables, and/or legumes.

Lunch: Moderate-to-heavy, with protein, vegetables, legumes, nuts, seeds, grain, and/or dairy.

Dinner: Moderate, with protein, vegetables, grain, legumes, nuts, seeds, and/or dairy.

DIETARY EMPHASIS

- Fruit should be consumed only in the morning or for bedtime snack.
- Eat more cooked than raw vegetables.
- For weight loss, eliminate refined sugar, alcohol, honey, and all artificial sweeteners, minimize breads and butter, and consume 20-25% of caloric intake as fats. Less than 15% inhibits weight loss. Avoid fruit juice, but may include fruit.
- For weight gain, simply increase the quantity of food intake.
- Vegetarian diets inadequate, as require 10-30% of caloric intake from dense protein.
- Fats, 20-25% of caloric intake from seeds, especially sesame tahini, and dense protein (chicken, turkey, fish, eggs, beef).

KEY SUPPORTS FOR SYSTEM

Music, as it allows for connection with body and emotions. Nature, sense of freedom – need to be in control of own life and environment.

COMPLEMENTARY GLANDULAR SUPPORT

Lymph, through daily movement such as walking; hypothalamus, through connecting feelings with intellect by nurturing and pampering self.

FOODS CRAVED

(When Energy is Low) Sweets, such as ice cream, chocolate (bittersweet), peanut butter cups, cookies, cinnamon rolls. Carbohydrates, like muffins, breads, grains. Spicy foods.

FOODS TO AVOID

Almonds, pasteurized milk, beer, and wine.

Thalamus

RECOMMENDED CUISINE

Mexican, Thai, Seafood. Moderate: Italian, Middle Eastern, Chinese.

PSYCHOLOGICAL PROFILE

ESSENCE

Just as the thalamus collects information and files it for storage in the cerebral cortex or brain, Thalamus body types collect and evaluate information. They like to be effective and tend to be perfectionists. Hearing is often their dominant sense, making them extremely sensitive to vibrations, and easily stressed by noise. Conversely, music is essential to them and can be used to shift out of their strong mental focus into a relaxing, creative, or nurturing mode. This is because music provides a direct link to their emotions. Just as they readily take in information, they are just as willing to let it go as new data becomes available, making them open-minded and willing to change.

CHARACTERISTIC TRAITS

Thalamuses are characterized by their sensitivity to and awareness of their physical and emotional surroundings. They will listen intently to what is going on around them and notice things that others miss, often simply storing the information in their well-organized memory banks. Even the minutest details are stored and filed away for future access.

Their superb organizational skills are reflected in their outer surroundings. They may even go so far as to have a filing cabinet in their bedroom to keep track of personal papers, articles and reference material that could be needed at some future date. Even as children, they like to have their toys neat and orderly.

Oriented to reality through the mind, they carefully deliberate over a problem before arriving at a clear decision as to how to solve it. They learn easily and enjoy studying subjects that interest them. Investigative and analytical, Thalamuses posses a high degree of intellectual curiosity and enjoy conversations that allow them to express the depth of their thoughts.

Curious and observant, Thalamuses are fairly adventurous and intrigued at the prospect of exploring new horizons. However, their daring is tempered by caution and they have a "look before you leap" attitude.

Thalamuses are generally people of substance and depth. They tend to be far more understanding of others than they are needing to be understood. While they tend to be more reserved, they can handle being the center of attention and enjoy lecturing, even though it's not a strong motivating factor. For them, it's more important to select activities and endeavors that are worthwhile, as this produces their greatest high and the most rewarding experiences.

Thalamus

MOTIVATION

Thalamuses have strong, active, inquiring minds, and relate to life by understanding how things work and why they are the way they are. Their ability to evaluate information and their highly developed powers of observation are their greatest strengths. There is an innate feeling that if they know what is going on and why, they will be safe and can feel secure.

Initially, Thalamuses are open and receptive, freely taking in new information without judging or censoring it. The next stage is a thorough mental analysis and skepticism, and then the decision. When they rely too heavily on their mind, they judge and categorize everything as black or white. The skeptical side begins to dominate and they get caught in the mental process or in over-analysis. It's when they are not in touch with their feelings or not trusting of their intuition that they are unable to integrate, and the decision process can become blocked. Procrastination occurs when there is a need for clarity, particularly when situations are vague or complicated.

Thalamuses are extremely sensitive to vibrations, particularly sound, and their hearing is often unusually acute. Music is particularly important as it provides a direct link to their emotions, and when stressed, Thalamus types will emotionally disconnect. Music is generally the quickest way to reconnect and let go of stress. Music allows them to shift their strong mental focus to more relaxing, nurturing, or creative modes. Not only is music used to calm and balance them or as a necessary catalyst for reflection, but also to stimulate or energize them. Music will get them motivated and activate their cells to get them going in the mornings.

The greater their insecurity, the greater the need to gather every possible piece of information, evaluate and re-evaluate all the data, constantly question, and even repeatedly ask the same question to make sure everything that is done is done perfectly.

"AT WORST"

When Thalamuses get too caught up in details, they become mentally tense and can be effectively immobilized (paralysis of analysis) or just lose their ability to progress at a satisfactory rate. Carried to the extreme, their caution and attentiveness becomes nit-picky. Sometimes they will swing to the opposite extreme and throw caution to the wind, becoming impatient and inattentive, or even impulsive and reckless. When they hold back from saying something that needs to be said, because of being wary of the consequences, they'll usually wind up having an outburst later from having stuffed their emotions.

Thalamuses will disconnect with their body, emotions, and/or inner knowing by ignoring pain, pushing their body, and failing to heed warning signs or not paying attention to where they are going. Getting side-tracked or circling around the problem without ever directly dealing with it is a way of not listening to themselves and their inner knowing. Another form of escape is to get caught in fantasy, going over and over every possible scenario while realizing that this is a waste of time and energy.

Thalamus

"AT WORST"

Super-critical of themselves, Thalamus types struggle with low self-esteem and are very susceptible to the "I'm not good enough" syndrome. Their lack of self-confidence can cause paralysis to the extent that they don't feel comfortable making major decisions or taking action, so they'll simply procrastinate, letting life or others set their course.

They can rely so heavily on the judgement and opinions of others, particularly authority figures, that they become immobilized. Anxieties about failure and lack of courage can cause them to spend so much time in research that they lose their effectiveness and never quite accomplish what they set out to achieve. Constantly seeking reassurance and support, they can become demanding and draining to those around them.

"AT BEST"

Thalamuses are very attentive to details and can handle technical work quite competently. They have excellent organizational skills, strive for excellence and work well independently, preferring to work at their own pace. They will examine a new pursuit carefully before actually embarking on it. They are quite dependable, and once a project is started, they maintain good momentum and can sustain their energy until the job is successfully completed.

The basic nature of Thalamuses is responsible, reliable and dependable, with a strong sense of loyalty. They have a sensitive nature and are relatively mild-mannered and easygoing with anger tending to be internalized rather than expressed directly. In relationships, they are gentle, giving and nurturing. With a strong social nature, they tend to be patient, compassionate, tactful, and sympathetic to others, placing a higher priority on people than on tasks.

When in tune with themselves, Thalamus types are self-reliant and personally responsible, taking excellent care of themselves. They are generally aware of their dietary and exercise needs and have the motivation and discipline to follow through on an appropriate health program.

Observant and thoughtful of the world around them, Thalamuses are also reflective about themselves. The more they've learned to accept and respect themselves through personal growth, the more they are willing to confront their own mistakes, take responsibility for some of the difficult situations they find themselves in, and make the changes they need to make. Being open-minded and adaptable, they are able to challenge their own behavior and beliefs, and change what no longer serves them.

Thalamus

FOOD LISTS

HEALTHY FOOD LIST

FREQUENTLY FOODS	3-7 meals per week – refers to each food, rather than category.
DENSE PROTEIN	Beef, beef broth, beef liver, buffalo; chicken, chicken broth, chicken livers, turkey, cornish game hen; anchovy, bonita, catfish, flounder, haddock, herring, perch, trout; clams, eel, lobsters, octopus, shrimp
DAIRY	Goat milk, buttermilk, yogurt (all), butter
CHEESE	Alleut, Colby, goat, Jack, Muenster, Romano, Rondele, Swiss
NUTS and SEEDS	Brazils, cashews (raw, roasted), cashew butter, water chestnuts, macadamia/cashew butter, filberts, hazelnuts, peanuts (raw, roasted), pine nuts (raw, roasted), walnuts (black, English), nut milks, raw or roasted seeds (caraway, pumpkin, sesame, sunflower), sesame seed butter, sunflower seed butter
LEGUMES	Beans (adzuki, black, garbanzo, kidney, lima [butter], navy, great northern, pinto, red, soy), black-eyed peas, split peas
GRAINS	Blue corn, blue corn tortilla, oats, oat bread, oat muffins, oat pancakes, rice (white or brown basmati, Japanese), rye, breads (rye [without wheat], sprouted rye, sprouted wheat), granola, sprouted grains
VEGETABLES	Artichokes, bamboo shoots, green beans, yellow wax beans, bok choy, broccoli, brussels sprouts, cabbage (green, napa, red), carrots, cauliflower, celery, chard, eggplant, garlic, peas, pumpkin, spinach, squash (acorn, banana, butternut, spaghetti, zucchini), tomatoes (canned, hot-house, vine-ripened), turnips
FRUITS	Bananas, blackberries, raspberries, strawberries, grapes (black, green, red), kiwi, oranges, peaches
FRUIT JUICES	Pineapple/coconut, cranapple
VEGETABLE OILS	Almond, avocado, canola, corn, olive, safflower, sesame, soy, sunflower
CONDIMENTS	Mustard, Hain™ safflower mayonnaise, garlic powder, herbs
SWEETENERS	Re-Vita®, stevia
CHIPS	Blue corn
BEVERAGES	Coffee with Re-Vita®, Constant Comment®tea
MODERATELY FOODS	1-2 meals per week – refers to each food, rather than category.
DENSE PROTEIN	Ham, pork, lamb, veal, venison, organ meats (heart, brain); duck; bass, cod, halibut, mackerel, mahi-mahi, orange roughy, salmon, sardines, shark, red snapper, sole, swordfish, tuna; abalone, calamari (squid), crab, mussels, scallops; eggs

Thalamus

DAIRY	Raw milk, half & half, sweet cream, sour cream, kefir, frozen yogurt, ice cream (Ben & Jerry's®, Dreyer's, Swensen's®)
CHEESE	American, blue, brie, Camembert, Cheddar, cottage, cream, Edam, feta, Gouda, kefir, Limburger, mozarella, Parmesan, ricotta
NUTS	Coconuts, macadamias (raw, roasted), macadamia butter, pecans, pistachios, peanut butter
LEGUMES	Hummus, miso, soy milk, tofu
GRAINS	Amaranth, barley, buckwheat, corn, corn bread, corn grits, corn tortillas, hominy grits, millet, popcorn, quinoa, rice (long or short grain brown, wild), rice bran, rice cakes, triticale, whole wheat, wheat bran, wheat germ, refined wheat flour, flour tortillas, breads (French, Italian, corn, corn/rye, garlic, kamut, potato, Poulsbo, rice, sourdough, multi-grain, 7-grain, whole wheat, white, sprouted grain), bagels, croissants, English muffins, crackers (saltines, oat, rye, wheat), pretzels, couscous, pasta, udon noodles, rice noodles, cream of rice, cream of rye, cream of wheat
VEGETABLES	Arugula, asparagus, avocados, lima beans, beets, broccoflower, cilantro, corn, cucumbers, greens (beet, collard, mustard, turnip), hominy, jicama, kale, kohlrabi, leeks, lettuce (Boston, butter, endive, iceberg, red leaf, romaine), mushrooms, okra, olives (green, ripe), onions (chives, green, brown, red, white, yellow, vidalia), parsley, parsnips, snow pea pods, bell peppers (green, red, yellow), mild chili peppers, pimentos, potatoes (red, russet, white rose, yukon gold, purple), sweet potatoes, radishes, daikon radishes, rutabaga, sauerkraut, seaweed (arame, dulse, kelp, nori, wakame), shallots, yellow (summer) squash, sprouts (alfalfa, clover, mung bean, radish, sunflower), watercress, yams
VEGETABLE JUICES	Celery, carrot, carrot/celery, parsley, spinach, tomato, V-8®
FRUITS	Apples (Golden or Red Delicious, Granny Smith, Jonathan, McIntosh, Pippin, Rome Beauty), apricots, blueberries, boysenberries, cranberries, gooseberries, cherries, grapefruits (white, red), guavas, kumquats, lemons, limes, loquats, mangos, melons (cantaloupe, casaba, crenshaw, honeydew, watermelon), nectarines, papayas, pears, persimmons, pineapples, plums (black, purple, red), pomegranates, rhubarb, tangelos, tangerines, dates, figs (fresh, dried), prunes, raisins
FRUIT JUICES	Apple, apple cider, apple/apricot, apricot, black cherry, red cherry, cranberry, grape (purple, red, white), grapefruit, guava, lemon, orange, papaya, pear, pineapple, prune, raspberry, tangerine, watermelon
VEGETABLE OILS	All-blend, flaxseed, peanut
SWEETENERS	Honey, molasses, sorghum, brown sugar, date sugar, raw sugar, refined cane sugar, barley malt syrup, corn syrup, maple syrup, brown rice syrup, fructose, succonant, saccharin, aspertame, Equal®, Sweet'n Low®, NutraSweet®
CONDIMENTS	Horseradish, barbecue sauce, pesto sauce, soy sauce, salsa, tahini, tamari, vinegar, salt, sea salt, Vege-Sal®, curry, Italian seasoning

Thalamus

SALAD DRESSINGS	Blue cheese, French, ranch, creamy Italian, creamy avocado, thousand island, vinegar and oil, lemon juice and oil
DESSERTS	Custards, tapioca, puddings, pies, cakes, chocolate, desserts containing chocolate, orange sherbet, raspberry sherbet
CHIPS	Bean, corn (white, yellow), potato
BEVERAGES	Coffee; herbal teas, black tea, green tea, Japanese tea, Chinese oolong tea; mineral water, sparkling water, lemonade; red wine, sake, barley malt liquor, champagne, gin, Scotch, vodka, whiskey; root beer, regular sodas
RARELY FOODS	No more than once a month
DENSE PROTEIN	Bacon, sausage; oysters
DAIRY	Pasteurized milk (whole, 2%, low fat, nonfat), most ice creams
NUTS	Almonds (raw, roasted), almond butter
LEGUMES	Lentils
GRAINS	Almond croissant
CONDIMENTS	Catsup, mayonnaise, margarine, hot chili peppers
BEVERAGES	White wine, diet soda

SENSITIVE FOOD LIST

FREQUENTLY FOODS	3-7 meals per week – refers to each food, rather than category.
DENSE PROTEIN	Beef; chicken, turkey; clams
DAIRY	Yogurt (all), butter
CHEESE	Goat
NUTS and SEEDS	Cashews (raw, roasted), cashew butter, macadamia/cashew butter, nut milks, raw and roasted seeds (caraway, pumpkin, sesame, sunflower), sesame seed butter, sunflower seed butter
LEGUMES	Beans (adzuki, black, navy, red)
GRAINS	Blue corn tortillas, oats, oat muffins, oat pancakes, rice (brown or white basmati, Japanese), granola, oat bread, rye bread (without wheat)
VEGETABLES	Green beans, carrots, celery, peas
FRUITS	Bananas, blackberries, raspberries, strawberries, grapes (black, green, red), kiwi, oranges, peaches
FRUIT JUICES	Pineapple/coconut
VEGETABLE OIL	Olive
CONDIMENTS	Mustard, garlic powder, herbs

Thalamus

MODERATELY FOODS	1-2 meals per week – refers to each food, rather than category.
DENSE PROTEIN	Beef broth, beef liver, buffalo, pork, ham, lamb, veal, venison, organ meats (heart, brain); chicken broth, chicken livers, cornish game hen, duck; anchovy, bass, bonita, catfish, cod, flounder, haddock, halibut, herring, mackerel, mahi-mahi, perch, orange roughy, salmon, shark, red snapper, sole, swordfish, trout, tuna; abalone, clams, crab, eel, lobster, octopus, mussels, scallops, shrimp; eggs
DAIRY	Raw milk, goat milk, buttermilk, half & half, sweet cream, sour cream, kefir, frozen yogurt
CHEESE	American, blue, brie, Camembert, Cheddar, Colby, cottage, Edam, feta, Gouda, Jack, kefir, Limburger, mozzarella, Muenster, Parmesan, ricotta, Romano, Swiss
NUTS	Brazils, water chestnuts, coconuts, filberts, hazelnuts, macadamias (raw, roasted), macadamia butter, pecans, pine nuts (raw, roasted), pistachios, walnuts (black, English)
LEGUMES	Beans (garbanzo, kidney, great northern, pinto, soy), black-eyed peas, split peas, hummus, soy milk, tofu
GRAINS	Amaranth, barley, buckwheat, corn, corn bread, corn grits, corn tortillas, hominy grits, millet, popcorn, quinoa, rice (long or short grain brown, wild), rice bran, rice cakes, rye, triticale, whole wheat, wheat bran, wheat germ, refined wheat flour, flour tortillas, breads (corn/rye, corn, garlic, rice, sprouted grain, Poulsbo), bagels, croissants, English muffins, crackers (saltines, oat, rye, wheat), couscous, pasta, udon noodles, rice noodles, cream of rice, cream of rye, cream of wheat
VEGETABLES	Artichokes, asparagus, bamboo shoots, yellow wax beans, lima beans, beets, bok choy, broccoflower, brussels sprouts, cabbage (green, napa, red), cauliflower, chard, cilantro, eggplant, greens (beet, collard, mustard, turnip), hominy, jicama, kale, kohlrabi, leeks, lettuce (Boston, butter, endive, iceberg, red leaf, romaine), mushrooms, okra, olives (green, ripe), onions (chives, green, brown, red, white, yellow, vidalia), parsley, parsnips, snow pea pods, bell peppers (green, red, yellow), mild chili peppers, pimentos, potatoes (red, white rose, yukon gold, purple), sweet potatoes, pumpkin, radishes, daikon radishes, rutabaga, sauerkraut, seaweed (arame, dulse, kelp, nori, wakame), shallots, sprouts (alfalfa, clover, mung bean, radish, sunflower), squash (acorn, banana, butternut, spaghetti, yellow [summer], zucchini), tomatoes (canned, hot-house, vine-ripened), turnips, yams
VEGETABLE JUICES	Celery, carrot, carrot/celery, parsley, spinach, tomato, V-8®
FRUITS	Apples (Golden or Red Delicious, Granny Smith, Jonathan, McIntosh, Pippin, Rome Beauty), apricots, blueberries, boysenberries, cranberries, gooseberries, cherries, grapefruits (white, red), guavas, kumquats, lemons, limes, loquats, mangos, melons (cantaloupe, casaba, crenshaw, honeydew, watermelon), nectarines, papayas, pears, persimmons, pineapples, plums

Thalamus

FRUITS (Continued)	(black, purple, red), pomegranates, rhubarb, tangelos, tangerines, dates, figs (fresh, dried), prunes, raisins
FRUIT JUICES	Apple, apple cider, apple/apricot, apricot, black cherry, red cherry, cranapple, cranberry, grape (purple, red, white), grapefruit, guava, lemon, orange, papaya, pear, pineapple, prune, raspberry, tangerine, watermelon
VEGETABLE OILS	All-blend, almond, avocado, canola, corn, flaxseed, peanut, safflower, sesame, soy, sunflower
SWEETENERS	Re-Vita®, stevia
CONDIMENTS	Hain™ safflower mayonnaise, salsa, tahini, vinegar, salt, sea salt, Vege-Sal®, curry, Italian seasoning
SALAD DRESSINGS	Vinegar and oil, lemon juice and oil
BEVERAGES	Herbal tea, Japanese tea, Chinese oolong tea; mineral water, sparkling water
RARELY FOODS	No more than once a month
DENSE PROTEIN	Bacon, sausage; sardines; calamari (squid), oysters
DAIRY	Pasteurized milk (whole, 2%, low fat, nonfat), ice cream
CHEESE	Alleut, cream, Rondele
NUTS	Almonds (raw, roasted), almond butter, peanuts (raw, roasted), peanut butter
LEGUMES	Lentils, lima (butter) beans, miso
GRAINS	Polished rice, breads (French, Italian, 7-grain, multi-grain, whole wheat, white, sourdough), almond croissants
VEGETABLES	Arugula, avocados, broccoli, corn, cucumbers, garlic, russet potatoes, spinach, watercress
SWEETENERS	Honey, molasses, sorghum, brown sugar, date sugar, raw sugar, refined cane sugar, barley malt syrup, corn syrup, maple syrup, brown rice syrup, fructose, succonant, saccharin, aspertame, Equal®, Sweet'n Low®, NutraSweet®
CONDIMENTS	Catsup, mayonnaise, margarine, soy sauce, tamari, hot chili peppers, horseradish, barbecue sauce, pesto sauce
SALAD DRESSINGS	Blue cheese, French, ranch, creamy Italian, creamy avocado, thousand island
DESSERTS	Custards, tapioca, puddings, pies, cakes, chocolate, desserts containing chocolate, orange sherbet, raspberry sherbet
CHIPS	Bean, corn (blue, white, yellow), potato
BEVERAGES	Coffee; black tea, green tea; lemonade; wine (white, red), sake, beer, barley malt liquor, champagne, gin, Scotch, vodka, whiskey; root beer, regular sodas, diet sodas

Thalamus

MENUS

DIETARY EMPHASIS :

- Eat more cooked than raw vegetables.
- Fruit should be consumed only in the morning or for bedtime snack.

WEIGHT LOSS:

- Eliminate refined sugar, alcohol, honey, and all artificial sweeteners.
- Avoid fruit juice, but may include fruit.
- Minimize breads and butter.
- 20-25% fats below 15% inhibits weight loss.

WEIGHT GAIN:

- Simply increase quantity of food intake.

VEGETARIAN DIET:

- Inadequate, as require 10-30% of calories from dense protein.

FATS:

- 20-25% of caloric intake. Best sources are from seeds, especially sesame tahini, and dense protein (chicken, turkey, fish, eggs, beef).

KEY

—all menus may be used by healthy persons.
( ) around foods means that they're optional
L denotes weight loss menus
S denotes sensitive menus
G denotes weight gain menus

BREAKFAST:
8-9 a.m. Light-to-moderate, with light protein, such as eggs, fruit, grain, nuts, seeds, dairy, vegetables and/or legumes.

L	S	G	Menu
L		G	Blackberries, blueberries, or boysenberries and cashews, sunflower seeds or hazelnuts
L	S	G	Banana or peaches
L		G	Granny Smith apples and pecans
	S	G	Strawberries or grapes w/cheese, cashews and Re-Vita®
L		G	Strawberries and rice – any variety
L	S		Plantain bananas
		G	Grapes and coconut w/Jack cheese
L		G	Mango and kiwi
L		G	Oatmeal and bananas or peaches
		G	Oatmeal w/dates and coconut
		G	Oatmeal w/butter and cashews or cashew milk
	S		Oatmeal or millet w/soy milk
L		G	Oatmeal w/Re-Vita® (butter)
L			Corn grits and okra or sunflower seeds
		G	Granola (Re-Vita®)
L			Couscous w/butter or Re-Vita®
		G	Oat muffins
L	S	G	Oat flour pancakes w/fresh peaches or apples
L		G	Oat flour pancakes w/Re-Vita®
		G	Blueberry pancakes w/butter
L		G	Pancakes, kiwi, and Re-Vita®
	S	G	Gluten-free pancakes w/eggs, blueberries, or Re-Vita®
	S	G	Banana-nut bread and eggs
	S		Banana-nut muffin made w/rice flour or gluten-free flour
L	S	G	Rice cakes (eggs)
		G	Rice cakes, cashew butter, and coleslaw
		G	Cornbread, butter, and pecans or Re-Vita®
		G	French toast w/Re-Vita®
		G	French or Italian bread toast w/banana and cashew butter
		G	Oat toast w/peanut or cashew butter, and Re-Vita® or honey
L	S		Scrambled eggs w/onions
		G	Eggs, potato, and turkey bacon
L	S	G	Eggs, brown rice, and butter
L		G	Eggs, rice, and peas
		G	Eggs and oat toast
L		G	Egg drop soup, pea pods, and steamed rice
L	S		Egg drop soup

Thalamus

S G	Corn tortillas (butter and eggs)
S	Corn tortillas w/sesame butter (celery)
S G	Artichoke noodles, butter, and boiled eggs
L G	Bell pepper, eggplant, and mild spices w/rice, rice cakes, or tofu
L G	Steamed potatoes w/parsley, corn, and broccoli or mixed vegetables
L G	Yellow and green squash, red pepper, onion, eggplant, and rice
L G	Steamed spinach w/carrots and tofu
L S	Acorn or banana squash w/butter
L S G	Yams and black walnuts
L G	Split pea soup
	WITH MEAL:
	Coffee w/Re-Vita® (cream)
	Black tea w/Re-Vita® and cream
L G	Cranberry concentrate w/berry Re-Vita®
L G	Cranberry juice
L G	Apple juice
	MID-MORNING SNACK: (Optional) 10:30-11 a.m. Nuts, seeds, grain, dairy, vegetables.
S	Cashew or sesame butter w/celery
S	Amaranth graham crackers or regular graham crackers w/sesame butter
S G	Rice cake and kefir cheese
	LUNCH: 12-2 p.m. Moderate-to-heavy, with protein, vegetables, legumes, nuts, seeds, grain, and/or dairy.
L G	Baked chicken stuffed w/carrots, celery, onions, and rice
L G	Chicken and lima beans
L G	Chicken, rice, and coleslaw or vegetables
G	Chicken and dumplings w/gravy
L G	Chicken breast w/spanish rice and green beans
L G	Stir-fry: chicken breast, celery, onions, carrots, broccoli, cauliflower, and squash
L G	Turkey meat loaf, potato, and asparagus
L G	Turkey, cranberries, and carrots
L S G	Lamb, potato, and coleslaw
L G	Lamb, parsnips, and broccoli
L S G	Lamb w/parsleyed potatoes (green beans)
L S G	Lamb stew: lamb, carrots, onions, potatoes, celery, and green peppers
G	Rib-eye beef steak marinated in onions, peppers, and sweet and sour sauce w/cabbage or coleslaw
L S G	Beef and green beans or coleslaw
L S G	Beef, potato, and peas (onions)
L S G	Green pepper stuffed w/rice and beef, lamb, chicken, or turkey
L S G	Tuna, pasta, and peas
S G	Tuna and pine nuts w/creamy Italian dressing (sprouts, spinach, and oat bread)
G	Tuna sandwich on oat bread, w/Hain™ Creamy Italian or Avocado dressing (tomato and lettuce)
	Baked potato w/Cheddar cheese or sour cream, butter, and chives
	Macaroni and cheese w/peas
L	Stir-fry vegetables w/basmati rice and soy sauce
S	Pinto beans w/lamb bones
G	Pinto beans w/lamb bones and tofu
L	Hummus and sunflower sprouts in rye pita bread
L	Juice – lettuce, celery, beet, and beet greens
S	Sesame tahini on celery sticks and flour tortilla
S	Pro-Gain® and goat milk (jicama)
	LUNCH or DINNER:
L G	Beef, potato or rice, and spinach (beets)
L	Beef and broccoli

Thalamus

L	S	G	
L		G	Lamb and green beans (potato, pasta, or rice)
L		G	Lamb, potato, and mint sauce (broccoli and/or cauliflower)
		G	Ham sandwich on potato bread and butter (zucchini soup)
		G	Ham, potato or potato bread, green beans or broccoli, and cauliflower or raw green bell peppers
		G	Chicken breast sandwich w/coleslaw
L	S	G	Chicken and baked beans
L			Chicken w/broccoli and carrots
L		G	Chicken and brussels sprouts (potatoes)
		G	Chicken, corn, and potato salad
L		G	Chicken, corn bread, and peas
L		G	Cashew chicken w/steamed rice
L	S	G	Chicken or turkey and green beans (potato)
L	S	G	Chicken or turkey w/pasta (spaghetti sauce)
L	S	G	Chicken, turkey, or beef w/potatoes and carrots
L		G	Chicken (dijon mustard sauce (potatoes, carrots, and onions) or broccoli
L	S		Chicken terriyaki
L		G	Turkey, mashed potatoes, gravy, and cranberry sauce (peas)
L		G	Turkey, rice, and cranberry sauce
L		G	Turkey and asparagus (spinach salad, pasta, or celery)
L	S		Turkey and cauliflower
L		G	Pork chop, potato, and broccoli
L		G	Orange roughy, rice, and broccoli and/or salad (lemon)
L		G	Fish and cauliflower (rice or pasta)
			Fish sticks, corn, and green beans
L	S	G	Tuna, noodles, and zucchini or green beans
L	S	G	Shrimp, rice, and peas
L	S		Halibut or snapper w/yellow squash and green onions
L	S	G	Sea bass or red snapper w/rice (asparagus or green beans)
L	S		Rice, squash, and carrots, or peas
L			Rice, chicken broth, and broccoli
	S	G	Bean burrito, salsa, and rice
	S	G	Pork and beans and corn bread
L	S		Hummus w/rice cakes, carrots, and string beans
L	S	G	Pasta and spaghetti sauce
L			Artichoke noodles w/spinach
	S	G	Green beans and cashews
	S		Sweet potato (butter)
	S		Mushrooms sauteed in butter and potato
	S	G	Taco salad on corn tortilla
	S	G	Tacos and carrots
L	S	G	Beef stew w/carrots and potato
L	S	G	Fish stew w/potatoes and onions
L			Chicken noodle soup
L	S		Chicken vegetable soup w/noodles
		G	Chili w/ground turkey and rye bread
	S	G	Pizza w/carrot juice
L			Tahini or hummus w/celery and/or cucumber, carrots, spinach, garlic, and lemon
L			Broccoli, yellow squash, okra, and onion
L			Potatoes – red or white – and broccoli
L			Spinach, carrots, and celery salad w/dressing soy sauce, apple cider vinegar, and peanut or olive oil
L			Spinach w/artichoke noodles (tofu)

MID-AFTERNOON SNACK:
(Optional) 4-5 p.m. Protein, grain, vegetables, nuts, seeds, dairy.

L	S	G	
L	S	G	Cashews w/jicama
L			Cucumber rolls
L			Rice cake
		G	Rice cake w/cream cheese and olives
L	S	G	Popcorn
	S		Sesame crackers (butter)

Thalamus

DINNER:
6-8 p.m. Moderate, with protein, vegetables, grain, legumes, nuts, seeds and/or dairy.

G Tamales, corn, and steamed broccoli w/rice
L S G Spaghetti w/ground turkey and tomato sauce
L S Vegetable pasta w/butter (romaine lettuce)
L S Artichoke noodles w/peas (curry sauce)
L S Sushi
L G Curried chicken and rice
L Chinese chicken salad
L S Broiled breast of chicken w/out skin, and salad: red and green leaf lettuce, tomato, and onion
L S G Ground turkey w/pasta (tomato sauce, romaine lettuce, and/or tomato and green onion salad)
L S G Turkey, noodles, and peas in turkey broth
L S Okra, spanish rice, tomatoes, and peppers
L Green beans, corn, and potato
L Black beans and spinach
L Beets, spinach, sunflower seeds, and green or red onions
L S Rice, steamed zucchini, onions, and dill weed
L S Steamed potatoes, mushrooms, onions, and carrots
L S Potatoes and carrots (parsley)
Sweet potatoes and cranberries
L Caesar salad
L S Okra gumbo: chicken broth, okra, celery, pepper, onion, and tomatoes
Greek salad w/pita bread
L S G Split pea soup w/lamb
G Split pea soup w/ham
S Peppers, onions, and celery in chicken broth w/Italian seasoning
Pasta w/pesto sauce
Cheese pizza and steamed carrots

EVENING SNACK:
(Optional) 9-12 p.m. Fruit, protein, grain, vegetables, nuts, seeds, dairy, legumes, sweets.

L S G Popcorn
Rye Krisp® and cheese
S G Blue corn tortilla chips (sesame seeds or guacamole)
L S Steamed corn tortillas w/sesame butter (celery)
S G Oatmeal cookie w/oat flour
G Fig bars
G Red licorice

DESSERTS
After lunch, dinner, mid-afternoon, or evening

G Coconut cream pie
G Pumpkin pie w/oat bran crust
G Apple pie w/cheese
L S Cashews or walnuts
L S G Cashew butter and jicama or celery
L S G Pumpkin, sesame, or sunflower seeds
L S G Prunes and walnuts
L S Frozen cherries
L S Apples, tangerines, watermelon, or strawberries
L S Applesauce
S White/green seedless grapes

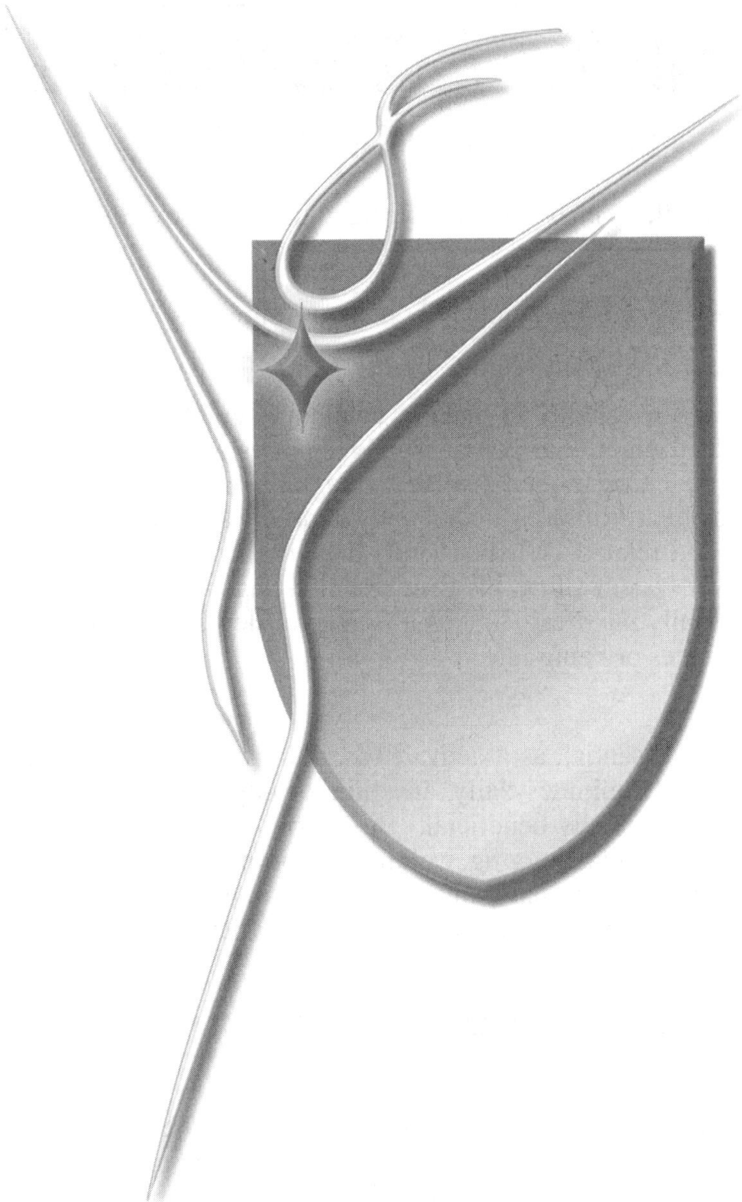

The "Thymus Body Type" is symbolized by a shield. Shielded from forces that could cause change, protected environments are stable and constant. Resisting change of any kind, Thymuses are loyal and responsible, committed to keeping their environment constant.

Thymus

BODY TYPE PROFILE

LOCATION	Upper middle of chest, below thyroid gland and above heart.
FUNCTION	Produces lymphocytes and antibodies for immune system.
POTENTIAL HEALTH PROBLEMS	Generally strong body. Typically, challenges emotional rather than physical. Unresolved emotional stress usually manifests structurally (as opposed to internally). Commonly involved areas are back, shoulder, nerves, and/or joints (as in arthritis). Metabolically, tend toward allergies, environmentally and/or food-related. When severely depleted, prone to autoimmune diseases. Digestive system often involved manifesting as constipation. Emotional stress usually manifests first as a feeling of depression; generally associated with finances or being idle.
RECOMMENDED EXERCISE	Exercise is essential, as it activates the immune system. Exercise should be for at least 15 minutes daily, any time of day. Needs sunlight, so outdoor activity is especially beneficial. Best forms of exercise include swimming, basketball, running, jogging, walking, low impact aerobics, and Tai Chi. Also recommended, stationary bike, or cross-country training. To strengthen upper body, moderate weight lifting. Most efficient exercise is callanetics.

WOMEN'S CHARACTERISTICS

DISTINGUISHING FEATURES	Tall to very tall, with long-limbed appearance. Well-meaning, take charge demeanor, which can be forceful, and sometimes perceived by others as controlling. Their strong sense of responsibility and loyalty coupled with their forceful presence allows them to bring stability into their environment.
ADDITIONAL PHYSICAL CHARACTERISTICS	Buttocks relatively flat-to-rounded. Low back curvature straight-to-average. Breasts small-to-average. Shoulders relatively even with hips. Waist straight-to-defined. Average to long-waisted. Height tall to very tall. Bone structure medium. Average, elongated musculature. Large, wide hands with long, slender fingers proportional to hands. Long arms. Average-to-long oval, or long rectangular face which often appears slender or small.
WEIGHT GAIN AREAS	Lower body with initial gain in lower abdomen, waist, possibly upper hips, and either entire upper 2/3rds of thighs or only upper inner thighs. Secondary gain in thighs, buttocks, upper and/or lower hips, and middle back. Alternative weight gain pattern is same except for minimal gain in thighs. May have difficulty gaining or maintaining adequate weight. When at ideal weight, generally have a stable weight pattern throughout life.

Thymus

DIETARY GUIDELINES

"HEALTHY"	SCHEDULING MEALS: Breakfast: Heavy, with protein, grain, vegetables, nuts, seeds, dairy, and/or legumes. Lunch: Moderate-to-heavy, with protein, grain, nuts, seeds, dairy, legumes, and/or vegetables. Dinner: Light-to-moderate, with legumes, grain, vegetables, fruit, nuts, seeds, eggs, dairy, and/or protein. Alternative Meal Schedule: If breakfast is light, can compensate by eating heavy lunch and/or dinner; although not preferred. Bulk of protein can be consumed at dinner if necessary.
"SENSITIVE"	Limit fruit to 2 times a week. • Protein, especially lamb and eggs, rye, seeds, nuts, vegetables, and olive oil. • Protein essential, ideally at breakfast and lunch, but if unable to do so, may consume bulk of protein at dinner. • For weight loss, eat dense protein for breakfast and lunch, eliminate refined sugar, particulatly sugary desserts and sweet drinks, including fruit juices and alcohol, minimize bread, and avoid all dairy products except butter. • For weight gain, consume 35% of daily calories from fats, include snacks, and exercise daily. • Vegetarian diets inadequate, since require 10-35% of calories from dense protein. To sustain on a vegetarian diet, essential to include protein powders or supplements, nuts and seeds, and especially 4 eggs a day, 7 days a week and 35% of calories from fats. • Fats, 25-35% of caloric intake, should be derived from dense protein (all), seeds, nuts (almonds, Brazils, peanuts, pine nuts), olive oil, and kefir. May derive 15-20% of fats from kefir.
KEY SUPPORTS FOR SYSTEM	Lamb and rye for thymus gland, protein, vegetables, and olive oil.
COMPLEMENTARY GLANDULAR SUPPORT	Adrenals, through consuming eggs, fish, chicken, fruits, and vegetables. Thalamus, through sunlight.
FOODS CRAVED	*(When Energy is Low)* Sweets and fats, like ice cream, chocolate, cookies, pastries, fruit. Protein, such as cheese and meat.

Thymus

FOODS TO AVOID

Sugary desserts and sweet drinks (including fruit juices), since sugar tends to stress immune system.

RECOMMENDED CUISINE

Chinese, Thai, Greek. Moderately: Mexican, Italian, Japanese; Seafood, pizza.

PSYCHOLOGICAL PROFILE

ESSENCE

Just as the thymus gland eliminates unknown protein – generally bacteria and viruses – to keep the body's internal environment safe, Thymus body types stabilize their environment. They are protective of their own and will go to great lengths to keep their environment constant, generally resisting change of any kind. Judging everything as good or bad, right or wrong, makes maintaining a constant, stable environment easier. Their initial response is usually negative as this eliminates the need for examining anything new further. Since being safe is generally associated with known situations, there is a deep seated fear of change. Their innate desire to protect and keep life constant gives rise to a sense of loyalty and responsibility that towers above most other types.

CHARACTERISTIC TRAITS

Thymus types are particularly strong-willed, forceful, and determined. Being very practical, they like things they can see and touch that preferably have been proven over time. Thymuses are most comfortable when their lives are steady and constant with the only changes being those they have instigated.

Preferring to stay with what they already know, or can see as clearly defined, Thymuses are reluctant to undertake anything that differs from what they are accustomed to. Their creativity tends to stay within familiar parameters, enhancing the tried and true.

Even though Thymuses tend to view things more from their heads than their hearts, they are not especially analytical in their approaches to problem-solving. The tendency is to take a broad overview, dive into the project, and deal with any difficulties that may arise – generally by trying to bulldoze their way through. Their basic attitude towards work is to take things as they come, and delegate the details whenever possible.

Known for having particularly high standards and high expectations, especially of themselves, Thymuses are often idealistic perfectionists. They like to be in charge, and will often control through their energy or presence. Generally tall, their size alone is often intimidating to people. Most have an extraordinarily high desire to be the center of attention and expect people to automatically accommodate them.

Thymus

MOTIVATION

Their primary concern is to protect themselves and those they care about. In their pursuit of self-protection, Thymus types strongly embrace the tried and true, and what's been established. They tend to see everything as either black or white, or one way or the other, with little consideration for in-betweens, degrees, shades, probabilities, or compromises.

They can be very one way about seeing or doing things, and that is usually their own way. Because of their single-minded intensity, giving up their own preferences or compromising can sometimes be very challenging. Thinking things through requires an effort, so they will often bypass the process once they have dichotomized something as right or wrong, and will put anything similar into these categories.

Thymuses usually respond to anything new in a negative way at least initially as they feel threatened by proposed changes. Their motivation for change is primarily physical pain, and because they are inclined to suppress their emotions, will often only realize a change is needed because of their physical condition. Since their nature is to be in control, they feel they should be able to handle everything. When things don't work as they had planned, the tendency is to blame others. Being more aware of their outside environment than their internal feelings, understanding themselves or others is difficult. Relationships are challenging as Thymuses have a strong need to control to feel secure.

Emotional stimulation produces a sense of power (even if destructive), heightening the feeling of being alive and allowing for a greater manifestation of energy flow. Manifestation of energy in a negative manner, however, makes them prone to mistakes. Unresolved emotional turmoil causes increasing irritability, intensifies areas of negativity, and results in injury to one's self anything from inadvertent self inflicted injury to self-sabotage.

"AT WORST"

Thymuses are the epitome of judgement, control, prejudice and rigidity. Their judgements are quick and fixed, and the one they judge most harshly is themselves. Their thinking is extremely rigid with a lot of "should's" and expectations of an ideal world. With a strong need to "be the best", Thymus types expect perfection in themselves and everything and everyone around them. Demanding perfection in this lifetime, and feeling they know best, they will usually react with anger or defensiveness when things don't go their way. When there's nothing more that can be done, they will internalize their anger and pout or become depressed.

With a "better than, less than" attitude, they are caught in a double bind of judging everyone as better than or less than themselves. If a person is judged as being better than, Thymuses feel inferior and will either beat themselves up or tear down the other person. When a person is judged as being less than, Thymus types expect that person to serve them. Since they can never relate to anyone on an equal basis, their expectations are never met and they drive people away, reinforcing their deep seated abandonment issues.

Thymus

"AT WORST" (Continued)

More demanding of attention than giving, they usually want to be centerstage. If an activity or event is not their show, they usually don't want to play. Men, more so than women, will often demand attention and if they don't get what they want, will withdraw and pout, or become even more forceful and direct, taking over the situation. Women tend to be more subtle and will control their environment by trying to control others' lives, in the guise of "this is what is best for you", or by blocking their own emotions.

"AT BEST"

Thymus types are stable, loyal, and dependable, and can be trusted to accomplish what they agree to do. They are rule abiding to the extent that the rules either are their own or support their purposes, but otherwise won't let rules interfere with their way of doing things. Thymuses are steady, consistent, and responsible, and have the stamina and endurance to fulfill their duties and honor their commitments, sometimes taking a well-deserved sense of pride in their self-control.

Thymuses have good leadership qualities, a natural "take charge" attitude and are able to meet challenges and direct others to effective action. Their ability to control gives them the opportunity to give others the external support they might need, as well as to gratify their own need for stability and protection. Change often comes slowly, but once committed to something, Thymuses will usually stay with it. They have a pronounced sense of loyalty and responsibility and can be very loving and protective toward those they care about. As they become more secure within themselves, they are able to identify with the feelings of others.

Motivated by succeeding at a personal challenge, true success comes when they can have genuine regard for themselves and others. This comes when they can consider others' feelings, allowing for more latitude rather than needing to make the world "perfect" as they see it. Rather than expecting and taking, there's an attitude of allowing and giving. Perfection is the realization that all is perfect and what appears as mistakes are merely learning experiences. Perfection requires taking total responsibility for what is going on in one's life by realizing that what each person experiences is what they have attracted. If they don't like the experience, they need to determine why, so they can clear the old belief structures or learn the lesson.

The ultimate for Thymuses is manifesting unconditional love for themselves and others, essentially reaching perfection in this lifetime. When they are able to release their judgements that keep them separate and resolve conflict through connecting with another's essence, they are able to integrate power and love and truly be an expression of love. This is when they can be the most powerful and influential of all the types.

Thymus

FOOD LISTS

HEALTHY FOOD LIST

FREQUENTLY FOODS	3-7 meals per week – refers to each food, rather than category.
DENSE PROTEIN	Beef, beef broth, beef liver, buffalo, lamb, pork, ham, bacon, sausage, venison, organ meats (heart, brain), game meats (all); chicken, chicken broth, chicken livers; bass, bonita, catfish, cod, flounder, haddock, mackerel, mahi-mahi, perch, roughy, sardines, shark, red snapper, sole, swordfish, yellowtail tuna, Chicken of the Sea® tuna; clams, eel, mussels, octopus, oysters; eggs
DAIRY	Milk (whole, 2%, low fat, nonfat, raw) goat milk, plain kefir, butter
CHEESE	Cheddar, Colby, pineapple cottage cheese, Jack, Muenster
NUTS and SEEDS	Cashew butter, cashew milk, coconuts, macadamias, macadamia/cashew butter, peanuts, pine nuts, black and English walnuts, seeds (pumpkin, sesame, sunflower), sesame butter
LEGUMES	Beans (black, garbanzo, kidney, lima [butter], soy), black-eyed peas, hummus, miso, soy milk, tofu
GRAINS	Oats, quinoa, rice, (brown or white basmati, long or short grain brown, wild, Japanese), rice cakes, rye, breads (oat, oat bran, rye, rye/pumpernickel), wheat/pumpernickel bagels, crackers (oat, rye, Rye Krisp®, graham), couscous, pasta, u*f*don noodles, rice noodles, cream of rice, cream of rye
VEGETABLES	Artichokes, asparagus, bamboo shoots, basil, yellow wax beans, bok choy, broccoli, brussels sprouts, carrots, cauliflower, celery, red chard, white corn, greens (beet, collard, mustard, turnip), kale, shitake mushrooms, onions (chives, green, white, yellow, vidalia), parsley, parsnips, peas, snow pea pods, red potatoes, radishes, rutabaga, seaweed (arame, dulse, kelp, nori, wakame) spinach, sprouts (alfalfa, clover, mung bean, radish, sunflower), squash (acorn, banana, butternut, spaghetti, yellow [summer], zucchini), pumpkin, stewed tomatoes, turnips
VEGETABLE JUICES	Carrot, tomato, V-8®
FRUITS	Apples (Red or Golden Delicious, Jonathan, McIntosh, Pippin, Rome Beauty, Granny Smith), bananas, blackberries, boysenberries, blueberries, cranberries, gooseberries, raspberries, cherries, green grapes, white grapefruits, kiwi, nectarines, oranges, lemons, limes, watermelons, papayas, peaches, pineapples, pomegranates, rhubarb, dates, prunes
FRUIT JUICES	Apple (raw, unfiltered), apple cider, apricot, apple/apricot, black cherry, red cherry, cranapple, cranberry, grape (purple, red, white), grapefruit, lemon, orange, papaya, pineapple, pineapple/coconut, prune, raspberry, watermelon
SWEETENERS	Re-Vita®, stevia
VEGETABLE OILS	All-blend, almond, avocado, canola, corn, flaxseed, olive, peanut, safflower, sesame, soy, sunflower
CONDIMENTS	Tabasco, medium or hot salsa
BEVERAGES	Flavored or plain mineral water, soda water

Thymus

MODERATELY FOODS	1-2 meals per week – refers to each food, rather than category.
DENSE PROTEIN	Veal; turkey, cornish game hen, duck; anchovy, halibut, herring, salmon, trout, tuna; abalone, calamari (squid), crab, lobster, scallops, shrimp
DAIRY	Lact-aid milk, buttermilk, half & half, sweet cream, sour cream, flavored kefir, plain or flavored yogurt, ice cream (Ben & Jerry's®, Dreyer's, Swensen's®)
CHEESE	American, blue, brie, Camembert, cottage, cream, Edam, feta, goat, Gouda, kefir, Limburger, mozzarella, Parmesan, ricotta, Romano, Swiss
NUTS and SEEDS	Almonds, almond butter, Brazils, cashews, water chestnuts, filberts, hazelnuts, macadamia butter, peanut butter, pecans, pistachios, seeds (caraway, poppy), sunflower seed butter
LEGUMES	Beans (adzuki, navy, great northern, pinto, red), lentils, split green peas, split yellow peas
GRAINS	Amaranth w/chicken broth, barley, buckwheat, corn, corn bread, corn grits, corn tortillas, hominy grits, millet, popcorn, rice bran, triticale, whole wheat, wheat bran, wheat germ, refined wheat flour, flour tortillas, breads (French Italian, sourdough, garlic, 7-grain, multi-grain, corn, corn/rye, rice, sprouted wheat, white, whole wheat), croissants, English muffins, bagels, crackers (saltines, wheat), cream of wheat
VEGETABLES	Arugula, avocados, green beans, lima beans, beets, cabbage (green, napa, red), capers, cilantro, yellow corn, cucumbers, eggplant, garlic, hominy, jicama, kohlrabi, leeks, lettuce (Boston, butter, endive, iceberg, red leaf, romaine), mushrooms, okra, olives (green, ripe), brown or red onions, peppers (green, red, yellow bell, jalapeno), pimentos, potatoes (white rose, russet, purple, yukon gold), sweet potatoes, daikon radishes, sauerkraut, shallots, raw tomatoes, watercress, yams
VEGETABLE JUICES	Celery, carrot/celery, parsley, spinach
FRUITS	Apricots, strawberries, grapes (black, red), pink grapefruits, guava, kumquats, loquats, mangos, melons (cantaloupe, casaba, crenshaw, honeydew), oranges, pears, Fuju persimmons, plums (black, purple, red), tangelos, tangerines, figs, raisins
FRUIT JUICES	Apple juice/water, guava, pear, tangerine
SWEETENERS	Honey, molasses, sorghum, brown sugar, date sugar, raw sugar, refined cane sugar, maple syrup, brown rice syrup, barley malt syrup, corn syrup, fructose, succonant
CONDIMENTS	Mayonnaise, horseradish, soy sauce, barbeque sauce, pesto sauce, cocoa, tahini, rice vinegar, salt, sea salt, Vege-Sal®
SALAD DRESSINGS	Blue cheese, French, ranch, creamy Italian, creamy avocado, thousand island, vinegar and oil, lemon juice and oil
DESSERTS	Custards, tapioca, puddings, pies, cakes, chocolate, chocolate, desserts containing chocolate, raspberry sherbet, orange sherbet

Thymus

CHIPS	Bean, corn (blue, white, yellow), potato
BEVERAGES	Herbal tea, black tea, green tea, Japanese tea, Chinese oolong tea; sparkling water, sparkling cider; sake, wine(white, red), champagne, beer, barley malt liquor, vodka, Scotch, gin, whiskey; root beer, regular sodas
RARELY FOODS	No more than once a month
DAIRY	Frozen yogurt, most ice creams
VEGETABLES	Broccoflower
SWEETENERS	Aspartame, saccharin®, Equal®, Sweet'n Low®, NutraSweet®
CONDIMENTS	Catsup, mustard, margarine
BEVERAGES	Coffee; diet sodas

SENSITIVE FOOD LIST

FREQUENTLY FOODS	3-7 meals per week – refers to each food, rather than category.
DENSE PROTEIN	Lamb, game meats (all); dark chicken; bass, sardines, shark, yellowtail tuna, Chicken of the Sea® tuna; clams, mussels; eggs
DAIRY	Plain kefir, butter
NUTS and SEEDS	Cashew butter, cashew milk, macadamia/cashew butter, pine nuts, sesame butter
LEGUMES	Soy milk
GRAINS	Oats, rice (brown or white basmati, Japanese), rice cakes, rye, Rye Krisp®, cream of rice, cream of rye
VEGETABLES	Broccoli, carrots, cauliflower, celery, shitake mushrooms, parsley, snow pea pods, radishes
MODERATELY FOODS	1-2 meals per week – refers to each food, rather than category.
DENSE PROTEIN	Beef, beef sausage, beef liver, beef broth, buffalo, pork, bacon, ham, sausage, veal, venison, organ meats (heart, brain); white chicken, chicken livers, chicken broth, turkey, cornish game hen, duck; anchovy, bonita, catfish, cod, flounder, haddock, halibut, herring, mackerel, mahi-mahi, perch, roughy, salmon, red snapper, sole, swordfish, trout; abalone, calamari (squid), crab, eel, lobster, octopus, oysters, scallops, shrimp
DAIRY	Lact-aid milk, half & half, sweet cream, sour cream, flavored kefir
CHEESE	Kefir

Thymus

NUTS and SEEDS	Almonds, almond butter, Brazils, cashews, water chestnuts, coconuts, filberts, hazelnuts, peanuts, peanut butter, pecans, pistachios, macadamias, macadamia butter, walnuts (black, English), seeds (caraway, sesame, pumpkin, sunflower) sunflower seed butter
LEGUMES	Beans (black, garbanzo, lima [butter], soy), lentils, black-eyed peas, split green peas, split yellow peas, hummus, miso, tofu
GRAINS	Amaranth w/chicken broth, barley, buckwheat, corn, corn bread, corn grits, corn tortillas, hominy grits, millet, popcorn, quinoa, wild rice, rice bran, triticale, whole wheat, wheat bran, wheat germ, refined wheat flour, flour tortillas, breads (rice, corn, corn/rye), bagels, croissants, English muffins, crackers (saltines, wheat, oat, rye), pasta, couscous, udon noodles, rice noodles, cream of wheat
VEGETABLES	Artichokes, asparagus, avocados, bamboo shoots, yellow wax beans, lima beans, beets, bok choy, brussels sprouts, cabbage (green, napa, red), capers, chard, cilantro, corn, cucumbers, eggplant, garlic, greens (beet, collard, mustard, turnip), jicama, kale, kohlrabi, leeks, lettuce (Boston, butter, endive, iceberg, red leaf, romaine), mushrooms, okra, olives (green, ripe), onions (chives, red, green, brown, white, yellow, vidalia), parsnips, peas, bell peppers (green, yellow, red), jalapeno peppers, pimentos, red potatoes, sweet potatoes, pumpkin, daikon radishes, rutabaga, sauerkraut, seaweed (arame, dulse, kelp, nori, wakame), shallots, spinach, sprouts (alfalfa, clover, mung bean, radish, sunflower), squash (acorn, banana, butternut, spaghetti, yellow [summer], zucchini), cooked tomatoes, turnips, yams
VEGETABLE JUICES	Celery, carrot, carrot/celery, parsley, spinach, tomato, V-8®
FRUITS	Apples (Golden or Red Delicious, Granny Smith, Jonathan, Pippin, Rome Beauty), apricots, bananas, blackberries, blueberries, boysenberries, cranberries, gooseberries, raspberries, strawberries, cherries, grapes (black, green, red, white), red grapefruits, guavas, kiwi, kumquats, loquats, mangos, melons (cantaloupe, casaba, honeydew, watermelon), nectarines, oranges, papayas, pears, peaches, Fuju persimmons, pineapples, plums (black, purple, red), pomegranates, prunes, rhubarb, tangelos, tangerines, dates, figs, prunes, raisins
FRUIT JUICES	Apple, apple cider, apple/apricot, apricot, black cherry, red cherry, cranapple, cranberry, grape (purple, red, white), grapefruit, guava, lemon, mango, orange, papaya, pear, pineapple, pineapple/coconut, prune, raspberry, tangerine, watermelon
VEGETABLE OILS	Almond, olive
SWEETENERS	Re-Vita®, stevia
CONDIMENTS	Medium or hot salsa, tahini, cumin seeds, vinegar, salt, sea salt, Vege-Sal®
SALAD DRESSINGS	Vinegar and oil, lemon juice and oil
BEVERAGES	Herbal tea, Japanese tea, Chinese oolong tea; Calistoga® flavored mineral water, sparkling water

Thymus

RARELY FOODS	No more than once a month
DENSE PROTEIN	Starkist® tuna
DAIRY	Milk (whole, 2%, low fat, nonfat, raw), goat milk, buttermilk, low fat plain yogurt, flavored yogurt, frozen yogurt, ice cream
CHEESE	American, blue, brie, Camembert, Cheddar, Colby, cottage, cream, Edam, feta, goat, Gouda, Jack, Limburger, Mozzarella, Muenster, Parmesan, ricotta, Swiss
LEGUMES	Beans (adzuki, kidney, navy, great northern, pinto, red)
GRAINS	Long or short grain brown rice, breads (French, Italian, sourdough, garlic, multi-grain, 7-grain, oat, rye, rye/pumpernickle, sprouted wheat, white, whole wheat), wheat/pumpernickle bagels, graham crackers
VEGETABLES	Arugula, green beans, broccoflower, potatoes (white rose, russet, purple, yukon gold), raw tomatoes, watercress
FRUITS	White grapefruits, lemons, limes, crenshaw melons
VEGETABLE OILS	All-blend, avocado, canola, corn, flaxseed, peanut, safflower, sesame, soy, sunflower
SWEETENERS	Honey, molasses, sorghum, refined cane sugar, date sugar, brown sugar, raw sugar, barley malt syrup, corn syrup, brown rice syrup, maple syrup, fructose, saccharin, succonant, aspartame, Equal®, Sweet'n Low®, NutraSweet®
CONDIMENTS	Catsup, horseradish, barbecue sauce, pesto sauce, Tabasco, mustard, mayonnaise, soy sauce, margarine
SALAD DRESSINGS	Blue cheese, French, ranch, creamy Italian, creamy avocado, thousand island
DESSERTS	Custards, tapioca, puddings, pies, cakes, chocolate, desserts containing chocolate, raspberry sherbet, orange sherbet
CHIPS	Bean, corn (blue, white, yellow), potato
BEVERAGES	Coffee; black tea, green tea; wine (white, red), sake, beer, barley malt liquor, champagne, gin, Scotch, vodka, whiskey; root beer, regular sodas, diet sodas

Thymus

MENUS

DIETARY EMPHASIS:

- Protein essential, ideally at breakfast and lunch, but if unable to do so, may consume bulk of protein at dinner.
- Protein, especially lamb and eggs (up to 4, 6x/week, for sensitive, up to 3, 4x/week – medium-boiled), rye, seeds, nuts, vegetables, and olive oil.

WEIGHT LOSS:

- Dense protein for breakfast and lunch.
- Eliminate refined sugar, particularly sugary desserts and sweet drinks, including fruit juices and alcohol.
- Minimize bread.
- Avoid all dairy products except butter.

WEIGHT GAIN:

- 35% of caloric intake should be from fats.
- Include snacks.
- Exercise daily.

VEGETARIAN DIET:

- Inadequate, since require 10-35% of calories from dense protein.
- To sustain on a vegetarian diet, use protein powders or supplements, nuts and seeds, and especially 4 eggs a day, 7 days a week and 35% of calories from fats.

FATS:

- 25-35% of caloric intake.
- Best sources are dense protein (all), seeds, nuts (almonds, Brazils, peanuts, pine nuts), olive oil, and kefir. May derive 15-20% of fats from kefir.

SENSITIVE:

•Limit fruit to 2 times a week.

KEY

—all menus may be used by healthy persons
( ) around foods means that they're optional
L denotes weight loss menus
S denotes sensitive menus
G denotes weight gain menus

L	S	G	**BREAKFAST**: 7-8 a.m. Heavy, with protein, grain, vegetables, nuts, seeds, dairy and/or legumes.
L	S		Omelette (salsa)
L	S		Eggs and lamb or turkey
		G	Eggs and lamb or beef steak (rye bread or toast)
			Eggs and rye toast or corn/rye toast
		G	Eggs and chicken or turkey (rye or date/nut/raisin bread or toast)
		G	Eggs, fillet of sole, and toast – rye, oat, wheat, corn/rye, or sourdough
		G	Eggs and Cheddar cheese (potatoes or rice and/or any toast)
	S		Eggs (any bread or toast w/nut butter – almond, cashew, macadamia/cashew or peanut)
L	S		Eggs and potatoes or rice
L	S		Eggs and oatmeal, brown basmati rice, cream of rice or cream of rye (butter)
L			Eggs w/corn grits or Mueseli®
		G	Eggs and buckwheat pancakes (Re-vita®)
L	S		Chicken and white basmati rice
L	S		Chicken and avocado on Rye Krisp®
	S		Turkey w/Rye Krisp®
L		G	Red snapper, eggs, and rice
L		G	Lamb, red potatoes, and peas
L		G	Steak, eggs, and potatoes
		G	Steak or hamburger sandwich on sourdough (A-1 Steak Sauce)
		G	Beef lasagna (green salad)
	S		Cream of rye w/butter
		G	Cream of rye w/butter and oat, rye, or wheat bread (almonds, cashews, pecans, or walnuts)
L			Cream of rice w/butter (almonds, cashews, pecans, walnuts, or peanuts)
	S		Puffed rice w/macadamia, cashew, or almond milk (almonds, cashews, pecans, walnuts, or peanuts,
	S	G	Corn or rye flakes and soy or nut milk (barley malt syrup)

Thymus

SNACK:
(Optional) 10 a.m. or 4 p.m.
Vegetables, dairy, nuts, seeds, grain.

	Avocado on Rye Krisp®
L	Carrots, celery, radishes, cauliflower, broccoli
L G	Almond butter and celery on Rye Krisp® cracker
S G	Rye Krisp® cracker and cashew butter or macadamia/cashew butter
S G	White or brown rice cakes and cashew butter or macadamia/cashew butter
S G	Kefir
G	Yogurt

LUNCH:
11:30 a.m. - 2:30 p.m. Moderate-to-heavy, with protein, grain, nuts, seeds, dairy, legumes and/or vegetables.

May be light or heavy depending on eating pattern of the day.

L S G	Chicken, baked potato, peas, and onions
L S G	Chicken burrito and white or brown basmati rice or salsa
G	Chicken enchilada and salsa
L	Chicken and tomato on Rye Krisp®
G	Chicken taco w/cheese, pinto beans, and rice
L S G	Oriental chicken, beef, or shrimp w/broccoli and white basmati rice
L S	Pasta (butter, and/or chicken or turkey)
L S G	Turkey or chicken, pasta, mushrooms, carrots, bell peppers, onions, and butter
G	Turkey sandwich on rye bread w/tomato or cheese, and avocado
L S G	Turkey tortellini (oil, and garlic), w/green beans and basil
L S	Turkey and avocado on rye crackers
L S G	Lamb curry and basmati rice
L S G	Lamb, mashed potatoes w/gravy, and lima beans
G	Lamb gyro sandwich (Greek feta cheese salad: olives, avocado, cucumber, feta cheese, olive oil, and lemon)
L S G	Red snapper, red potatoes, and green beans
L S G	Salmon, basmati rice, zucchini, onions, and carrots
L S G	Salmon, basmati rice, and asparagus
G	Sardines w/lemon on rye/pumpernickel bread and salad
L S G	Scallops and pasta w/mushrooms, carrots, bell peppers, and butter
L S G	Sea bass or sole, and basmati rice (salad: romaine lettuce, carrots, red onions, mushrooms, eggs, and roquefort dressing)
L S G	Shrimp, basmati rice, and peas
L S G	Shrimp, pasta, and green beans
	Shrimp and avocado on rye bread or crackers
L S G	Sole and basmati rice (artichokes)
L S G	Trout, broccoli, and squash
	Trout w/cole slaw
L S G	Tuna and pasta w/butter and raw celery
G	Tuna on rye bread w/tomato and broccoli
S	Tuna and avocado on rye crackers
	Tuna on oatmeal bread w/avocado and poppy seed dressing
L	Tuna on oatmeal bread w/avocado
L S G	Tuna, avocado, celery, onion, and avocado dressing
L S G	Clams and pasta w/marinara sauce, clam sauce, or olive oil
L G	Clam chowder, fish, and rice
	Egg salad sandwich and tomatoes (lettuce)
L	Pinto beans w/rice, romaine lettuce salad w/other vegetables, and fruit
L S G	Pinto beans, rice, salsa, guacamole, and corn tortilla

LUNCH or DINNER:

L	Oriental chicken, beef, or shrimp w/broccoli and rice
L S	Chicken taco (salsa and refried beans)
L S	Bean burrito and spanish rice (salsa)
L S	Black bean burrito
G	Bean burrito w/Jack cheese(rice and/or salsa

Thymus

L S G Pinto beans, basmati rice, salsa, guacamole, and corn tortilla

L Tofu w/Chinese vegetables and rice

L S Lentils, brown basmati rice, and peas

L S Vegetarian chili (couscous)

Cottage cheese w/pineapple and spinach salad spinach leaves and feta cheese

L Vegetable pot pie w/tofu cheese

L S Mashed potatoes (butter) and zucchini, broccoli, cauliflower, beets, or carrots

L G Lasagna and broccoli, peas, carrots, and/or cauliflower

S Meatless franks w/steamed broccoli

Soy cheese pizza w/vegetables on whole wheat crust

MID-AFTERNOON SNACK:
(Optional) 4 p.m. Fruit, vegetables, dairy, nuts, seeds, grain.

G Pears and cottage cheese

G Bagels, lox, cream cheese, and tomato

G Papaya juice in smoothie w/yogurt

G Peach or raspberry kefir or smoothie

G Apple, oranges, pineapples, peaches, green grapes, blueberries, or cantaloupe

DINNER:
6-9 p.m. Light-to-moderate, with legumes, grain, vegetables, fruit, nuts, seeds, eggs, dairy and/or protein. May be heavy if insufficient protein has been consumed during the day.

L S Plain pasta w/basil pesto or marinara sauce and artichokes (parsley)

G Plain pasta w/olive oil, basil pesto, or marinara sauce and parsley, turkey tortellini w/parmesan cheese, oil, and garlic, green beans w/basil, and raspberries

L S Pasta primevera

G Pasta w/tomato or marinara sauce and Parmesan cheese

L S Rye or rice cereal w/butter (egg)

L S Corn grits (egg)

G Cheese omelette (rye or oat toast)

G Egg salad sandwich and tomatoes (lettuce)

L G Black beans, rice w/Spike®, and flour tortilla (avocado)

L S G Split pea soup and Rye Krisp® (peaches)

L S G Vegetable beef soup and Rye Krisp® (apple)

L S G Chicken noodle soup and Rye Krisp® (orange)

L S G Clam chowder, then apple

G Oriental stir fry: broccoli/chicken or vegetable/chicken w/1 cup rice, chicken livers w/mustard, and baked apple

L Cucumber roll and vegetable tempura

G Spinach salad: spinach leaves, feta cheese, eggs, sesame oil

L S Yam (butter)

Orange juice smoothie w/pineapple and banana

G Cottage cheese w/pineapple, and spinach salad: spinach leaves and feta cheese

G Cottage cheese and apple sauce

G Fruit shake w/nuts and protein powder (toast and nut butter)

S Apple w/cashew butter

EVENING SNACK:
(Optional) 10 p.m.-1 a.m. Fruit, protein, vegetables, grain, nuts, seeds, dairy, sweets.

L Blueberries, blackberries, or raspberries

G Pumpkin, apple, or berry pie

G Pro Gain (oatmeal)

G Ben & Jerry's®, Dreyer's, or Swensen's® ice cream

Baked apple

Fruit and toast (macadamia nuts)

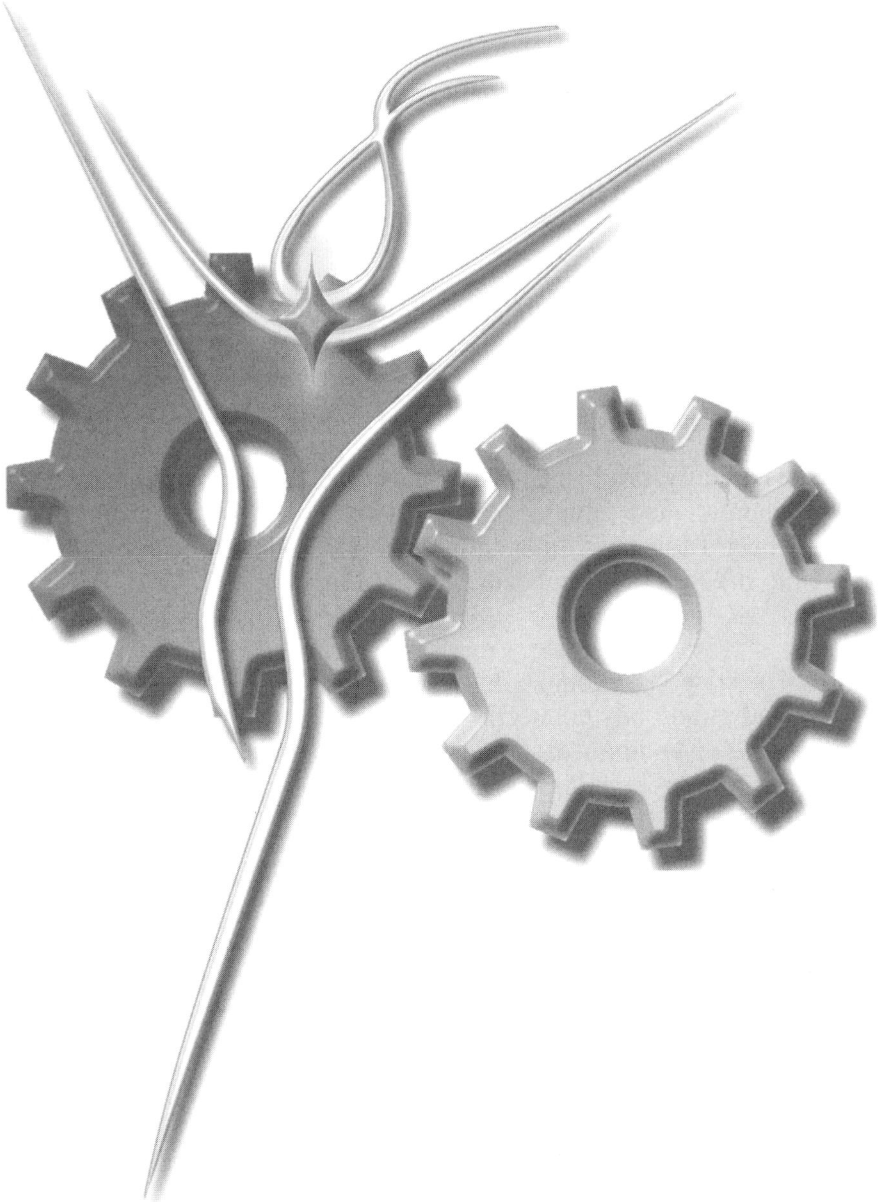

The "Thyroid Body Type"
is symbolized by gears. Synchronized movement is essential to getting things done. Bridging the gap between the theoretical and practical, they thrive on doing things that are worthwhile.

Thyroid

BODY TYPE PROFILE

LOCATION	Front center of throat.
FUNCTION	Secretes hormones that regulate metabolism, particularly those that cause rapid mobilization of fats, controls basal metabolic rate, and during childhood affects growth. Is activated by anterior pituitary gland.
POTENTIAL HEALTH PROBLEMS	Generally bright and alert, sensitive, mentally quick, and intuitive. Good stamina and endurance. Digestive sensitivity or distress with tendency toward constipation or sluggishness. Chronic acne or facial blemishes. Prone to nervous tension, headaches, and fatigue.
RECOMMENDED EXERCISE	Exercise is optional. Its benefit is physical for muscle tone, figure control, and mind/body connection. Activities such as callanetics, dance, and hiking develop endurance, stamina, and muscular strength. Aerobic exercise such as walking, rebounding, or trampoline are good for developing muscle.

WOMEN'S CHARACTERISTICS

DISTINGUISHING FEATURES	Body well-proportioned with delicate or slender hands, long, tapered fingers, and narrow feet. Graceful mannerisms, often with delicate appearance. Eyes reveal brightness and sensitivity. Known for being able to see what needs to be done and getting it done.
ADDITIONAL PHYSICAL CHARACTERISTICS	Buttocks relatively flat-to-rounded. Low back curvature straight-to-average. Breasts average; may increase with age and/or weight gain. Shoulders relatively even with hips. Waist defined to well-defined. Average to long-waisted. Height, petite-to-tall. Bone structure small-to-medium. Average, elongated musculature. Shapely legs, with muscular, well-defined calves. Hair generally thick-to-average, healthy, and abundant. V-shaped jaw on either average oval or heart-shaped face.
WEIGHT GAIN AREAS	Lower body with initial gain in lower abdomen, waist, upper hips, and entire upper 2/3rds of thighs, including upper inner, inner knees, and middle back. Secondary weight gain extends into entire abdomen, upper arms, entire back, thighs extending to knees, face, under chin, breasts, and buttocks.

Thyroid

DIETARY GUIDELINES

SCHEDULING MEALS

"HEALTHY"

Breakfast, Lunch, and Dinner: Light-to-heavy, with protein, nuts, seeds, grain, vegetables, legumes, dairy, and/or fruit. Keep combinations simple. Size of meals, as well as number, are flexible depending on lifestyle and the day's activities.

"SENSITIVE"

Breakfast: Moderate, with protein, grain, vegetables, and/or fruit.

Lunch: Light-to-moderate, with protein, nuts, vegetables, grain, and/or fruit.

Dinner: Light-to-heavy, with protein, grain, vegetables, and/or fruit.

Those who work with energy during the day often find they do best with moderate breakfast consisting of protein and grain, grain and vegetable, grain followed by fruit juice, or combination of protein, vegetables, and grain. Lunch often light, with vegetables, nuts, protein, grains, or fruit or vegetable juices, or any combination thereof. Foods may be eaten singularly. Dinner ranges from light-to-heavy, with more substantial protein eaten at this time, often consisting of protein, grain, and vegetables, possibly with fruit or fruit juice or Kombucha tea afterwards.

Addition of 4th meal (mid-afternoon snack) common, especially if late dinner. Time and quantity of dinner often dictates breakfast size.

DIETARY EMPHASIS

- Consume minimum of 2 oz. of dense protein (chicken, turkey, eggs, or fish) with grain such as rice or pasta: 5 meals a week. May have up to 2 eggs, 4-6 meals a week and breads, 2 meals a week. Fruit or fruit juice after protein often assists digestion. Eat more cooked than raw vegetables.
- For weight loss, consume 20-30% of calories from dense protein, limit snacks to evening, avoid dairy except butter, breads, refined sugar, and limit fruit to 2 meals per week. When at ideal weight, breads, dairy, sugar, and fats will increase weight.
- For weight gain, consume 25-35% of calories from dense protein. May have fruit up to 2 times per day.
- Vegetarian diets inadequate since they require 10-30% of calories from dense protein.
- Fats, 20% of caloric intake. Best sources are almonds and dense protein (chicken, turkey, eggs, fish).

KEY SUPPORTS FOR SYSTEM

Basmati rice and protein. Almonds support the heart. Beets and/or beet greens cleanse liver and stimulate bowel function. Kombucha tea (preferably made with Misty Mango, Chinese oolong, or green tea) after meals aids digestion, assimilation, and regulation of bowels.

Thyroid

COMPLEMENTARY GLANDULAR SUPPORT	Lungs, through nurturing self and/or others, and nervous system through connecting with various aspects of self.
FOODS CRAVED	*(When Energy is Low)* Sweets and carbohydrates like pastries, cookies, muffins, breads, croissants, chocolate, ice cream, cherries, and raspberries. Food stimulates thyroid function, so tend to eat when energy is low. Caffeine often used as stimulant.
FOODS TO AVOID	Sugars, whole wheat breads, sweets, artificial sweeteners, and caffeine. Limit sweet fruit because it contains too much thyroid-stimulating simple sugar.
RECOMMENDED CUISINE	Thai, Chinese, Seafood. Simple foods and combinations with mild to moderate seasonings.

Thyroid

PSYCHOLOGICAL PROFILE

ESSENCE

Just as the thyroid gland regulates the metabolism, ensuring the adequate release of energy into the body, Thyroid types are known for manifestation or getting things done. Extremely responsible, they will go to great lengths to fulfill their obligations, often at their own expense. Thyroids thrive on doing things that are worthwhile and are often idealistic, wanting to make a contribution to their world. With an affinity for both the theoretical and the practical, Thyroids are constantly formulating theories, then testing and refining them based on their practical application. Bridging the gap between the head and the body, or the mind and the emotions, Thyroids are able to see both sides of an issue, distill it, and communicate its essence.

CHARACTERISTIC TRAITS

The sensitivity of the Thyroid type is often apparent in their eyes. There is brightness and a presence that reveals an openness and availability. Thyroids characteristically have a strong compassion and empathy for others. With a multi-faceted nature, Thyroids are capable of understanding and relating to all the other body types.

Being intimately connected to both head and body, Thyroids can bridge the gap between the mental and the sensuous. Many have an intense interest in gaining knowledge as their whole orientation to life is intellectual, while at the same time having a keen awareness of their body and sensory perceptions. Their senses are very finely tuned, especially the tactile, with a heightened sense of touch. They frequently demonstrate an intense interest in things aesthetic, whether it be music, theater, or fine art.

When a subject captures their attention, Thyroids will use their strong mental capacities to study it in depth and intuitive abilities to capture its essence. By looking at the whole picture, they are able to see and categorize ideas and theories into a completely new pattern. They will then express, test, and modify based on practical application until they either refine its application and usefulness or discard it.

Thyroid types can be quite sociable and gregarious, fitting in well with others and enjoying their company. While talkative, open, and receptive, there's generally a sense that there's still a whole lot more that's not being expressed. Being exceptionally self-contained, they can also be soft-spoken and reserved, even to the point of appearing aloof, secretive, or withdrawn. Internalizing rather than assertively expressing their feelings and attitudes, Thyroids have a definite code of privacy and independence about them – an air of dignity.

MOTIVATION

Motivated by their desire for self-realization, Thyroids seek personal growth and deal with what's not working in their lives on an ongoing basis. Because of their intensity and lack of fear when exploring spiritual and emotional realms, they can access areas that most people around them don't understand. Consequently, they generally have less of a need to share what's going on in their lives than most other types.

Thyroid

MOTIVATION (Continued)

Typically as children, Thyroid types were aware of being different and misunderstood, so they learned to be emotionally self-sufficient and responsible for themselves. Generally in touch with their feelings, Thyroids can also be quite aware of the feelings of others. Not wanting to do anything to hurt someone else's feelings or to suffer from being belittled, betrayed, or misunderstood, Thyroids often exercise restraint in expressing themselves, controlling their emotions, or evading areas of potential conflict.

In their attempt to discover ways to speak their truth in an acceptable manner, Thyroids often hold back, reviewing what they want to say in their minds, even to the point of waiting until the appropriate moment for expression has passed. When dealing one-on-one, Thyroids can swing to the opposite extreme, telling long, detailed stories and losing the point in their wanderings. Mentally adept and able to see both sides, Thyroids have the ability to dive in, identify the problem and its cause, formulate a viable solution or theory, and speak clearly and directly.

Sensitive to the emotional environment around them and not wanting to upset their equilibrium or the harmony they value with others, Thyroids are likely to avoid dealing with conflict and disharmony. Having discovered as children that directly speaking their truth was difficult for those around them to handle and not having the skills to solve the problem, Thyroids tend to stuff their feelings. By not discussing areas of conflict, preferring to smooth things over or letting them slide, they often hold back communication that could be valuable. When they do have to face conflict, Thyroids tend to do so gingerly and indirectly.

"AT WORST"

It's easy for Thyroids to fall into a pattern of self-denial, putting other things and people first, taking things too seriously, and taking on too much. Seeing themselves as capable and responsible, they will often get caught in helping others so much that they deplete their energy or overextend themselves to the point that there's not enough time left for their own needs.

Thyroids can become irritable or depressed and withdrawn when they don't feel they are doing something worthwhile or that their efforts are making any real difference in the world. Needing to be productively engaged in something meaningful, they may become obsessed with trying to fulfill this deeply felt need, which is closely related to their own self-nurturing and fulfillment.

By nature one of the most reserved types, Thyroids can come across as cold, unfeeling, distant, or detached. Being overly focused on one of their various mental pursuits, they can close themselves off to others and become almost oblivious to their emotional concerns. They can become mentally rigid, particularly once they've reached a decision on something, making it very difficult for them to consider anyone else's viewpoint.

Thyroid

Mental rigidity occurs when they become overly linear and bogged down by details, losing touch with their spiritual connection. Dogmatism, self-righteousness, and victimhood may appear when they let themselves become plagued by worry, self-doubt, and a belief in lack and limitation.

"AT BEST "

Thyroids become truly empowered when they connect with their feelings and verbally communicate in a manner others can relate to, hear, and accept. Maintaining their own inner peace, Thyroids excel when they're doing something that is worthwhile or making a contribution. Hardworking, strong-willed, and idealistic about their chosen pursuits, Thyroids have a sense of dedication that almost guarantees success in whatever endeavors they choose to undertake.

Thoughtful, reflective, and observant, Thyroids are very good at seeing and understanding all sides of an issue and tend to make decisions carefully and methodically. They take pride in their ability to figure out what needs to be done in any given situation, have the courage and fortitude to set it in motion, and the competence and determination to carry it through to completion. Once Thyroids make up their mind to do something, they do whatever it takes to accomplish the goal, persevering long after others would have given up.

There's a "quiet passion" in the way Thyroids operate, which others typically see as their intensity. It's really their unconditional commitment to doing whatever it takes to accomplish their mission, whether it be self-realization or assisting someone else. By balancing their mental acuity with their spiritual connection and creative expression, Thyroids are able to be successful in whatever they undertake and make significant contributions to the world. Utilizing their ability to connect the theoretical with the practical and distill its essence along with their talent for formulating and implementing theories, combined with the flexibility to adjust them as needed, Thyroids are able to transform ideas into reality, bringing peace and understanding to the world.

Thyroid

FOOD LISTS

HEALTHY FOOD LIST

FREQUENTLY FOODS	3-7 meals per week – refers to each food, rather than category.
DENSE PROTEIN	Chicken, chicken broth, chicken livers, cornish game hen, turkey; bonita, flounder, haddock, halibut, perch, orange roughy, salmon, sardines, shark, red snapper, sole, swordfish, tuna; abalone, calamari (squid), crab, clams, eel, mussels, octopus, scallops; eggs
DAIRY	Butter
NUTS	Almonds (roasted unsalted or raw soaked), almond butter
GRAINS	Oats, popcorn, white or brown basmati rice, short grain brown rice, brown rice flour, rice cakes, oat flour, oat crackers
VEGETABLES	Artichokes, asparagus, bamboo shoots, beets, steamed broccoli, carrots, green peas, snow pea pods, bell peppers (green, red, yellow), nori seaweed
FRUITS	Apples (Granny Smith, Jonathan, Pippin), apricots (fresh or unsulphured), cranberries, gooseberries, raspberries, cherries, lemons, mangos, persimmons, pomegranates
FRUIT JUICES	Apple, apple/apricot, black cherry, cherry cider, cranberry, pineapple/ coconut, raspberry
SWEETENERS	Re-Vita®, stevia
BEVERAGES	Herbal tea
MODERATELY FOODS	1-2 meals per week – refers to each food, rather than category.
DENSE PROTEIN	Beef broth, beef liver, buffalo, lamb, veal, venison, organ meats (heart, brain); duck; anchovy, bass, catfish, cod, herring, mackerel, mahi–mahi, trout; lobster, oysters, shrimp
DAIRY	Milk (whole, 2%, low fat, nonfat, raw), goat milk, half & half, sour cream, kefir, plain or flavored yogurt, ice cream (Ben & Jerry's®, Dreyer's, Swensen's®)
CHEESE	American, blue, brie, Camembert, Cheddar, Colby, cream, cottage, Edam, feta, goat, Gouda, Jack, kefir, Limburger, mozzarella, Muenster, Parmesan, ricotta, Romano, Swiss
NUTS and SEEDS	Brazils, cashews, cashew butter, water chestnuts, coconut, coconut milk, filberts, hazelnuts, macadamias, macadamia butter, macadamia/cashew butter, peanuts, peanut butter, pecans, pine nuts, pistachios, walnuts (black, English), seeds (caraway, pumpkin, sesame, sunflower), sesame seed butter, sunflower seed butter

Thyroid

LEGUMES	Beans (adzuki, black, garbanzo, kidney, lima [butter], navy, great northern, pinto, red, soy), split peas, black–eyed peas, lentils, hummus, miso, soy milk
GRAINS	Amaranth, barley, corn, corn grits, corn bread, corn tortillas, hominy grits, millet w/chicken broth, quinoa, rice (long grain brown, Japanese, wild), rice bran, rye, triticale, wheat bran, flour tortillas, refined wheat flour, breads (French, Italian, sourdough, garlic, oat, corn, rice, corn/rye, rye, sprouted grain, white) croissants, bagels, English muffins, crackers (saltines, oat, rye), couscous, semolina pasta, sesame pasta, udon noodles, rice noodles, cream of rice, cream of rye, cream of wheat
VEGETABLES	Arugula, avocados, green beans, yellow wax beans, lima beans, bok choy, raw broccoli, broccoflower, brussels sprouts, cabbage (green, napa, red) cauliflower, celery, chard, cilantro, corn, cucumbers, eggplant, garlic, greens (beet, collard, mustard, turnip), jicama, kale, kohlrabi, leeks, okra, mushrooms, green or ripe olives, onions (chives, green, brown, red, white, yellow, vidalia), parsley, parsnips, chili peppers, pimentos, potatoes (all varieties)), pumpkin, radishes, daikon radishes, rutabaga, sauerkraut, seaweed (arame, dulse, kelp, wakame), shallots, spinach, sprouts (alfalfa, sunflower, clover), squash (acorn, banana, butternut, yellow [summer], spaghetti), turnips, watercress, yams
VEGETABLE JUICES	Carrot, carrot/beet/celery, carrot/celery/parsley/spinach, tomato, V-8®
FRUITS	Apples (Golden or Red Delicious, McIntosh, Rome Beauty), canned apricots, bananas, blackberries, blueberries, boysenberries, strawberries, grapes (black, green, red), grapefruits (white, red), guavas, kiwi, kumquats, limes, loquats, melons (cantaloupe, crenshaw, honeydew, watermelon), nectarines, oranges, papayas, peaches, pears, pineapples, plums (black, purple, red), rhubarb, tangelos, tangerines, dates, figs, prunes, raisins
FRUIT JUICES	Apple cider, apricot, red cherry, cranapple, grape, (purple, red, white), grapefruit, guava, lemon, orange, papaya, pear, pineapple, prune, tangerine, watermelon
VEGETABLE OILS	All-blend, almond, avocado, canola, corn, flaxseed, olive, peanut, safflower, sesame, soy, sunflower
SWEETENERS	Honey, molasses, sorghum, brown sugar, date sugar, raw sugar, barley malt syrup, corn syrup, maple syrup, brown rice syrup, fructose, succonant, saccharin
CONDIMENTS	Mustard, horseradish, soy sauce, barbecue sauce, pesto sauce, paprika, salsa, tahini, vinegar, Morton's® Lite salt, sea salt, Vege–Sal®
SALAD DRESSINGS	Blue cheese, French, ranch, creamy Italian, creamy avocado, thousand island, vinegar and oil, lemon juice and oil
DESSERTS	Custards, tapioca, puddings, pies, cakes, chocolate, desserts containing chocolate, raspberry sherbet, orange sherbet
CHIPS	Bean, corn (blue, white, yellow), potato

Thyroid

BEVERAGES	Coffee, coffee with Re-Vita®; green tea, black tea, Japanese tea, Chinese oolong tea; Cafix®; mineral water, sparkling water; wine (red, white), sake, gin, vodka; root beer, regular sodas
RARELY FOODS	No more than once a month
DENSE PROTEIN	Beef, pork, ham, bacon, sausage
DAIRY	Buttermilk, sweet cream, frozen yogurt, most ice creams
LEGUMES	Tofu
GRAINS	Buckwheat, whole wheat, wheat germ, breads (whole wheat, 7-grain, multi-grain), whole wheat crackers, 7-grain cereal
VEGETABLES	Lettuce (all varieties), sweet potatoes, sprouts (mung bean, radish), tomatoes, zucchini
FRUITS	Casaba melons
SWEETENERS	Refined cane sugar, aspartame, Equal®, Sweet'n Low®, NutraSweet®
CONDIMENTS	Catsup, mayonnaise, margarine
BEVERAGES	Beer, barley malt liquor, champagne, Scotch, whiskey; diet sodas

SENSITIVE FOOD LIST

FREQUENTLY FOODS	3-7 times per week – refers to each food, rather than category.
DENSE PROTEIN	Chicken, turkey; eggs
DAIRY	Butter
NUTS	Almonds (roasted unsalted or raw soaked), almond butter
GRAINS	Oats, oat flour, popcorn, rice (white or brown basmati, short grain brown), brown rice flour, rice cakes
VEGETABLES	Artichokes, bamboo shoots, beets, steamed broccoli, carrots, green peas, snow pea pods
FRUITS	Apricots (fresh or unsulphured), raspberries, cherries, lemons, mangos
MODERATELY FOODS	1-2 times per week – refers to each food, rather than category.
DENSE PROTEIN	Beef broth, buffalo, lamb, venison, organ meats (brain, heart); chicken broth, chicken livers, cornish game hen, duck; bass, bonita, catfish, cod, flounder, haddock, halibut, herring, mackerel, mahi-mahi, perch, orange roughy, salmon, sardines, shark, red snapper, sole, swordfish, tuna, trout; abalone, calamari (squid), clams, crab, eel, lobster, mussels, octopus, oysters, scallops, shrimp

Thyroid

NUTS	Brazils, cashews, cashew butter, water chestnuts, coconuts, coconut milk, filberts, hazelnuts, macadamias, macadamia butter, macadamia/cashew butter, pecans, pine nuts, pistachio
LEGUMES	Split peas
GRAINS	Barley, corn, corn bread, corn grits, corn tortillas, oatmeal, quinoa, rice (Japanese, wild), rice bran, rye, couscous, oat pasta, semolina pasta, udon noodles, rice noodles, cream of rice, cream of rye
VEGETABLES	Asparagus, avocados, green beans, bok choy, celery, chard, cucumbers, eggplant, garlic, greens (beet, collard, mustard, turnip), jicama, kale, kohlrabi, leeks, mushrooms, okra, onions (brown, red, white, yellow, vidalia), parsley, parsnips, bell peppers (green, red), pimentos, potatoes (all varieties), pumpkin, daikon radishes, seaweed (arame, dulse, kelp, nori, wakame), shallots, spinach, yams
VEGETABLE JUICES	Carrot, carrot/celery/parsley/spinach
FRUITS	Apples (Granny Smith, Pippin, Jonathan), canned apricots, blackberries, boysenberries, cranberries, gooseberries, grapefruits (red, white)
FRUIT JUICES	Apple cider, apple/apricot, apricot, black cherry, red cherry, cherry cider, lemon, pineapple/coconut
SWEETENERS	Re-Vita®, stevia
SALAD DRESSINGS	Vinegar and oil, lemon juice and oil
BEVERAGES	Herbal tea, Japanese tea; mineral water, sparkling water
RARELY FOODS	No more than once a month
DENSE PROTEIN	Beef, beef liver, veal, pork, ham, bacon, sausage; anchovy
DAIRY	Milk (whole, 2%, low fat, nonfat, raw), goat milk, buttermilk, half & half, sweet cream, sour cream, plain or flavored yogurt, kefir, frozen yogurt, ice cream
CHEESE	American, blue, brie, Camembert, Cheddar, Colby, cottage, cream, Edam, feta, goat, Gouda, Jack, kefir, Limburger, mozzarella, Muenster, Parmesan, ricotta, Romano, Swiss
NUTS and SEEDS	Peanuts, peanut butter, walnuts (black, English), seeds (caraway, pumpkin, sesame, sunflower) sesame seed butter, sunflower seed butter
LEGUMES	Beans (adzuki, black, garbanzo, kidney, lima [butter], navy, great northern, pinto, red, soy), lentils, black-eyed peas, hummus, miso, soy milk, tofu
GRAINS	Amaranth, buckwheat, hominy grits, millet, long grain brown rice, triticale, whole wheat, wheat bran, wheat germ, flour tortillas, refined wheat flour, breads, bagels, croissants, English muffins, crackers, 7-grain cereal, cream of wheat

Thyroid

VEGETABLES	Arugula, lima beans, yellow wax beans, raw broccoli, broccoflower, brussels sprouts, cabbage (green, napa, red), cauliflower, chives, cilantro, corn, lettuce (all varieties), olives (green, ripe), green onions, bell peppers (purple, yellow), chili peppers, radishes, rutabaga, sauerkraut, sweet potatoes, sprouts (alfalfa, clover, mung bean, radish, sunflower), squash (acorn, banana, butternut, spaghetti, yellow [summer], zucchini), tomatoes, turnips, watercress
VEGETABLE JUICES	Celery, green juice, tomato, V8®
FRUITS	Apples (Golden or Red Delicious, Rome Beauty, McIntosh), bananas, blueberries, strawberries, grapes (black, green, red), guavas, kiwi, kumquats, limes, loquats, melons (casaba, cantaloupe, crenshaw, honeydew, watermelon), nectarines, oranges, papayas, peaches, pears, persimmons, pineapples, plums (black, purple, red), pomegranates, rhubarb, tangelos, tangerines, dates, figs, prunes, raisins
FRUIT JUICES	Apple, cranapple, cranberry, raspberry, grape (purple, red, white), grapefruit, guava, orange, papaya, pear, pineapple, prune, tangerine, watermelon
VEGETABLE OILS	All-blend, almond, avocado, canola, corn, flaxseed, olive, peanut, safflower, sesame, soy, sunflower
SWEETENERS	Honey, brown sugar, raw sugar, refined cane sugar, date sugar, molasses, sorghum, barley malt syrup, corn syrup, maple syrup, brown rice syrup, fructose, succonant, saccharin, aspartame, Equal®, Sweet'n Low®, NutraSweet®
CONDIMENTS	Catsup, margarine, mayonnaise, mustard, horseradish, barbecue sauce, pesto sauce, paprika, salsa, Morton's® Lite salt, sea salt, soy sauce, tahini, tamari, Vege-Sal®, vinegar
SALAD DRESSINGS	Blue cheese, French, ranch, creamy Italian, creamy avocado, thousand island
DESSERTS	Custards, tapioca, puddings, pies, cakes, chocolate, desserts containing chocolate, raspberry sherbet, orange sherbet
CHIPS	Bean, corn (blue, white, yellow), potato
BEVERAGES	Coffee (regular or decaffeinated), coffee with Re-Vita®; black tea, green tea, Chinese oolong tea, raspberry iced tea; Cafix®, Postum®; wine (red, white), sake, beer, barley malt liquor, champagne, vodka, Scotch, gin, whiskey; root beer, regular sodas, diet Pepsi®, diet sodas

Thyroid

MENUS

DIETARY EMPHASIS:

- Consume minimum of 2 oz. dense protein (chicken, turkey, eggs, or fish) with grain such as rice or pasta, 5 meals a week.
- May have up to 2 eggs 4-6 meals a week, bread 2 meals a week.
- Almonds as they support the heart.
- Limit sweet fruit, because it contains too much thyroid-stimulating simple sugar.
- Fruit or fruit juice after protein often assists digestion.
- Consume more cooked than raw vegetables.
- Beets and/or beet greens cleanse the liver and stimulate bowel function.
- Kombucha tea after meals aids digestion.

WEIGHT LOSS:

- 20-30% of calories from dense protein.
- Limit fruit to 2 meals per week.
- Limit snacks to evening.
- Avoid breads, refined sugar, and dairy except butter.
- When at ideal weight, breads, dairy, sugar, and fats will increase weight.

WEIGHT GAIN:

- Consume 25-35% of calories from dense protein.
- May have fruit up to 2 times per day.

VEGETARIAN DIET:

- Inadequate, since require 10-30% of caloric intake from dense protein.

FATS:

- 20% of caloric intake.
- Best sources are almonds and dense protein (chicken, turkey, eggs, fish).

KEY

—	all menus may be used by healthy persons
( )	around foods means that they are optional
L	denotes weight loss menus
S	denotes sensitive menus
S*	denotes very sensitive menus
G	denotes weight gain menus

BREAKFAST:

7-8 a.m. Light-to-heavy, with protein, nuts, seeds, grain, vegetables, legumes, dairy and/or fruit.

SENSITIVE: Moderate, with protein, grain, vegetables and/or fruit.

L	S	G	Menu
L	S*		Scrambled egg and broccoli
L	S*	G	Scrambled egg and rice
L		G	Scrambled eggs w/turkey or mussels (cherry cider)
		G	Eggs and potatoes (black cherry juice)
L	S*	G	2 soft-boiled eggs w/steamed broccoli or unsalted peas
		G	Eggs, pancakes, and blackberries w/ blackberry syrup
	S		Baked yukon gold potato or yam (butter) (peas)
L	S*	G	Calamari steaks and rice
	S		Basmati or short grain brown rice in chicken broth
	S*		White basmati rice w/steamed carrots and broccoli
L	S		Rice and green peas
L		G	Cream of rice w/dry roasted almonds
		G	Sweet rice w/coconut milk and mango
	S		Oatmeal, butter, and Re-Vita® (oat flour)
L		G	Oat treat: raw oatmeal, oat flour, butter, and Re-Vita® (apple/apricot juice
L	S	G	Oatmeal w/Re-Vita® (carrot juice)
		G	Oatmeal w/oat bran and honey or cream and carrot juice
L		G	Oatmeal and egg, then cherry cider, pineapple/coconut, apple/apricot, or cranberry juice
L		G	Cream of rice w/Re-Vita® and/or almond butter
L		G	Corn grits w/butter (pineapple/coconut juice)
			Prunes and couscous
		G	Pineapple/coconut juice
			Grapefruit
			Mango – frozen, dried, or fresh

Thyroid

	BREAKFAST or LUNCH:
L S G	Turkey, white or dark and white basmati rice
S G	Chicken and baked yukon gold potato (reg. sour cream)
L S G	Calamari sauteed in butter (parsley) and white basmati rice
L S G	Game hen and peas
L S G	Scallops and carrots, onions, and broccoli
	BREAKFAST, LUNCH or DINNER:
L S*G	Canned crab, rice, and nori seaweed
	Tea with honey – up to 4 cups per day w/ meals or alone
	MID-MORNING SNACK:
	(Optional) 10-11 a.m. Vegetables, nuts, protein.
S G	Avocado
L S	Bok choy w/tahini
S	Raw, soaked almonds
L G	Roasted, unsalted almonds (carrots or bell peppers)
L G	Carrot juice
L G	Carrot/beet/spinach juice
L S G	Berry Re-Vita® w/cranberry concentrate
L G	Hard-boiled egg
	LUNCH:
	12–2 p.m. Light-to-heavy, with protein, nuts, seeds, vegetables, grain, legumes, dairy and/or fruit.
	SENSITIVE: Light-to-moderate, with protein, nuts, vegetables, grain and/or fruit.
L S G	Turkey and cranberry sauce
L S	Turkey and cucumber
G	Turkey and avocado (mustard) on rye bread
L S G	Turkey, rice, and peas
L S G	Chicken, rice, and broccoli
L S G	Salmon and spinach souffle
L G	Split pea soup
L G	Mushroom barley soup
L G	Chicken rice soup
L	Onion soup
G	Yogurt (flavored) and almonds
L G	Rice cakes w/almond butter
L	Salad: spinach, red cabbage, red peppers, broccoli, cauliflower, and vinaigrette dressing
L S	Beets, carrots, or red bell pepper
L	Carrot/celery/parsley juice
L	Carrot/beet/spinach juice
	Raspberries
	MID-AFTERNOON SNACK:
	(Optional) 4-5 p.m. Fruit or fruit juices, vegetables, grain, nuts.
L G	Juices: pineapple/coconut, apple/apricot, cherry/apple, or apple
L S G	Berry Re-Vita® w/cranberry concentrate
G	Almond butter w/apple
	Rice cake
L G	Hard-boiled egg
L S G	Fruit: apricots, cherries, raspberries, tart apple, grapefruit, or mango
L S	Raw carrots, bell peppers, or cucumber
	LUNCH or DINNER:
G	Turkey, rice dressing, potatoes, gravy, cranberry sauce, and steamed broccoli, carrots, and brown onions
L G	Turkey or chicken and baked potato
L G	Turkey, basmati or short grain brown rice, and green beans
L G	Turkey, pasta, and raw carrots
L G	Scallops or calamari, rice, and peas (onions)
L G	Chicken, yukon gold potato, raw red or green bell pepper, and/or steamed broccoli
L S G	Chicken, pasta, and broccoli
G	Chicken, potatoes, and corn
L S*	Chicken soup w/carrots, celery, onions, potatoes, and parsley

Thyroid

L Calamari, rice, and beets (beet greens w/lemon juice, raw carrots)

L G Calamari, lemon pasta w/garlic butter, and basil

L G Orange roughy or sole, rice, and peas

L S G White fish, rice, and asparagus

L S G Salmon and rice or pasta

L G Scallops in stir-fry w/snow pea pods, bamboo shoots, carrots, onions, and mushrooms over rice

S* Scallops and basmati rice

L G Scallops or calamari, rice, and artichokes w/lemon juice

L G Shrimp scampi, rice, asparagus, and/or raw carrots

L G Shrimp w/lemon juice, rice, and raw spinach

L G Tuna, avocado, and carrots

L G Tuna and noodles or pasta

L S California roll w/rice and avocado, carrots, cucumber, jicama, and/or bell peppers

G Cottage cheese w/pineapple

L G Eggs, broccoli, rice, and mushrooms

L Hard-boiled egg and raw bell pepper

L G Egg salad w/celery (carrots, bell peppers, and/or potato)

L S G Roasted almonds, raw bell pepper, and/or carrot

L G Almond butter w/Pippin or Granny Smith apple

L G Almond butter on rice cake w/raw carrots and/or bell pepper

L Stir-fry: broccoli, onions, and mushrooms w/rice and noodles

S* Spinach, yukon gold potato, onion, celery, and eggplant

L S* Squash and rice

L S Acorn squash w/Re-Vita® (butter)

L Sauteed eggplant w/Italian spices and rice (beets)

L S* Eggplant stuffed w/rice and spices

L S Beet pasta and steamed broccoli

G Lemon pasta w/garlic butter, basil, and Parmesan and Romano cheeses

L Rice, peas, carrots, and onions

L S*G Short grain brown rice in chicken broth

L G Artichokes and short grain brown rice in chicken broth

L Carrot/beet/spinach juice

L Yams and peas

L Salad: spinach, beets, and lemon juice

L G Salad: spinach, beets, peas, red onions, green onions, eggs, cucumbers, green peppers, carrots, broccoli, green beans, and ranch dressing

L S Bell pepper, carrots, cucumber, jicama, and/or avocado

L S* Artichokes, rice, peas, carrots, and onions

G Plain yogurt w/Re-Vita® and carrot

L G Mussel, oyster, or clam chowder (jicama and bell pepper)

DINNER:

7-9 p.m. Light-to-heavy, with protein, nuts, seeds, grain, legumes, vegetables, fruit and/or dairy.

SENSITIVE: 7-8 p.m. Light-to-heavy with protein, grain, vegetables and/or fruit.

L S* Hard-boiled egg and steamed broccoli

L S*G Sea bass, rice, and steamed or cooked carrots

L G Baked tuna, rice, and carrots

L G Perch, rice, and peas

G Miso soup, scallops, rice, and broccoli

L G Turkey, white rose potatoes, cranberry sauce, and raw bell peppers

L G Oriental almond chicken: snow pea pods, bell peppers, carrots, shitake mushrooms, chicken, almonds, and basmati or brown rice

L S*G Chicken and wild rice (asparagus)

L S*G Chicken, carrots, and broccoli (potatoes)

L S*G Chicken (dark) and peas

L S*G Chicken, potatoes, and cooked carrots

L G Chicken, fish, turkey, shellfish, or organ meats, raw or steamed vegetables, and rice or plain pasta

Thyroid

L G Chicken or mussels and pasta (butter), green peas, and raw carrots

L S G Rice and broccoli or peas

L S G Baked yam (butter) and seasoned broccoli, or peas

L S G Millet cooked in chicken broth, steamed vegetables, or raw vegetables, such as carrots, cucumbers, bell peppers, jicama, and/or avocado

L Butternut squash and steamed broccoli or peas

L G Butternut squash and couscous (butter, seasoning, and/or onions)

EVENING SNACK:
(Optional) 9-12 p.m. Fruit, fruit juice or sweets, nuts, grain, dairy, vegetables.

S* Watermelon or grapefruit

L S Fresh or frozen mango

L Frozen cherries

L S G Dried cranberries

L S G Plain or sesame unsalted rice cake

L S*G Air-popped popcorn – anytime

S G California roll

L S*G Hard-boiled egg

S G Roasted, unsalted almonds

S*G Almond butter on rice cakes

G Pastry, ice cream, yogurt or kefir

S* Protein drink or chicken broth

G Warm whole milk w/honey

SNACK:
(Optional) 3 a.m. Protein.

Roasted, unsalted almonds

Hard-boiled egg or deviled egg

Resources

RECOMMENDED BOOKS, TAPES & SEMINARS

Deal, Sheldon C., N.D., D.C., *Life Through Nutrition*, New Life Publishing Co., Tucson, AZ (1974)
— *New Life through Natural Methods*, New Life Publishing Co., Tucson, AZ (1979)

Diamond, John D., M.D., *Your Body Doesn't Lie*, Harper & Row, New York, NY (1979)
— *Life Energy*, Harper Collins Publishing, New York, NY (1979)

Durlacher, James V., D.C., *Freedom From Fear Forever*, Compulsive behavior, how to effectively eliminate fears and phobias, Van Ness Publishing Co., Tempe, AZ (1995)

Grudermeyer, David, Ph.D., Grudermeyer, Rebecca, Psy.D., Patrick, Lerissa Nancy, *Sensible Self-Help* The First Road Map for the Healing, Emotional Healing, Willingness Works Press, San Diego (1996)

Hawkins, David R. M.D., *Power Versus Force:* An Anatomy of Consciousness, the hidden determinents of human behavior, Veritas Publishing (1995)

Hope, Larry, *Recovery of the Human Spirit*, a tape set with book. Reawaken the human spirit into perpetual consciousness, enliven your inner potential into unbounded awareness. Seminars: Celebration Trainings, Enlightened Vacation, 5757 Westheimer Ste. 3-307, Houston, TX 77057 (713) 592-0300, Fax (713) 592-9333, 1 (800) 935-2001

Jorgensen, Richard D., *What you don't know about relationships might be killing them* (discovering a true self-identity). Logical solutions to emotional events through learning technology by Awareness Communication technology, Home Video Seminars, San Diego

Moreton, Valerie Seeman, N.D, *A New Day in Healing!* unresolved emotions, a healing guide, Kalos Publishing, San Diego, CA (1992)

Myss, Caroline M., Ph. D., *Anatomy of the Spirit* , Crown Publishers, New York, NY (1996)

Thie, John, D.C., *Touch For Health* (1975). Seminars: 6-day therapy training from John Thie, D.C. Learn to balance your energies, enabling the spirit/mind/emotions/physical body to nourish, support and heal one another. Touch For Health Education Seminars, Dr. John F. Thie, 6162 La Gloria Drive, Malibu, CA 90265 (310) 589-5269

TPN's Success & Personal Development channel. Shows designed to help viewers become more successful in every aspect of their life, broadcasts 24 hours a day, 7 days a week. Carried on Primestar Satellite TV with over 160 channels. Charlie Tyack, (619) 695-1624

Resources

SPECIAL FOODS AND NUTRITIONAL SUPPLEMEMENTS

Re-Vita® – by Re-Vita®, Inc.

Spirulina that has been fed minerals and contains all 22 of the amino acids. May be used as a supplement or as a meal replacement once or twice a day. It comes in syrup form and is sweet. The average serving is 1 tablespoon. Flavors include berry, butternut, vanilla, and chocolate. Adding approximately 1/8 teaspoon of the chocolate flavor to a cup of coffee will often neutralize the negative affect of coffee on the body.

Pro-Gain® – by Metagenics®

Easy to digest, milk-based, protein supplement. Originally developed for athletes and used in hospitals to rebuild muscle mass.

Sunrider® Products

These products have an herbal base which detoxifies the body, as well as supports and rebuilds it. Skin types, who tend to be nutritionally depleted, do especially well with this diet as do Stomach types. Benefit and suitability for other types varies, so products should be assessed on an individual basis.

Sunny Dew™ – Stevia, concentrated liquid dietary supplement. Can also be used as a sweetener.

Nu Plus™ – Combination of 50 food-grade herbs which strengthen the body's system by nourishing tissues and cells. Good source of complex carbohydrates. Great for recovery after exercise.

Quinary™ – Concentrated food-grade herbs designed to balance the body's 5 main systems: digestive, immune, endocrine/hormonal, circulatory, and respiratory.

Fortune Delight™ **Herb Beverage** – Low calorie herbal beverage designed to assist the body's natural elimination process, helping to remove impurities that may be stored in fat cells.

Sun Bar® – Snack bar. High in concentrated herbs and complex carohydrates. Great before and after exercising.

Essential Fatty Acids

Chlorophyll Complex Perles, Cataplex F Perles, Linium B6, Super EFF, or Sesame Seed Oil Perles by Standard Process, Inc.

Bioctasol Forte, or Flax Seed Oil by Biotics Research Corp.

Chlorotene by Metagenics® or Ethical Nutrients®

SuperBlue/Green™ Algae – by Cell Tech

Plant protein, particularly supportive for Lymph types and often Medullas. Others may use it on a short term basis.

Noni™ – by Morinda™ Inc.

Good for digestive problems, constipation. Regulates blood sugar levels and enhances the immune system. Used for bacterial and viral infections, influenza, the common cold, malaria, tuberculosis, sinus problems, chronic fatigue, menstrual problems, migraine headaches, arthritis, senility, and high or low blood pressure. Its active ingredient, proxeronine, acts as a pain reliever. Consequently, Noni can be applied topically to areas of severe back pain, skin and flesh wounds, cuts, bruises, boils, and infections. It is also available in cream and oil form.

Resources

Corrected Salt™ – by Life Plus™
Balances sodium with chloride, sulphur, and magnesium.

Spiru-tein Bars® – by Nature's Plus®

PRODUCTS

Harmonizer – by Rainbow Crossings

Contains specially formulated distilled water, which amplifies energy. This product offers protection from toxins and chemicals usually found in water, food, or air.

Polarizer (International Patent) – by Springlife Polarity Research

Contains a formulation of kelp and minerals which amplifies positive energy. Offers protection from toxins and chemicals found in water, food, or air.

EXERCISE

Fitness Ball – The easiest way to exercise. Incorporate exercise into your lifestyle by using a fitness ball as a chair. The weakest point of the body is the pelvis which results in weakness of the lower abdominal muscles and low back pain. Sitting on the ball forces you to use your pelvic and lower abdominal muscles. This improves posture, reduces wrist problems, and stimulates cerebral-spinal fluid movement, resulting in increased alertness and mental clarity.

SynergySystems™ exercise videos based on the work of J.F. Pilates, by Cathie Murakami, Del Mar, CA (619) 792-5675, e-mail: catsynergy@aol.com.

"Blisswork" by Juawayne Hope, San Diego, CA (619) 576-7073

COOKING

Cooking classes and SaladMaster Cookware Low heat, vacuum cooking system. Provides a new concept in cooking that takes advantage of the latest in nutritional research and actually shortens cooking time by 50%. It preserves at least 98% of the vitamins, minerals, and enzymes, and prevents shrinkage of everything you cook, from meats to vegetables. Carol Dysart, (619) 421-8085 or page at 800-617-8166 and enter your number.

Heebner, Lesa, *Cooking With the Seasons,* Garlic & Sapphires®, Del Mar, CA (1994) (619) 755-7773
—— *Calypso Bean Soup & Other Savory Recipes,* Collins, San Francisco, CA (1996)

To order or for additional information contact your health care professional, nutritionist, local distributor or call: (619) 756-3704, 1(888) 2MY-TYPE or 1 (888) 269-8973, Fax (619) 756-6933, Web site at http://www.bodytype.com

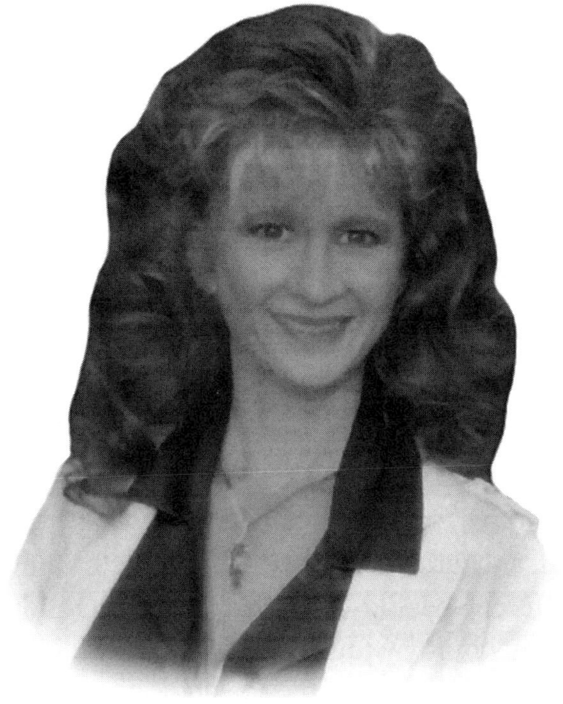

About the Author

Dr. Carolyn L. Mein began her private practice using applied kinesiology in 1974, and is a charter member diplomate of the International College of Applied Kinesiology. In addition to her Chiropractic Degree, she holds a B.A. in Bio-Nutrition, is Certified in Acupuncture, and is a Fellow of the American Council of Applied Clinical Nutrition.

Research-oriented, Dr. Mein's focus has been to optimize a person's health and vitality in the most effective and efficient ways possible. Realizing that optimal health and happiness requires balance, support and integration of all areas, Dr. Mein developed a technique known as Transpersonal Physiology to correct and stabilize the structure, neuro-emotional reprogramming, and a body typing system.

Studying the vast field of nutrition, Dr. Mein quickly became aware of the apparent contradictions in the information. While there are general principles that are true for everyone, she found too many questions that needed to be answered on an individual basis. Fortunately, her research lead her to discover a common ground – body typing. Having 25 different types answered the question of how people could be so different, yet explained why certain people had a unique similarity.

In her desire to make a worthwhile contribution to the world by improving the quality of the lives of individuals, Dr. Mein put together "The 25 Body Typing System". It is designed to provide people with specific dietary information and the essence of what they need to know about themselves to be personally responsible for their own health, growth and well-being.

Dedicated to the betterment of mankind, Dr. Mein lectures, writes and maintains an active practice in Rancho Santa Fe, CA.

Body Typing Guides

BOOKS

"Different Bodies, Different Diets" Women's Edition & Men's Edition. Complete guide to determining your body type with photos and profiles of all the 25 types. Provides a life-time eating plan consisting of your ideal diet. Designed to help you achieve optimal health and vitality as well as normalize your weight, whether you are over, under, or just want to maintain. Based on over 20 years of research, *The 25 Body Type System* is more than a diet. Each body type has certain disease tendencies, particular exercise requirements, and a specific psychological profile.

BOOKLETS

"25 Body Type Photos" Women's Version & Men's Version. Explains the fundamentals of body typing using key physical characteristics so you can determine your body type. Photos of real-life people show 8 different people of each type at their ideal weight, overweight and underweight through full body photos with front, side, and back views for each of the 25 body types. It also contains all of the Essences of the Psychological Profiles.

"Body Type Essences" Contains the 2-page color photo of both men and women of all 25 types plus their icons. It describes how to determine body type through the Area of Attention and from the psychological Points of Connection. Also included are the Essences of each of the 25 types."

"Questionnaire" Women's Version & Men's Version. Consists of detailed questions with photos of the various physical characteristics to help you discover your type.

"Muscle Testing" Contains a step-by-step guide to muscle testing both with a partner and on your own. This technique is very useful in determining your body's response to foods. The "Key Indicator Foods By Type" chart contains a list of key foods that can be used to identify and verify body types.

"Microwaves & Dietary Myths" Reveals the truth about the most common dietary beliefs and the truth about microwave cooking.

"Advanced Dietary Guide" A guide to fasts, cleansing diets, and common diet programs. Not all diets are good on a long-term basis for all types, some can even be detrimental. Many diets can be helpful when followed on a short-term basis – 1 day to 2 weeks. This guide identifies which diets are effective for your body type and how to use them.

"Body Type Profile & Diet" Available for each one of the 25 types. Food lists containing the most common foods are divided into three groups, "Frequently", "Moderately", and "Rarely". All menus are simple and practical, developed to support each specific type. There are 20-60 different menu suggestions for each meal plus snacks. An implementation guide, physical characteristics and complete psychological profiles are included for each type.

VIDEO

"Different Bodies, Different Diets Video"
An introduction to body typing hosted by Dr. Mein (approximately 35 minutes).

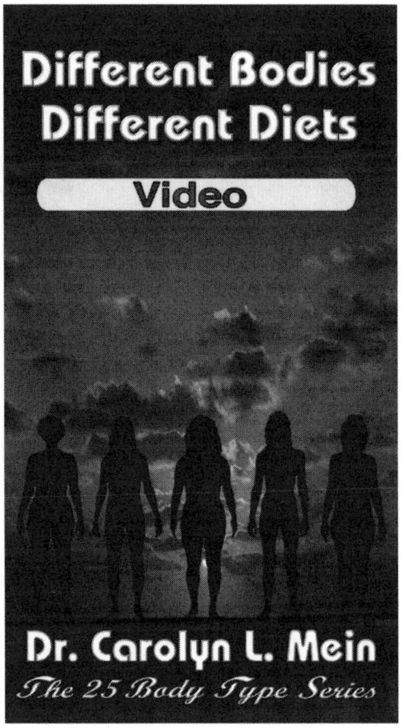

COMPUTER

"Different Bodies, Different Diets CD-ROM"
This program guides you step-by-step so you can determine your body type through an interactive test section featuring Dr. Mein in full motion video. The CD contains hundreds of color photos, music and narration. Body type your friends and family, then print out a custom diet menu for them. Available in Windows Version and Macintosh Version.

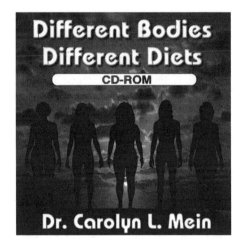

Our Web site is located at **http://www.bodytype.com**

Quantity discounts are available

Order: 1(888) 269-8973

Fax: (619) 756-6933

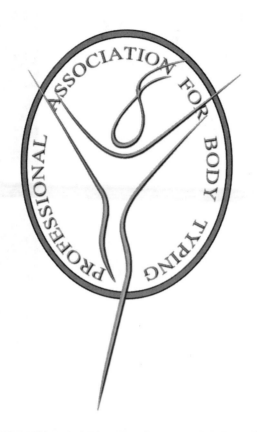

Professional Association for Body Typing

Health care professionals certified in body typing are available to assist you. These doctors, nurses, nutritionists, psychologists, and counselors have followed a rigorous certification process in body typing. Each brings a speciality that he or she will use in conjunction with body typing to create a comprehensive program to assist people in reaching their goals. To find the certified professional for body typing in your area:

Call our referral hot line at
1 (888) 2MY-TYPE

1 (888) 269-8973

http://www.bodytype.com

The 25 Body Type System Order Form

Carolyn L. Mein, D.C. • P.O.Box 8112 • Rancho Santa Fe, CA 92067
(619) 756-3704 • Fax (619) 756-6933 • 1 (888) 2MY-TYPE

☐ Mr.
☐ Mrs. Name ______________________________ Date ________
☐ Ms.

Address ____

City __________________________ State _______ Zip ______

Phone _(_____)________________ Fax _(_____)_____________

E-mail ____

☐ **I would like to receive a FREE Body Type Newsletter**

- In depth interviews and actual case histories
- Prepublication specials
- Hot updates of new breakthroughs
- Discounts on health products

or register at our Web site
http://www.bodytype.com

TITLE	QTY	COST	TOTAL
Different Bodies, Different Diets: Women's Edition		**$29.95**	
Different Bodies, Different Diets: Men's Edition		**$29.95**	
Different Bodies, Different Diets: Video		**$19.95**	
Different Bodies, Different Diets: CD-ROM		**$49.95**	
Body Type Essences		**$ 9.95**	
Women's Body Type Photos		**$ 9.95**	
Men's Body Type Photos		**$ 9.95**	
Women's Body Type Questionnaire		**$ 4.95**	
Men's Body Type Questionnaire		**$ 4.95**	
Muscle Testing		**$ 4.95**	
Microwaves & Dietary Myths		**$ 4.95**	
Advanced Dietary Guide		**$ 4.95**	
Profile & Diet Body Type: ______________		**$ 9.95**	
Profile & Diet Body Type: ______________		**$ 9.95**	
Profile & Diet Body Type: ______________		**$ 9.95**	
For Postage & Handling add:			**$ 5.00**
(CA residences add 7.75% sales tax)			
Make checks payable to: **Carolyn L. Mein, D.C.**	**TOTAL**		

We'd like to hear from you, your experience, questions and comments:

Body Type ______________ Occupation ________________________ Age _____